Dental Materials and Their Selection

Dental Materials and Their Selection

Second Edition

William J. O'Brien, PhD, FADM
Professor
Department of Biologic and Materials Sciences
Director, Specialized Materials Science Research Center
School of Dentistry
The University of Michigan
Ann Arbor, Michigan

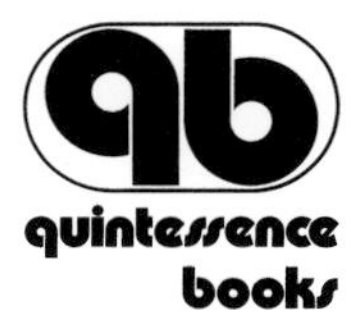

Quintessence Publishing Co, Inc
Chicago, Berlin, London, Tokyo, Paris, Barcelona,
São Paulo, Moscow, Prague, and Warsaw

Library of Congress Cataloging-in-Publication Data

Dental materials and their selection / [edited by] William J. O'Brien.
-- 2nd ed.
p. cm.
Rev. ed. of: Dental materials / edited by William J. O'Brien.
Includes bibliographical references and index.
ISBN 0-86715-297-4
1. Dental materials. I. O'Brien, William J. (William Joseph), 1940– . II. Dental materials.
[DNLM: 1. Dental materials. WU 190 D4158 1997]
RK652.5.D454 1997
617.6'95--dc21
DNLM/DLC
for Library of Congress 96-48070
CIP

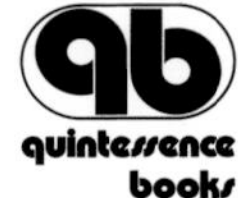

Quintessence Publishing Co, Inc
551 North Kimberly Drive
Carol Stream, IL 60188

Editor: Elizabeth M. Solaro
Production: Eric S. Przybylski
Cover design: Chris Jung and Lisa A. Ream
Cover photo: Photomicrograph showing the intermetallic compounds formed during the setting of dental amalgam.

Printed in the United States of America

Contents

Contributors *vii*

Foreword *ix*

Preface *xi*

Acknowledgments *xii*

1 A Comparison of Metals, Ceramics, and Polymers *1*

2 Physical Properties *13*

3 Color and Appearance *25*

4 Surface Phenomena and Adhesion to Tooth Structure *39*

5 Gypsum Products *51*

6 Polymers and Polymerization: Denture Base Polymers *79*

7 Polymeric Restorative Materials: Composites and Sealants *97*

8 Abrasion, Polishing, and Bleaching *115*

9 Impression Materials *123*

10 Waxes *147*

11 Dental Cements *151*

12 Structure and Properties of Metals and Alloys *175*

13 Dental Amalgams *187*

14 Direct Gold Filling Materials *203*

15 Precious Metal Casting Alloys *215*

16 Alloys for Porcelain-Fused-to-Metal Restorations *225*

17 Casting *237*

18 High-Temperature Investments *249*

19 Base Metal Casting Alloys *259*

20 Orthodontic Wires *273*

21 Dental Porcelain *287*

22 Soldering, Welding, and Electroplating *303*

23 Dental Implant Materials *315*

Appendix A – Tabulated Values of Physical and Mechanical Properties *331*

Appendix B – Periodic Chart of the Elements *405*

Appendix C – Units and Conversion Factors *406*

Appendix D – Longevity of Restorations Commonly Used in Dentistry *407*

Index *409*

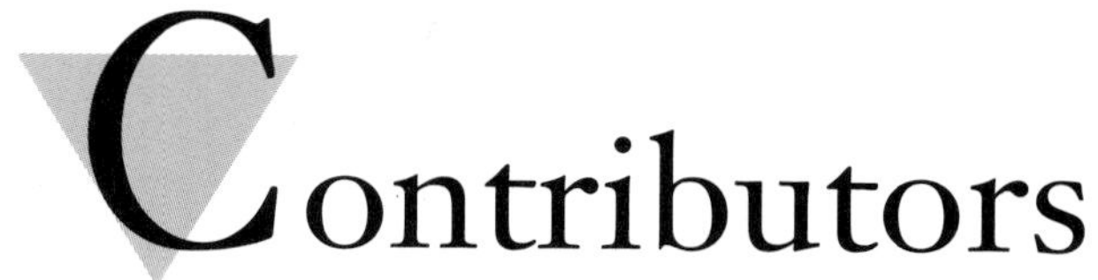

Contributors

Raymond L. Bertolotti, DDS, PhD
Clinical Professor
Restorative Dentistry
School of Dentistry
University of California
San Francisco, California
Alloys for Porcelain-Fused-to-Metal Restorations

William A. Brantley, PhD
Professor
Department of Prosthetic Dentistry
Ohio State University College of Dentistry
Columbus, Ohio
Orthodontic Wires

Gordon Christensen, DDS, MSD, PhD
Senior Consultant
Clinical Research Associates
Provo, Utah
Longevity of Restorations

Richard G. Earnshaw, PhD, MDSc
Reader in Prosthetic Dentistry Emeritus
Faculty of Dentistry
University of Sydney
Sydney, Australia
Gypsum Products

Pui L. Fan, PhD
Director
Research Institute
American Dental Association
Chicago, Illinois
Color and Appearance

Evan H. Greener, BMetE, MS, PhD
Professor Emeritus
Department of Basic Sciences
Northwestern University Dental School
Chicago, Illinois
Dental Amalgams

Carole L. Groh, BS, MBA
Research Associate
Department of Biologic and Materials Sciences
School of Dentistry
University of Michigan
Ann Arbor, Michigan
Impression Materials

Eugene F. Huget, BS, DDS, MS
Professor
Department of Biologic and Diagnostic Sciences
College of Dentistry
University of Tennessee
Memphis, Tennessee
Base Metal Casting Alloys

David H. Kohn, PhD
Associate Professor Department of Biologic and Materials Sciences
School of Dentistry
Department of Bioengineering
School of Engineering
University of Michigan
Ann Arbor, Michigan
Dental Implant Materials

Valerie A. Lee, DDS, PhD
Research Associate
Department of Biologic and Materials Sciences
School of Dentistry
University of Michigan
Ann Arbor, Michigan
Polymers: Chemistry and Denture Base Polymers
Polymeric Restorative Materials

J. Rodway Mackert, Jr., DMD, PhD
Professor of Dental Materials
Department of Restorative Dentistry
School of Dentistry
Medical College of Georgia
Augusta, Georgia
A Comparison of Metals, Ceramics, and Polymers
Physical Properties

Peter C. Moon, MS, PhD
Professor of Restorative Dentistry
School of Dentistry
Medical College of Virginia
Virginia Commonwealth University
Richmond, Virginia
Structure of Properties of Metals and Alloys

Osamu Okuno, PhD
Professor and Chair
Department of Dental Material Science
School of Dentistry
Tohoku University
Sendai, Japan
High-Temperature Investments

Stephen T. Rasmussen, PhD
Research Associate
Department of Biologic and Materials Sciences
School of Dentistry
University of Michigan
Ann Arbor, Michigan
Soldering, Welding, and Electroplating

Rodrigo Reis, DDS, MS
Professor of Dentistry and Clinical Research Director
School of Dentistry
Unigranrio University
Rio de Janeiro, Brazil
Polymeric Restorative Materials

Harold E. Schnepper, DMD, MSD
Professor
Department of Restorative Dentistry
School of Dentistry
Loma Linda University
Loma Linda, California
Direct Gold Filling Materials

Dennis C. Smith, MSc, PhD, FRIS
Professor Emeritus
Faculty of Dentistry
University of Toronto
Toronto, Ontario, Canada
Dental Cements

Kenneth W. Stoffers, DMD, MS
Associate Professor
Cariology, Restorative Sciences, and Endodontics
School of Dentistry
University of Michigan
Ann Arbor, Michigan
Clinical Decision-Making Scenarios

John A. Tesk, BS, MS, PhD
Coordinator
Biomaterials Program Polymers Division
National Institute of Standards and Technology
Gaithersburg, Maryland
High-Temperature Investments

Mathijs M. A. Vrijhoef, PhD
Clinical Consultant
3M Sante
Malakoff, France
Dental Amalgams

Foreword

For many students, the study of dental materials presents a major difficulty. Many treat the subject as a "basic science obstacle" to be forgotten once it has been removed. For educators, the sequencing of the dental materials course in the curriculum is a problem. For some, its placement in the first year provides a foundation for other restorative dentistry courses. Others believe that dental materials have most relevance in the third year, after students have been exposed to some restorative dentistry. Regardless of its placement in the curriculum, the subject has often been treated as a separate entity with the hope that the student will integrate the knowledge into dental practice. Unfortunately, most graduates have not applied their knowledge to clinical situations in a customized fashion.

In view of the enormous amount of information that has become available and the rapid changes that occur, the student must learn to integrate materials information and dental practice while in school to become an effective dentist. Students must learn to apply principles of materials science to problem solving and bring their knowledge into comprehensive patient care. The implication of this approach to dental education is that dental materials is taught in the context of developing dental skills.

For practicing dentists, the fast pace of development of new materials means that they are called upon to evaluate and integrate an ever-growing mass of research information into practice. The dentist has to remain informed about controversial issues related to the safety of various dental materials and constantly answer patients' questions. To be effective requires a commitment to lifelong learning, with continuing education and ready access to a reference text with information that is easy to understand.

Dental Materials and Their Selection, Second Edition, provides a tool for such integration of dental materials into dental practice for the student, as well as a reference for the dentist. Throughout the book—even in the often dreaded discussions of physical properties of materials—clinical applications and examples are provided. This approach addresses the questions of relevance and applicability, which are not immediately obvious to students. The principles of materials science that shape restorative dentistry practices, as well as considerations for materials selection for different restorative techniques, are emphasized. A glossary at the end of each chapter, a carryover from the previous edition, and clinical decision scenarios, a new feature in this edition, are helpful to the beginning dentist. Questions and answers at the end of each chapter allow students to measure their progress. The troubleshooting tips provided are also helpful for practicing dentists using a material for the first time.

The book is a welcome addition to the tools available to teachers of dental materials and dental practitioners in their efforts to integrate knowledge of materials into dental practice.

Francis K. Mante, BDS, MS, PhD, DMD
Assistant Professor
Director of Biomaterials
Department of Restorative Dentistry
School of Dental Medicine
University of Pennsylvania
Philadelphia, Pennsylvania

Dedicated to the memory of Dr Gunnar Ryge, 1916–1991,

dental materials pioneer, mentor to many, and humanitarian

Preface

This edition has a number of features that we hope will improve its usefulness as a text for dental students and a reference for dentists.

First, this edition includes updated tree diagrams for classifying dental materials. These diagrams are invaluable in visualizing the types of dental materials available under broad clinical categories. As dental materials products have evolved, a variety of different formulations are available at any one time. The result is a plethora of products. These tree diagrams are particularly helpful for students, who are new to dentistry, in distinguishing product classifications.

Decision-making tables are included in chapters involving clinical materials as a second feature of this edition. These tables address the application of basic information, a major concern in dental education and clinical practice. All of us who teach dental materials have found that students and clinicians often have difficulty in applying basic information to clinical decisions. Today, the most frequently asked question is, "Which material should I use for a specific application?" These simple decision-making tables make it possible to make rational decisions based upon basic information about two materials and identification of the criteria in a given situation. The best choice depends on the characteristics of the two materials and the context in which they are being used. The use of this process in class discussions and exercises will provide training in the skill of rational decision making, which is valuable in a clinical setting.

A third feature that has been updated in this edition is the appendix on physical properties. Because the dental materials field involves a considerable amount of data scattered throughout the literature, these tables provide a valuable resource. This database will be continuously updated, and may be accessed on the World Wide Web by pointing a web browser to:

http://www.lib.umich.edu/libhome/Dentistry.lib/Dental_tables/intro.html

Anyone with published data of his or her own or from other sources is urged to submit material to the database as described in the database introduction.

Finally, the main feature of this book that has been maintained in this edition is the use of questions in many of the chapters. Questions and answers are provided to improve understanding on important points. One useful practice in teaching is to assign discussion questions to think about before a lecture. New to this edition are discussion questions in most of the chapters. These thought-provoking questions are suitable for discussion in the classroom or self-study; no answers have been provided to stimulate as many ideas as possible.

Acknowledgments

First, I would like to thank the many contributors to the second edition who have helped to make this book as up-to-date as possible in this dynamic field. I am also thankful to contributors to the first edition, including J. David Eick, R. Roydhouse, K.F. Leinfelder, B.E. Causton, C.L. Suarez, L.N. Johnson, M. Rosenblum, G.A. Zarb, A. Smith, W.N. von der Lehr, and M.D. Jendresen.

I greatly appreciate the many people who contributed data to the biomaterial tables and to Carole Groh who patiently organized the new data into the many categories. Gratitude is also due to John Powers who organized the original database. This new edition would not have been possible without the help of Chris Jung who prepared many illustrations. Elizabeth Rodriguiz, the biomaterials secretary, did an excellent job of proofreading the page proofs with her eagle eye.

I would also like to acknowledge Drs. Waletha Wasson, Gisele de Faria Neiva, and David E. Wacker for contributing excellent decision-making tables, as well as Bill Johnston and Donald Hunkel for their collaboration on the study from which the cover photo was taken. It is impossible to thank everyone individually, and my gratitude goes to those whom I may have overlooked.

Chapter 1

A Comparison of Metals, Ceramics, and Polymers

When a dentist considers the type of restoration to place in a patient's mouth, the choice may be between different varieties of the same material, for example, different types of amalgam. Or perhaps the choice will involve a decision between two different kinds of the same basic material, such as two different kinds of metals—amalgam and cast gold. With the rapid developments in dental materials over the past several years, it is becoming increasingly more common that the dentist's choice is between two different basic materials, such as between a metal amalgam and a polymer-and-ceramic composite, or between a metal crown and an all-ceramic crown.

A wide spectrum of properties is present within each basic material type; nevertheless, there is a "family resemblance" among the varieties of each material type. For example, although metals exhibit a wide range of strengths, melting ranges, and so on, they resemble one another in their ductility, thermal and electrical conductivity, and metallic luster. Similarly, ceramics can be characterized as strong yet brittle, and polymers tend to be flexible (low elastic modulus) and weak. These "family traits" of the three basic materials are more easily understandable, and thus more easily remembered, if we know the reasons behind them. In fact, simply understanding one key concept for each of the three basic materials gives us significant insight into how each class of materials behaves as a restorative dental material, as well as an idea of the potential of these materials if some of their limitations can be overcome. The relationships among the three basic materials is shown in Fig 1-1.

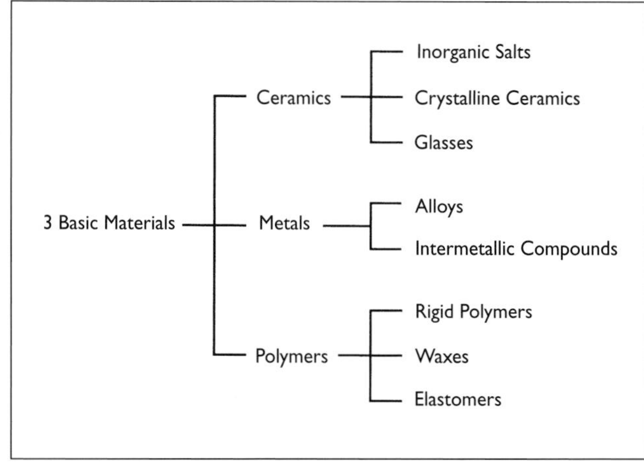

Fig 1-1 A tree diagram classifying the three basic materials.

Selection among various materials

Table 1-1 summarizes the general behaviors of the various types of materials discussed in this chapter. Certain inherent properties of materials will influence their selection for use in dentistry. For example, metals are inherently strong, in general, and have good stiffness (modulus of elasticity). These properties would tend to recommend them as restorative materials. On the other hand, metals conduct heat rapidly and are opaque (non-

Table 1-1 A comparison of the properties of metals, ceramics, and polymers

	Metals		Ceramics			Polymers	
Properties	Alloys	Intermetallic compounds	Inorganic Salts	Crystalline	Glasses	Rigid	Rubbers
Hardness	Medium to hard	Hard	Medium to hard	Hard	Hard	Soft	Very soft
Strength	Medium to high	Medium	Medium	High	High	Low	Low
Toughness	High	Low	Low	Most low, some high	Low	Low	Medium
Elastic modulus	High	High	High	High	High	Low	Very low
Electrical conductivity	High	High	Low	Low	Low	Low	Low
Thermal conductivity	High	High	Low	Low	Low	Low	Low
Thermal expansion	Low	Low	Low	Low	Low	High	High
Density	High	High	Medium	Medium	Medium	Low	Low
Translucency	None	None	Medium	High	High	High	Low
Examples	Gold-copper	Amalgam phases	Gypsum, zinc phosphate	SiO_2, Al_2O_3	Dental porcelain	Poly(methyl methacrylate) (PMMA)	Impression materials

esthetic), limiting their usefulness in restorative dentistry. Ceramics and polymers are thermally insulating and tend to be more translucent. Hence, these materials insulate the pulp from extremes of heat and cold and offer the potential of more lifelike esthetics. They tend to have lower toughness than metals, however, and polymers have much lower strength.

Because no one class of materials possesses all the desired properties, it is not surprising that materials tend to be used in combination. The porcelain-fused-to-metal restoration combines the strength and ductility of metal with the esthetics of dental porcelain. A ceramic or polymer base is used to insulate the pulp from a thermally conducting metallic restoration. A high thermally expanding, low-strength, low-elastic-modulus polymer is reinforced with a low thermally expanding, high-strength, high-elastic-modulus ceramic filler to form a dental composite resin material. An understanding of the advantages and limitations of the various types of materials enables us to make selections based on the best compromise of desired properties versus inherent limitations.

Predicted versus actual strengths

It is possible to predict the strength of a material from the strengths of the individual bonds between the atoms in the material. The values of strength obtained by such a prediction are typically 1 million to 3 million pounds per square inch (psi), or about 7 to 21 GPa. Actual strengths of most materials are ten to 100 times lower.

Why do materials fail to exhibit the strengths one would expect from the bonds between atoms? Why do ceramics break suddenly without yielding, whereas metals often yield and distort to 120% or more of their original length before fracturing? Why are polymers so much weaker and more flexible than metals and ceramics? Why do metals conduct heat and electricity, whereas polymers and ceramics do not? As will be seen in this chapter, many of the answers to these questions can be understood by knowing only a few things about the structures of these materials. There is one key concept, for example, that will not only explain the tendency for ceramics to be brittle, but will also explain all of the methods used to strengthen ceramics. Similarly,

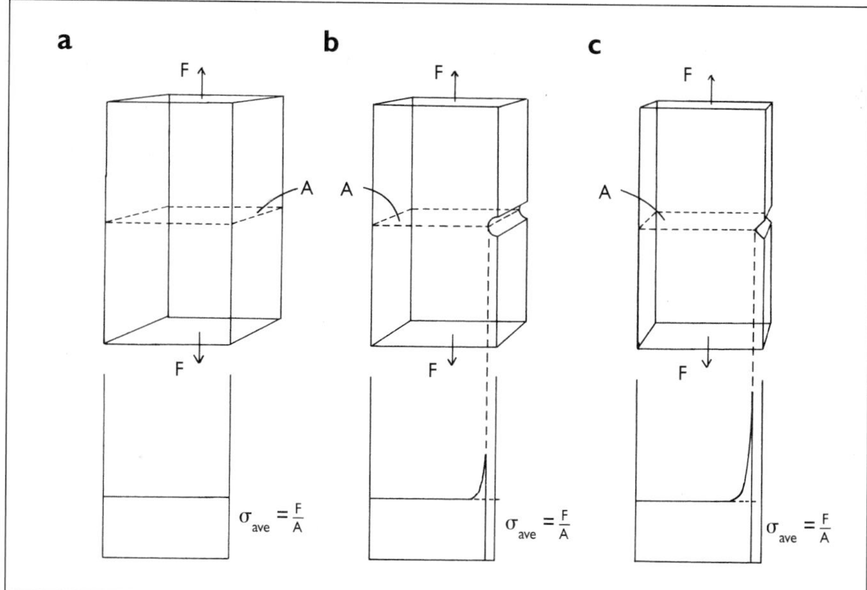

Fig 1-2 Stress raisers and the effect of their shape on stress concentration. (a) If no stress raiser is present, the stress is constant across cross section A. (b) If a rounded notch is present, the stress is constant over most of the cross section. (c) As the notch becomes sharper, the stress concentration becomes greater.

one key concept will explain why polymers expand about ten times as much as metals or ceramics when heated the same amount, why polymers are generally weak, why they are ten times more flexible than metals or ceramics, and why they tend to absorb water and other fluids.

Ceramics

Consider a block of material as depicted in Fig 1-2a. If this block is stretched by applying a force, F, the stress at any point on cross section A is the same as the average stress, σ_{ave}. For example, if the cross-sectional dimensions of the block are ½ in. ½ in. = ¼ in.^{2} (1.27 cm × 1.27 cm = 1.61 cm^2), and a force of 3,000 lb (13 kN) is applied, the average stress along cross section A is 12,000 psi, or 83 MPa. However, if a semicircular groove were machined across one side of the block of material, as depicted in Fig 1-2b, the stress at each point across a plane passing through this groove would not be the same as the average stress. The stress would be constant over most of the cross section, but near the groove, the stress would suddenly rise and reach a maximum right at the edge of the groove. This phenomenon occurs around any irregularity in a block of material. The groove or other irregularity is called a *stress raiser*. The stress around a stress raiser can be many times higher than the average stress in the body.

The amount the stress is increased depends upon the shape of the stress raiser. For example, if the stress raiser in our block of material were a sharp notch rather than a semicircular groove, the stress would increase greatly at the tip of the sharp notch, as shown in Fig 1-2c. As the tip of the notch becomes smaller (ie, the notch becomes sharper), the stress concentration at the tip of the notch becomes greater.

The minute scratches present on the surfaces of nearly all materials behave as sharp notches whose tips are as narrow as the spacing between atoms in the material. Thus, the stress concentration at the tips of these minute scratches causes the stress to reach the theoretical strength of the material at relatively low average stress. When the theoretical strength of the material is exceeded at the tip of the notch, the bonds at the notch tip break, as shown in Fig 1-3a. The adjacent bonds now are at the tip of the notch and thus are at the point of greatest stress concentration, as shown in Fig 1-3b. As the crack propagates through the material, the stress concentration is maintained at the crack tip until the crack moves completely through the material.* This stress concentration phenomenon

* Actually, the exceeding of the theoretical strength of the material at the crack tip is a necessary but insufficient condition for crack propagation. The remaining condition involves a balance between the surface energy required to form the two new surfaces of the crack, and the elastic strain energy arising from the applied stress. This is called the Griffith energy balance, discussion of which is beyond the scope of this book.

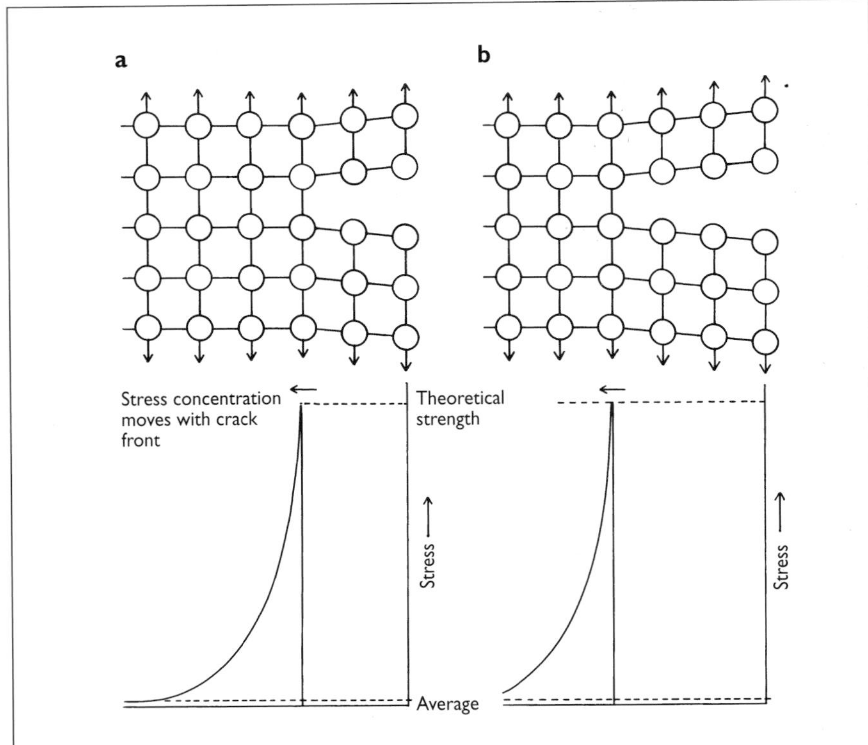

Fig 1-3 Role of stress raisers in achieving localized stresses as great as the theoretical strength of the material. The stress at the tip of the notch reaches the theoretical strength of the material even though the average stress is many times lower. As the most highly stressed bond breaks (a), the stress is transferred to the next bond (b).

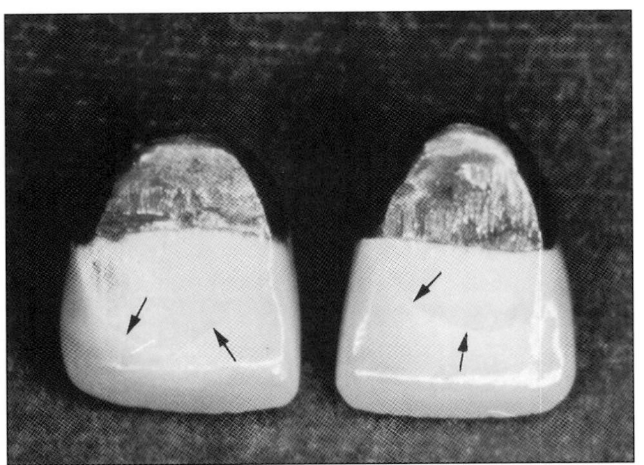

Fig 1-4 Brittle fracture *(arrows)* of ceramic (dental porcelain) owing to mismatch in the coefficient of thermal expansion between porcelain and metal. (Photo courtesy of R. P. O'Connor, DMD.)

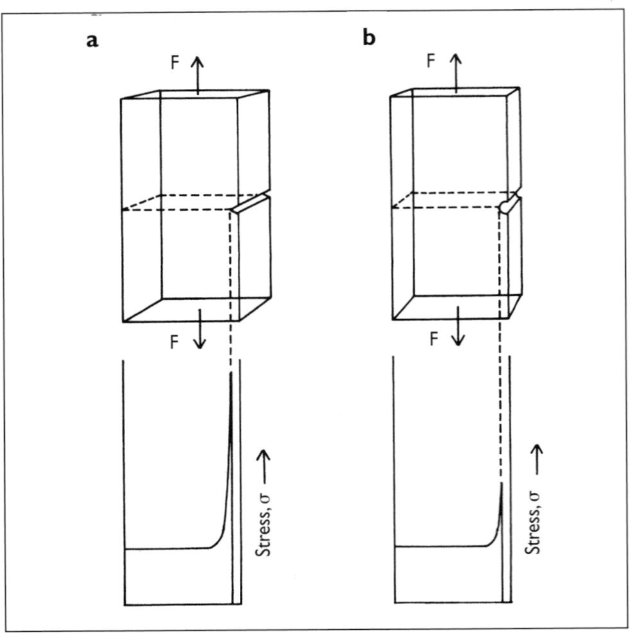

Fig 1-5 Rounding or blunting of stress raisers that occurs in ductile materials. Stress concentration is self-limiting in ductile materials because the region under greatest stress, the tip of the sharp stress raiser (a), yields to round or blunt the stress raiser and lower the stress (b).

enables us to understand how materials can fail at stresses far below their expected strength. This situation exists in the cutting of glass. When glass is cut, a line is scribed on one surface with a diamond point or a hardened steel glass-cutting wheel. This scribed line is a very shallow scratch or crack in comparison to the thickness of the piece of glass, but it acts as a stress raiser to concentrate the stress at the tip of the crack, as described above.

Understanding the effect of stress concentration is the key to understanding the failure of brittle materials, such as ceramics, which influences their selection as dental materials and dictates the design of restorations fabricated from these materials.

The tendency for ceramics to fail in a brittle manner at stresses which are far below the theoretical strengths of these materials can be understood in light of the concept of stress concentration at surface scratches and other defects. Most of the techniques for strengthening ceramics can also be understood by virtue of this concept.

Clinical applications of ceramics

Ceramics are inherently brittle and must be used in such a way so as to minimize the effect of this property. Ceramic restorations must not be subjected, for example, to large tensile stresses to avoid catastrophic failure. A method for reducing the influence of the brittleness of ceramics is to fuse them to a material of greater toughness (eg, metal), as is done with porcelain-fused-to-metal (PFM) restorations. Ceramics also may be reinforced with dispersions of high-toughness materials, as is the case with the alumina (Al_2O_3)-reinforced porcelain used in porcelain jacket crowns. Figure 1-4 shows brittle fractures that occurred in the porcelain of two PFM crowns owing to the mismatch in thermal expansion between the porcelain and metal.

Metals

Effect of ductility on stress concentration

As discussed in the previous section, stress raisers at the surface of a material can cause the stress in a localized region around the tip of the stress raiser to reach the theoretical strength of the material. When this happens in a brittle material, a crack propagates through the material, resulting in fracture (see the footnote on p. 3). In a ductile material, something happens before the theoretical strength of the material is reached at the tip of the stress raiser that accounts for the tremendous difference in behavior between, for example, a glass and a metal. As discussed previously, the magnitude of the stress concentration at the tip of a notch, surface scratch, or other stress raiser is determined by the sharpness of the stress raiser. If a sharp notch or scratch is present in the surface of a brittle material, the stress concentration around this notch would be something like that shown in Fig 1-5a. If such a stress raiser is initially present in a ductile metal, the material at the tip of the stress raiser deforms under stress so the sharp notch becomes a rounded groove, as shown in Fig 1-5b. Because the tip of the stress raiser is now rounded rather than sharp, the stress concentration at the tip of this stress raiser is much lower. There are two important facts to recognize in this process:

1. As with brittle materials, the actual strengths of ductile materials are many times less than those predicted from strengths of bonds between atoms.
2. Unlike the behavior around the notch in a brittle material, the stress concentration blunts the sharp tip of the stress raiser, thus lowering the stress concentration effect.

Mechanism of ductile behavior

What, then, is responsible for the ductile behavior of a metal? Consideration of what is happening on an atomic level provides insights into the difference between brittle materials and ductile ones. A schematic of the arrangement of atoms in a piece of metal is shown in Fig 1-6. If this piece of metal is subjected to a tensile stress as shown, this stress can be resolved into two components when considered relative to the plane A-A′. One component tends to move the rows of atoms on either side of the plane A-A′ apart from each other, and the other component tends to cause the planes to slide past one another along the plane A-A′.

The component of the stress that tends to cause the planes to slide past one another is the one that causes a material to deform plastically. Scientists are able to calculate, from the bond strengths between the atoms, the stresses that would be required to make one plane of atoms slide past another plane; these stresses

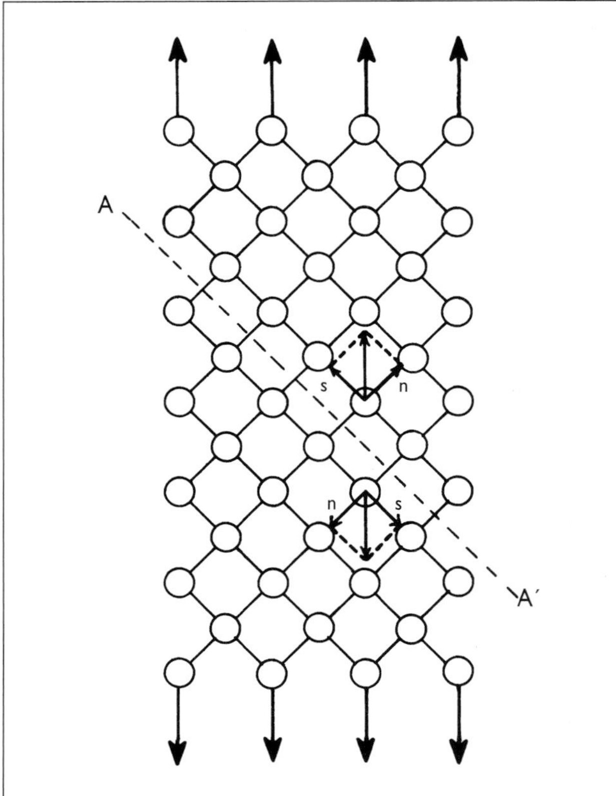

Fig 1-6 Tensile stress on a piece of material can be considered stress normal (n) (perpendicular) to plane A-A′, together with stress parallel (s) to plane A-A′. The stress parallel to plane A-A′ tends to cause the atoms along plane A-A′ to slide (shear) past each other.

are 100 or more times higher than those actually observed. If, however, the bonds were to break one at a time and re-form immediately with the adjacent atom, one plane could move past the other at very low stress levels.

The mechanism of this process is shown in Fig 1-7. Figures 1-7a through 1-7f show how, by breaking and re-forming bonds, an extra plane of atoms can move along plane A-A′ until this "ripple" in the crystal lattice passes completely through the material. Multiple repetitions of this process along many planes similar to A-A′ allow a metal to yield to an applied stress without fracturing. This ripple in the lattice structure is called a *dislocation*, and it is responsible for the ductile behavior of metals.

Metals can be hardened and strengthened by a variety of treatments that make it more difficult for dislocations to move through the metal lattice. Alloying, cold-working, and formation of second phases in a metal are all ways of impeding dislocation motion. Some crystal structures of metals, such as intermetallic compounds, make it difficult for dislocations to move. The passage of a dislocation through the ordered structure of an intermetallic compound would result in an unfavorable atomic arrangement, so dislocations move only with difficulty.

With metals, it is important to remember that their ability to yield without fracturing, as well as all of the methods for making metals harder and stronger, is understandable in light of the concept of dislocations in the metal structure.

Other properties of metals, such as their electrical and thermal conductivity, can be understood as resulting from the *metallic bond*. In the metallic bond some of the electrons are free to move rapidly through the lattice of metal ions. This unusual aspect of the metallic bond enables metals to conduct heat and electricity.

The electronic structure of the metallic bond also accounts for the opacity of metals. Figure 1-8 illustrates the metallic bond with its lattice of positively charged metal ion cores and electrons that are free to move between the ion cores.

Dislocations in ceramic materials and in intermetallic compounds

Why do ceramic materials not yield in the same manner as metals? The answer to this question involves consideration of two types of ceramic materials:

1. Amorphous materials (glasses)—Glassy materials do not possess an ordered crystalline structure as do metals. Therefore, dislocations of a crystalline lattice cannot exist in glassy materials. Thus, glasses have no mechanism for yielding without fracture.
2. Crystalline ceramic materials—Dislocations exist in crystalline ceramic materials, but their mobility is severely limited, because their movement would require that atoms of like charge be brought adjacent to one another, as seen in Fig 1-9. The energy required to do this is so large that dislocations are essentially immobile in crystalline ceramic materials.

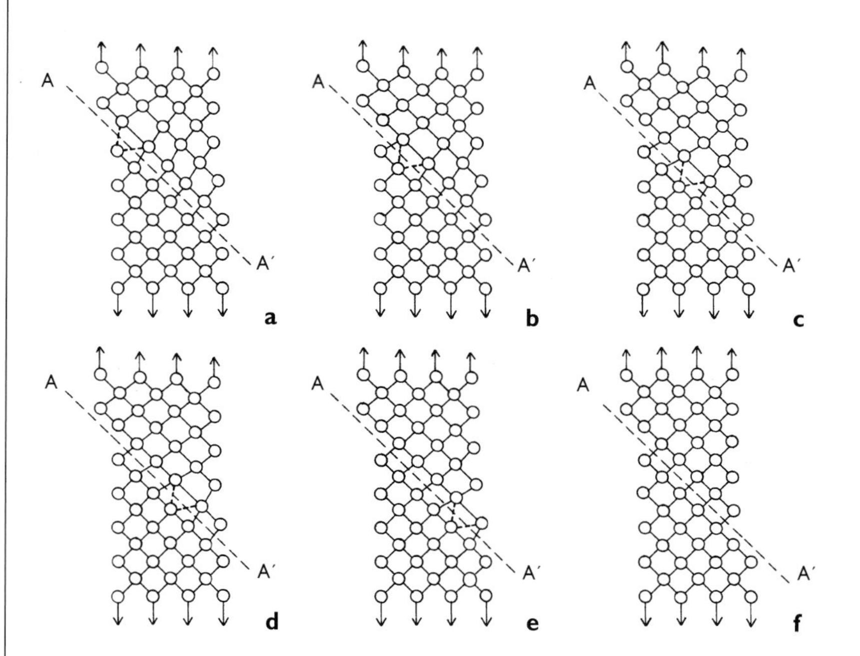

Fig 1-7 Figures 1-7a through 1-7f show how the shearing stress can cause a dislocation to pass through the network of atoms, breaking only one row of bonds at a time. For the atoms along plane A-A′ to slide past one another all at once would require enormous stress. The fact that metals yield to stresses much lower than expected is explained by the breaking of only one row of bonds (perpendicular to the page) at a time.

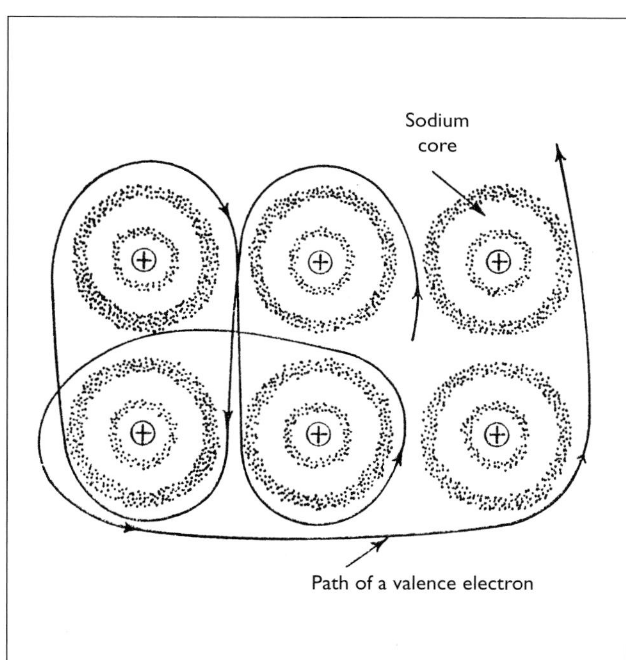

Fig 1-8 Representation of the metallic bond showing the metal ion cores surrounded by free electrons. (After Lewis TJ, Secker PE. Science of Materials. New York: Reinhold, 1965.)

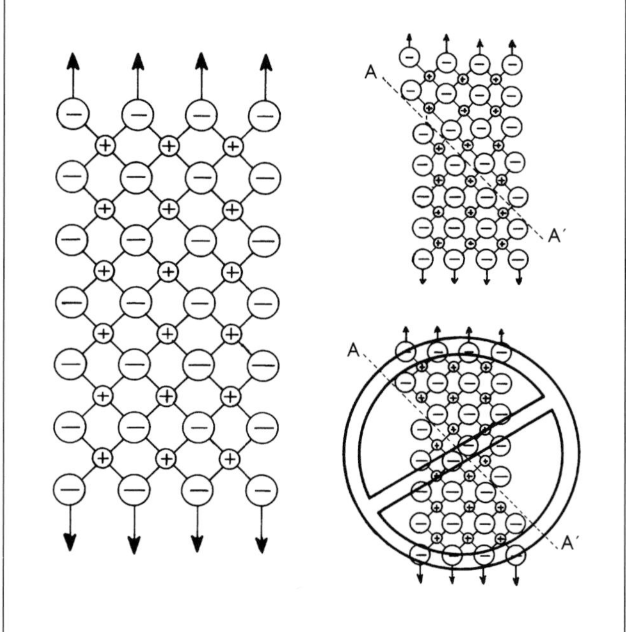

Fig 1-9 The alternating charges of an ionic structure (crystalline ceramic) do not allow dislocations to move along plane A-A′. If a dislocation were to pass through such a structure, it would result in ions of like charge coming into direct contact, which would require too much energy.

Intermetallic compounds, unlike ordinary metal alloys, have a specific formula (eg, Ag_3Sn, the main component of dental amalgam alloy powder) and an ordered arrangement of atoms. The movement of a dislocation through this ordered structure would produce a disruption of the order similar to that shown in Fig 1-9 for crystalline ceramic materials. Hence, dislocations move only with difficulty in intermetallic compounds, and this property renders them more brittle than ordinary metal alloys.

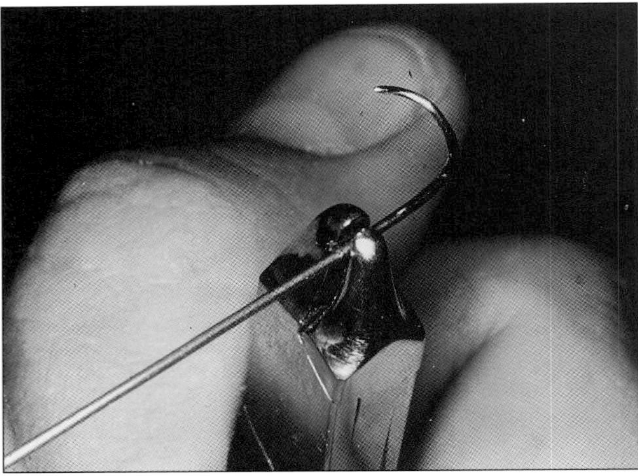

Fig 1-10 Ductility of metal as illustrated by the adaptation (bending) of a partial denture wrought wire clasp.

Clinical applications of metals

Metals are generally ductile and tough when compared to ceramics, although a few types of metals, such as dental amalgams, are markedly more brittle than others. This ductility allows the margins of castings to be burnished, orthodontic wires to be bent, and partial denture clasps to be adjusted. Figure 1-10 shows how the ductility of metal allows the wire clasp for a partial denture framework to be bent permanently to provide the desired retention. The ductile behavior of the partial denture alloy can be contrasted with the brittle behavior of the intermetallic material, dental amalgam, as shown in Fig 1-11.

Polymers

The behavior of polymers is fundamentally different from both ceramics and metals. To understand this difference, it is useful to consider the modulus of elasticity and the strength of polymers at a molecular level.

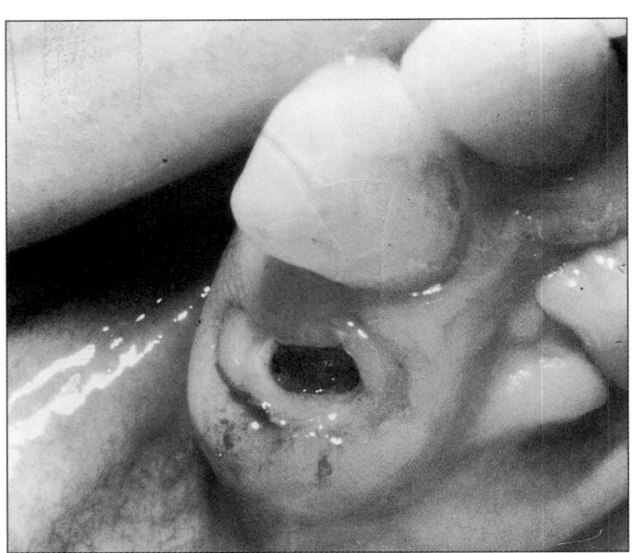

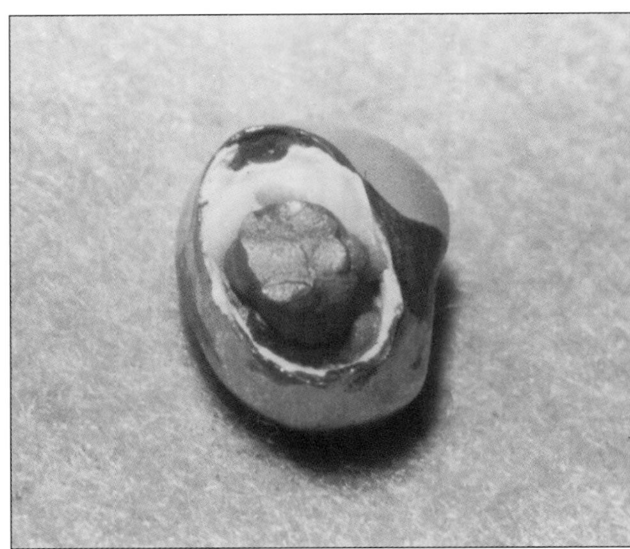

Fig 1-11 Brittle fracture of an amalgam post and core that had supported a PFM crown. Set dental amalgam is a mixture of several intermetallic compounds. Intermetallic compounds tend to be brittle rather than ductile. (Photo courtesy of R. P. O'Connor, DMD.)

Modulus of elasticity

When chains of polyethylene are aligned parallel to one another and are subjected to a tensile stress along their long axes as shown in Fig 1-12a, the stress required to stretch the atoms in the chains farther apart is found to be surprisingly high. In fact, the modulus of elasticity of polyethylene when measured in this way is 30 million psi, about the same as steel! However, if the applied stress is perpendicular to the long axes of the chains, as shown in Fig 1-12b, the modulus of elasticity is only about 0.5 million psi. The high modulus of elasticity (30 million psi) in the first case results from the strong bonds between the atoms *within* polymer chains. The low elastic modulus (0.5 million psi) in the second case results from the weak bonds between atoms in *adjacent* chains.

Bulk polymers have their polymer molecules in a more random, tangled arrangement, and hence there are somewhat fewer secondary bonds between chains than when the chains are perfectly aligned. The tangling and coiling of the polymer molecules make polymers even more flexible, because of the lower stress required to straighten out a coiled molecule compared to the stress necessary to stretch the atoms in a molecule further apart.

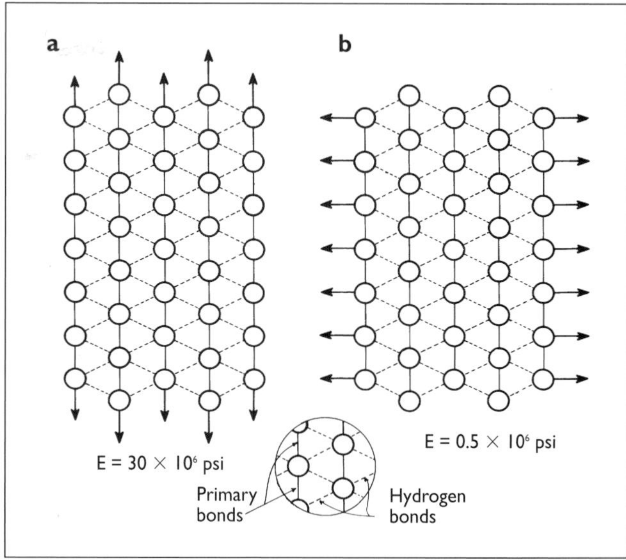

Fig 1-12 (a) Strong (primary) bonds between atoms within a polymer chain result in a high stiffness (modulus of elasticity) when aligned chains are stretched along their lengths. (b) Weak (hydrogen) bonds between atoms in adjacent chains result in a low modulus of elasticity when aligned chains are stretched perpendicular to their lengths.

Strength

The low strength of polymers when compared to ceramics and metals can also be understood in terms of the strong bonds within polymer chains, and the weak bonds between polymer chains. If the rule-of-thumb value for theoretical strength, $0.1E$, is applied to the oriented polyethylene fiber shown in Fig 1-12a, a value of 3 million psi is obtained for the theoretical strength of polyethylene. Typical bulk polymers, however, seldom have tensile strengths of more than 10,000 psi. The weak secondary bonds between polymer chains allow these chains to slide past one another at much lower stresses than those required to break the bonds within the chains.

Thermal expansion

The increase of the temperature of a material as the result of increased atomic vibration within it is a familiar concept. This atomic vibration is limited by the bonds between atoms in a material such that when strong bonds are present between atoms, the atoms vibrate over a small amplitude, and when weak bonds are present, the atoms vibrate over a large amplitude. Ceramics and metals are characterized by strong bonds between atoms, and the secondary bonds play an insignificant role in their properties. As a result, most ceramics and metals expand a relatively small amount when heated—that is, their coefficients of thermal expansion are relatively low. Polymers, however, are characterized by strong bonds within polymer chains and weak bonds between polymer chains. Thus, the vibration of carbon atoms within the polymer chain is restricted in the directions parallel to the long axis of the chain, but the atoms are free to vibrate in the two directions perpendicular to the long axis of the polymer chain. As a result, when a polymer is heated, the chains must move further apart to allow for the larger-amplitude vibration, which occurs perpendicular to the long axes of the polymer chains. This phenomenon accounts for the large coefficient of thermal expansion exhibited by polymers. Figure 1-13 illustrates the different thermal expansion behaviors of a polymeric material and a crystalline material.

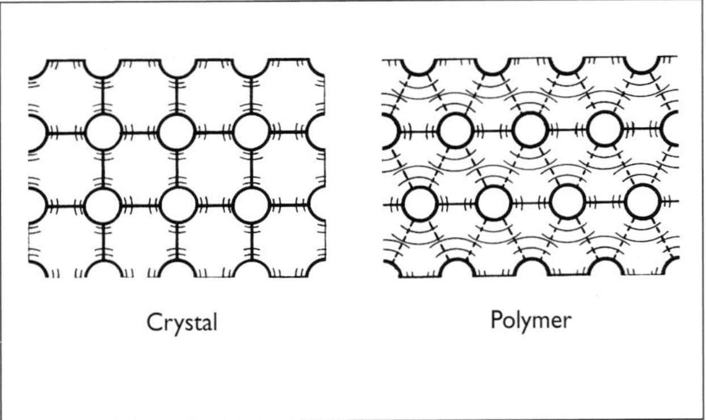

Fig 1-13 The different thermal expansion behaviors of a polymeric material and a crystalline material.

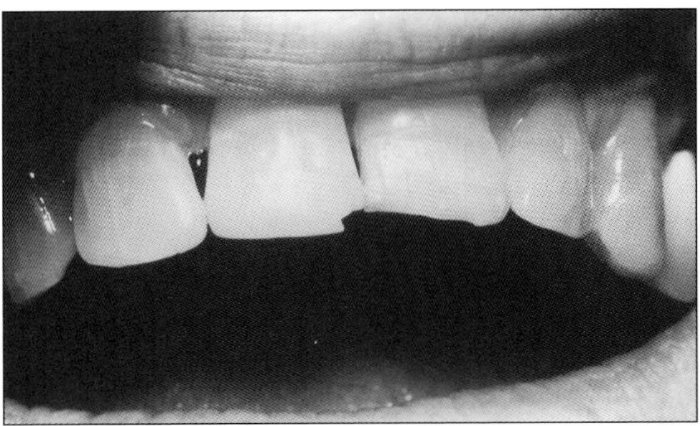

Fig 1-14 Fracture of a Class IV microfilled composite restoration. The low filler content of most microfills leaves the polymer matrix bearing the majority of the stress. Polymers are generally too weak for bearing large stresses. (Photo courtesy of C.D. Smith, DDS.)

Water absorption

Because of the weak secondary bonds in polymer materials, water molecules are able to penetrate between the polymer chains in a process called *water absorption*. Water absorption has both positive and negative aspects. On the positive side, it is the main factor in correcting the 0.5% processing shrinkage that occurs during the fabrication of heat-cured denture bases. When the acrylic polymer absorbs water the polymer molecules are forced apart slightly, causing the denture base to expand. This expansion during water absorption compensates for the processing shrinkage.

On the negative side, water is responsible for the hydrolytic degradation of polymers. In addition, the ions carried by the water may cause the polymer to break down more quickly or to become stained or malodorous.

Effect of cross-linking

Because many of the undesirable properties of polymers are due to weak bonds between polymer chains, it would seem that a way to improve them would be to link chains together with primary chemical bonds. In fact, this method, called *cross-linking*, is widely used to improve the strength, resistance to water absorption, abrasion resistance, and other properties of polymers. Because of the small number of primary bonds in a given volume of polymer material when compared to ceramics or metals, however, polymer properties remain generally inferior even with cross-linking.

The key to understanding polymers is that the low strengths and elastic moduli of polymers, as well as many other distinctive properties, can be seen in light of the concept of strong bonds within polymer chains and weak bonds between polymer chains.

Clinical applications of polymers

Polymers have had limited use as restorative materials by themselves because of their low strength and high thermal expansion. Some of the unfavorable properties of polymers have been mitigated by the incorporation of inorganic fillers to form composite materials. Modification of the polymer resins themselves to make them hydrophobic has improved their resistance to water absorption. The properties of polymers may be further improved by increasing their crystallinity, but the bonds between chains in crystalline polymers are still only secondary bonds. The intrinsic weaknesses of polymers will probably continue to limit their use as restorative materials. The incisal fracture of a Class IV microfilled composite restoration is shown in Fig 1-14. Microfilled composite resins tend to have considerably lower levels of the stronger inorganic filler, and so the stresses are borne more heavily by the weaker resin matrix. In Class IV restorations, microfills generally have insufficient strength to withstand the stresses that may be encountered.

Glossary

alloy A material that exhibits metallic properties and is composed of one or more elements—at least one of which is a metal. For example, steel is an alloy of iron and carbon, brass is an alloy of copper and zinc, and bronze is an alloy of copper and tin.

ceramic In the broadest sense, a compound of metallic and nonmetallic elements. By this definition, materials ranging from aluminum oxide (Al_2O_3) to table salt (NaCl) are classified as ceramics. In dentistry, gypsum ($CaSO_4 \cdot 2H_2O$), many dental cements (eg, zinc phosphate), and porcelains are examples of ceramic materials.

crystalline Having atoms or molecules arranged in a regular, repeating three-dimensional pattern. Metals are nearly always crystalline; ceramics and polymers can be crystalline or noncrystalline (amorphous).

dislocation A defect in a crystal that is caused by an extra plane of atoms in the structure (see Fig 1-7). The movement of dislocations is responsible for the ability of metals to bend without breaking.

intermetallic compound A chemical compound whose components are metals. The gamma phase of amalgam, Ag_3Sn, is an example of an intermetallic compound.

metal A crystalline material that consists of positively charged ions in an ordered, closely packed arrangement and bonded with a cloud of free electrons. This type of bond, called a *metallic bond*, is responsible for many of the properties of metals—electrical and thermal conductivity, metallic luster, and (usually) high strength.

polymer A material that is made up of repeating units, or *mers*. Most polymers are based upon a carbon (–C–C–C–C–) backbone in the polymer chain, although a silicone (–O–Si–O–Si–O–) backbone is important in many polymers.

stress raiser An irregularity on the surface or in the interior of an object that causes applied stress to concentrate in a localized area of the object. Other things being equal, the sharper the stress raiser, the greater the localized stress around it.

Discussion questions

1. Although metals have had a long history of application as restorative materials, which properties of metals are causing a decline in their use? Which properties will promote their use for dental applications for many more years?
2. Which physical properties are related to the large differences in wear resistance of polymers and ceramics?
3. Although the strength values of materials based upon testing given in research publications are often high, dental devices may fail at low levels of stress. Explain and indicate how materials need to be used in dentistry to achieve the full strength potential of the materials used.
4. Why are the mechanical properties of materials so important in restorative dentistry?
5. How does the atomic bonding of materials determine many of the observed properties of materials?

Questions and answers

1. **Characterize the three basic materials (metals, ceramics, and polymers) in regard to modulus of elasticity, strength, ductility, and coefficient of thermal expansion.** (See Table 1-1.)
2. **Describe the relationship between the shape of a stress raiser and the concentration of stress around it.** The sharper the stress raiser, the greater the concentration of stress around it.
3. **Discuss the key concept for each of the three basic materials and show how it explains the properties of each.**

   Ceramics—Stress concentration at surface scratches and other defects causes ceramics to fail at stresses far below their theoretical strengths.

   Metals—The ability of crystal defects called dislocations to move within the crystal structure of metals gives them their ability to bend without fracturing.

   Polymers—Strong bonds within the polymer chains and weak bonds between polymer chains are responsible for the low strengths and elastic moduli of polymers.

Recommended reading

Davidge RW. Mechanical Behavior of Ceramics. Cambridge: Cambridge University Press, 1979.

Dieter GE. Mechanical Metallurgy, 2nd ed. New York: McGraw-Hill, Inc, 1976.

O'Brien WJ, Ryge G. An Outline of Dental Materials and Their Selection. Philadelphia: WB Saunders Co, 1978.

Ruoff AL. Materials Science. Englewood Cliffs, NJ: Prentice-Hall, Inc, 1973.

Schultz J. Polymer Materials Science. Englewood Cliffs, NJ: Prentice-Hall, Inc, 1974.

Chapter 2

Physical Properties

Physical properties of materials can be considered as the ways that materials respond to changes in their environments. The relationships among the various properties are classified according to the scheme in Fig 2-1.

Mechanical properties

The concepts of stress, strain, modulus of elasticity, plastic deformation, and other properties were introduced in chapter 1. Because of the unfamiliarity and abstruse nature of many of these concepts, they will be discussed here in somewhat greater depth, and some additional concepts will be introduced as necessary to understand the physical behavior of materials.

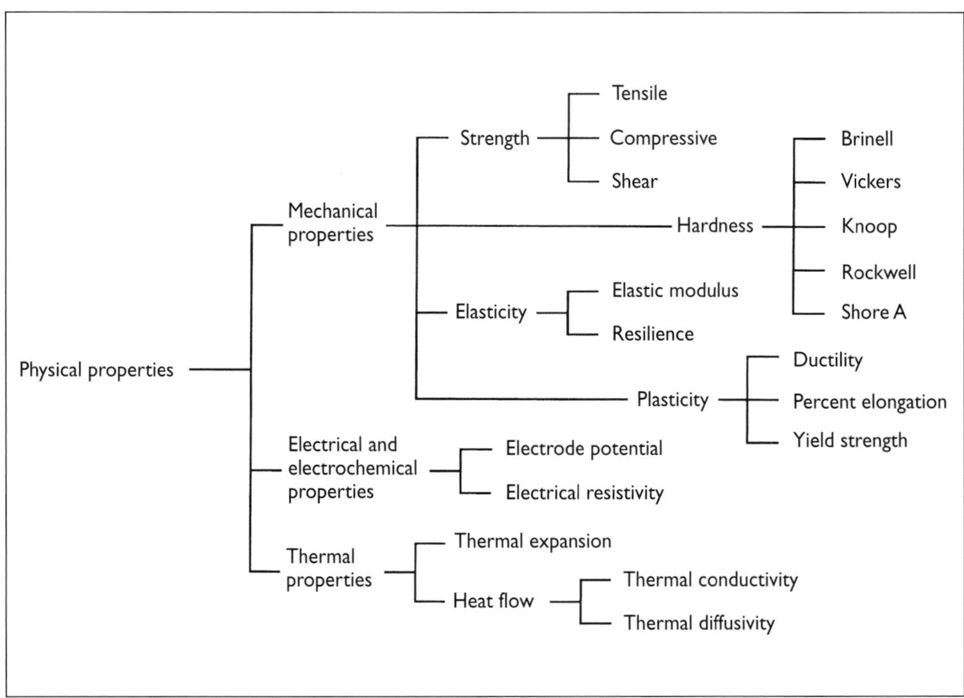

Fig 2-1 A tree diagram classifying physical properties.

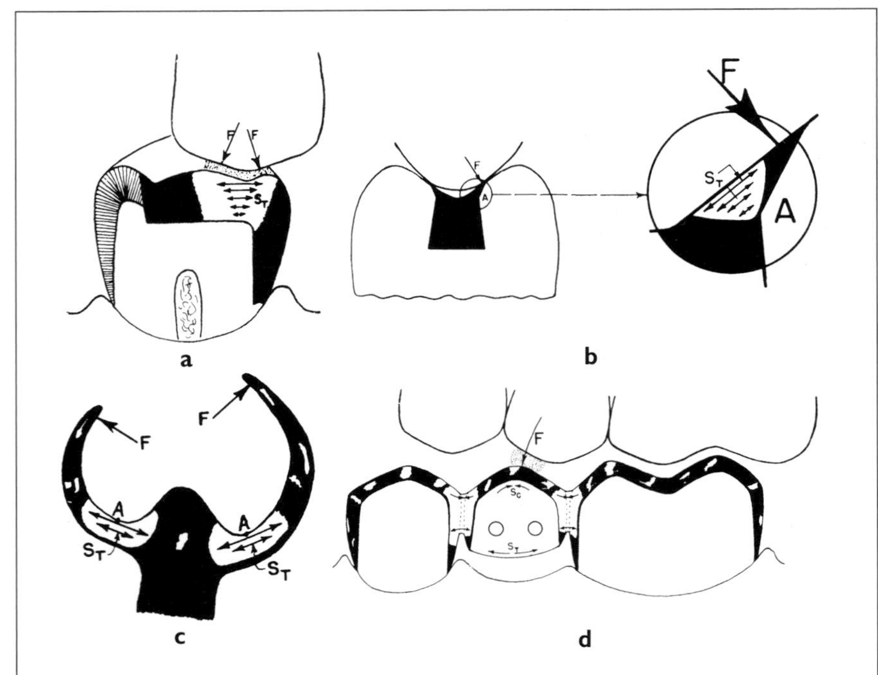

Fig 2-2 (a) Tensile stress (S_T) at the isthmus of a two-surface amalgam restoration. (b) Tensile stress at the occlusal surface of a beveled amalgam restoration. (c) Tensile stress at the junctions of a partial denture clasp. (d) Tensile and compressive stresses in a soldering bridge. *F* = force; *A* = area. (From Mahler, 1958. Reprinted with permission.)

Stress

Consider again the block of material described in the previous chapter that was ½ in. × ½ in. (1.27 cm × 1.27 cm) in cross section and was subjected to a 3,000-lb (about 13 kN) load. As we pointed out in that example, the stress experienced by that block—determined by dividing the force by the cross-sectional area of the block—is 12,000 psi, or 83 MPa. Stress (σ) is the force (*F*) divided by the cross-sectional area (*A*):

$$\sigma = \frac{F}{A}$$

Now consider a similar block, but with smaller dimensions— ¼ in. × ¼ in. (about 0.6 cm × 0.6 cm) in cross section (area of $\frac{1}{16}$ in.^{2} or about 0.4 cm^2). If this new block is subjected to the same 3,000-lb (13-kN) tensile load, the stress in this case is 3,000 lb (13 kN) divided by $\frac{1}{16}$ in.^{2} (about 0.4 cm^2) = 48,000 psi (about 330 MPa).

Thus, the usefulness of the concept of *stress* is apparent. It is not sufficient merely to state the load or force that is being applied to a dental material, because the stress that is produced in the material depends just as much on the cross-sectional area on which the load is acting as it does upon the load itself. If the block that measured ¼ in. × ¼ in. in cross section is subjected to a load of 12,000 lb (about 53 kN) instead of 3,000 lb (about 13 kN), the stress is 48,000 psi (about 330 MPa). Thus it is apparent that the stress in a material depends as much upon the cross-sectional area on which the load is acting as it does upon the load itself. If the cross-sectional area is made 4 times smaller (¼ as large), or if the load is made 4 times larger, the stress is increased by a factor of 4. Thus, the stress is said to be inversely proportional to the cross-sectional area and directly proportional to the load.

It is rare that an object will be subject to the pure tensile, compressive, or shear stresses experienced by test specimens in a materials testing laboratory. As shown in Fig 2-2, however, wherever bending forces are present, tensile stresses are present in critical areas, which could result in failure. The basic types of stresses produced in dental structures under a force are *tensile*, *compressive*, and *shear*. All three are present in a beam loaded in the center. If the value of these stresses exceeds the strength of the material, the structure will fail. It is therefore important to know the strength values of materials.

Strain

When a block of material is subjected to a tensile stress as described in the preceding section, it temporarily becomes longer by a certain amount. This temporary increase in length is called *strain.* A few examples will illustrate how strain is described. Consider the block with the cross section of ¼ in. × ¼ in. = 1/16 in.^{2} (0.6 cm × 0.6 cm = 0.4 cm^2) and assume it has a length of 10 in. (25.40 cm) when no load is applied. If the length is measured while the 3,000-lb (13-kN) load is being applied and the new length is 10.016 in. (25.441 cm), the strain is computed by dividing the increase in length (0.016 in., 0.041 cm) by the original length (10.000 in., 25.40 cm) to obtain 0.0016. Strain is a dimensionless quantity because we are dividing unit length by unit length, but sometimes it is written as "in./in." or "cm/cm." Strain can also be expressed in a percentage, in which case the dimensionless value is multiplied by 100%. In the given example, the strain would be 0.16%.

If a piece of the same material with the same cross section but 11 in. (27.940 cm) long were subjected to the same load (3,000 lb, about 13 kN), and the length of the block of material were measured while the load was being applied, it would be 11.0176 in. (27.9847 cm). To compute the strain produced, the change in length (0.0176 in., 0.0447 cm) is divided by the original length (11.0000 in., 27.9400 cm), and the strain is determined to be 0.0016 (or 0.16%), the same value obtained above for the block of material measuring 10 in. (25.4 cm). Thus, it can be seen that strain is independent of the length of the specimen.

Now consider a bar of high-strength steel, ¼ in. × ¼ in. = 1/16 in.^{2} (0.6 cm × 0.6 cm = 0.4 cm^2) in cross section and 10 in. (25.4 cm) long, that is capable of supporting a tensile load of 6,000 lb (about 27 kN). If the length of this bar were measured while it is under this 6,000-lb (27-kN) load, it would be 10.032 in. (25.4813 cm). If the strain is computed as before, the change in length (0.032 in., 0.0813 cm) divided by the original length (10.000 in., 25.4 cm) is found to be 0.0032 or 0.32%. Hence, it can be seen that if the cross-sectional area of the block of material is kept the same and the load applied is doubled, the strain experienced by the material is doubled.

Elasticity

The preceding examples showed that both stress and strain are directly proportional to the load applied when the cross-sectional area is kept the same. Hence, if the load is doubled, both the stress and the strain likewise will be doubled. It can be seen that the ratio between stress (σ) and strain (ϵ) is the same, thus:

$$\frac{\sigma}{\epsilon} = \frac{2\sigma}{2\epsilon} = \frac{3\sigma}{3\epsilon}$$

The property of having a constant ratio of stress to strain is called *elasticity*, and the constant that is the ratio of stress to strain is called the *modulus of elasticity*. To gain a clearer understanding of the concept of elasticity and to see what it means for two materials to have different moduli of elasticity, it is helpful to consider the analogy of two springs of different stiffnesses as shown in Fig 2-3. Spring 2 is stiffer than spring 1; hence, when they support equal weights the stiffer

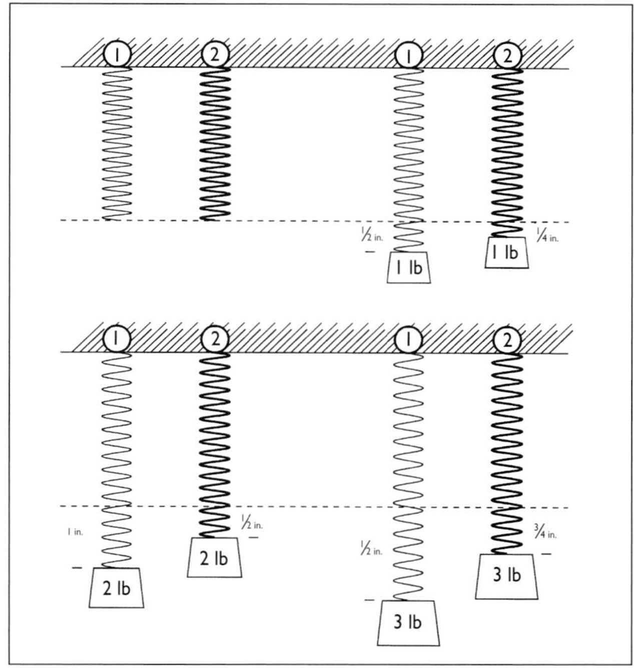

Fig 2-3 The concept of modulus of elasticity using the analogy of springs. Spring 1 is a flexible spring, representing a material with a low modulus of elasticity. Spring 2 is a stiff spring, representing a material with a high modulus of elasticity. When the same load is applied to both springs, they stretch different amounts. The weight applied to the spring is analogous to the stress (σ), the amount the spring stretches is analogous to the strain (ϵ), and the stiffness of the spring is analogous to the modulus of elasticity (E).

spring is extended a smaller amount. Increasing the load from 1 lb (4.4 N) to 2 lb (8.9 N) causes each spring to extend twice as much as it did under the 1-lb (4.4-N) load. Subjecting both springs to a 3-lb (13-N) load causes each one to extend 3 times as much as it did under a 1-lb (4.4-N) load, and so on. It can be seen that, irrespective of the load applied for either spring 1 or spring 2, the ratio of the extension to the load is a constant for that spring. However, the constants for the two springs are different. In this analogy, the extension of the spring corresponds to strain, the load or weight on the spring corresponds to stress, and the spring constant corresponds to the modulus of elasticity.

It is obvious that more weight cannot be added to a spring indefinitely and still have the extension increase proportionately. At some point the spring will become "stretched out" and will not return to its original size when the weight is removed. In the same way, when a material is stressed above a certain point, stress is no longer proportional to strain. The highest stress at which stress is proportional to strain is called the *elastic limit*, or the *proportional limit*. Because this stress is difficult to determine precisely, as it would entail looking for an infinitely small deviation from proportionality, it is customary to designate a certain permanent deformation or *offset* (usually 0.002, or 0.2%) and to report the *yield strength* of the material at this strain. Thus the terms "elastic limit" and "proportional limit" are synonymous, whereas "yield strength" has a slightly different meaning. The yield strength of a material is always slightly higher than the elastic limit.

If a material continues to have more and more weight applied to it, it will of course eventually break. If the material is being stretched (tensile loading), the stress at breakage is called the *ultimate tensile strength* (UTS). When many metals are stressed above their proportional limits, they undergo a process called *work hardening*, and actually become stronger and harder. But with the increased strength provided by work hardening comes increased brittleness. It is thus very important to avoid overdoing it when bending a wire or a partial denture clasp—too much bending of the metal back and forth will make it harder and more brittle.

The modulus of elasticity is an inherent property of the material and cannot be altered appreciably by heat treatment, work hardening, or any other kind of conditioning. This property is called *structure insensitivity*, because it is not sensitive to any alteration to the structure (meaning the microstructure) of the material. The modulus of elasticity is one of the few properties that is not sensitive to any alteration of the structure of the material. The yield strength of a material, for example, is sensitive to work hardening and will increase with increasing amounts of work hardening.

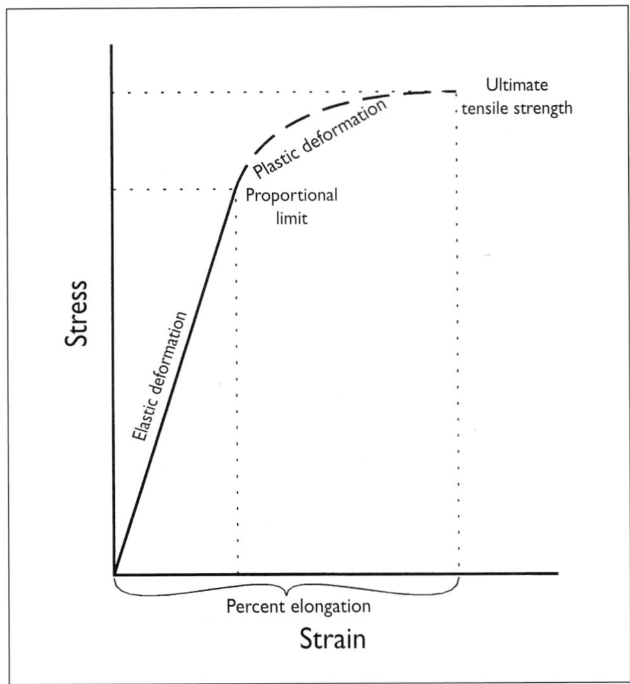

Fig 2-4 Measurement of stress and strain on an object being stretched. In the region labeled "elastic deformation," stress is proportional to strain, whereas in the region labeled "plastic deformation," stress and strain are no longer proportional (strain increases faster than stress does). The highest stress at which stress and strain are still proportional is called the proportional limit, and the maximum stress just before the object breaks is called the ultimate tensile strength. The total amount that the object stretches (ie, the total strain), which is the sum of the elastic deformation and the plastic deformation, is called the percent elongation.

Plasticity

When the elastic or proportional limit is exceeded in a material, it is said to exhibit *plastic* behavior. (The term "plastic" means "moldable," but the term has come to be associated with polymers.) Materials that experience a large amount of plastic behavior or permanent deformation are said to be *ductile*. Materials that undergo little or no plastic behavior are said to be *brittle*. If stress is plotted against strain, with stress as the ordinate (y axis) and strain as the abscissa (x axis), a diagram such as the one in Fig 2-4 is the result. It can be seen that stress is proportional to strength up to the elastic (or proportional) limit. Above this stress, stress and strain are no longer proportional. If a material is stressed into the plastic region or region of permanent deformation and then the stress is removed, the material will have a permanent *set*, or deformation. If stress is continuously increased, the material will undergo more and more plastic deformation and will ultimately fracture. The highest stress achieved during this process is called the ultimate tensile strength of the material, as mentioned previously. The total strain at fracture (elastic strain + plastic strain) is called the *elongation*. Elongation of metals is important in several situations in dentistry. When one is burnishing the margin of a crown, the property that most comes into play is the elongation, although the yield strength is also important. For example, gold alloys are generally easy to burnish because they have a lower yield strength. Nickel-chromium and cobalt-chromium alloys may have adequate elongation for burnishing, but their yield strengths are so high that they make burnishing difficult. Another example of the importance of elongation is the bending of a partial denture clasp to adjust the retention.

The integrated area under the entire stress–strain curve is a measure of the energy required to fracture the material, or its *toughness*. The integrated area under only the elastic region of the stress-strain curve is a measure of the ability of the material to store elastic energy (the way a compressed spring does). This ability is called the *resilience* of the material.

Tabulated data for (Young's) modulus of elasticity, yield strength, ultimate tensile strength, percent elongation, and other mechanical properties are listed in Appendix A.

Fatigue

When materials are subjected to cycles of loading and unloading, as during mastication, they may fail due to fatigue at stresses below the ultimate tensile strength. Usually, small cracks at the surface or within the material gradually grow larger upon cycling, and eventually the material fails. Fatigue curves, such as the one shown in Fig 2-5, show the experimentally determined number of cycles to failure at different stress levels. The higher the stress placed on and off the material, the fewer the number of cycles until failure.

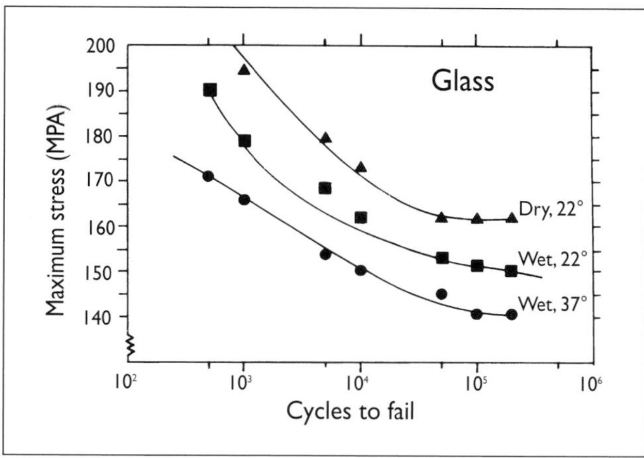

Fig 2-5 Fatigue curves for glass-filled composite resin restorative material. (Courtesy of R.A. Draughn, PhD.)

Viscous flow

Many dental materials are in a fluid state when they are formed, and viscous flow phenomena are important considerations. Our understanding of the behavior of impression materials and amalgam involve viscoelastic phenomena. When shear stress–strain rate (flow rate) plots are obtained, they enable viscous materials to be classified in several ways. A newtonian fluid shows a constant viscosity, η, which is independent of strain rate:

$$\eta = \frac{\sigma}{\epsilon} = \text{constant}$$

where η is the viscosity in poise, σ is the shear stress acting on the fluid, and ϵ is the strain, or flow rate.

Actual fluids differ from these in their flow responses to the level of stress applied. Plastic fluids (eg, putty) don't flow at all until a minimum stress is applied. Pseudoplastic fluids (eg, fluoride gels) show an instantaneous decrease in apparent viscosity or consistency (become more free-flowing) with increasing shear rate. Dilatant fluids (eg, fluid denture base resins) show an increase in rigidity as more pressure is applied. Thixotropic fluids (eg, fluoride gels, house paints) flow more freely when vibrated, shaken, or stirred than if allowed to sit undisturbed. Formulation of the various suspensions and gels used in dentistry to impart one or more of these properties can make them easier to handle. For example, impression materials that do not run off impression trays but are less viscous under pressure in a syringe have a definite advantage.

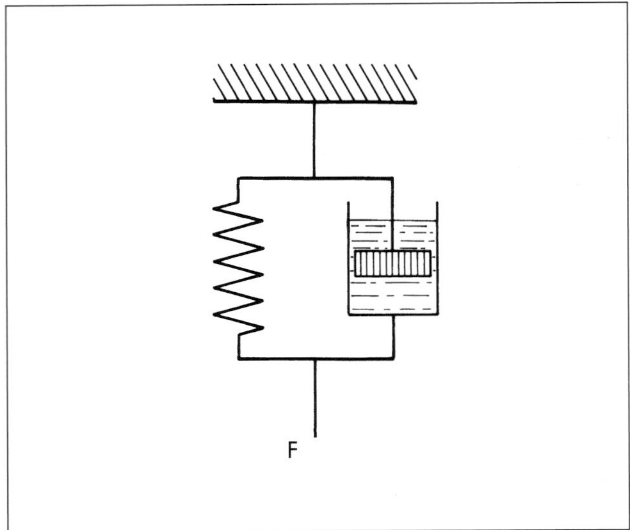

Fig 2-6 Model of a viscoelastic material.

Viscoelastic behavior

Many materials, including elastic impression materials, waxes, and even hardened amalgam, show a combination of elasticity and viscous flow. Figure 2-6 is a model of how a viscoelastic material acts under stress, the so-called spring-and-dashpot (or Voigt) model. (A *dashpot* is an oil-filled cylinder with a loosely fitted piston—most automobile shock absorbers are of a dashpot design.) As the model is stretched, the spring component on the left stretches and the piston of the dashpot also moves through the viscous liquid. The strain under stress and after release of the stress is time-dependent. The strain gradually builds up until the release of stress, and then it gradually goes back to zero as the spring element returns to its original length but is dampened by the dashpot element. Elastic impression materials are viscoelastic; initially they are strained upon removal from the mouth and require a short period of time to recover before models or dies are poured.

Hardness

The resistance of a material to indentation or penetration is called *hardness*. The technical definition of hardness varies little, if at all, from the familiar definition, with the possible exception that the technical definition carries with it the connotation of a method of measurement. Most of the methods for measuring hardness consist of making a dent in the surface of a material with a specified force in a controlled and reproducible manner and measuring the size of the dent. For the measurement methods discussed in this section, as the hardness increases, the respective hardness number increases also. For example, Figure 2-7 indicates the relative positions of a variety of dental and other materials on a Knoop hardness scale ranging from soft on the left to hard on the right. The positions of the different materials on the line indicate their relative hardnesses.

Brinell hardness number (BHN)

The indenter for the Brinell hardness test is a small hardened-steel ball, which is forced into the surface of a material under a specified load. This indentation process leaves a round dent in the material, and hardness is determined by measuring the diameter of the dent. Brinell hardness values for selected metals are listed in Appendix A.

Vickers hardness number (VHN) or diamond pyramid hardness (DPH)

The Vickers hardness indenter is a square, pyramid-shaped diamond, which leaves a square, diamond-shaped indentation in the surface of the material being tested. Hardness is determined by measuring the diagonals of the square and taking the average of the two dimensions. The Vickers hardness test is also called the *diamond pyramid hardness test*.

The Brinell and Vickers hardness tests are both used to measure the hardness of dental alloys, and hardness values on alloy packages are expressed in either Vickers or Brinell hardness numbers. To compare Vickers and Brinell numbers, use the following relationship:

$$\text{VHN} = 1.05 \times \text{BHN},$$

$$\text{or BHN} = \frac{\text{VHN}}{1.05}$$

For example, if a package of casting alloy lists a Vickers hardness of 242 and you want to compare it with a different brand that lists the Brinell hardness, you would divide the VHN by 1.05 to obtain a BHN of 230. Diamond pyramid (Vickers) hardness values for several types of materials are listed in Appendix A.

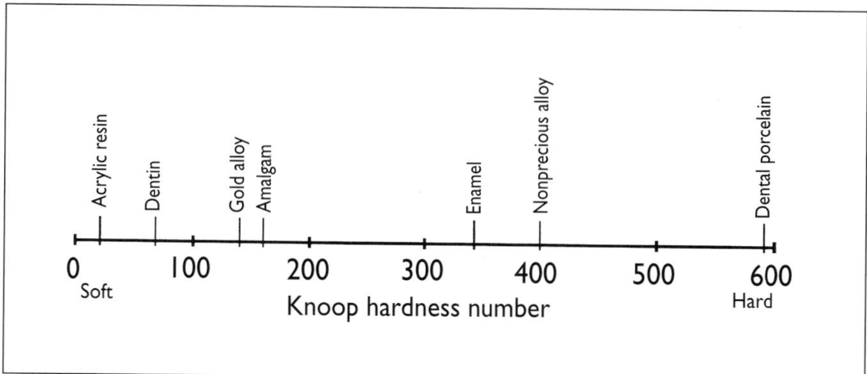

Fig 2-7 Relative hardnesses of a variety of dental materials and tooth substances. The positions of the different materials on the line indicate their relative hardnesses.

Knoop hardness (KHN)

The indenter for the Knoop hardness test is also made of a diamond, but its outline is somewhat different from the Vickers indenter; although it is diamond shaped, one diagonal is much longer than the other. Only the long diagonal is measured to determined the Knoop hardness number. Knoop hardness numbers for a variety of materials are listed in Appendix A.

Rockwell hardness (R_A, R_B, . . . R_G)

The Rockwell hardness test is used primarily for determining the hardnesses of steels and is the most widely used hardness test in the United States. The Vickers, Brinell, and Knoop hardness tests are more commonly used for dental materials, however. Rockwell uses different hardened steel balls or diamond cones and different loads. Each combination forms a specific Rockwell scale (A, B, and C scales are the most common). The different scales are used for materials of different hardness ranges.

Shore A durometer

The Shore A hardness test is used to measure the hardness of rubbers and soft plastics. The Shore A scale is between 0 and 100 units, with penetration of the material by the indenter yielding a value of 0, and no penetration yielding a value of 100. Shore A hardness values for several polymeric materials are listed in Appendix A.

Thermal properties

Heat flow through a material

Metals tend to be good conductors of heat, and this property must be taken into consideration when placing metallic restorations. Dentin is a thermal insulator (poor conductor of heat); thus, when a sufficient thickness of dentin is present, the patient feels no sensitivity to heat and cold through a metallic restoration. However, when only a thin layer of dentin remains, some thermal protection must be provided for the pulp. A good rule of thumb in determining the thickness of cement base necessary in a given situation is to visualize how much dentin would have to be present in the excavation site so no base would be necessary and to apply base up to this level. The rate at which heat flows through a material is expressed as *thermal conductivity* or *thermal diffusivity*. The difference between these two terms is described in the following subsections.

Thermal conductivity

Thermal conductivity (k) is a measure of the speed at which heat travels (in calories per second) through a given thickness of material (1 cm), when one side of the material is maintained at a constant temperature that is 1°C higher than the other side. Thermal conductivity is expressed in units of cal cm/cm^2 sec °C. Thermal conductivity values for a variety of materials are listed in Appendix A.

Thermal diffusivity

Whereas thermal conductivity gives an idea of the relative rates at which heat flows through various materials, it fails to take into account the fact that various materials require different amounts of heat (calories) to raise their temperatures an equal amount. For example, 1 gram of water requires 1.000 calorie to raise its temperature 1°C, whereas 1 gram of dentin requires only 0.28 calorie, and 1 gram of gold requires only 0.031 calorie to produce a 1°C temperature increase. Thus, thermal conductivity alone will not tell

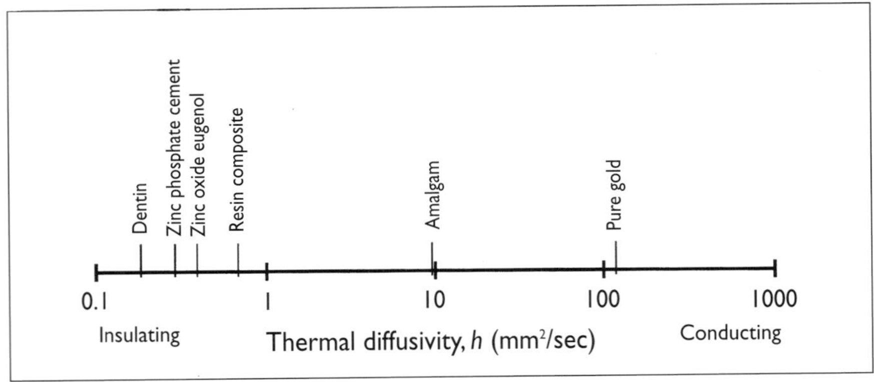

Fig 2-8 Thermal diffusivities of restorative materials.

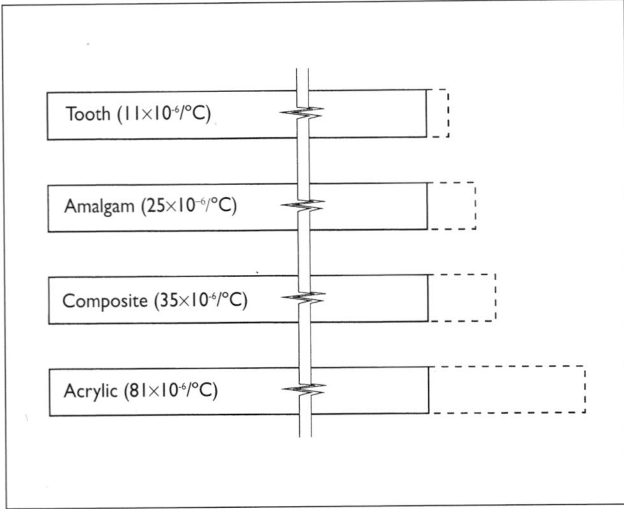

Fig 2-9 Relative thermal expansions of several restorative materials and tooth structure. The relative amounts the materials expand when heated the same amount are represented by the dashed lines. The amount of expansion is magnified to make it visible for comparison of the materials.

us, for instance, how rapidly the interior surface under a crown will heat up when the exterior surface is heated. To know how quickly the interior of the crown will approach the temperature of the exterior, we need to know the thermal diffusivity of the alloy. The thermal diffusivity (h) of a material (expressed in units of mm^2/sec) is dependent on its thermal conductivity, heat capacity (C_p), and density (ρ):

$$h = \frac{k}{(C_p \times \rho)}$$

The relative thermal diffusivities of several dental materials are shown in Fig 2-8, and tabular data on a variety of materials are included in Appendix A.

Thermal expansion

There are several situations in dentistry in which the thermal expansion of materials is important. Thermal cycling of restorations with markedly different expansion coefficients from tooth structure can cause percolation as discussed previously. The porcelain and metal in a porcelain-fused-to-metal (PFM) restoration must contract at the same rate upon cooling from the porcelain firing temperature if the build-up of large residual stresses is to be avoided. The cooling of a denture base from the processing temperature to room temperature is primarily responsible for the processing shrinkage that occurs. The thermal expansion behavior of dental wax, gold alloy, investment, and so on, are all important in producing properly fitting castings. Figure 2-9 illustrates the relative values of coefficient of thermal expansion for tooth, amalgam, composite, and acrylic resin. The diagram is only schematic—the expansion has been magnified to make it visible—the actual thermal expansion would be too small to see. The thermal expansion coefficients, or the fractional changes in length per °Celsius, are given in parentheses. Tabular thermal expansion data on a variety of materials are included in Appendix A.

Electrical and electrochemical properties

Electrode potentials

An electrochemical series is a listing of elements according to their tendency to gain or lose electrons in solution. The series is referenced versus the potential of a standard hydrogen electrode, which is arbitrarily

Table 2-1 Standard electrode potentials

Half-reaction	E^0 (volts)
$Li^+ + e = Li$	–3.04
$K^+ + e = K$	–2.93
$Ca^{2+} + 2e = Ca$	–2.87
$Na^+ + e = Na$	–2.71
$Mg^{2+} + 2e = Mg$	–2.37
$Al^{3+} + 3e = Al$	–1.662
$Zn^{2+} + 2e = Zn$	–0.762
$Cr^{3+} + 3e = Cr$	–0.744
$Fe^{2+} + 2e = Fe$	–0.447
$Ni^{2+} + 2e = Ni$	–0.257
$Sn^{2+} + 2e = Sn$	–0.1375
$Pb^{2+} + 2e = Pb$	–0.1262
$Fe^{3+} + 3e = Fe$	–0.037
$H^+ + e = H$	0.000 (reference)
$Cu^{2+} + 2e = Cu$	+0.342
$Cu^+ + e = Cu$	+0.521
$Ag^+ + e = Ag$	+0.800
$Hg^{2+} + 2e = Hg$	+0.851
$Pt^{2+} + 2e = Pt$	+1.118
$Au^+ + e = Au$	+1.692

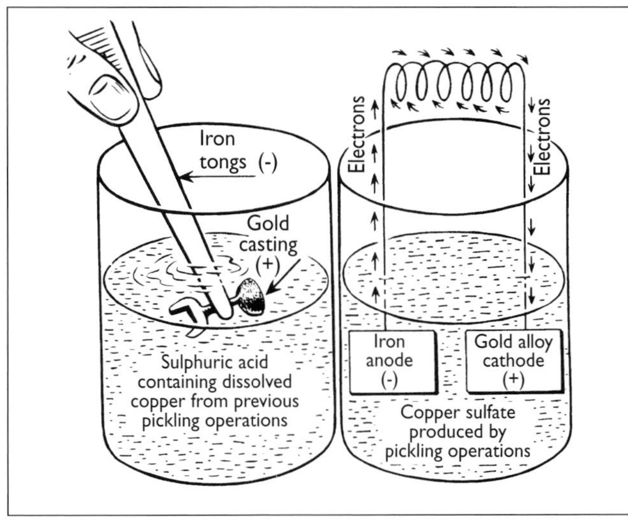

Fig 2-10 Accidental plating of copper during pickling of gold casting. The model of the cell is formed by iron tongs and gold alloy *(right)*. (From O'Brien, 1962. Reprinted with permission.)

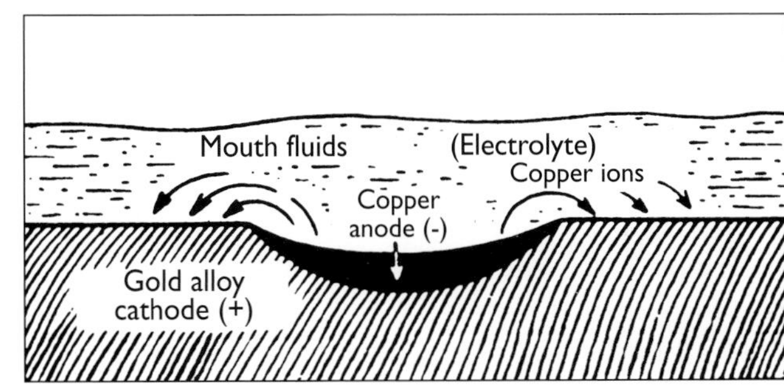

Fig 2-11 Corrosion cell set up around surface pit containing copper not removed by polishing (see Fig 2-10). (From O'Brien, 1962. Reprinted with permission.)

assigned a value of 0.000 volts. If the elements are listed according to the tendency of their atoms to lose electrons, the potentials are termed *oxidation potentials*. If they are listed according to the tendency of their ions to gain electrons, the potentials are termed *reduction potentials*. Reduction potentials at 25°C and 1 atmosphere of pressure are termed *standard electrode potentials* (see Table 2-1). Metals with a large positive electrode potential, such as platinum and gold, are more resistant to oxidation and corrosion in the oral cavity. If there is a large difference between the electrode potentials of two metals in contact with the same solution, such as between gold and aluminum, an electrolytic cell may develop. If this occurs in the mouth, the patient may experience discomfort.

The exact nature of tarnish and corrosion of restorative materials in vivo is extremely complex and involves much more than electrode potentials of materials. A possible source of the corrosion of gold alloys is accidental contamination of the surface with copper during pickling, and subsequent electrochemical action in saliva (Figs 2-10 and 2-11).

Table 2-2 Electrical resistivity of several materials

Material	Resistivity (ohm-cm)
Copper	1.7×10^{-6}
SiO_2 (glass)	$> 10^{14}$
Human enamel	$\sim 4 \times 10^{6}$
Human dentin	$\sim 3 \times 10^{4}$
Zinc phosphate cement	2×10^{5}
Zinc oxide–eugenol	5×10^{9}

Electrical resistivity

Electrical resistivity measures the resistance of a material to the flow of an electrical current. The relationship between the resistance (R) in ohms, the resistivity (ρ), the length (l), and the cross-sectional area, (A) is as follows:

$$R = \rho \left(\frac{l}{A} \right)$$

Electrical resistivity values for several materials are given in Table 2-2. The low resistivity of metallic restorative materials is responsible for discomfort to the pulp if dissimilar metals generate a voltage. The insulating properties of cements help to reduce this problem.

Glossary

anelastic Deviating from a proportional relationship of stress and strain.

compression Two forces applied toward one another in the same straight line.

diametral tensile strength The ultimate tensile strength of a brittle material measured by compressing a cylindrical specimen across its diameter.

ductility Ability of a material to be plastically strained in tension.

dynamic creep A slow deformation under cyclic stresses below the normal yield strength.

elastic Capable of sustaining deformation without permanent change in size or shape.

elastic modulus Stiffness of a material within the elastic range. Numerically, it is the ratio of stress and strain.

electrical resistivity Ability of a material to resist conduction of an electric current.

elongation Overall deformation (elastic + plastic) as a result of tensile force application.

fatigue Tendency to fracture under cyclic stresses.

fracture strength Strength at fracture based on the original dimensions of the specimen. Also called ultimate strength.

hardness Resistance to permanent indentation on the surface.

linear coefficient of thermal expansion Change in length per unit original length for a 1°C temperature change.

proportional limit The maximum stress at which the straight-line relationship between stress and strain is valid.

resilience Energy needed to deform a material to the proportional limit.

shear Two sets of forces applied toward one another but not in the same straight line.

strain (nominal) Change in length per unit original length.

stress (nominal) Force per unit area.

tension Two sets of forces applied away from one another in the same straight line.

thermal conductivity The quantity of heat passing through a material 1 cm thick with a cross section of 1 cm^2, having a temperature difference of 1°C.

thermal diffusivity Measure of the heat transfer of a material in the time-dependent state.

toughness Amount of energy needed for fracture.

ultimate strength The maximum strength obtained based on the original dimensions of the sample.

viscoelastic Having both elastic and viscous properties.

viscous Resistant to flow (referring to a fluid).

yield strength Strength measured at the stress at which a small amount of plastic strain occurs. Also called yield point.

Discussion questions

1. What is galvanic action in the mouth and how can it be minimized?
2. Why is thermal diffusivity more relevant to the insulation of the pulp than thermal conductivity?
3. Explain why dental bridges may fail under tensile stresses when under biting forces that appear to be compressive?
4. How is the leakage of mouth fluids around a composite restoration related to the coefficient of thermal expansion and temperature changes in the mouth?
5. Why is time so important in the behavior of viscoelastic materials such as impression materials and waxes?

Questions and answers

1. **Discuss why a knowledge and understanding of the physical and mechanical properties of biomaterials is important in dentistry.** Knowledge and understanding of physical and mechanical properties help the dentist predict how a material will behave in vivo and how it should be manipulated.
2. **Explain why the thermal diffusivity of a material is more applicable to behavior in vivo than is its thermal conductivity.** Thermal diffusivity is a time-dependent property, and, since the temperature of the oral cavity changes dramatically within a few seconds (drinking hot coffee versus eating ice cream), it predicts the behavior of materials under more realistic conditions. Thermal conductivity, on the other hand, is a steady-state property, and the temperature of the mouth is not constant over time.
3. **Draw and label a stress-strain diagram including the proportional limit, yield point, and ultimate tensile strength.** See Fig 2-4.
4. **Define hardness and its relation to other mechanical properties.** Hardness is the resistance of a material to permanent indentation in its surface. It involves complex stresses, so it cannot be directly related to any other physical property.
5. **Compare materials *a* and *b* on the basis of the following two stress–strain curves, obtained by pulling the materials in tension.**

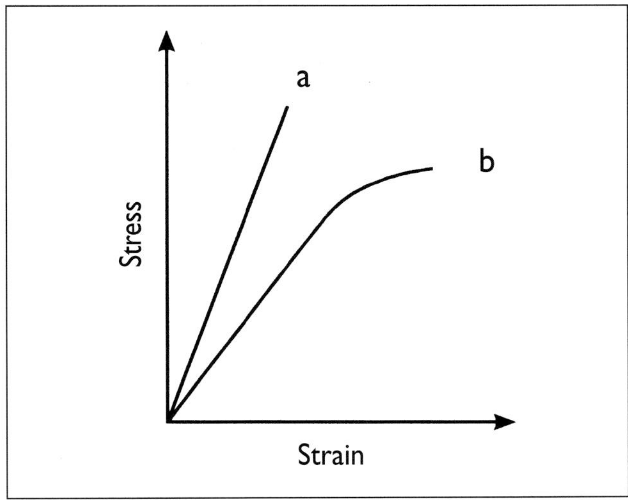

a is brittle	*a* is stiffer than *b*
b is ductile	*a* is stronger than *b*
	b is tougher than *a*

Recommended reading

Mahler DB, Terkla LG. Analysis of stress in dental structures. Dent Clin North Am Nov 1958.

O'Brien WJ. Electrochemical corrosion of gold alloys. Dent Abstracts 7:46, 1962.

Chapter 3

Color and Appearance

Among the important factors that influence esthetic appearances of restorations are color, translucency, gloss, and fluorescence. Each of these factors, as perceived by an observer such as a dentist, technician, or patient, is influenced by (*1*) the *illuminant* (light source), (*2*) the *inherent optical parameters* of the restorative materials that dictate the interaction of the light from the illuminant with the material, and (*3*) the *interpretation* of the observer (Fig 3-1). An understanding of these factors in restorative materials, and proper consideration and communication of this information, greatly assist the choice and fabrication of esthetic restorations.

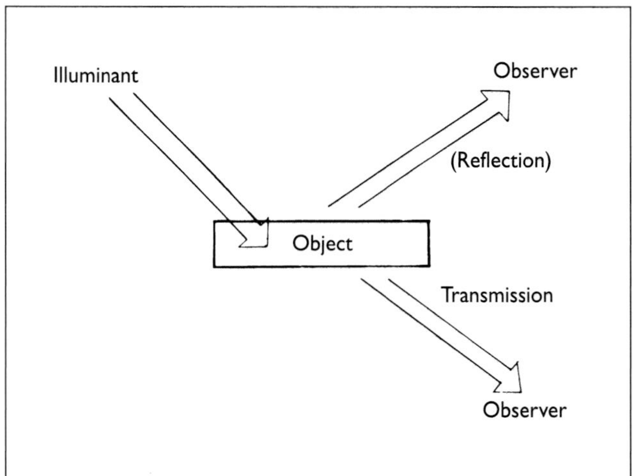

Fig 3-1 Illuminant, object, and observer interaction.

Illuminant

Light waves emitted from the illuminant interact with the object and are perceived by the observer. The color content of the illuminant interacts with the object being perceived. The color content of the illuminant is the intensity of light emitted at each wavelength (spectral distribution). This is dependent on the type of illuminant. The wavelengths of light are associated with hues—commonly referred to as *color* (Fig 3-2). White light contains a mixture of wavelengths (colors). It is dispersed into components when it passes through a prism, as shown in Fig 3-3. Different illuminants have different intensity distributions with respect to wavelength; examples are the differences in illuminant A and fluorescent light illustrated in Figs 3-4a and 3-4b.

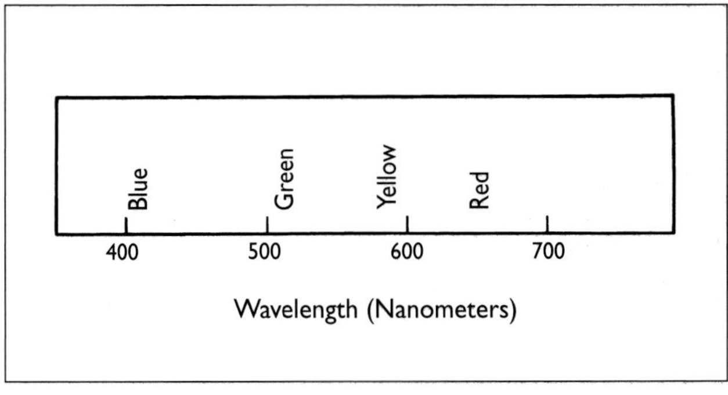

Fig 3-2 Wavelength and hue. (Adapted from Billmeyer and Saltzman, 1960.)

Illuminants are sometimes described by their color temperature (in degrees kelvin). This is based on the equivalence of the illuminant as compared to a radiating body with a temperature equal to the color temperature.

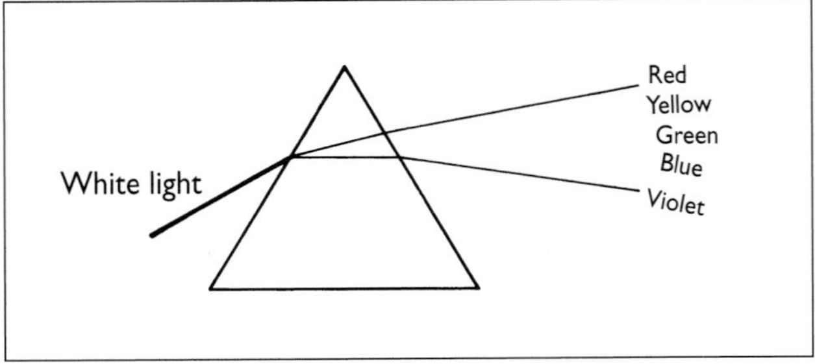

Fig 3-3 Dispersion of white light by a prism.

The characteristics of an illuminant are important in color evaluation because the intensity distribution, with respect to wavelength, identifies the light spectrum available to interact with the object and then be perceived by the observer. In any color description the type of illuminant used needs to be defined. Furthermore, the appropriate illuminant needs to be used in shade selection and shade matching. Illuminants that closely approximate daylight are preferred because color considerations for restorations, when seen under these illuminants, are close to those seen under natural light. Several "daylight" sources intended for use in dental operatories are available. Representative spectral distributions of some of these illuminants are shown in Figs 3-5a and 3-5b.

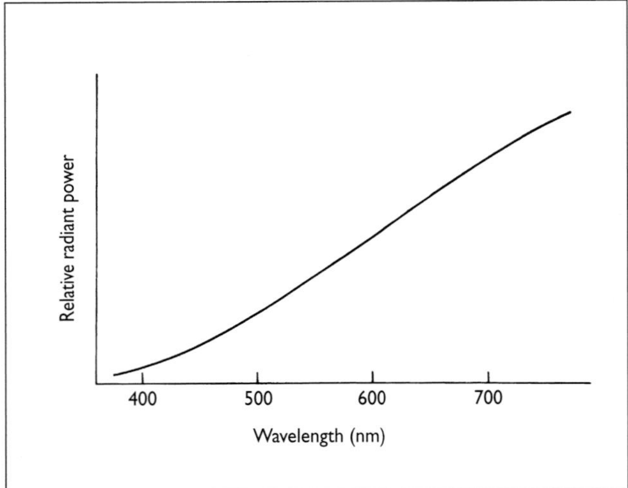

Fig 3-4a Intensity distributions of illuminant A.

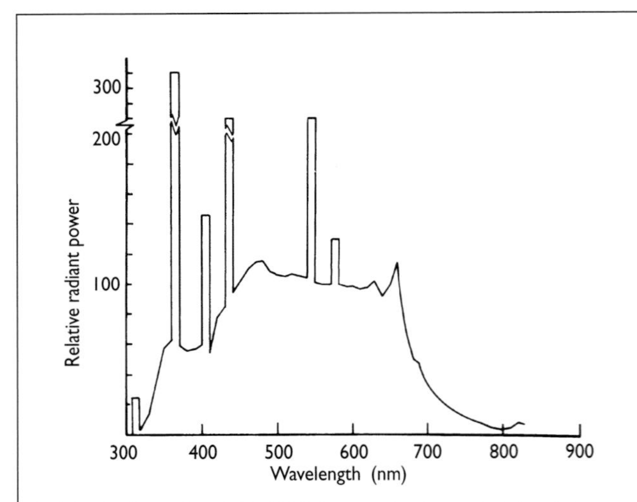

Fig 3-4b Intensity distributions of fluorescent light.

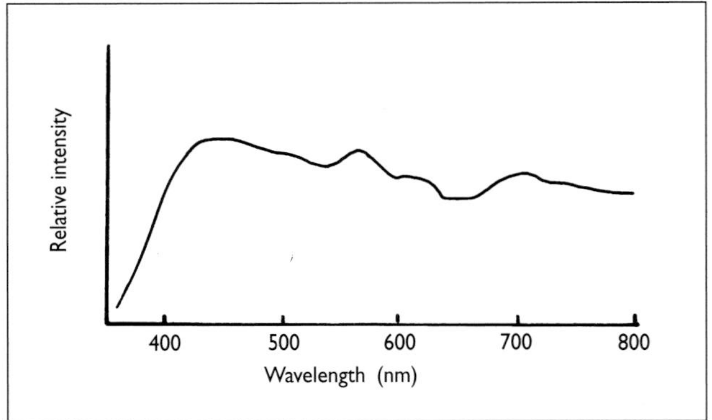

Fig 3-5a Spectral distribution of Neylite (J.M. Ney Co.).

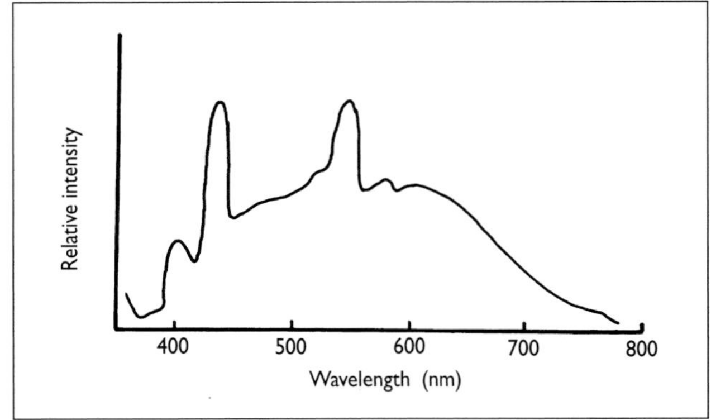

Fig 3-5b Spectral distribution of Vita-Lite (Duro Test Corp.).

Color-rendering index

Another parameter used in characterizing an illuminant is the color-rendering index. Color rendering of a light source is the effect that the source (illuminant) has on the color appearance of objects in comparison with their color appearance under a reference source. The color-rendering index is a measure of the degree to which the illuminant can impart the color of an object as compared to the reference source. A color-rendering index of 100 is considered ideal. For an adequate color-matching environment, the illuminant should have a color-rendering index of 90 or above (Preston et al, 1978). A summary of color-rendering indices of some illuminants used in dentistry is shown in Table 3-1.

Surroundings in a dental operatory may modify the actual light reaching the object. Colors of walls, clothing, and soft tissues such as lips contribute to the color of the light incident on teeth, shade guides, and restorative materials.

Object

The inherent color property of an object is its characteristic interactions with the light from the illuminant. These interactions include reflection, transmission, and the absorption involved in both processes.

Reflection

A material gains its reflective color by reflecting that part of the spectrum of light incident upon it and absorbs the other parts of the light spectrum. A blue surface reflects only the blue part of the light spectrum and absorbs all other colors (Fig 3-6). A white surface reflects all incident wavelengths. A black object absorbs all wavelengths and reflects none. An object also appears black when no light is reflected from it; for example, a blue object appears black when viewed in red light. Materials of different reflected color have different color reflectance (Fig 3-7). Reflection spectra of objects are usually obtained using a spectrophotometer.

Table 3-1 Color-rendering indices of illuminants

Illuminant (Manufacturer)	Color-rendering index
Chroma 50 (General Electric Co.)	92
Chroma 75 (General Electric Co.)	94
Cool white (General Electric Co.)	65
Hanau Viewing Lamp (Teledyne Hanau)	93
Neylite (J.M. Ney Co.)	98
Verilux (Verilux, Inc.)	93
Vita-Lite (Duro Test Corp.)	87, 91

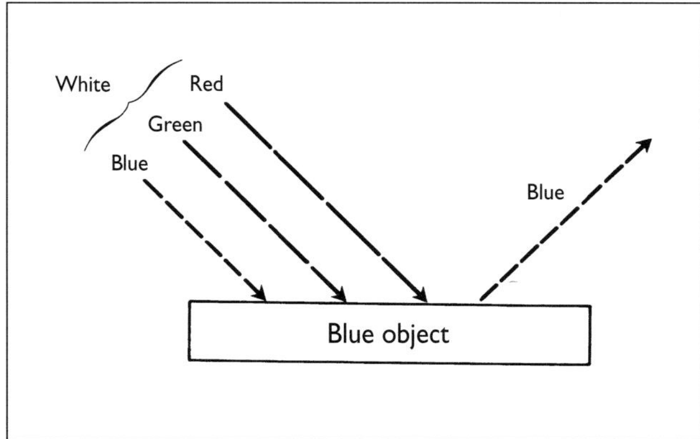

Fig 3-6 Reflected color. A blue object reflects only blue light and absorbs all other colors.

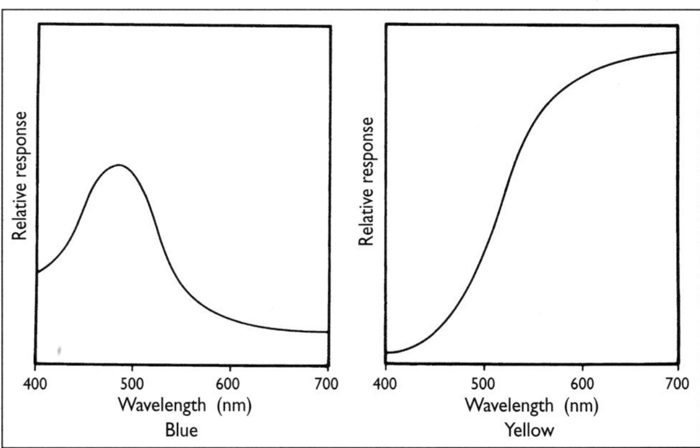

Fig 3-7 Color reflectance of a blue object and a yellow object. (Adapted from Billmeyer and Saltzman, 1960.)

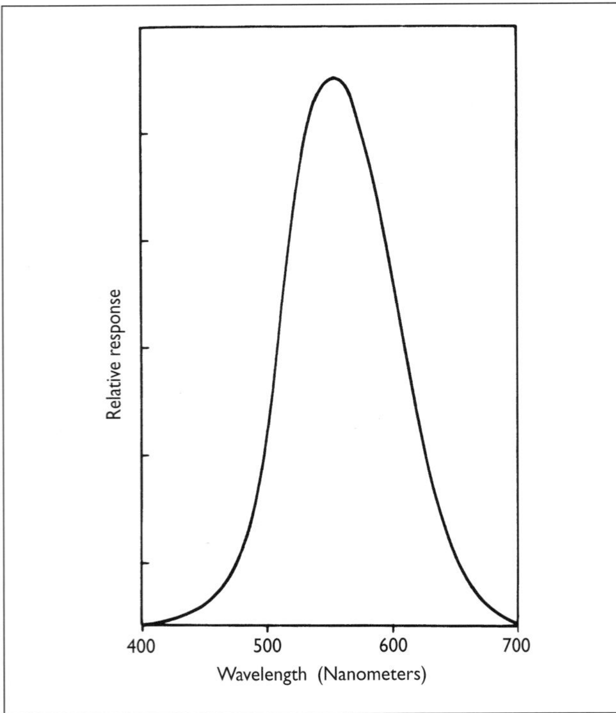

Fig 3-8 Relative response of a human eye at different wavelengths. (Adapted from Billmeyer and Saltzman, 1960.)

Mixing of reflected colors

In order to obtain a desired esthetic appearance for a restoration, it is often necessary to use more than one colorant. Each colorant has its own characteristic reflected color because of its reflection spectrum and its absorption of other parts of the spectrum. The mixing of two colorants with different reflected colors, and therefore different absorptions, results in a reflection of the part or parts of the light spectrum common to both colorants. In other words, each colorant will absorb the part of the light spectrum as if it were by itself. The parts of the light spectrum that are not absorbed by either colorant are, therefore, the resultant reflected color of the mixture of the two.

Transmission

A material gains its transmitted color by the resultant spectrum it transmits. Wavelengths that are not transmitted are absorbed. For example, a green filter transmits light in the green wavelength region of the light spectrum and absorbs all other wavelengths.

Observer

The observer receives the light reflected or transmitted by the object and then interprets the results. In many cases, the observer uses the human eye as the detector. Eye responses vary among individuals. The human eye response varies with wavelength. It is most sensitive in the green color region (Fig 3-8). The human eye is best in detecting color differences by comparison.

The detection of color by the human eye results from stimuli received by cone-shaped cells in the retina. Color blindness—the inability to distinguish certain colors—is due to abnormalities in these cells. Constant stimulus of one color decreases the response of the eye to that color. This is sometimes known as *color fatigue*. After removal of the stimulus, a complementary color image may persist.

In color measurements and parametric color determinations, the CIE (Commission Internationale de l'Eclairage) Standard Colorimetric Observer is often referenced.

Other detectors may be used as an observer in place of the human eye. These are usually photodetectors, such as spectrophotometers or colorimeters. The response of photodetectors varies among types, and they differ from the response of the human eye. Color-measuring devices are designed to minimize the effect of photodetector responses.

Color systems

Color systems are used to describe the color parameters of objects. The following are examples of some color systems used in describing the color of dental materials.

Munsell color system

The Munsell color system uses a three-dimensional system with hue, value, and chroma as coordinates (Fig 3-9).

Hue is commonly referred to as color: examples are blue, yellow, and red. Hue is also associated with the wavelengths of the light observed.

Value is the lightness or darkness of a color. A tooth of low value appears gray and nonvital. Value is the most important color factor in tooth color matching.

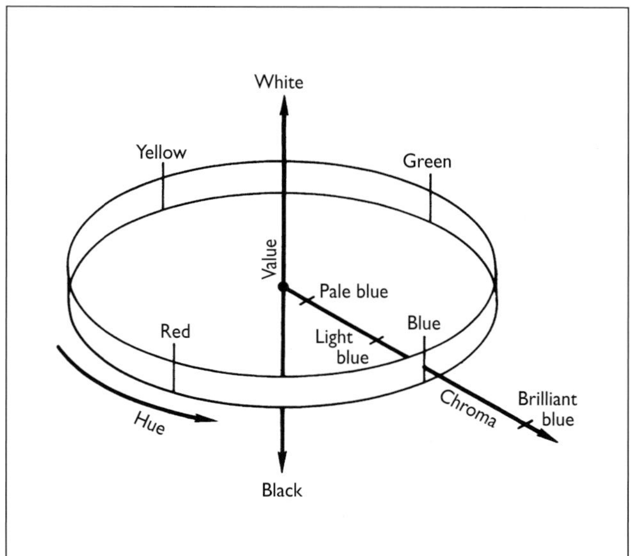

Fig 3-9 A color system with hue, value, and chroma as coordinates.

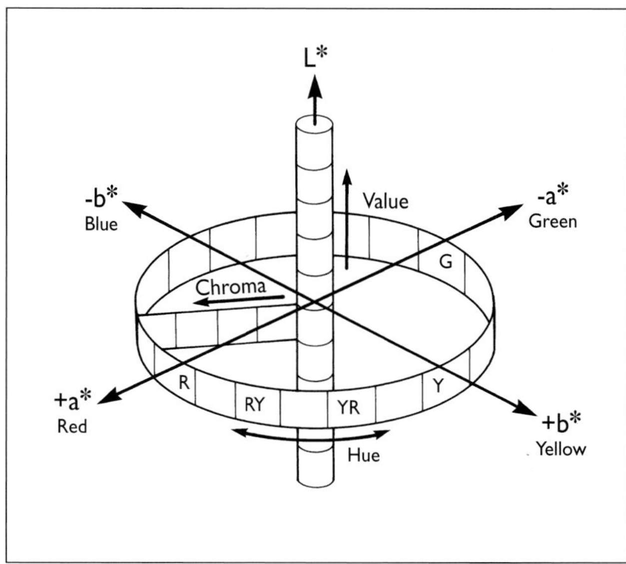

Fig 3-10 CIE and Munsell color arrangements. (From Seghi et al, 1986. Reprinted with permission.)

Chroma is a measurement of color intensity; that is, the amount of hue saturation in a color. An example is a beaker of water containing one drop of colorant; it is lower in chroma than a beaker of water containing ten drops of the same colorant.

CIE color systems

The CIE tristimulus values system used three parameters, X, Y, and Z, which are based on the spectral response functions defined by the CIE observer. A CIE chromaticity diagram is also sometimes used to define color.

Another CIE color system (CIE L*a*b*) uses the three parameters L*, a*, and b* to define color. The L*, a*, and b* values can be calculated from the tristimulus X, Y, and Z values. The advantage of this color system is that its arrangement is an approximately uniform three-dimensional color space whose elements are equally spaced on the basis of visual color perception. A unit change in each of the three color parameters is approximately equally perceived. The quality L* correlates to lightness, similar to the value in the Munsell system. The a* and b* coordinates describe the chromatic component (Fig 3-10).

Table 3-2 Clinical color-matching tolerances

Color difference, ΔE	Clinical color match
0	Perfect
0.5–1	Excellent
1–2	Good
2–3.5	Clinically acceptable
> 3.5	Mismatch

The color difference, ΔE, in the CIE L*a*b* system is defined as

$$\Delta E^* = [(\Delta L^*)^2 + (\Delta a^*)^2 + (\Delta b^*)^2]^{1/2}$$

where ΔL*, Δa*, and Δb* are the differences between the CIE L*a*b* color parameter of two samples. An advantage of CIE L*a*b* ΔE is that it can serve as a tolerance for color matching. Clinical color matching between teeth and restorations may be rated according to ΔE values, as given in Table 3-2, based on clinical studies. Shade guides are held to a tolerance of a ΔE of 2 according to an American Dental Association (ADA) standard. Although these ΔE values can serve as

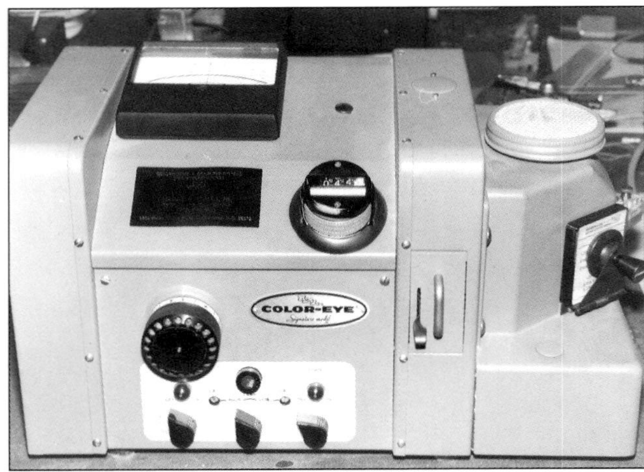

Fig 3-11 IDL Color-Eye.

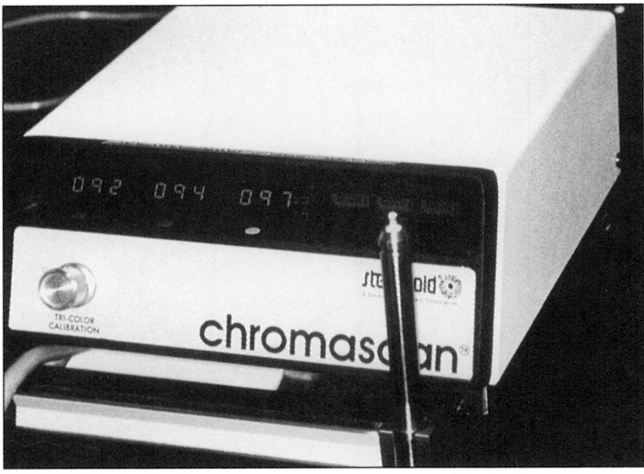

Fig 3-12 Chromascan clinical colorimeter.

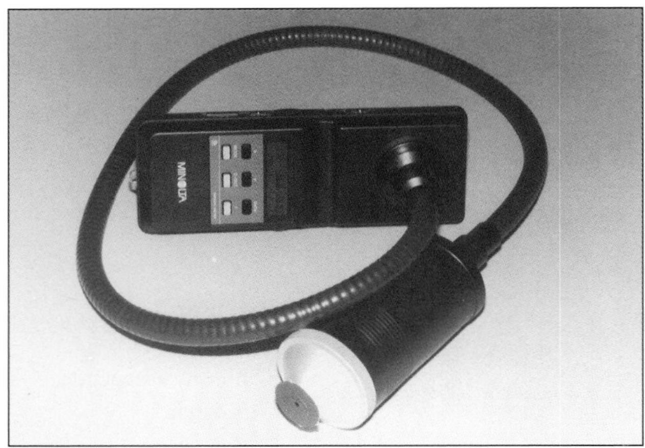

Fig 3-13 Minolta Chroma-Meter.

approximate tolerances, some individuals perceive color differences as low as 0.5, whereas others do not see differences of 4. This is often a source of disagreement among patients, dentists, and laboratory technicians.

Color measurements

Apart from visual comparison using color standards such as Munsell color chips, color measurements are made using either spectrophotometric or colorimetric methods.

Spectrophotometers measure the amount of light reflected at each wavelength. A double-beam spectrophotometer compares the responses from the object and a reference standard. From the spectral response, color parameters for the object can be calculated. Spectrophotometric measurements have been used to evaluate the color parameters for restorative resins, denture teeth, porcelains, shade guides, and color changes in dental materials.

Colorimeters measure the amount of light reflected at selected spectral responses. The selections are based on the CIE tristimulus value standard observers. There are several instruments available, and applications of their measurement methods for dental materials have been reported (Powers et al, 1980; O'Brien et al, 1983; Stanford et al, 1985). The instruments give readings in tristimulus values (X, Y, Z) or CIE L*a*b* values. Some of these instruments are the IDL Color-Eye (Instrument Development Laboratories, Inc.), shown in Fig 3-11; the Chromascan (Sterndent Corp.), shown in Fig 3-12; and the Minolta Chroma-Meter (Minolta Corp.), shown in Fig 3-13.

Metamerism

The change in color matching of two objects under different light sources is called metamerism. Two objects that are matched under one light source but not under other light sources form a *metameric pair*

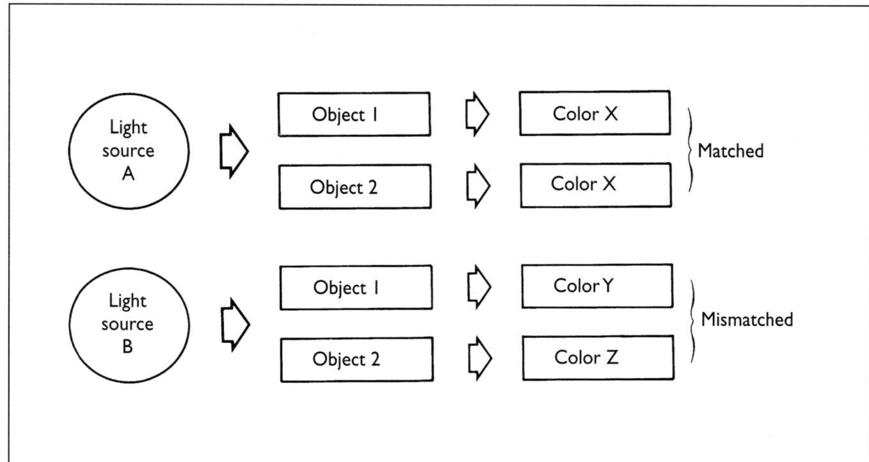

Fig 3-14 Metamerism. Objects 1 and 2 are matched under light source A but do not match under light source B.

(Fig 3-14). They have different color reflectance curves. An example of metamerism is when a shade-guide tooth matches the tooth under fluorescent light but not under incandescent light. Metamerism results from possible differences in illumination between the dental clinic and the dental laboratory, causing poor matching in a fabricated restoration such as a porcelain crown.

Standardization of illuminations (usually similar to the patient's environment) in color matching diminishes the effect of metamerism in shade matching. The ideal situation, of course, is to have the objects possess the same color reflectance curve. The objects are then an *isomeric pair*; they are color matched under all light sources.

Translucency

The translucency of an object is the amount of incident light transmitted and scattered by that object. A high translucency gives a lighter color appearance. A more translucent material will show more effect of the backing on the color and appearance. Translucency decreases with increasing scattering within the material.

The opposite of translucency is opacity. Light scattering in a material is the result of scattering centers that cause the incident light to be scattered in all directions. Examples of scattering centers are air bubbles and opacifiers such as titanium dioxide. Another example is the filler particles in a composite resin matrix. The effect of scattering is dependent on the size, shape, and number of scattering centers. Scattering is also dependent on the difference in refractive indices between the scattering centers and the matrix in which the centers are located.

A more in-depth treatment of translucency involves the consideration of absorption and scattering using the theory of Kubelka and Munk. The applications of this theory to dental materials include restorative resins and dental porcelains.

Measurements of translucency may be performed using transmission spectrophotometers, reflection spectrophotometers, light meters, or colorimeters. Measurements of translucency of dental porcelains and human enamel are published in the dental literature (O'Brien et al, 1985; Brodbelt et al, 1980; Spitzer and ten Bosch, 1975; Brodbelt et al, 1981).

Gloss

Surface gloss is the optical property that produces a lustrous appearance. Contrast gloss, or *luster*, is the proportion of specular reflection to diffuse reflection (Fig 3-15). Another consideration for gloss is the amount of collimated incident light that is specularly reflected. In specular reflection, the angle of incidence is equal to the angle of reflectance. When the incident

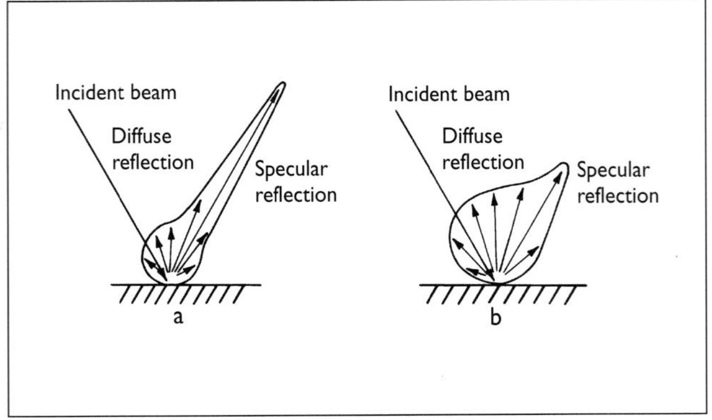

Fig 3-15 Schematic diagram of diffuse and specular reflection: (a) high gloss; (b) low gloss. (From O'Brien et al, 1984. Reprinted with permission.)

beam is scattered by the object, there is a decrease in gloss as a larger portion of the incident beam is diffuse-scattered.

A high surface gloss is usually associated with smooth surfaces. In composite restorative resins, surface gloss decreases with increasing surface roughness. Gloss is an important appearance property of dental restorative materials. Differences in gloss between restorations or between restorations and teeth are easily detectable even in colors that are matched. In addition, high gloss reduces the effect of a color difference, because the color of the reflected light is more prominent. In a restorative material, high gloss also lightens the color appearance.

Fluorescence

Fluorescence is the emission of light by an object at different wavelengths from those of the incident light. The emission ceases immediately upon removal of the incident light. Natural teeth fluoresce in the blue region when illuminated by ultraviolet light. Dental porcelains are also fluorescent under ultraviolet light. The quality of the fluorescence depends on the brand of porcelain, some of which fluoresces in colors different from those of natural teeth.

Double layer effects on esthetics

The color of a tooth is strongly influenced by the thickness of the enamel and the color of the underlying dentin. Similar considerations apply to restorations that are of layered structure. Examples are porcelain restorations that are composed of body porcelain over an inner opaque porcelain (Fig 3-16) and composite resins over more opaque resins. In these layered structures, esthetic appearances are no longer just simple considerations of the factors previously described but also involve diffuse reflectance and the relation between the translucency and thickness of the outer layer and the color and reflectance of the inner layer. The outer translucent layer acts as a light-scattering filter over the inner layer (Fig 3-17). As the thickness of the outer layer increases, the effect of the inner layer is diminished. Similar situations also exist when the translucency of the outer layer decreases. Considerations of models of diffuse reflectance in dental porcelain systems using the Kubelka-Munk equation have shown excellent agreement between experimentally observed and theoretically calculated color parameters (O'Brien et al, 1985).

Dental shade guides

Shade guides are used in determining the color of natural teeth so that artificial substitute restorations will possess similar color and esthetics. Preferred properties in a shade guide include logical arrangements and adequate distribution in color space, matching with natural teeth, inherent consistency among shade guides, and matching between shade guides and the dental materials such as porcelains and composite resins or denture teeth. Not all these properties are met by the shade guides currently available. Furthermore, not all shade guides are fabricated from the dental materials to which they are to be matched.

Most shade guides use a designation to denote the shade and color. The same designation may not be comparable among brands. The distribution of shades within a shade guide is not necessarily evenly partitioned in color space. Some attempts have been made to use a more logical approach and an even distribution in shade guides, but only a limited number follow this approach (Preston, 1985).

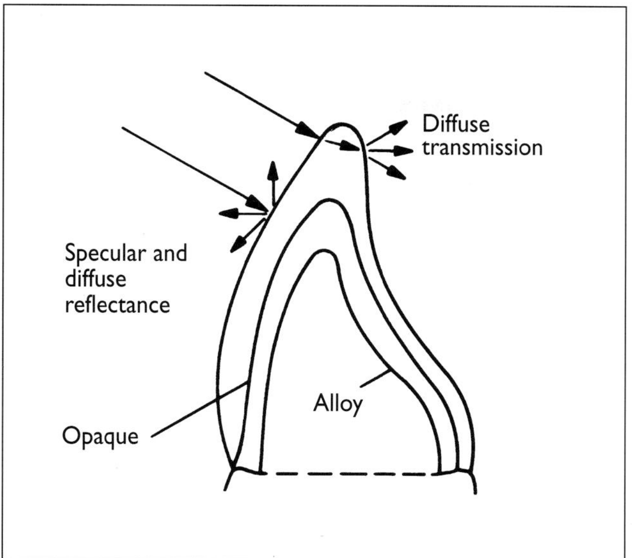

Fig 3-16 Optical considerations for a porcelain-fused-to-metal restoration. (From O'Brien et al, 1985. Reprinted with permission.)

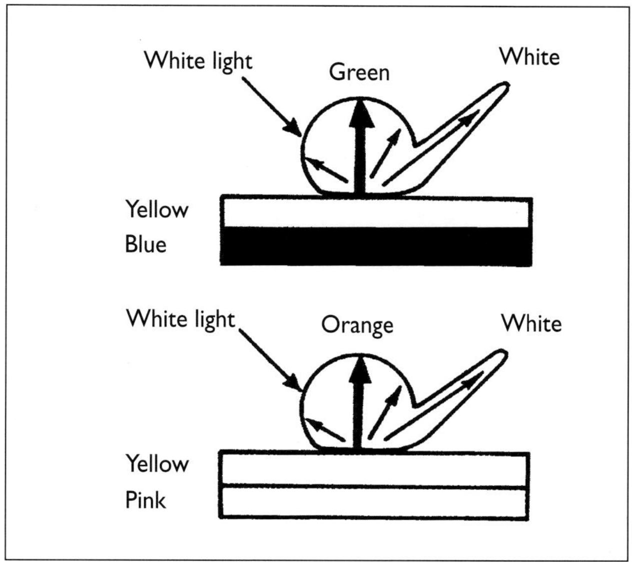

Fig 3-17 Double layer effect. (From O'Brien, 1985. Reprinted with permission.)

Shade matching in the dental operatory

Shade matching is a complex situation. It is important to remember the triadic interactions of illuminant, object, and observer described previously. Considerations should also include metamerism, gloss, translucency, and fluorescence. Recognition of the factors influencing shade match improve the result of the match.

The most important factor in shade matching is the *illuminant*. This is the lighting in the dental operatory used in shade matching. A color-corrected light source with a color temperature of 5,500 K and a color-rendering index of 90 or above is recommended. If possible, the shade matching should also be checked under a different light condition, for example, a warm white fluorescent light. In cases where the patients may have specific requirements, such as extensive activity under some lighting conditions, shade-matching checks under those conditions are also recommended. The color environment of the dental operatory is another important factor in shade matching. A neutral, light gray background color reduces modification of color perception.

Some recommendations in shade matching are as follows:

1. Shade match under lights of similar spectral distribution and intensity, both in the dental operatory and the laboratory. Lighting conditions should be similar to daylight, and the color-rendering index should be at least 90.
2. Consider the effects of translucency and position. A high translucency and a more distal position in the natural dentition cause a darker gray appearance.
3. Use the manufacturer's shade guide for fabricating the restoration.
4. Follow the manufacturer's recommendations for preparing the surface of the tooth for shade matching. A diffuse-reflection condition is usually used.
5. Remove the individual shade tab from the guide and hold it close to the tooth for shade matching.
6. The surface texture of the restoration should match that of the remaining dentition as closely as possible.

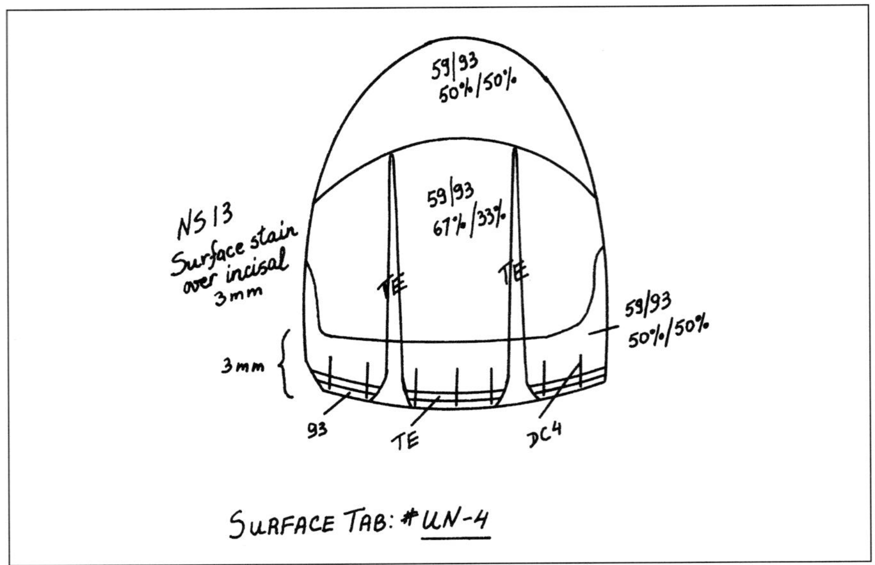

Fig 3-18 Illustration of a map supplied to a ceramist to communicate color. (From Seluk and LaLonde, 1985. Reprinted with permission.)

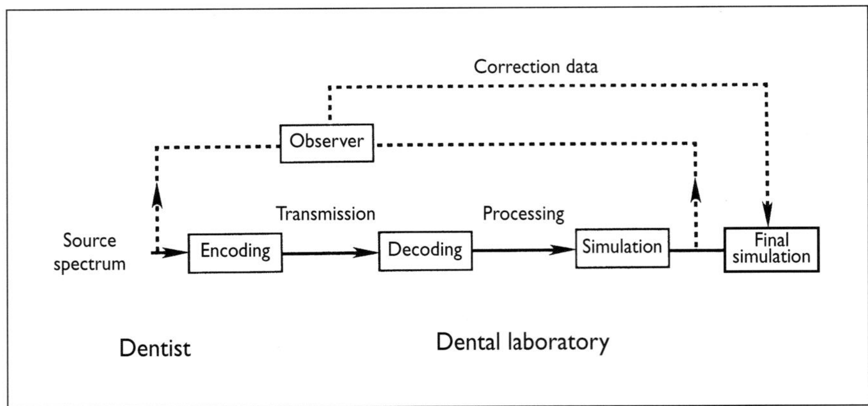

Fig 3-19 Schematic illustration of transmission of shade-matching information.

Communication of shade-matching information to the laboratory

The shade tab used for shade matching should be transmitted to the laboratory and should be specifically for the material to be used to fabricate the restoration. The type of lighting used for shade matching should be included in the communication to decrease the effect of metamerism. The prescription should accurately transmit the shade information as well as any characterization. An example of a map indicating the approximate shade, its depth, and information about its location is shown in Fig 3-18.

The sequential steps in the overall transmission of shade-matching information and the final clinical acceptance of the fabricated restoration have been described by O'Brien (1987). A schematic illustration is shown in Fig 3-19. The *source spectrum* is the color and translucency information of the tooth to which the fabricated restoration is to be matched. The shade taking is the *encoding* process. The information is *decoded* in the dental laboratory. The *simulation* is the fabricated restoration, which is then delivered to the dentist *observer* for evaluation for acceptance. If necessary, additional correction data to enhance the matching are communicated back for further simulation until the *final simulation* is reached. This is the fabricated restoration with necessary corrections to attain a clinically acceptable degree of shade matching to adjacent teeth.

Glossary

black object An object that reflects no incident color lights.

chroma Color intensity.

color content Relative intensity at each wavelength.

color fatigue Decrease in response to one color owing to constant stimulus.

color reflectance Relative amount of each color reflected.

color system A three-dimensional system for defining color.

color transmittance Relative amount of each color transmitted.

fluorescence Glow of an object when illuminated.

gloss Shininess; relative amount of light reflected.

hue Commonly called color (eg, blue, yellow). It is associated with wavelength.

isomeric pair Two objects that match color under different light sources.

metameric pair Two objects that exhibit metamerism.

metamerism Change in color matching of two objects under different light sources.

opacity $\text{Opacity} = \dfrac{\text{Intensity of incident light}}{\text{Intensity of transmitted light}}$

High opacity is associated with low intensity of transmitted light.

reflected color Color reflected by an object.

refractive index

$$\text{Refractive index } (n) = \frac{\text{Velocity of light in air}}{\text{Velocity of light in medium}}$$

Refractive index of dental porcelain is 1.5. Refractive index of tin dioxide (an opacifier) is 2.0.

translucency Amount of light transmitted; the rest of the light is scattered.

value Lightness or darkness of a color; a measurement of the amount of gray.

white object An object that reflects all incident color lights.

Discussion questions

1. How would a dental clinic need to be changed in order to be a better environment for color matching?
2. Why is it not necessary that a dental restoration match adjacent tooth structure exactly? About how far off in color can it be?
3. Why is it necessary to send the selected shade guide sample to the dental laboratory rather than just the shade guide number?
4. Beside color, which other appearance properties are important in creating an esthetic restoration?

Questions and answers

1. **Give an example of the variables in color definition.** Hue, value, and chroma; X, Y, and Z tristimulus values; L*, a*, and b*.
2. **A porcelain crown may appear gray and nonvital; which variable is involved?** A crown that appears gray and nonvital has a low value.
3. **Name the coordinates required to define a color in a color system.** Hue, value, and chroma; X, Y, and Z tristimulus values; L*, a*, and b*.
4. **Why does a green object appear black in blue light?** The green object absorbs the blue light. As no light is reflected, the object appears black.
5. **What are the factors affecting color appearance?** The source, the surroundings, and the observer.
6. **How does translucency affect color appearance?** A high translucency gives a lighter color appearance.
7. **What does gloss do to color appearance?** A high gloss lightens color appearance.
8. **What is metamerism?** The change in color matching of two objects under different light sources.
9. **How does metamerism affect the appearance of dental restorations?** Metamerism may cause a restoration to have a good color match under one lighting condition but a poor color match under another lighting condition.
10. **Why do dental porcelains appear different under different lighting environments?** Dental porcelains are fluorescent in some lighting environments.

Recommended reading

American Dental Association. Council on Dental Materials, Instruments and Equipment. How to improve shade matching in the dental operatory. J Am Dent Assoc 102:209–210, 1981.

Bergen SF, McCasland J. Dental operatory lighting and tooth color discrimination. J Am Dent Assoc 94:130–134, 1977.

Billmeyer FW Jr, Saltzman M. Principles of Color Technology. New York: Interscience, 1960.

Brodbelt RHW, O'Brien WJ, Fan PL. Translucency of dental porcelains. J Dent Res 59:70–75, 1980.

Brodbelt RHW, O'Brien WJ, Fan PL, Frazier-Dib JG, Yu R. Translucency of human dental enamel. J Dent Res 60:1749–1753, 1981.

Cook WD, Chong MP. Color stability and visual perception of dimethacrylate based dental composite resins. Biomaterials 6:257–264, 1985.

Cook WD, Vryonis P. Spectral distributions of dental colour-matching lamps. Aust Dent J 30:15–21, 1985.

Dennison JB, Powers JM, Koran A. Color of dental restorative resins. J Dent Res 57:557–562, 1978.

Dickson G, Forziati AF, Lawson MS, Schoonover IC. Fluorescence of teeth: a means of investigating their structure. J Am Dent Assoc 45:661–667, 1956.

Ecker GA, Moser JB, Wozniak WT, Brinsden GJ. Effect of repeated firing on fluorescence of porcelain-fused-to-metal porcelains. J Prosthet Dent 54:207–214, 1985.

Hall JB, Hefferen JJ, Olsen H. Study of fluorescence characteristics of extracted human teeth by the use of a clinical fluorometer. J Dent Res 49:1431–1436, 1978.

Johnston WM, O'Brien WJ, Tien TY. The determination of optical absorption and scattering in translucent porcelain. Color Res and Application 11:125–130, 1986.

Johnston WM, O'Brien WJ, Tien TY. Concentration additivity of Kubelka-Munk optical coefficients of porcelain mixtures. Color Res and Application 11:131–137, 1986.

Jørgenson MW, Goodkind RJ. Spectrophotometric study of five porcelain shades relative to the dimensions of color, porcelain thickness and repeated firings. J Prosthet Dent 42:96–105, 1979.

Judd DB, Wyszecki G. Color in Business, Science and Industry. New York: John Wiley & Sons, Inc, 1975.

McPhee ER. Light and color in dentistry. I. Nature and perception. J Mich Dent Assoc 60:565–572, 1978.

McPhee ER. Extrinsic coloration of ceramometal restorations. Dent Clin North Am 29:645–666, 1985.

Miller L. Organizing color in dentistry. J Am Dent Assoc (special issue): 26E–40E, 1987.

Miyagawa Y, Powers JM, O'Brien WJ. Optical properties of direct restorative materials. J Dent Res 60:890–894, 1981.

O'Brien WJ. Double layer effect and other optical phenomena related to esthetics. Dent Clin North Am 29:667–672, 1985.

O'Brien WJ. Fraunhofer diffraction of light by human enamel. J Dent Res 67:484–486, 1988.

O'Brien WJ. Optical phenomena at interfaces. IADR Symposium on Biomaterials and Interfaces. Chicago, 1987.

O'Brien WJ. Research in esthetics related to ceramic systems. Ceramic Eng Sci 6:57–65, 1985.

O'Brien WJ, Boenke KM, Groh CL. Coverage errors of two shade guides. Int J Prosthodont 4:45–50, 1991.

O'Brien WJ, Groh CL, Boenke KM. A new, small-color-difference equation for dental shades. J Dent Res 69:1762–1764, 1990.

O'Brien WJ, Groh CL, Boenke KM. A one-dimensional color order system for dental shade guides. Dent Mater 5:371–374, 1989.

O'Brien WJ, Johnston WM, Fanian F, Lambert S. The surface roughness and gloss of composites. J Dent Res 63:685–688, 1984.

O'Brien WJ, Johnston WM, Fanian F. Double-layer color effects in porcelain systems. J Dent Res 64:940–943, 1985.

O'Brien WJ, Kay K-S, Boenke KM, Groh CL. Sources of color variation on firing porcelain. Dent Mater 7:170–173, 1991.

O'Brien WJ, Nelson D, Lorey RE. The assessment of chroma sensitivity to porcelain pigments. J Prosthet Dent 49:63–66, 1983.

Peplinski DR, Wozniak WT, Moser JB. Spectral studies of new luminophors for dental porcelain. J Dent Res 59:1501–1506, 1980.

Powers JM, Dennison JB, Koran A. Color sensitivity of restorative resins under accelerated aging. J Dent Res 57:964–970, 1978.

Powers JM, Dennison JB, Lepeak PJ. Parameters that affect the color of direct restorative resins. J Dent Res 57:876–880, 1978.

Powers JM, Fan PL, Raptis CN. Color stability of new composite restorative materials under accelerated aging. J Dent Res 59:2071–2074, 1980.

Powers JM, Yeh CL, Miyagawa Y. Optical properties of composites of selected shades of white light. J Oral Rehabil 10:319–324, 1983.

Preston JD. Current status of shade selection and color matching. Quintessence Int 16:47–58, 1985.

Preston JD, Ward LC, Bobrick M. Light and lighting in the dental office. Dent Clin North Am 22:431–451, 1978.

Seghi RR, Johnston WM, O'Brien WJ. Spectrophotometric analysis of color differences between porcelain systems. J Prosthet Dent 56:35–40, 1986.

Seluk LW, La Londe TD. Esthetics and communication with a custom shade guide. Dent Clin North Am 29:741–751, 1985.

Shotwell JL, Johnston WM, Swarts RG. Color comparison of denture teeth and shade guides. J Prosthet Dent 56:31–34, 1986.

Spitzer D, ten Bosch JJ. The absorption and scattering of light in bovine and human enamel. Calcif Tissue Res 17:129–137, 1975.

Spitzer D, ten Bosch JJ. The total luminescence of bovine and human dental enamel. Calcif Tissue Res 20:201–208, 1976.

Sproull RC. Color matching in dentistry. I. The three-dimensional nature of color. J Prosthet Dent 29:416–424, 1973.

Sproull RC. Color matching in dentistry. II. Practical applications of the organization of color. J Prosthet Dent 29:556–566, 1973.

Sproull RC. Color matching in dentistry. III. Color control. J Prosthet Dent 31:146–154, 1974.

Stanford WB, Fan PL, Wozniak WT, Stanford JW. Effect of finishing on color and gloss of composites with different fillers. J Am Dent Assoc 110:211–213, 1985.

Woolsey GD, Johnston WM, O'Brien WJ. Masking power of dental opaque porcelains. J Dent Res 63:936–939, 1981.

Wozniak WT, Fan PL, McGill SB, Stanford JW. Color comparisons of composite resins of various shade designations. Dent Mater 1:121–123, 1985.

Wozniak WT, Moore BK. Luminescence spectra of dental porcelain. J Dent Res 57:971–974, 1978.

Wyszecki G, Stiles WS. Color Science. New York: John Wiley & Sons, Inc, 1967.

Yeh CL, Powers JM, Miyagawa Y. Color of selected shades of composites by reflection spectrophotometry. J Dent Res 61:1176–1179, 1982.

Chapter 4

Surface Phenomena and Adhesion to Tooth Structure

Surface phenomena include surface tension, wetting, adsorption, capillary action, and adhesion. Applications include capillary penetration around restorations, dentures, and teeth, and adhesion to tooth structure by sealants and restorative materials.

Surface energy

Atoms and molecules at the surfaces of liquids and solids possess more energy than do those in the interior. In the case of liquids, this energy is called *surface tension*. As illustrated in Fig 4-1, the molecules at the surface are farther apart owing to loss of molecules by evaporation. From Fig 4-2 it can be seen that this greater average separation leads to a net attraction between molecules and a higher energy of attraction. This results in a surface contractile force or surface tension, which causes the liquid to form drops and to exhibit a surface skin that resists extension or penetration.

The surface energies of several substances are given in Table 4-1. It can be seen that the surface energies of oxides and metals are greater than those of liquids. In general, the higher the bond strength of a substance, the greater the surface energy. Since metallic bonds are much stronger than the van der Waals bonds of liquids, metals have higher surface energies. The units of surface energy are $ergs/cm^2$, but the surface tension of liquids is often expressed in the equivalent units of dynes/cm. The total surface energy of a system is the product of the surface energy of the material and the total area. Therefore, a high total surface energy exists if a material is finely divided (powder or colloid) to provide a large surface area, especially if the material has a high surface energy per unit area (eg, metals or ionic crystals).

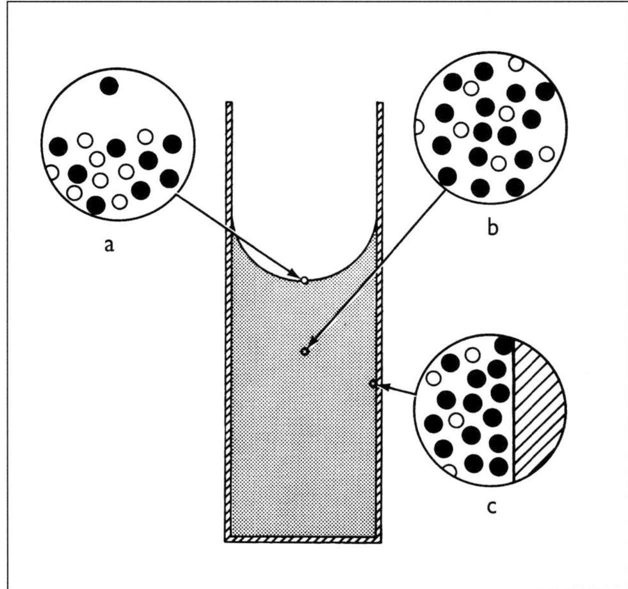

Fig 4-1 Distribution of vacancies (*open circles*) within isolated capillary liquid. More vacancies are present at the surface (a) as compared to the bulk (b). Fewer vacancies are found at the liquid/solid interface (c). (From O'Brien, 1970. Reprinted with permission.)

Table 4-1 Surface energies of various substances

Substance	Surface energy (erg/cm²)	Temperature (°C)
Water	72	20
Benzene	29	20
Olive oil	36	20
Saliva	56	23
NaCl crystal	300	25
Dental porcelain	365	1,000
Copper, solid	1,430	1,080
Silver, solid	1,140	750

Table 4-2 Contact angles of liquids on solids

Solid	Liquid	Contact angle (degrees)
Amalgam alloy	Water	80
Silicate cement	Water	10
Acrylic	Water	75
Teflon	Water	110
Ag_3Sn	Mercury	140
Gold alloys	Porcelain enamel	40–50
Nickel alloys	Porcelain enamel	80–100
Hydron	Water	0
Etched enamel	Pit and fissure sealants	0

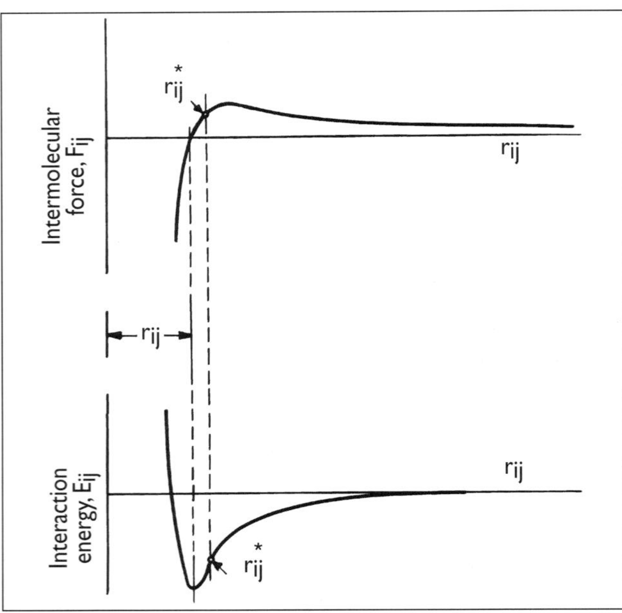

Fig 4-2 Relations between intermolecular forces, intermolecular energies, and distance as affected by distance (r_{ij}) between molecules. Departure from equilibrium distance r_{ij} causes repulsion or attraction. (From O'Brien, 1970. Reprinted with permission.)

Sintering

This is a densification process in which finely divided particles are heated in contact. The firing of porcelain is a sintering process used for forming artificial teeth and porcelain-fused-to-metal crowns. The driving force for this process is the reduction of total surface area and, thus, total surface energy.

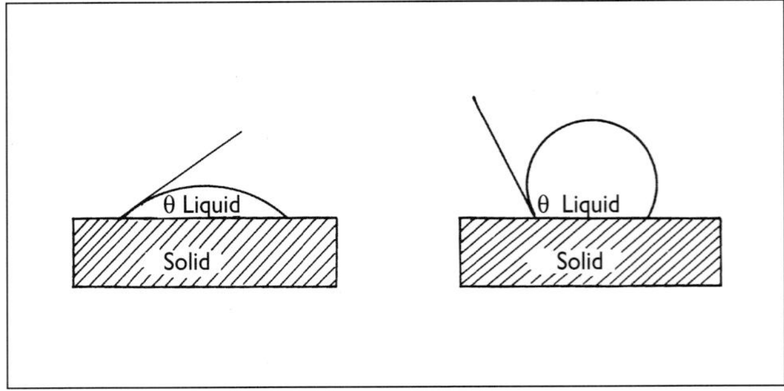

Fig 4-3 Wetting: low contact angle and good wetting (*left*); high contact angle and poor wetting (*right*). (From O'Brien and Ryge, 1965b. Reprinted with permission.)

Wetting

Wetting is defined in terms of the degree of spreading of a liquid drop on a solid surface. The contact angle (θ), formed by the liquid surface and the interface separating the liquid and solid, is used as a measure of the degree of wetting (Fig 4-3). A 0-degree contact angle indicates complete wetting, and low values correspond to good wetting. Values above 90 degrees indicate poor wetting. Table 4-2 gives contact angles for several systems. Good wetting promotes capillary penetration and adhesion and indicates strong attraction between the liquid and solid surface molecules. Good wetting is important in soldering and is a factor in better denture retention. A more natural appearance is achieved if restorative materials are wetted by a thin film of saliva.

Hydrophobic substances are those that exhibit high contact angles with water (eg, Teflon, silicone coatings) as shown in Figs 4-4 and 4-5.

Adsorption

In order to reduce surface energy, atoms and molecules that are mobile will concentrate at high energy surfaces. For example, finely divided charcoal will adsorb quantities of several gases; detergent (or soap) molecules will concentrate at the surface of water, leading to a large reduction in surface energy. Adsorption is strongest when there is large energy saving (high surface energy material and large surface area) and slows down as the surface is covered.

Adsorption occurs only at the surface, whereas absorption involves penetration and uptake by the interior of the material (as in swelling of hydrocolloid impression materials in water). Gold foil adsorbs gases readily and must be degassed before use.

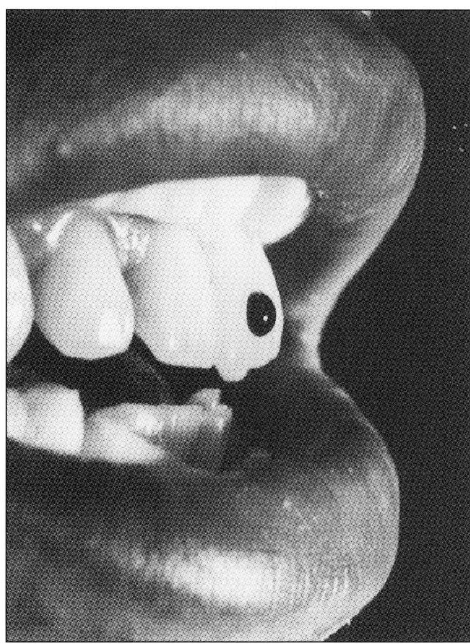

Fig 4-4 Hydrophobic film of fluorinated polymer on enamel giving high contact angle. (From O'Brien, 1973a. Reprinted with permission.)

Colloids

Colloids contain material that is present in particles larger than ordinary atoms or molecules but still invisible to the unaided eye (ie, 10 to 10,000 Å). There are three types of colloidal systems.

Insoluble dispersed particles

These are called *lyophobic*, since the materials are insoluble in a liquid medium (eg, sulfur in water). The fine particles acquire electrical charges that keep them in suspension. Table 4-3 gives a classification of the types of lyophobic systems. As one example of such a system, colloidal gold is used to form a gold coating on alloys to be bonded to porcelain. Although lyophobic systems may last for many years, they are unstable and can be precipitated by electrical methods (smokes) or gravity (emulsions).

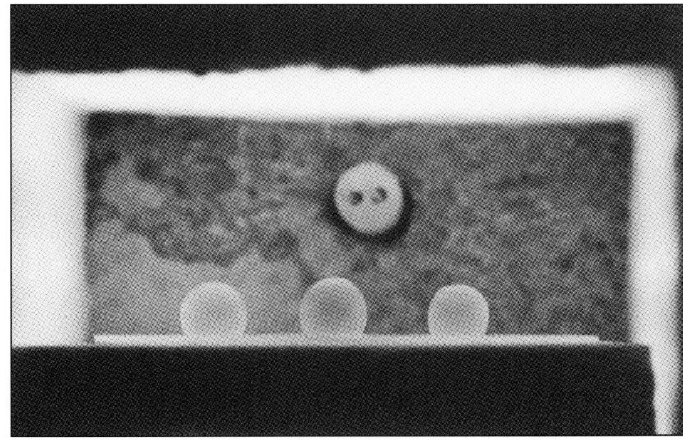

Fig 4-5 Poor wetting shown by porcelain enamel drops on nongold alloy at 1,040°C. The furnace thermocouple is seen above the drops. (From O'Brien and Ryge, 1965a. Reprinted with permission.)

Table 4-3 Classification of colloids

Dispersed phase	Continuous phase	Type
Solid	Liquid	Sol
Solid	Gas	Aerosol (smoke)
Liquid	Liquid	Emulsion
Liquid	Gas	Aerosol (fog)
Gas	Liquid	Foam
Gas	Solid	Foam

Large molecules

These systems are true solutions in which the dispersed molecules are of colloidal dimension. They are stable, but the large size of the macromolecules pre-

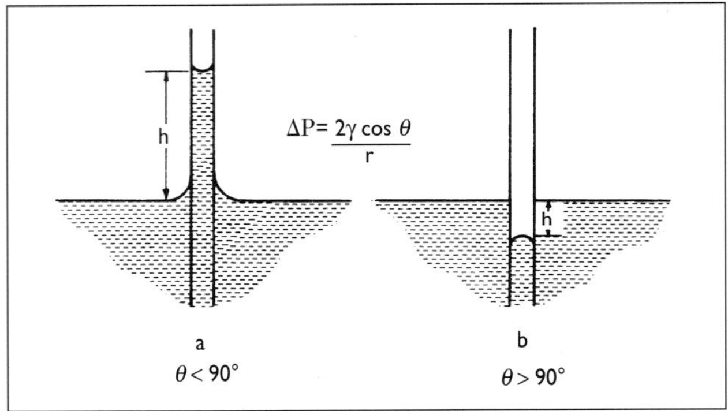

Fig 4-6 Effect of contact angle on capillary penetration: (a) capillary elevation; (b) capillary depression. ΔP is the capillary pressure. (From O'Brien et al, 1968. Reprinted with permission.)

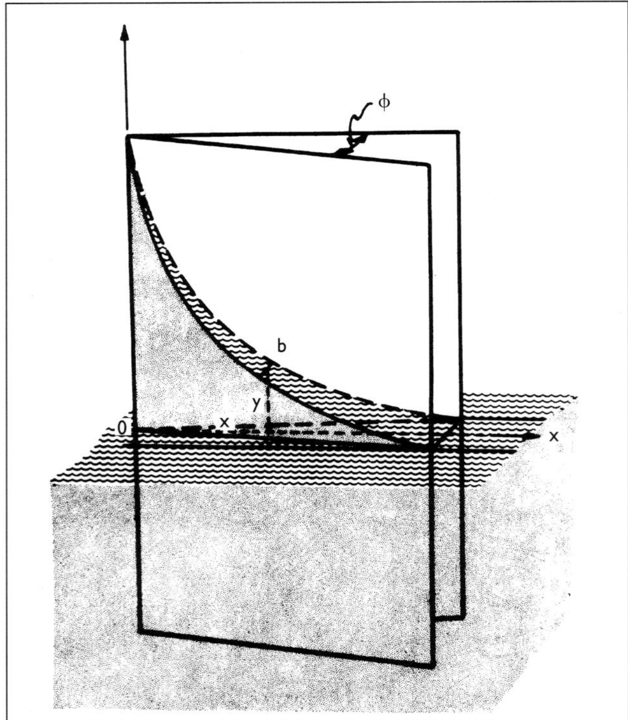

Fig 4-7 Effects of gap distance b and distance from the vertex x on capillary elevation y between two plates at an angle. (From O'Brien, 1973b. Reprinted with permission.)

sent gives the solutions properties similar to those of lyophobic systems.

Dental materials consisting of such solutions include agar and alginate hydrocolloid impression materials. These materials aggregate to form gels, owing to van der Waals bonding between the long chain molecules. Gels undergo imbibition and syneresis (absorption and exudation of solvent) with resulting swelling and shrinkage, respectively. This behavior is responsible for the dimensional instability of these impression materials. As with other colloidal systems, the liquid state is called the sol state.

Association colloids

These are aggregates of smaller molecules that achieve colloidal size. Surface active agents, such as soaps and detergents, are examples. Each molecule consists of a long chain hydrocarbon with a small charged polar group at one end (eg, sodium palmitate). The aggregates formed by these molecules, called *micelles*, often are spherical; in aqueous systems, the hydrocarbon ends gather in the center of the micelle and the polar groups are exposed on the outside. This system is useful in cleaning because grease and other organic films are dissolved in the interior of the micelles and held in suspension.

Capillary penetration

The surface energy of a liquid creates pressure that drives the liquid into crevices, narrow spaces, and thin tubes. Saliva penetration around restorations (leakage) and around teeth are important examples. Capillary penetration of saliva is also partially responsible for denture retention.

Capillary rise

If a glass tube is immersed in a liquid (Fig 4-6, a), the capillary rise, h, is given by the formula:

$$h = 2\gamma \cos \theta / rdg,$$

where γ is the surface tension, θ is the contact angle, r is the tube radius, d is the liquid's density, and g is the gravitational constant, 980 dynes/g. If the contact angle is less than 90 degrees, as in water-glass and saliva-enamel systems, elevation of the liquid occurs. However, if the contact angle exceeds 90 degrees (eg, mercury on glass or water on Teflon), depression takes place and pressure must be applied to force the liquid into the space (Fig 4-6, b). The effect of gap distance is shown in Fig 4-7 for two plates at an angle. In order

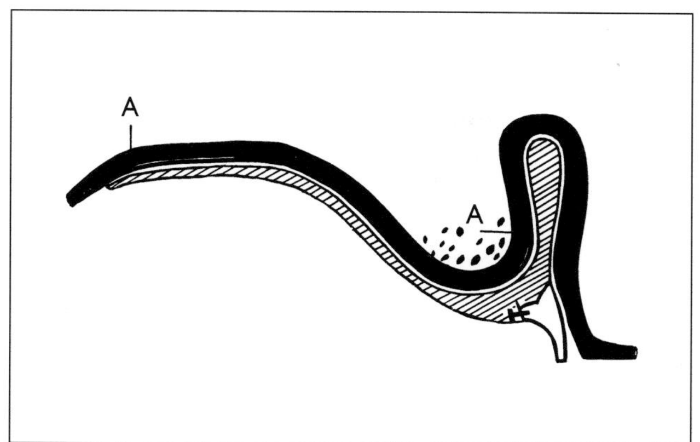

Fig 4-8 Capillary space between denture and mucosa. A = capillary.

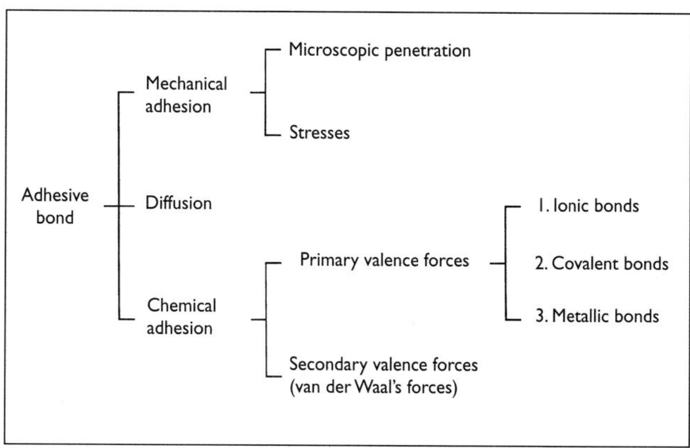

Fig 4-9 Classification of bonding mechanisms.

to increase the penetration of saliva around acrylic dentures, surface coatings of silica are applied to reduce the contact angle. The main factor here, however, is maintenance of a small gap distance (ie, close adaptation between denture and mucosa), as shown in Fig 4-8.

Penetration coefficient

The rate of movement of a liquid into a capillary space is related to the surface tension (γ), contact angle (θ), and viscosity (η), as given by the penetration coefficient (PC):

$$PC = \gamma \cos \theta / 2\eta$$

Therefore, a liquid with low viscosity, high surface tension, and low contact angle (ie, good wetting) will penetrate faster than one with the opposite combination of properties. This is important in adhesives such as pit and fissure sealants, which must penetrate into surface roughness and crevices quickly for good bonding.

Table 4-4 is a table of penetration coefficient values for some pit and fissure sealants.

Table 4-4 Penetration coefficients of five commercial materials

Material	Penetration coefficient
Adaptic Bonding Agent	12.8
Delton	10.0
Concise Enamel Bond	4.8
Nuva Seal	3.0
Adaptic Glaze	0.62

Adhesion

Adhesion is the attachment of materials in contact that resists the forces of separation. Adhesive phenomena are critical in many areas of dental materials, including the bonding of porcelains to metals and the adhesion of resins to tooth structure. Several types of adhesive bonds may be identified according to the classifications in Fig 4-9. Mechanical adhesion depends upon mechanical interlocking of the two phases and may include microscopic attachments, as in the case of resin bonding to etched enamel or hoop stresses of a porcelain around a metal core. Chemical adhesion relies on chemical bonding between two phases. Diffusion bonding results when one phase penetrates by diffusion into the surface of a second phase and forms a "hybrid" layer, which is a composite of the two materials.

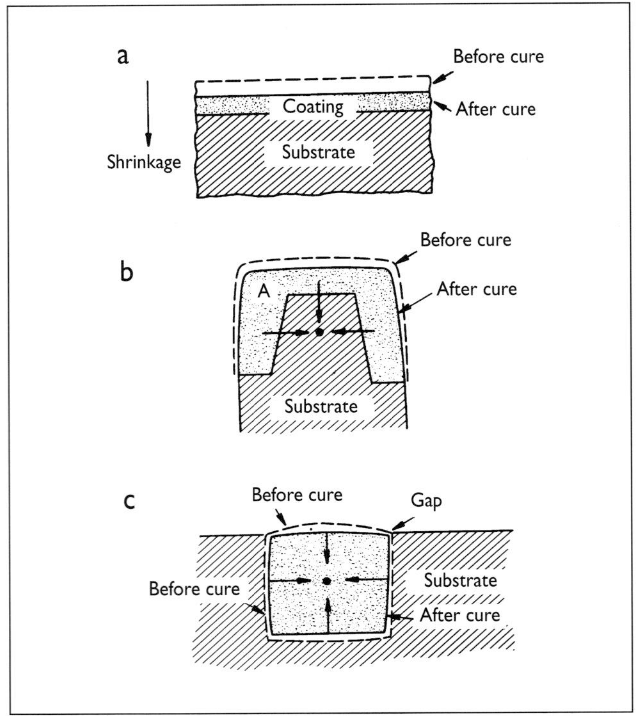

Fig 4-10 Shrinkage of adhesive toward center of mass during curing: (a) film, (b) crowns, (c) filling; A = adhesive. (From Lee, 1973. Reprinted with permission.)

Several factors affect the strength of an adhesive bond:

1. *Cleanliness.* The surfaces to be attached should be free of debris and contamination.
2. *Penetration of surface.* Liquid adhesives (eg, sealants and bonding agents) must penetrate into crevices created by acid etching of enamel and dentin. The penetration coefficient of the liquid was discussed in the preceding section.
3. *Chemical reactions.* The formation of strong chemical bonds across an interface will increase the number of attachment sites. This is believed to occur between porcelain enamels and the oxides of tin, indium, and iron formed on the surfaces of alloys containing high proportions of precious metals. On the other hand, a weak compound may be formed by a chemical reaction, resulting in a weak boundary layer (eg, certain oxides) rather than attachment sites.
4. *Shrinkage of adhesive.* Liquid adhesives solidify by processes such as solvent evaporation and polymerization, and shrinkage results. The adhesive may then pull away from the substrate, or stresses may be created that weaken the bond. Shrinkage is toward the center of the adhesive mass (Fig 4-10). However, shrinkage in light-cured systems occurs toward the light source.
5. *Thermal stresses.* If the adhesive and substrate have different thermal expansion coefficients, changes in temperature will produce stresses in the bond. For example, porcelain enamels are bonded to alloys at high temperatures and then cooled to room temperature. Close matching of the thermal expansion coefficients of porcelain enamel and alloy is required to minimize stresses.
6. *Corrosive environment.* The presence of water or corrosive liquid or vapor will often lead to the deterioration of an adhesive bond. For example, acrylic resins will initially adhere to clean unetched tooth enamel, but the bond deteriorates upon storage in water.

Adhesion to enamel and dentin

Enamel

Enamel is highly mineralized tissue composed of hydroxyapatite (about 96%), water (about 4%), and collagen (about 1%). Treatment with 35% to 50% phosphoric acid results in selective demineralization of exposed enamel rod ends, leaving a surface with increased area and high energy (Fig 4-11). High surface energy permits efficient wetting by the hydrophobic resin, which penetrates to form tags (Fig 4-12) and provides bond strength through mechanical interlocking. Contamination of the dry, etched surface by saliva or water, or incomplete removal of the etching agent or dissolved minerals adversely affects the long-term stability of the bond. The acid-etch technique produces shear bond strengths during laboratory testing of 20 to 22 MPa, on average above those produced at the composite/enamel interface by shrinkage due to polymerization (~18 MPa).

Acid-etching of enamel is a widely accepted clinical procedure and has increased the life of composite resin restorations by decreasing the possibility of marginal staining, secondary caries, and postoperative sensitivity due to sealing of the enamel margins. The acid-etch technique allows the use of a more conservative cavity preparation and, to a certain extent, restores fracture resistance to the bonded structure.

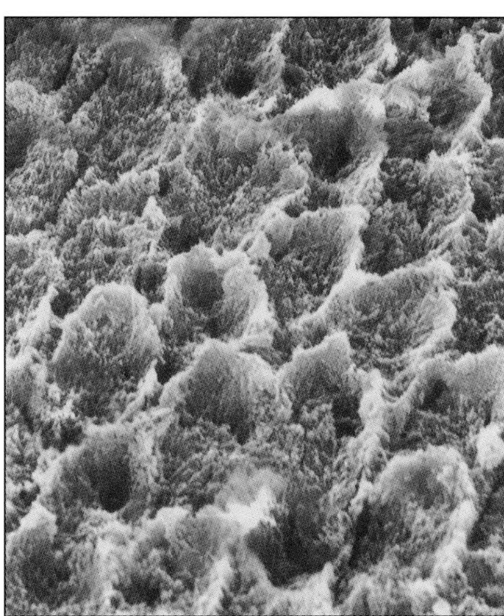

Fig 4-11 Microstructure of enamel etched with phosphoric acid. (Original magnification ×4,100.)

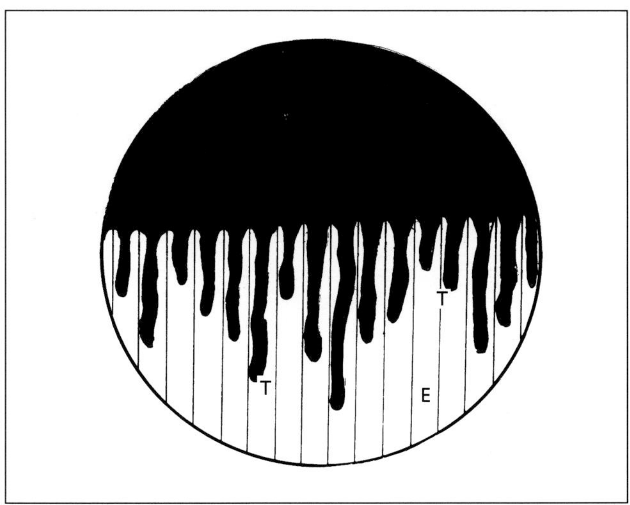

Fig 4-12 Attachment sites of polymer tags (T) in etched enamel (E).

Dentin

Human dentin is composed of hydroxyapatite (45%), water (25%), and organic matrix (30%). Bonding to dentin is routinely achieved by etching and the diffusion of hydrophilic primers, followed by application of bonding resins. Composite restorative materials are then bonded to the resin layer with laboratory bond strengths of 22 to 35 MPa. The stages of conditioning and resin impregnation are illustrated in Figure 4-13. In the first stage, the conditioning dissolves the smear layer of debris on the dentin surface and in tubules, partially decalcifies the dentin to an optimum depth of around 5 µm, and opens dentinal tubules. In the second stage, hydrophilic primer coupling agents such as hydroxyethylmethacrylate (HEMA), 4-methyloxy ethyl trimelletic anhydride (4-META), and glutaraldehyde are applied and penetrate into both the tubules and the decalcified intertubular dentin. The primer stabilizes collagen and facilitates the penetration of the bonding resins, which are bisphenol A-glycidyl methacrylate (Bis-GMA) or urethane-dimethacrylate (UDMA) monomers that are applied and polymerized.

There are two main types of conditioner components in current use. First there are the *strong acids* (phosphoric and citric acids). These acids attack the layer of debris on the dentin as the smear layer and dentin nonselectively and expose the tubules (Fig 4-14). Other acids (10% maleic acid) are used to dissolve both inorganic and organic tissues, but they are less aggressive. The second type of conditioner is *weak acids* (eg, polyacrylic acid), which are used to dissolve only the smear layer without demineralizing dentin.

The layer of resin penetration is known as the *hybrid zone* and may extend from 1 to 5 µm deep (Fig 4-15). If there is a layer of decalcified dentin below the hybrid zone, it acts to weaken the bond due to the resin being absent. This can be avoided by limiting the depth of etching with shorter etching times or less concentrated acids. Excessive drying of the dentin layer before primer application is not desirable, since it leads to collapse of the surface collagen layer and reduces primer diffusion. Lateral penetration into peritubular dentin may also take place from resin that has penetrated first into the tubules. Figure 4-16 shows a scanning electron micrograph (SEM) of a fractured hybrid layer with tags that have been plucked from the tubules during bond testing. Resin tags in tubules are not strongly anchored due to polymerization shrinkage and dentinal fluid. Commercial dentin bonding agents are shown in Figs 4-17 and 4-18.

Bond-strength values of materials to enamel and dentin are given in Table 4-5. The variation of laboratory bond-strength values to dentin are significantly higher than those reported for enamel. Therefore, bonding to dentin is less reliable.

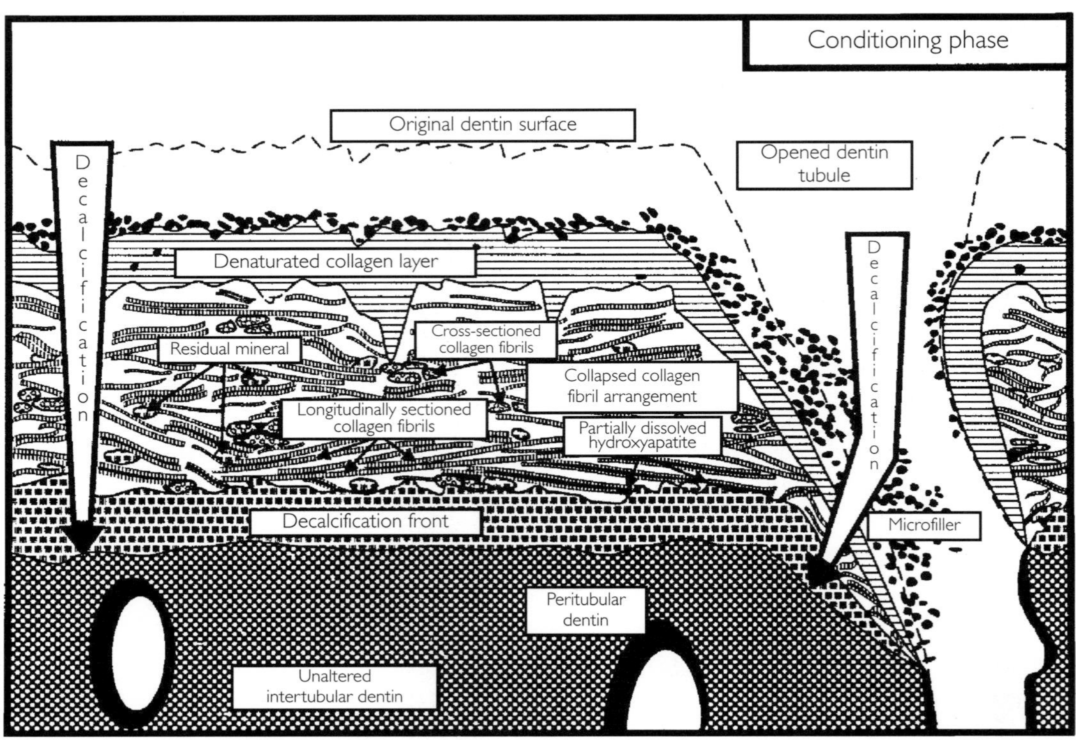

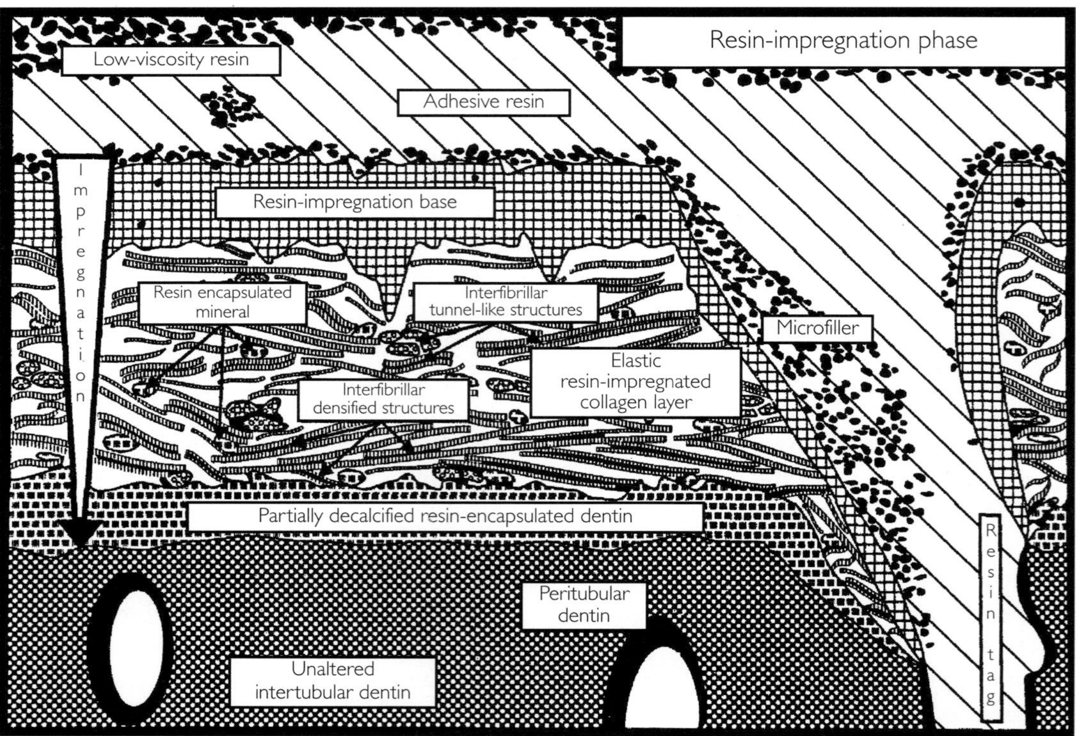

Fig 4-13 Schematic representation of the resin-dentin interdiffusion zone at (a) the conditioning phase and (b) the resin-impregnation phase. (From Van Meerbeek, 1993.)

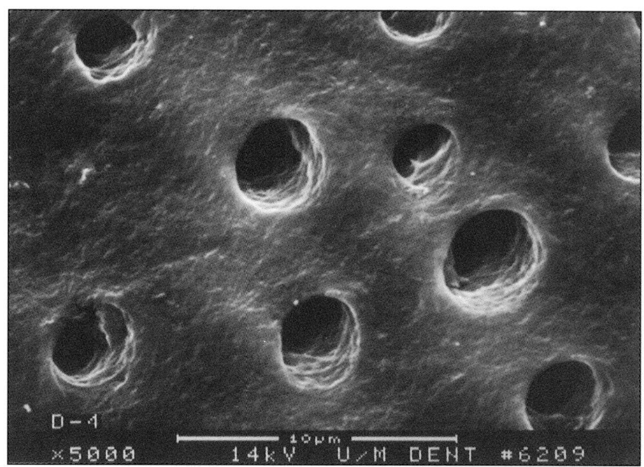

Fig 4-14 Dentin after deep etching with 20% phosphoric acid for 2 minutes. (Original magnification × 5,000.)

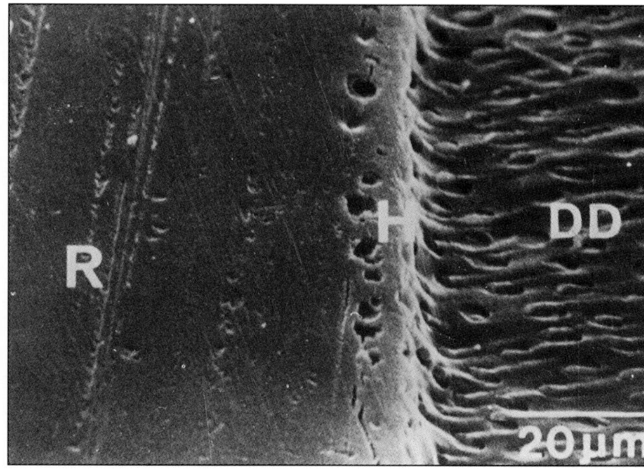

Fig 4-15 Cross-sectional view of resin-etched bovine dentin interface showing resin (R), the hybrid zone (H), and demineralized dentin (DD). (From Wang and Nakabayashi, 1991.)

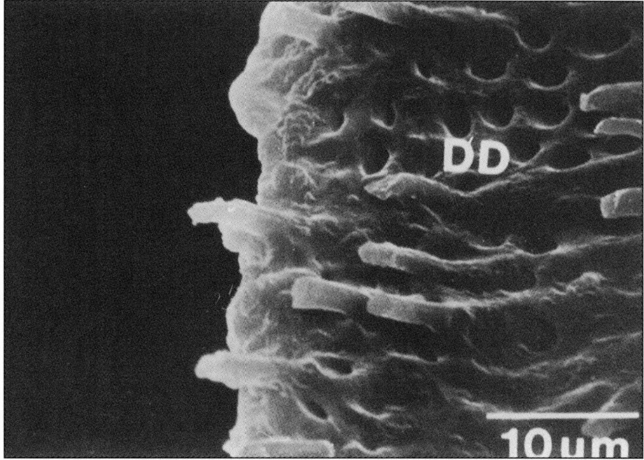

Fig 4-16 Scanning electron micrograph of a fractured resin-dentin interface showing resin tags plucked from tubules. (From Wang and Nakabayashi, 1991.)

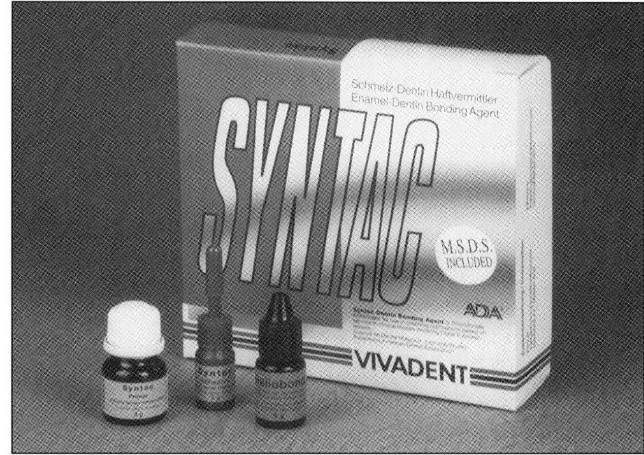

Fig 4-17 An enamel dentin bonding agent.

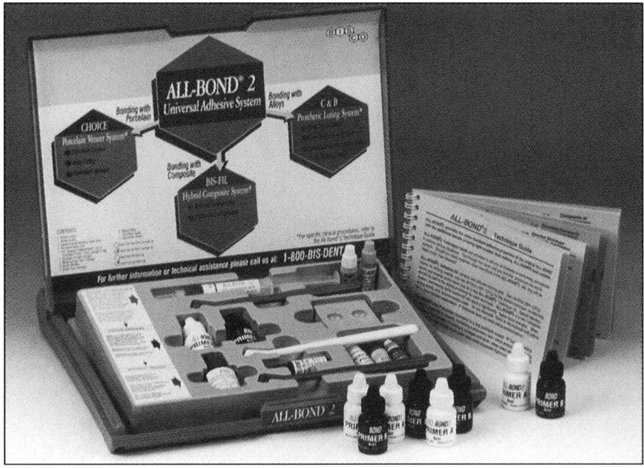

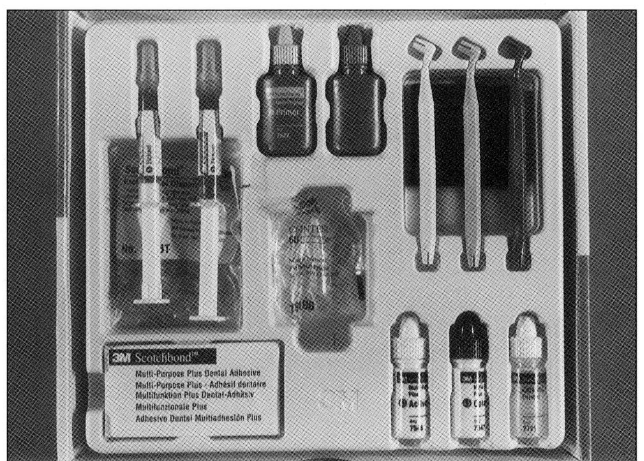

Figs 4-18a and b Two general-purpose dental adhesives.

Table 4-5 Tensile bond strengths obtained between various restorative materials and tooth substance*

Bonding couple	Bond strength (MPa)
Acid-etched enamel + resin (eg, Bis-GMA)	16–20
Enamel + glass ionomer	5
Dentin + glass ionomer	1–3
Dentin + glass ionomer (light cured)	3–11
Enamel + NPG-GMA	5
Enamel + NPG-GMA	2
Dentin + 4-META	2
Dentin + mordant ion + 4-META	18
Dentin + phosphate esters of Bis-GMA	3–5
Acid-etched enamel + phosphate esters of Bis-GMA	20
Dentin + maleic acid/HEMA + HEMA/Bis-GMA	18
Acid-etched enamel + HEMA/Bis-GMA	23
Dentin + isocyanate	4
Dentin + glutaraldehyde/HEMA	18

*Derived from McCabe, JF. Applied Dental Materials. London: Blackwell, 1990.

Glossary

adhesion Surface attachment of two materials (as opposed to cohesion, which is the bonding within a single material).

capillary penetration Movement of a liquid into a crevice or tube because of capillary pressure.

colloid Material in which a constituent in a finely divided state that is invisible to the eye but capable of scattering light is suspended. Although colloids are not true solutions, many have long-term stability.

contact angle Angle formed between the surface of a liquid drop and the solid surface on which it rests. Usually designated by the Greek letter Θ and used as a measure of wetting.

hydrophobic Water repellent; showing a high contact angle.

penetration coefficient Combination of the properties of viscosity, surface tension, and contact angle that promotes rapid capillary penetration.

sintering Densification process in which solid particles are fused together, usually at high temperatures.

surface energy Extra energy that atoms or molecules on the surface of a substance have over those in the interior. The units are erg/cm^2. The surface energy of a liquid is referred to as surface tension.

wetting The spreading of a liquid drop on the surface of a solid.

Discussion questions

1. Why is wetting by an adhesive so important to bonding to tooth structure or any other material?
2. Why is the strength of enamel and dentin a limiting factor in the adhesive bond strength?
3. What is the essential role that hydrophilic primer coupling agents play in the formation of the hybrid layer?
4. How does the geometry of a restoration affect the final bond strength to tooth structure?

Questions and answers

1. **Why does surface tension exist in liquids?** The molecules at the surfaces of liquids exert a greater intermolecular force on each other than do interior molecules, owing to their greater average separation. This attraction, or pull, results in a contractile surface stress.
2. **How does wetting affect capillary penetration of a liquid?** The degree of capillary penetration decreases as the contact angle increases. Above a contact angle of 90 degrees, a liquid will not penetrate and depression occurs (eg, mercury in a glass tube).
3. **How do absorption and adsorption differ?** Adsorption involves the uptake of one substance at the surface of another. Absorption involves the penetration of one substance into the interior of another.
4. **Name three colloidal systems of importance to dental materials.** Agar and alginate impression materials, colloidal gold, and detergents.
5. **Which properties affect the penetration rate of liquids into capillaries?** The penetration coefficient includes viscosity, surface tension, and contact angle as follows (PC in cm/sec):

$$PC = \frac{\gamma \cos \theta}{2\eta}$$

Recommended reading

Adamson AW. Physical Chemistry of Surfaces. New York: Interscience Publishers, Inc, 1960.

Asmussen E. Clinical relevance of physical, chemical and bonding properties of composite resins. Oper Dent 10:61–73, 1985.

Asmussen E, Antonucci JM, Bowen RL. Adhesion to dentin by means of Gluma resin. Scand J Dent Res 96:584–589, 1988.

Asmussen E, Munksgaard EC. Bonding of restorative resins to dentine: Status of dentine adhesives and impact on cavity design and filling techniques. Int Dent J 38:97–104, 1988.

Baran G, O'Brien WJ. The wetting of silver-tin phases by mercury in air. J Am Dent Assoc 94:898–900, 1977.

Bayne SC, et al. Contributing co-variables in clinical trials. Am J Dent 4:247–250, 1991.

Berry EA III, von der Lehr WN, Herring HK. Dentin surface treatments for the removal of the smear layer: an SEM study. J Am Dent Assoc 115:65–67, 1987.

Bowen RL. Bonding agents and adhesives: reactor response. Adv Dent Res 2:155–157, 1988.

Bowen RL, Cobb EN, Rapson JE. Adhesive bonding of various materials to hard tooth tissues: Improvement in bond strength to dentin. J Dent Res 61:1070–1076, 1982.

Bowen RL, Eichmiller FC, Marjenhof WA. Glass-ceramic inserts anticipated for megafilled composite restorations. J Am Dent Assoc 122:71–75, 1991.

Bryant RW, Mahler DB. Modulus of elasticity in bonding of composite and amalgams. J Prosthet Dent 56:243–248, 1986.

Brannstrom M. Smear layer: pathological and treatment considerations. Oper Dent Suppl 3:35–42, 1984.

Douglas WH. Clinical status of dentine bonding agents. J Dent 17:209–215, 1989.

Duke ES, Lindemuth J. Variability of clinical dentin substrates. Am J Dent 4:241–246, 1991.

Duke ES, Lindemuth J. Polymeric adhesion to dentin: contrasting substrates. Am J Dent 3:264–270, 1990.

Duncanson MG Jr, Miranda FJ, Probst RT. Resin dentin bonding agents—rationale and results. Quintessence Int 17:625–629, 1986.

Fan PI. Dentin bonding systems: An update. J Am Dent Assoc 114:91–95, 1987.

Fan PI, O'Brien WJ. Penetrativity of sealants. J Dent Res 54:262–264, 1974.

Fan PI, O'Brien WJ. Strain resulting from adhesive action of water in capillary bridges. Nature, Aug 21, 1975.

Gaberolglio R, Brannstrom M. Scanning electron microscopic investigation of human dentinal tubules. Arch Oral Biol 21:355–362, 1976.

Glantz PO. On wettability and adhesiveness. Odontol Rev 20, (Suppl 17), 1969.

Heymann HO, et al. Examining tooth flexure effects of dentinal adhesives in class V cervical lesions. J Am Dent Assoc 116(2):179–183, 1991.

Jörgensen KD, Asmussen E, Shimokobe H. Enamel damage caused by contracting restorative resins. Scand J Dent Res 83:120–122, 1975.

Jörgensen KD, et al. Deformation of cavities and resin fillings in loaded teeth. J Dent Res 84:46–50, 1976.

Lambrechts P, et al. Evaluation of clinical performance for posterior composite resins and dentine adhesives. Oper Dent 12:53–78, 1987.

Lee H. Adhesion of polymeric materials to tooth structure. In H Moskowitz (ed). Proc Symposium on Adhesive Dental Materials. New York: New York University, 1973.

Lewis AF, Natarajan RT. The attachment site theory of adhesive joint strength. In LH Lee (ed). Adhesion Science and Technology. Part B. New York: Plenum Press, 1975; 563–575.

McGuckin RS, et al. Shear bond strength of Scotchbond in vivo. Dent Mater 7(1):50–53, 1991.

Morin DL, et al. Biophysical stress analysis of restored teeth: experimental strain measurement. Dent Mater 4:41–48, 1988.

Morin DL, et al. Cusp reinforcement by the acid-etch technique. J Dent Res 63:1075–1078, 1984.

O'Brien WJ. Capillary Penetration of Liquids Between Solids. Doctoral Dissertation. Ann Arbor: University of Michigan, 1967.

O'Brien WJ. Surface energy of liquid isolated in narrow capillaries. Surface Sci 19:387, 1970.

O'Brien WJ. Capillary effects on adhesion. In H Moskowitz (ed). Proc Symposium on Adhesive Dental Materials. New York: New York University, 1973a.

O'Brien WJ. Capillary action around dental structures. J Dent Res 52:533–549, 1973b.

O'Brien WJ. Effects of capillary penetration and negative pressure at sites of caries susceptibility. In HM Stiles, et al (eds). Microbial Aspects of Dental Caries. Washington, DC: Information Retrieval Inc, 1976.

O'Brien WJ, Craig RG, Peyton FA. Capillary penetration around a hydrophobic filling material. J Prosthet Dent 19:399–405, 1968.

O'Brien WJ, Fan PL. Capillary adhesion. In LH Lee (ed). Adhesion Science and Technology. Part B. New York: Plenum Press, 1975; 621–633.

O'Brien WJ, Ryge G. Contact angles of drops of enamel on metals. J Prosthet Dent 15:1094–1100, 1965a.

O'Brien WJ, Ryge G. Wettability of poly(methyl methacrylate) treated with silicone tetrachloride. J Prosthet Dent 15:304–308, 1965b.

Pashley DH. Dentin bonding: overview of the substrate with respect to the adhesive material. J Esthet Dent 3(2):46–50, 1991.

Pashley DH. In vitro simulations of in vivo bonding conditions. Am J Dent 4:237–240, 1991.

Pashley DH. Smear layer: physiological consideration. Oper Dent Suppl 3:13–29, 1984.

Pashley DH, et al. Regional resistances to fluid flow in human dentine in vitro. Arch Oral Biol 23:807–810, 1978.

Perdigão J. An Ultra-Morphological Study of Human Dentin Exposed to Adhesive Systems. Leuven, Belgium: University of Leuven; 1995. Thesis.

Selna LG, et al. Finite element analysis of dental structures: axisymmetric and plane stress idealizations. J Biomed Mater Res 9:237–244, 1975.

Tao L, et al. Effect of different types of smear layers on dentin and enamel shear bond strengths. Dent Mater 4:208–216, 1988.

Thresher RW, Saito GE. The stress analysis of human teeth. J Biomech 6:443–449, 1973.

Van Meerbeek, et al. Factors affecting adhesion to mineralized tissues. Oper Dent Supp 5;111–124, 1992.

Wang T, Nakabayashi N. Effect of 2-(Methacryloxy) ethyl phenyl hydrogen phosphate on adhesion to dentin. J Dent Res 70(1):59–66, 1991.

Yettram AL, et al. Finite element stress analysis of the crowns of normal and restored teeth. J Dent Res 55:1004–1011, 1976.

Ziemiecki TL, et al. Clinical evaluation of cervical composite resin restorations placed without retention. Oper Dent 12:27–33, 1987.

Chapter 5

Gypsum Products

In general, the term *gypsum products* refers to various forms of calcium sulfate, hydrous and anhydrous, manufactured by the calcination of calcium sulfate dihydrate ($CaSO_4 \cdot 2H_2O$), which occurs as the mineral gypsum. Calcination can be controlled to produce partial or complete dehydration. Gypsum products can also be obtained by calcining "synthetic" or "chemical" gypsum, a by-product of the manufacture of phosphoric acid. Industrially, all these materials are known as gypsum plasters.

Although not directly employed in dental restorations, gypsum products are important accessory materials used in many clinical and laboratory procedures. Their correct use contributes to the success of these procedures. They are classified by the International Standards Organization (1983) into four types:

Type 1: Impression plaster
Type 2: Plaster
Type 3: Stone
Type 4: Stone, high strength

This classification is illustrated in Fig 5-1. Both types of plaster are based on ordinary commercial gypsum plaster (plaster of Paris), while both types of stone are based on high-strength gypsum plasters. Type 4

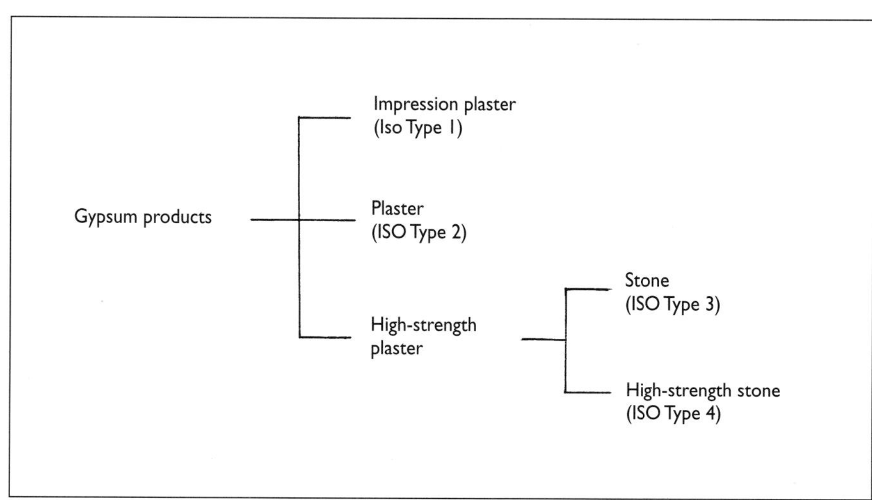

Fig 5-1 Classification of gypsum products.

stones are commonly referred to as die stones. Table 5-1 lists typical materials.

The term gypsum products can be extended to include gypsum-bonded investments, used as mold materials for casting dental gold alloys, because calcium sulfate hemihydrate is an essential component, forming the bond in the set material. These materials will be dealt with separately later in this chapter.

Table 5-1 Typical gypsum products

Impression plaster (ISO Type 1)	Impression plaster (Modern Materials Manufacturing Co)
Plaster (ISO Type 2)	Snow White Plaster No. 1 (Kerr/Sybron)
Stone (ISO Type 3)	Microstone (Whip Mix Corp)
High-strength stone (ISO Type 4)	Vel Mix Stone (Kerr/Sybron)

Plaster and Stone

These are both the result of partial dehydration of gypsum, which produces calcium sulfate hemihydrate ($CaSO_4 \cdot {}^1/_2H_2O$). Differences in properties result from differences in the physical nature of the powders, which in turn is a result of differences in manufacturing methods.

Chemistry

In the temperature range 20° to 700°C, which is of importance in the dental manipulation of gypsum products, three phase transformations occur in the $CaSO_4 \cdot H_2O$ system. The first two represent the two stages in the dehydration of gypsum, and these are followed by a further transformation into anhydrous calcium sulfate:

$$CaSO_4 \cdot H_2O \xrightleftharpoons{40^\circ\text{–}45^\circ C} CaSO_4 \cdot {}^1/_2H_2O \text{ (+ water)}$$

calcium sulfate hemihydrate

$$\xrightleftharpoons{90^\circ\text{–}100^\circ C} \gamma\text{-}CaSO_4 \text{ (+ water)}$$

hexagonal calcium sulfate (soluble anhydrite)

$$\xrightarrow{300^\circ\text{–}400^\circ C} \beta\text{-}CaSO_4$$

orthorhombic calcium sulfate (insoluble anhydrite)

It is not possible to give unequivocal temperatures for these transformations; the ranges given summarize the results of several different determinations.

For the first transformation, from dihydrate to hemihydrate, the temperature limits were determined by weight loss measurements on specimens heated isothermally in dry air for 2.5 years (Andrews, 1951) and would represent an equilibrium value.

Thermogravimetric measurements of the temperature for the second transformation, calcium sulfate hemihydrate to hexagonal calcium sulfate, have involved isothermal heating for periods only up to a maximum of 22 days (Khalil et al, 1971; Weiser et al, 1936), so the true equilibrium temperature for this transformation is probably a little lower than shown. Gay (1965) has identified hexagonal calcium sulfate by X-ray diffraction in specimens of hemihydrate heated in the range 75° to 105°C. Hexagonal calcium sulfate is unstable below about 80°C, and, if cooled to lower temperatures, it rapidly rehydrates, even in the presence of water vapor, to form the hemihydrate. The temperature range given for the third transformation, hexagonal to orthorhombic calcium sulfate, is based on measurements made on specimens heated at a rate of 5 K/min (Earnshaw and Mori, 1985), so again the true equilibrium temperature for this transformation would be lower than shown here. Orthorhombic calcium sulfate is the stable anhydrous form in this system and exists as the mineral insoluble anhydrite.

Theoretically, hemihydrate is the stable hydrous form of calcium sulfate only in the approximate temperature range of 45° to 90°C. It exists as a metastable phase under dry conditions at lower temperatures, including ambient, although it has been shown that hydration can occur if particles are exposed to the atmosphere under conditions where the water vapor pressure is high (Torrance and Darvell, 1990).

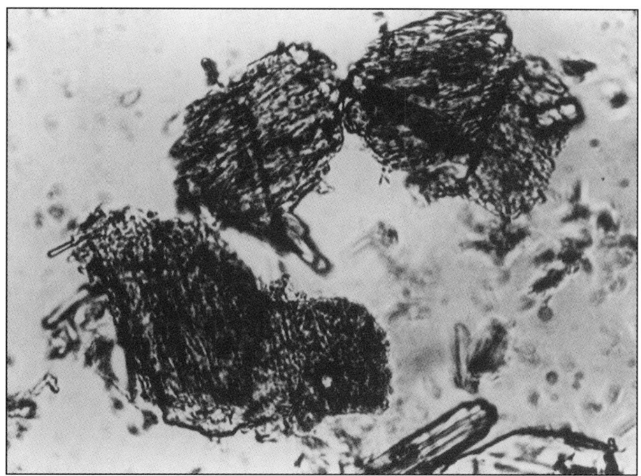

Fig 5-2 Particles of plaster. (Original magnification × 400.)

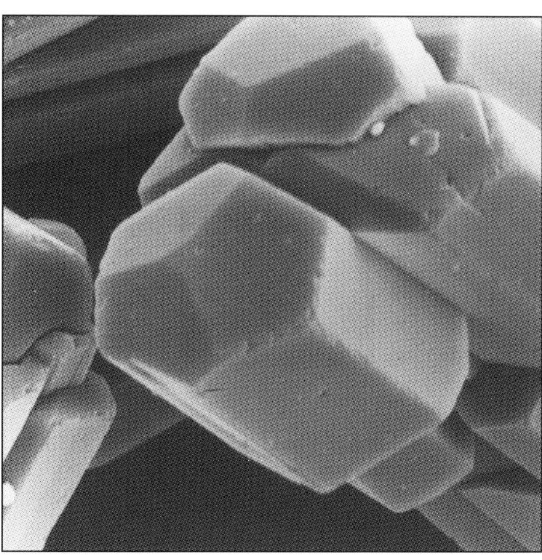

Fig 5-3 Crystals of wet-calcined gypsum plaster before grinding. (Scanning electron micrograph, original magnification × 3,000.)

Manufacture

From the transformation temperatures given in the previous section, it can be seen that calcium sulfate hemihydrate would be produced by heating gypsum to temperatures in the range of 45° to 90°C. However, at these temperatures the reaction is slow; even at 90°C, substantially complete conversion takes about 12 hours (Khalil et al, 1971). Therefore, in commercial processes temperatures higher than this are used for shorter times. The stable phase at these higher temperatures is hexagonal calcium sulfate, so the initial product of calcination is partly or very largely this anhydrous form. However, on cooling to temperatures below 80°C and exposure to the atmosphere, the hexagonal calcium sulfate rehydrates to form the hemihydrate.

Plaster of Paris

This is the traditional hemihydrate plaster produced by the dry calcination of ground gypsum in open containers (pans, kettles, or rotary kilns) at temperatures in the range of 120° to 180°C. In the absence of liquid water, there is no opportunity for reorganization of crystal morphology, so, although the crystal structure of the final product after exposure to air is that of calcium sulfate hemihydrate, the powder particles retain the rough irregular shape of the original ground gypsum. Loss of water under dry conditions leaves parallel channels in these particles (Fig 5-2), so hemihydrate plasters produced by dry calcination are powders with a low apparent density, a high relative surface area, and a poor packing ability.

Medium- and high-strength plasters (stones)

Plasters giving a stronger set mass are manufactured by wet calcination. Here sufficient liquid water is present to allow through-solution conversion, so recrystallization produces dense prismatic crystals of hexagonal calcium sulfate. These rehydrate to the hemihydrate on cooling in air, but this secondary conversion cannot be accompanied by recrystallization. The final powder particles are pseudomorphic, having the monoclinic crystal structure of hemihydrate, but retaining the hexagonal crystal habit of the anhydrous calcium sulfate precursor (Fig 5-3).

Hemihydrate powders produced by wet calcination therefore have a higher apparent density and a smaller relative surface area than those resulting from dry calcination. A controlled amount of grinding rounds off the crystals and produces a proportion of fines, both factors improving the packing ability of

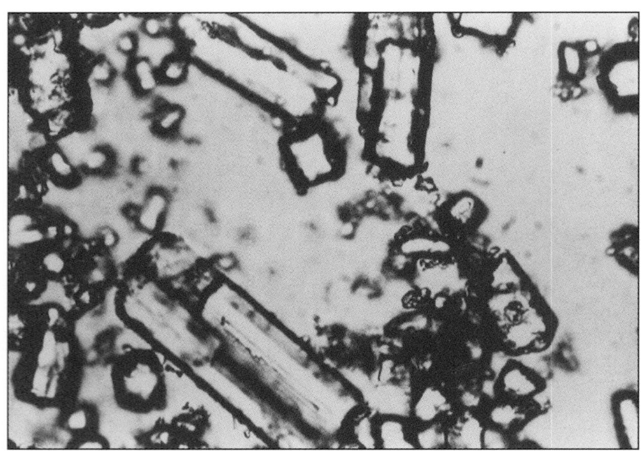

Fig 5-4 Particles of high-strength stone. (Original magnification × 400.)

the powder and so increasing the apparent density still further. Particles of a typical dental stone are shown in Fig 5-4.

Medium-strength plasters

These are typified by Hydrocal (United States Gypsum Co), which is the basis of many ordinary dental stones. It is produced by autoclaving lump gypsum in superheated steam, at a pressure of 117 kPa, giving a temperature of 123°C, for 5 to 7 hours. After drying at 100°C or higher and grinding, a hemihydrate powder is produced that gives a set mass considerably stronger than that produced by dry-calcined materials.

High-strength plasters

Modifications to the wet process yield hemihydrate powders giving even stronger set products. These are typified by Densite (Georgia-Pacific) and Crystacal (British Gypsum Ltd). Here wet calcination takes place in the presence of crystal habit modifiers, producing crystals that are shorter and thicker than those resulting from autoclaving in steam. After controlled grinding these powders have even higher apparent densities and yield even stronger set masses than Hydrocal-type stones: they form the basis of most dental die stones. Densite is produced by boiling lump gypsum in a 30% calcium chloride solution and Crystacal by autoclaving finely ground gypsum in the presence of small amounts (less than 1%) of sodium succinate.

Apparent density

The apparent density of a powder is the reciprocal of its bulkiness and so gives a measure of its packing ability. The low apparent density of hemihydrate powders produced by dry calcination is caused in part by the rough irregular shapes of the individual particles (see Fig 5-2). A more important factor, however, is a high adhesion of particles to their neighbors, caused by a high surface free energy resulting from crystal imperfections and adsorption of gases during calcination (Gregg, 1965). This adhesiveness of particles makes it likely that they will stick together at first contact, establishing bridges in the powder and creating a structure with many voids and a low apparent density. In contrast, powder particles produced by wet calcination are smooth and dense (see Fig 5-4). They show less crystallographic strain and therefore have a lower surface free energy, so they have a better packing ability and a higher apparent density.

The setting process

The setting reaction

When the hemihydrate powder is mixed with water in the correct proportions, it forms a thick slurry. The hemihydrate is sparingly soluble in water (6.5 g/L at 20°C), so only a small amount can dissolve. Initially, therefore, the mix is a two-phase suspension of hemihydrate particles in a saturated aqueous solution. The stable hydrate at temperatures below 40°C is the dihydrate (gypsum), which is even less soluble (2.4 g/L at 20°C) than the hemihydrate. The aqueous phase is therefore supersaturated with respect to the dihydrate, which crystallizes out at suitable nucleation centers in the suspension. These gypsum crystals normally are acicular in habit and often radiate out from nucleation centers in the form of spherulitic aggregates.

These nucleation centers may be impurities (eg, residual gypsum particles), particles of gypsum added as seeds to accelerate setting, or strained areas on undissolved hemihydrate particles. The consequent depletion of calcium and sulfate ions in the aqueous phase allows more hemihydrate to go into solution and, in turn, to precipitate out as gypsum. The setting process is therefore one of heterogeneously nucleated recrystallization, characterized by a continuous solution of hemihydrate, diffusion of calcium and sulfate ions to nucleation centers, and the precipitation of microscopic gypsum crystals. The setting reaction is the reverse of the first stage of dehydration and so is exothermic. It is represented by the following equation:

$$2CaSO_4 \cdot {}^1/_2H_2O + 3H_2O \rightarrow 2CaSO_4 \cdot H_2O$$

Water requirement

The differing water requirements of plaster, stone, and high-strength stone are the result mainly of differences in the apparent density of the powder. The factors that promote adhesiveness of the particles in the dry powder persist when they are suspended in water (Ridge, 1961). For this reason dry-calcined plaster, with its low apparent density, produces a flocculated suspension and needs a relatively high proportion of mixing water to give a mix of workable viscosity. Water/powder (W/P) ratios of 0.5 to 0.6 are usual. Hemihydrate powders produced by wet calcination, because of their higher apparent densities, require less mixing water; typical W/P ratios are 0.30 to 0.33 for ordinary dental stones and 0.20 to 0.25 for high-strength stones.

In setting, 100 g of hemihydrate combines with 18.6 g water. Therefore at the completion of the reaction in normal mixes there is always some excess unreacted water (as a saturated solution of calcium sulfate) remaining in the set mass. This residual water weakens the cast. It can be removed by low-temperature drying but leaves microscopic porosity that weakens the dry cast. Both wet and dry strengths of the set material depend on the relative amount of unreacted water remaining after setting, and so on the W/P ratio of the original mix. The relative amount of residual water is least in high-strength stone, which therefore gives the strongest set mass.

Stages in setting

The setting process is continuous from the beginning of mixing until the setting reaction is complete, by which time the material has reached its full wet strength. However, important physical changes can be recognized during this process. Initially there is a continuous aqueous phase present, and the mix is a viscous liquid, exhibiting pseudoplasticity so that it flows readily under vibration; in this stage the mix has a glossy surface giving specular reflections. As the setting reaction proceeds, gypsum crystals continue to grow at the expense of the aqueous phase, and the viscosity of the mix increases. When the clumps of growing gypsum crystals interact, the mix becomes plastic; it will not flow under vibration but can readily be molded. At this time the glossy surface disappears as the aqueous phase is drawn into pores formed when the growing gypsum crystals thrust apart. Continued crystal growth converts the plastic mass into a rigid solid, weak and friable at first but gaining strength as the relative amount of solid phase increases.

These four stages may be designated (*1*) fluid, (*2*) plastic, (*3*) friable, and (*4*) carvable.

Volume changes during setting

The setting reaction causes a decrease in the true volume of the reactants, and under suitable conditions this contraction can be observed early in the setting process, when the mix is still fluid. However, once the mix begins to attain rigidity (marked by the loss of surface gloss) an isotropic expansion is observed, resulting from growth pressure of the gypsum crystals that are forming. There is therefore a decrease in apparent density of the mix during the latter stages of setting, accompanied by the formation of microscopic voids separating individual crystals in the aggregate.

The initial contraction is unlikely to affect the important dimensions of a gypsum cast, because in the still-fluid mix it will occur mainly in a vertical direction. Gravity will keep the mix adapted to the anatomical portion of an impression. The expansion that is observed after the mix attains rigidity takes place in all directions and will affect the dimensions of the cast. The point at which the initial contraction ceases is used as zero in laboratory measurements of effective setting expansion.

Rate of the setting reaction

Within wide limits, the rate of hydration during setting is independent of the W/P ratio (Lautenschlager et al, 1969). However, the rate at which the associated physical changes described earlier occur is highly dependent on the W/P ratio of the mix, because these changes result from interaction of clumps of gypsum crystals growing from nucleation centers in the slurry.

Thick mixes (low W/P ratios) harden more quickly because available nucleation centers are concentrated in a smaller volume; interaction of the growing solid phase occurs earlier and is more effective in promoting expansion.

The effect of additives

Many salts and colloids are known to alter the setting characteristics of hemihydrate plasters by their effect on the rate of the setting reaction. They have been used in the formulation of dental plasters and stones for many years, mainly on an empirical basis, because their modes of action are not always completely understood.

Finely powdered gypsum is an efficient accelerator, which acts by providing seeds for heterogeneous nucleation. In low concentrations soluble sulfates and chlorides are accelerators, apparently acting by increasing the rate of solution of the hemihydrate. However, salts of relatively low solubility, such as sodium chloride and sodium sulfate, act as retarders in higher concentrations, because as setting proceeds the amount of free water in the mix decreases and the concentration of the additive increases. When the limit of solubility is exceeded, the salt precipitates on nuclei of crystallization, thus poisoning them. Acetates, borates, citrates, and tartrates are retarders, which may act by nuclei poisoning, by reducing the rate of solution of hemihydrate, or by inhibiting the growth of dihydrate crystals. Reaction of some additives with hemihydrate can occur; soluble tartrates and citrates precipitate calcium tartrate and citrate, respectively. Colloids are effective retarders, presumably acting by nuclei poisoning.

Many accelerators and retarders reduce the setting expansion, sometimes by changing the crystal habit of growing gypsum crystals from acicular to a more compact form and inhibiting spherulite formation (Koslowski and Ludwig, 1984); both factors reduce the effect of the crystals' growth pressure. This is accompanied by a reduction in the strength of the set material.

The microstructure of cast gypsum

The set material consists of a tangled aggregate of monoclinic gypsum crystals, usually acicular in shape, with lengths in the range of 5 to 20 μm. The aggregate exhibits two distinct types of inherent porosity on a microscopic scale:

1. Microporosity caused by the presence of residual unreacted water. These voids are roughly spherical and occur between clumps of gypsum crystals.
2. Microporosity resulting from growth of gypsum crystals. These voids are associated with setting expansion and are smaller than the first type; they appear as angular spaces between individual crystals in the aggregate.

The effect of W/P ratio

The relative amounts of both types of porosity are affected by the W/P ratio of the mix, but in opposite ways:

1. A low W/P ratio (thick mix) leaves less residual water in the set mass and so decreases the amount of the first type of porosity.
2. A low W/P ratio increases the effect of crystal growth during setting, because available nucleation centers are concentrated in a smaller total volume of mix; interaction of growing gypsum crystals occurs earlier and is more effective so the amount of the second type of porosity is increased.
3. In any W/P ratio, the total proportion of inherent porosity in the set mass is the sum of these two types. The effect of the first type predominates, so for any given plaster or stone there is always a decrease in the total inherent porosity of the set mass (ie, an increase in apparent density) as the W/P ratio of the mix is reduced. Inherent porosity represents about 40% of the total cast volume at a W/P ratio of 0.50 and about 20% at a W/P ratio of 0.25 (Lautenschlager and Corbin, 1969).

Typical microstructures of casts made from plaster mixed in a W/P ratio of 0.50 and high-strength stone mixed in a W/P ratio of 0.25 are shown in Fig 5-5. The second type of microporosity described here (resulting from residual water) shows clearly in the micrograph of

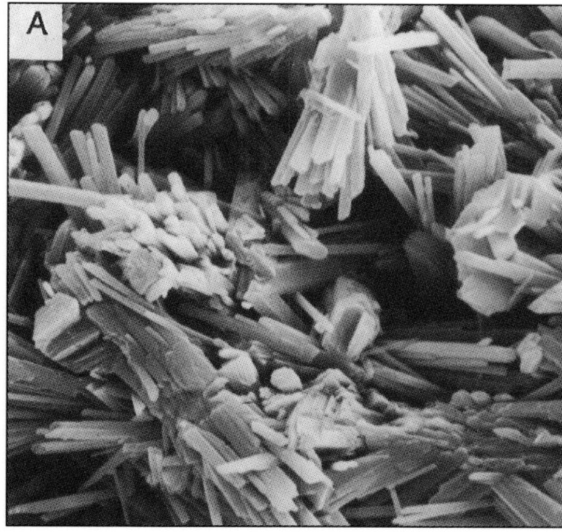

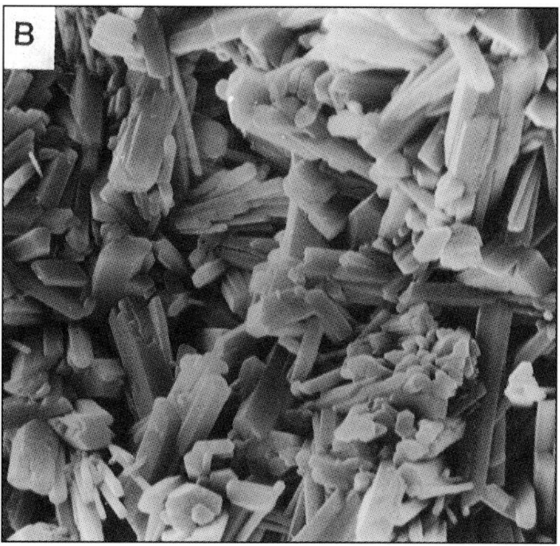

Fig 5-5 Fracture surface of cast gypsum. (Scanning electron micrographs, original magnification × 3,000.) (A) Plaster, W/P = 0.50; (B) high-strength stone, W/P = 0.25. (From Bever, 1986. Reprinted with permission.)

set plaster, where the voids occur between spherulitic clumps of gypsum crystals. The higher apparent density of the set high-strength stone is obvious.

Properties

Rate of setting

Manipulation time Recognition of the physical changes occurring in the mix during setting is important in the manipulation of plaster and stone.

1. When casting (eg, pouring casts or dies), manipulation must be completed before the mix loses fluidity. The change is marked by the disappearance of the glossy surface from the mix.
2. When molding (eg, taking impressions or jaw registrations, articulating casts, flasking wax pattern dentures), manipulation must be completed before the mix loses plasticity and enters the friable stage. There is no recognized objective method of measuring this time.

Setting time An arbitrary setting time (initial set) can be determined by using suitable penetrometers (eg, Gillmore or Vicat initial needles; both give approximately the same initial setting time). Measured in this way, the initial set is a guide to the time when the rigid material is strong enough to handle and, in particular, when it can be carved or trimmed to the final shape.

If a dental manufacturer specifies a setting time, it will be a Gillmore or Vicat initial set. Both the setting reaction and strength increase continue for some time after this initial set. Gillmore and Vicat final needles may be used to establish a final setting time, but this is not usual in dental technology.

Control of rate of setting

1. *The use of additives.* In formulating dental products, manufacturers adjust the rate of setting of raw hemihydrates by adding accelerators and retarders, often as a balanced mixture. Typical accelerators are potassium sulfate and potassium sodium tartrate (“Rochelle salts”). Typical retarders are sodium citrate and sodium tetraborate decahydrate (borax). The action of accelerators and retarders has already been discussed.
2. *W/P ratio.* It has already been pointed out that changing the W/P ratio has a marked effect on the rate at which the physical changes associated with setting of the mix occur. These changes take place more rapidly as the W/P ratio is reduced. Manipulation and setting times are thus directly proportional to W/P ratio.

Table 5-2 Linear setting expansions of typical dental gypsum products (setting in air)

Type	W/P ratio	Setting expansion
Impression plaster	0.60	0.13
Plaster	0.50	0.30
Stone	0.30	0.12
High-strength stone	0.23	0.10

Setting expansion

Typical values for setting expansion for the four types of dental gypsum plaster are given in Table 5-2. These are the results of laboratory measurements on four widely used materials, setting in air.

The observed expansion that occurs when dental plaster or stone sets is a volumetric one. In dental testing a value is determined for linear setting expansion, and the assumption is made that the expansion is isotropic. This assumption is not always justified; if restraint is imposed in some directions but not others (eg, by a rigid impression), setting expansion can be far from isotropic.

Effect of immersion Gypsum products exposed to additional water while setting (eg, by immersion) show a greater expansion than when setting in air, a phenomenon commonly (but inaccurately) called hygroscopic expansion. When expansion begins, externally available water is drawn into pores forming in the setting mass, and this maintains a continuous aqueous phase in which crystal growth takes place freely. Under dry conditions this additional water is not available, and as expansion occurs the aqueous phase in the mix is reduced to a film over the growing gypsum crystals. Surface tension forces in this liquid film restrain further crystal growth, thereby reducing the observed setting expansion of the mix (Mahler and Ady, 1960). Thus the so-called hygroscopic expansion is simply an enhanced setting expansion that occurs in the presence of additional water.

Control of setting expansion

1. *Use of additives.* A low setting expansion is desirable in applications where dimensional accuracy is important (eg, in impression taking and pouring working casts and dies). Many accelerators and retarders of setting also reduce setting expansion. Manufacturers can reduce setting expansion and at the same time control setting time by adding a balanced blend of accelerator and retarder to the raw hemihydrate. Typical combinations are potassium sulfate–borax and potassium sodium tartrate–sodium citrate.

   These additives also reduce the strength of the set material. This is not a disadvantage in impression plasters, but in stones, strength as well as dimensional accuracy is important; formulation of the latter materials therefore involves striking a compromise between a desirable reduction in setting expansion and an undesirable reduction in strength.

   Although normally, in the interests of dimensional accuracy, die stones in particular are formulated to have a low setting expansion, there are exceptions. High-expanding die stones are available with setting expansions as high as 0.30%. Their higher expansions result from a lower concentration of modifying additives, so these materials also achieve higher compressive strengths when set. They are intended for use in indirect casting techniques, when investment expansion alone may be insufficient to compensate fully for alloy casting shrinkage. Here the setting expansion of the die stone is intended to contribute to the total mold expansion by producing an oversized pattern (Fusayama, 1964), but it is important that the impression be soft and flexible enough for isotropic setting expansion to occur.

2. *W/P ratio.* For any given gypsum product, reducing the relative amount of aqueous phase in the mix allows more effective interaction of growing gypsum crystals during setting, thus increasing the setting expansion. Setting expansion is therefore inversely proportional to the W/P ratio. Because of their lower water requirement, the raw hemihydrates used to produce stones and die stones have a higher inherent setting expansion in normal mixes than does plaster. This effect is masked, however, by the additives used in their formulation (Fig 5-6).

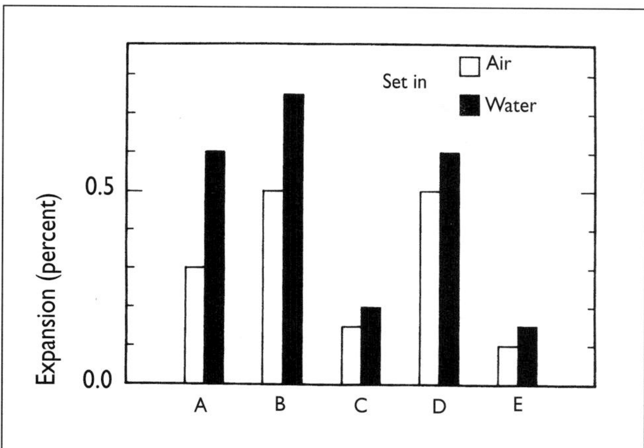

Fig 5-6 Linear setting expansion in air and in water of various types of gypsum products. (A) Plaster (W/P = 0.50); (B) unmodified stone (Hydrocal B, W/P = 0.32); (C) a commercial stone based on Hydrocal (W/P = 0.32); (D) unmodified high-strength stone (Densite K5, W/P = 0.24); (E) a commercial high-strength stone based on Densite (W/P = 0.24).

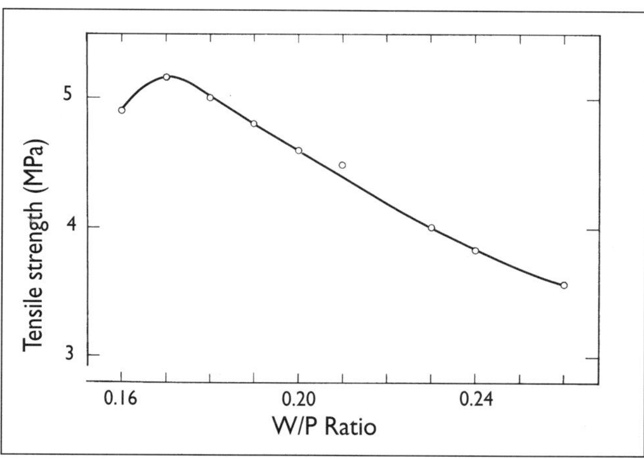

Fig 5-7 The effect of W/P ratio on the wet tensile strength of a high-strength stone. (From Selby, 1979.)

Table 5-3 Strength properties of typical dental gypsum products (the materials tested were the same as those in Table 5-2)

		Tensile strength (MPa)		Compressive strength (MPa)	
Type	W/P ratio	Wet	Dry	Wet	Dry
Impression plaster	0.60	1.3	—	5.9	—
Plaster	0.50	2.3	4.1	12.4	24.9
Stone	0.30	3.5	7.6	25.5	63.5
High-strength stone	0.23	4.3	9.9	40.7	80.7

Strength

Cast gypsum is a brittle material and so is weaker in tension than in compression. Materials with the highest compressive strengths are the most brittle, and their tensile strengths are proportionally lower. For set plaster, the tensile strength is about 20% of the compressive strength; for set high-strength stone, about 10%. Since fracture of cast gypsum typically occurs in tension, tensile strength is a better guide to fracture resistance. However, compressive strength gives a better indication of surface hardness. Values for tensile and compressive strengths of four typical dental gypsum plasters are shown in Table 5-3. The materials tested were the same as those listed in Table 5-2.

1. *The effect of W/P ratio.* In general, strength properties are inversely related to W/P ratio and so to the total amount of inherent porosity (Fig 5-7). Therefore when maximum strength is required, a given material should be mixed in as low a W/P ratio as practicable. The limiting factor is the viscosity of the mix, because it increases with decreasing W/P ratio and can become so high that the ability to pour sound casts is prejudiced.

   In high-strength stones mixed even in normal W/P ratios, there is little water present in excess of the theoretical W/P ratio (0.186) required for complete conversion of hemihydrate to dihydrate. Since the setting reaction depends on diffusion of ions, it may not proceed to completion in standard mixes, and residual hemihydrate particles are often seen in micrographs of set high-strength stone. The content of unreacted hemihydrate becomes much greater in very thick mixes, but as Fig 5-7 shows this does not adversely affect the strength until the W/P ratio is well below that theoretically needed for complete hydration. Such thick mixes would be impossible to manipulate successfully in most dental applications.

With any plaster or stone, using a low W/P ratio to obtain maximum strength properties also gives an increased setting expansion, which must be accepted. But in applications where dimensional accuracy is more important than strength (eg, impressions), higher W/P ratios can be used.

2. *The effect of drying.* Removal of all uncombined water from cast gypsum by low-temperature drying approximately doubles strength properties (see Table 5-3), but there is no strength increase until the last 2% of free water is removed. This strength increase on drying is reversible; soaking a dry cast in water reduces its strength to the original level.

Gypsum is stable only below about 40°C. Drying at higher temperatures must be carefully controlled; loss of water of crystallization occurs rapidly at 100°C or higher and causes shrinkage and a reduction in strength.

Solubility

Because gypsum is sparingly soluble in water, long-term immersion is contraindicated. If dried gypsum casts have to be soaked, it is better to use a saturated solution of calcium sulfate.

Disinfection of gypsum casts

To prevent cross-infection, the practice of disinfecting impressions is becoming increasingly common. However, prolonged immersion in disinfectant solutions can cause unacceptably large dimensional changes in hydrocolloid (Bergman et al, 1985; Olsson et al, 1987) and polyether (Johnson et al, 1988) impressions. Moreover, during subsequent clinical procedures, casts or dies can become reinfected with pathogenic organisms, which can then be transferred to technical staff. As an alternative, the addition of disinfectants to the mixing water when casts are poured has been investigated; 5% phenol (McGill et al, 1988) and 2% glutaraldehyde (Ivanovski et al, 1995) have proved to be effective, and did not adversely affect the properties of the set material. However, both are known tissue irritants. Dental stones are available which contain a disinfectant (Donovan and Chee, 1989; Schutt, 1989). Alternatively, casts and dies may be treated by immersion in a disinfecting solution after each clinical stage.

Autoclave sterilization of casts has been suggested (Whyte and Brockhurst, 1996). Some loss of strength and surface hardness and an increase in dimensions occur, but it is claimed that under carefully controlled conditions the casts retain adequate properties for ordinary laboratory use.

Gypsum-bonded investments

Gypsum-bonded investments are the mold materials most commonly employed in the casting of dental gold alloys with liquidus temperatures no higher than 1,080°C, which are normally used for gold inlays, crowns, and fixed and removable partial dentures. Because of their tendency to decompose at high temperatures, these investments are not suitable for casting high-melting gold alloys, palladium alloys (used for copings in alloy-ceramic restorations), or most base-metal alloys, such as nickel-chromium and cobalt-chromium. Gypsum-bonded investments are classified by the International Standards Organization (1990) as

Type 1: Thermal expansion type, for casting inlays and crowns
Type 2: Hygroscopic expansion type, for casting inlays and crowns
Type 3: For casting complete and partial denture bases

This classification is illustrated in Fig 5-8, and typical materials are listed in Table 5-4. Some materials, classified by their manufacturers as "universal," are claimed to be suitable for casting all gold-alloy restorations.

Composition

All gypsum-bonded investment powders consist basically of a refractory filler and a binder. There may also be small amounts (less than 5%) of important modifying agents present.

Refractory

The refractory component is either cristobalite or quartz (or occasionally a mixture of the two), present usually in the range of 55% to 75%. These components are both polymorphs of silica (SiO_2).

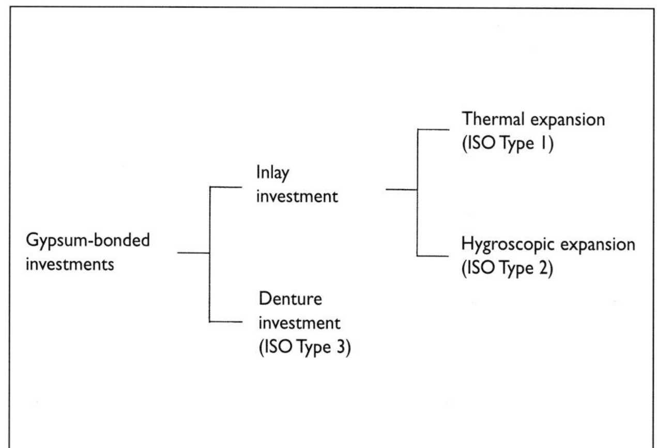

Fig 5-8 Classification of gypsum-bonded investments.

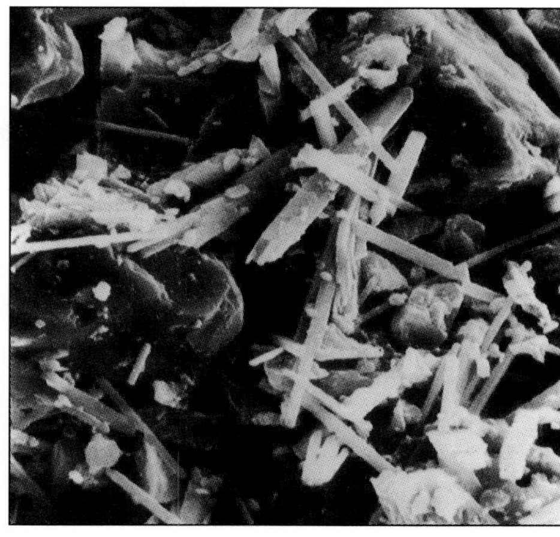

Fig 5-9 Microstructure of a set gypsum-bonded investment (Kerr Cristobalite Inlay); W/P = 0.38. The large particles are cristobalite; the small acicular crystals are gypsum formed during setting. (Scanning electron micrograph of fracture surface, original magnification × 3,000.)

Table 5-4 Typical gypsum-bonded investments

Type	Example
Inlay investment, thermal expansion (ISO Type 1)	Cristobalite Inlay (Kerr/Sybron)
Inlay investment, hygroscopic expansion (ISO Type 2)	Beauty-Cast (Whip Mix Corp)
Denture investment (ISO Type 3)	R & R Gray (York Div., Dentsply International, Inc)

Binder

In the investment powder, the binder is calcium sulfate hemihydrate, either plaster or stone. When the investment sets, the silica is unaffected; the hemihydrate binder combines with water to form dihydrate (gypsum) as in the setting of other gypsum products. The setting reaction is therefore the same as that shown in the equation given previously. The set investment consists of fine particles of silica embedded in an interlocking aggregate of smaller acicular gypsum crystals (Fig 5-9). The continuous porosity characteristic of cast gypsum provides the necessary mold venting to assist in the production of sound castings.

Modifying agents

Small amounts of modifying agents are added to many commercial gypsum-bonded investments. These may be accelerators or retarders to control the rate of setting, reducing agents such as powdered graphite or copper to protect embedded gold alloy components in "casting-on" techniques, or additives to increase the thermal expansion of the investment. Typical additives of the last type are boric acid and soluble halide salts, particularly those of alkali or alkaline earth metals.

Effect of composition on setting and thermal behavior

Refractory

Although silica is referred to as the refractory component, cast gypsum itself is sufficiently heat-resisting to be used as a mold material, because it can be heated to temperatures as high as 1,000°C without decomposing (Gutt and Smith, 1967). In fact, adding silica reduces its heat resistance, because in such mixtures at temperatures above 900°C, the following reaction occurs:

$$CaSO_4 + SiO_2 \rightarrow CaSiO_3 + SO_3$$

At high temperatures, the sulfur trioxide liberated by this reaction causes rapid corrosion of the casting.

Crystalline silica is used in dental investments not to improve their heat resistance but to control dimensional changes on heating. When heated, cast gypsum shows a marked contraction, and because both quartz and cristobalite have high expansions when heated, they offset the shrinkage of the binder and can provide a positive thermal expansion if this is needed.

Silica exists in 22 different condensed phases. Five of these are amorphous, and 17 are crystalline; the latter are the polymorphs of silica. Of this group, only one phase, low-temperature quartz, is thermodynamically stable at normal temperature and pressure. Two more, tridymite S-1 and low-temperature cristobalite, exist under normal atmospheric conditions as metastable (but actually long-lived) phases.

Only two polymorphs of silica are of importance in dental investments: quartz and cristobalite. Quartz is a common mineral; cristobalite occurs naturally as a rare mineral but is normally manufactured by prolonged heating of quartz at high temperatures to induce the appropriate slow inversion. Both quartz and cristobalite exist in low-temperature (α) and high-temperature (β) phases, and in both materials the change between low- and high-temperature phases is rapid and readily reversible on cooling. This change is known as the high-low inversion.

In both quartz and cristobalite the high-temperature phase is less dense than the low, so the $\alpha \rightarrow \beta$ inversion is accompanied by an isothermal expansion. This is added to the normal thermal expansion to give a large overall expansion at high temperatures.

As in all crystalline materials, single crystals of quartz and cristobalite show anisotropy of physical properties, including their coefficients of thermal expansion. However, in dental investments they are used as a fine powder with random orientation of individual particles, so in the aggregate they behave isotropically, and properties such as the coefficient of thermal expansion have a uniform average value.

Typical linear thermal expansion curves for powdered quartz and cristobalite are shown in Fig 5-10. Specimens were made by densely compacting the powders into aggregates with a minimum amount of binder in the interstices, so the thermal expansion of the specimens was essentially that of the silica component in dental investments.

The temperature of the $\alpha \rightarrow \beta$ inversion of cristobalite varies according to the source of the sample and its previous thermal history; in the manufactured cristobalite used in dental investments it is about 250°C (Fig 5-10, curve A). The inversion gives an isothermal expansion of about 1.3%, and the total expansion at 700°C is about 2.2%. Dental investments designed to have a high thermal expansion usually contain cristobalite as the refractory.

Quartz (Fig 5-10, curve B) undergoes its $\alpha \rightarrow \beta$ inversion at 573°C, producing an isothermal expansion of about 0.7%. The high-temperature form has a negative coefficient of thermal expansion, and the overall total expansion at 700°C is about 1.6%.

Binder

When the set investment is heated, the cast gypsum binder shows a marked contraction, which occurs in several stages. In the early stages of heating, a contraction accompanies loss of water of crystallization, as the dihydrate reverts to hemihydrate and then to hexagonal calcium sulfate. A large contraction then accompanies its $\gamma \rightarrow \beta$ transformation, which occurs in the approximate temperature range 300° to 400°C. A further large contraction begins at about 650°C, which is probably the result of densification by sintering. The total linear contraction of cast gypsum prepared from plaster (W/P = 0.50) and heated to 700°C can be as high as 3%; the corresponding shrinkage for cast gypsum prepared from a high-strength stone (W/P = 0.25) is about 1%. The latter is usually preferred as a binder in gypsum-bonded investments, not only because of its lower shrinkage on heating but because its superior strength when set allows a higher concentration of silica to be used in the investment, thereby reducing still further the effect of binder contraction.

Effects of varying composition

Within practical limits, increasing the proportion of silica in the investment powder increases the manipulation time (given by the time of loss of fluidity) and the initial setting time (Fig 5-11), the setting expansion, both in air and in water, and the thermal expansion (Fig 5-12) and reduces the compressive strength (Fig 5-13). The rate of the setting reaction itself is unchanged; the

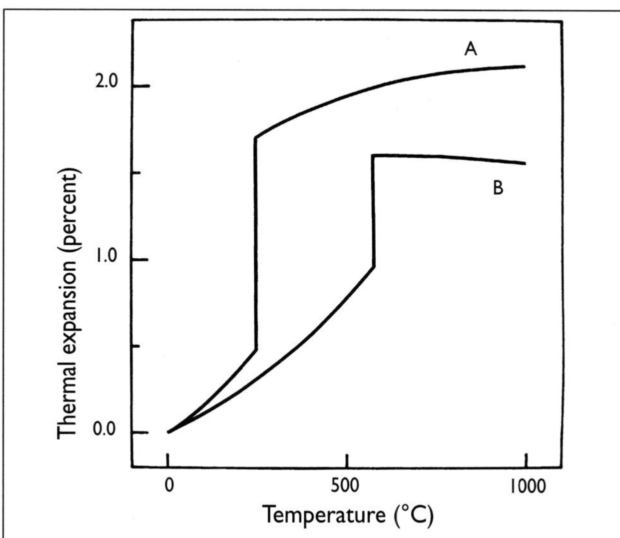

Fig 5-10 The linear thermal expansion of cristobalite (curve A) and quartz (curve B). The specimens were aggregates of fine powders, united with a minimum amount of binder; their thermal behavior was thus similar to that of the refractory component of dental casting investments. Cristobalite undergoes inversion at about 250°C, quartz at 573°C.

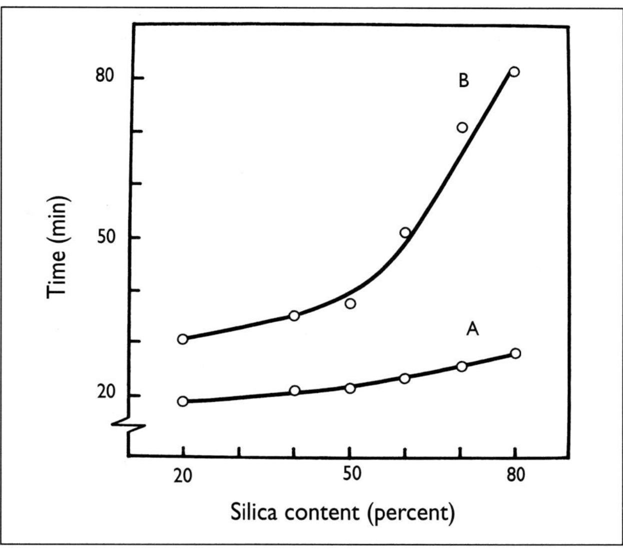

Fig 5-11 The effect of silica content on the manipulation time (curve A) and setting time (curve B) of experimental investments. Manipulation time was determined by the time of loss of gloss, which indicates loss of fluidity; setting time by the Vicat initial set. The investments were mixtures of cristobalite and a high-strength stone, and all specimens were mixed in a W/P ratio of 0.40.

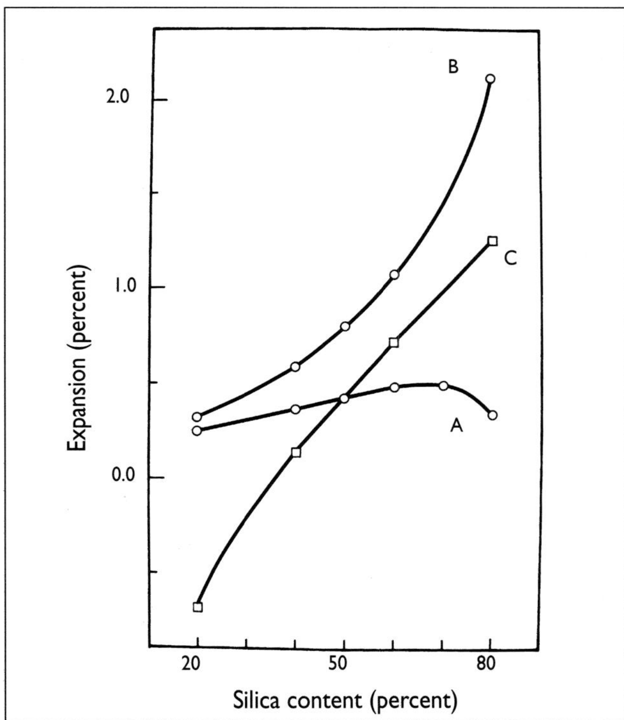

Fig 5-12 The effect of silica content on the setting expansion in air (curve A), the setting expansion in water (curve B), and the thermal expansion (curve C) of experimental investments (compositions and W/P ratio as in Fig 5-11). Setting expansions were recorded 2 hours after mixing, and thermal expansions after heating to 700°C.

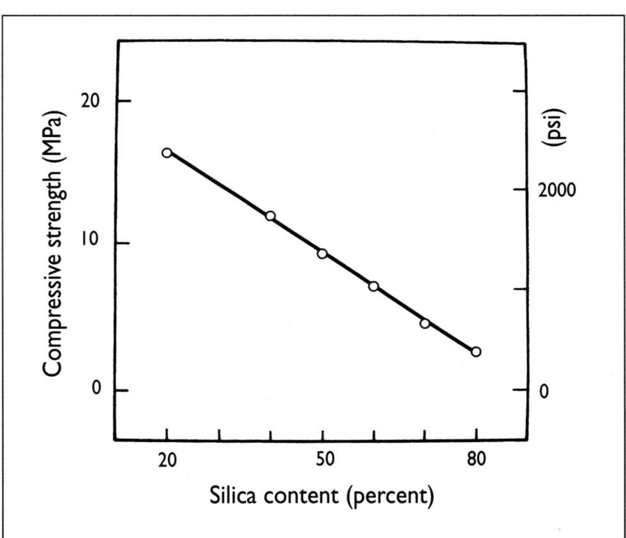

Fig 5-13 The effect of silica content on the compressive strength of experimental investments (compositions and W/P ratio as in Fig 5-11). Tests were made on wet specimens, 2 hours after mixing.

increases in observed manipulation and setting times occur because the particles of refractory filler interfere with the interlocking of growing gypsum crystals, making this less effective in developing a solid structure. The compressive strength of the set investment is reduced for the same reason. Setting expansion is increased when interlocking of growing gypsum crystals is inhibited by the refractory particles, because more of the crystal growth is directed outward. Thermal expansion is increased because, at any temperature, it is given by summing the binder contraction and the refractory expansion; increasing the proportion of the expanding component increases the observed expansion.

Effects of modifying agents

Important modifying agents are those added to some commercial investments to increase their thermal expansion. These include boric acid and soluble halide salts of alkali or alkaline earth metals. All of them act mainly by reducing the two large contractions of the gypsum binder that occur on heating to temperatures above 300°C.

Boric acid, when heated above 150°C, forms a viscous liquid with a composition intermediate between metaboric acid and boron oxide; this viscous liquid impedes the evaporation of the last traces of water, delaying the $\gamma \rightarrow \beta$ transformation of calcium sulfate (Mori, 1986). The presence of the viscous liquid phase also reduces the high-temperature contraction that results from sintering, because it stabilizes the original contacts formed between the gypsum crystals and silica during setting (Mori, 1982).

The presence of halide anions greatly reduces the first major shrinkage and completely eliminates the second. The reason for this is not yet understood. If alkali metal or alkaline earth cations are also present (eg, as halide salts), the effect of the halide anion is nullified at temperatures above 650°C and a rapid contraction occurs; this is probably the result of accelerated sintering. This large high-temperature shrinkage of the binder is not observed in gypsum-bonded investments containing alkali metal or alkaline earth halides, because at a concentration of 50% or more of silica the silica particles in the set investment form a continuous "skeleton" that resists overall shrinkage.

The presence of modifiers added to increase the thermal expansion also affects the strength changes of the investment that occur on heating, again because of their effects on the calcium sulfate binder.

On heating, gypsum-bonded investments without these additives show a rapid increase in compressive strength of about 100% in the range of 100° to 175°C; this is the result of drying and is analogous to that occurring in cast gypsum. Between 175° and 225°C there is an equally rapid decrease in compressive strength, attributable to the dehydration reaction dihydrate → hemihydrate, bringing the strength back to about that of the original wet specimens. Relatively minor strength fluctuations occur during subsequent heating to higher temperatures, attributable to (*1*) further phase changes in the binder, (*2*) the $\alpha \rightarrow \beta$ inversion in the refractory, and (*3*) sintering of the binder (Ohno et al, 1982). Investments of this type, heated to temperatures in the range of 670° to 700°C, show compressive strength changes ranging from +10% to –40%, compared with the wet strength at ambient temperatures.

Investments containing boric acid, when heated to the same temperatures show increases in compressive strength ranging from +40% to +50%, the result probably of the effect of the viscous liquid phase stabilizing contacts between calcium sulfate and silica particles. Investments containing halides of alkali metals and alkaline earths (eg, sodium, barium, and strontium chlorides) show a marked strength decrease on heating to 700°C, ranging from – 50% to – 85%. This is probably the result of the increased sintering contraction of the binder at temperatures over 650°C. The silica skeleton resists shrinkage of the investment as a whole, so the high sintering contraction occurs independently in the binder, reducing the strength of its bond with the silica particles.

Properties

Particle size of the powder

The particle size affects the smoothness of the mold cavity surface (and thus of the casting) and also the inherent porosity of the mold (thus the venting of the mold cavity). Only the particle size of the refractory filler is of practical importance. It is the major constituent and remains unchanged in the set investment. The gypsum crystals formed during setting of the binder are much smaller than the silica particles (see Fig 5-9).

Excessive surface roughness of the casting can interfere with its fit; a refractory with a fine particle size ensures a smooth mold surface and a smooth casting. In gypsum-bonded investments, venting of the mold cavity is normally provided by the continuous porosity inherent in the set material. This is at a maximum when packing of the silica particles is least dense, which in turn is achieved by ensuring that the particle size is uniform.

Therefore, the refractory powder used in making the investment should have a uniform, fine particle size. A particle size of no more than 75 μm is usual.

Rate of setting

The same physical changes that occur during the setting of gypsum plasters can also be recognized when gypsum-bonded investments set.

Manipulation time Investing the wax pattern or pouring the investment cast must be completed while the mix is still fluid. As with gypsum plasters, loss of fluidity is indicated by the disappearance of the glossy surface from the mix.

Setting time This is usually given as a Gillmore or Vicat initial set. It indicates when the investment is strong enough for the sprue base and sprue former to be removed. Preferably mold heating should be delayed until setting expansion is complete (usually between 1 and 2 hours from the start of mixing).

Expansion

Inlay investments currently available have total expansions, measured under laboratory conditions, in the range 1.5% to 2.5%. Denture investments gain increased strength by having a higher content of hemihydrate binder, at the expense of the refractory component, so their total expansions are less; the lower figure for the expansion range is about 1.3%. It is, however, by no means certain that such figures show the expansion of the mold cavity that can be expected under practical conditions.

Modern methods of casting small restorations can be classified into two groups.

1. In *hygroscopic expansion techniques*, all or most of the mold expansion is gained when the investment sets; the setting expansion is greatly increased by exposure to additional water. Thermal expansion of the investment is relatively low.
2. In *thermal expansion techniques*, both setting and thermal expansion contribute importantly to mold expansion.

Setting expansion

1. *Setting expansion in air.* Linear setting expansions of most inlay investments, measured under dry conditions, are in the range of 0.1% to 0.6%.
2. *Setting expansion in water (hygroscopic setting expansion).* Inlay investments show a much greater setting expansion if exposed to additional water during setting (eg, by immersion in a water bath). The phenomenon is the same as that described for gypsum plasters, but the effect on setting expansion is much greater because of the presence of the refractory particles (see Fig 5-12). If no constraint is imposed, the linear setting expansion of inlay investments can be as high as 4%. But even a small restraining force causes a large reduction, and when measured under usual laboratory conditions, the hygroscopic setting expansion of most inlay investments is in the range of 0.3% to 2.0%. Investments specifically designed for use in hygroscopic expansion techniques have setting expansions, when immersed in water, of at least 1.3%.
3. *The effect of the casting ring liner.* In most casting techniques the investment mold sets and is heated in a casting ring made of heat-resisting alloy. The need for a soft ring liner, to eliminate or at least reduce restraint to investment expansion by the ring, was first recognized by Souder (Hollenback, 1962), who advocated the use of asbestos tape to provide the necessary cushioning. Since asbestos readily absorbs water, the liner was prewetted to prevent its absorbing water from the unset investment mix.

The technique of lining a casting ring with wet asbestos was first described in 1930 by Taylor and coworkers, and from then until recent times, the use of a wet asbestos ring liner has been a standard procedure. This makes additional water available to the setting investment and causes an increased setting expansion. Even when the investment mold sets in air, as in thermal expansion techniques, some hygroscopic setting expansion occurs. Investments used in thermal expansion techniques have a relatively high silica content, so the increase in setting expansion produced by exposure to water is high (see Fig 5-12). Because this high setting expansion is uncontrollable and likely to be nonuniform, techniques have been developed in which a dry, waterproofed asbestos ring liner is used (Fusayama, 1959, 1964) or the use of the rigid casting ring with its liner is avoided (Finger and Jørgensen, 1980).

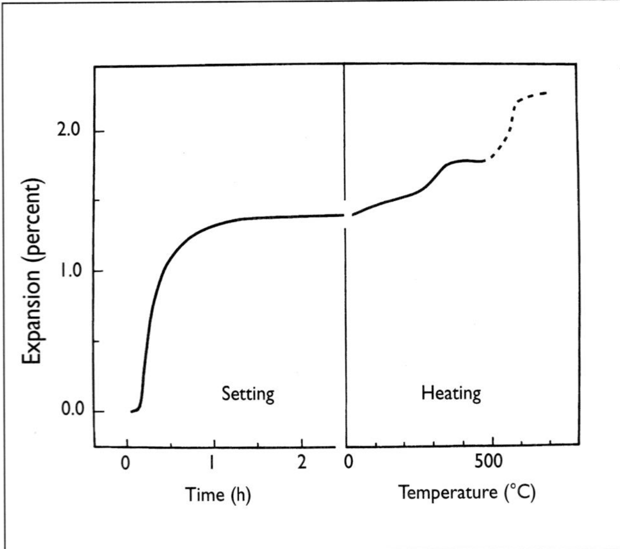

Fig 5-14 Setting and thermal expansion of a typical investment of the hygroscopic expansion type (Whip Mix Beauty-Cast, W/P = 0.30). The specimen was immersed in room-temperature water during setting and was then heated to 480°C. This investment is based on quartz and contains a halide, which gives it a small positive thermal expansion, uniform over a range of about 150°C. The dashed continuation of the curve shows the effect of heating the investment to 700°C.

Recently, attention has been drawn to the danger that asbestos fibers in casting-ring liners could cause asbestosis or mesothelioma (Priest and Horner, 1980). It is claimed that the acceptable threshold limit for asbestos fibers in air can be considerably exceeded when castings are removed from asbestos-lined casting rings (Yli-Urpo et al, 1982). For this reason, and because of the increasing unavailability of asbestos products, asbestos as a casting-ring liner has been almost completely replaced by alternative materials. There are two types: (*1*) cellulose, which readily absorbs water and, like asbestos, must be prewetted; and (*2*) ceramic materials which at atmospheric pressure will not absorb water and are normally used dry. The ceramic materials are made from fibers of an aluminosilicate glass derived from kaolin; these are formed into sheets by means of standard paper-making techniques (Barnard, 1981). The major components in the glass are alumina (47% to 65%) and silica (38% to 50%), which makes the material highly heat-resistant. On the other hand, the cellulose materials burn if heated in air, and at a burnout temperature of 700°C they disappear completely from the casting ring. However, if liners are kept short of both ends of the ring, the investment mold is retained in place during casting.

Cellulose liners have a water uptake similar to asbestos, and a similar effect on the setting expansion of the investment.

Although they absorb negligible amounts of water when immersed at atmospheric pressure, ceramic liners absorb it readily under vacuum. This occurs during vacuum investing; since the previously dry liners obtain the water from the investment mix, the W/P ratio of the unset investment is greatly reduced. The combination of a low W/P ratio and a wet liner considerably increases the investment's setting expansion; the total expansion is higher than when prewetted asbestos or cellulose liners are used with normal W/P ratios.

Thermal expansion After it has set, the investment mold is heated to the recommended temperature for casting. This is necessary to dry the investment, to melt and burn out the wax pattern, to oxidize residual carbon from the mold, and to prevent premature freezing of thin sections when the alloy is cast. Heating also causes thermal expansion of the mold and, therefore, of the mold cavity.

1. *Hygroscopic expansion techniques.* With these techniques, the mold is heated to about 480°C, at which temperature its thermal expansion is relatively low (Fig 5-14). Investments for use in these techniques are based on a quartz refractory that does not undergo inversion until heated to 573°C (see Fig 5-10).

   A mold temperature as low as 480°C has the advantage of ensuring a fine grain structure in the solidified casting, though this is not an important consideration if the alloy contains grain-refining elements. It has the disadvantage that carbon remaining from burnout of the wax pattern is oxidized very slowly. Excessive carbon deposits interfere with venting of the mold cavity, so prolonged heating at the casting temperature (preferably 1 hour) is needed to ensure that casting defects caused by inadequate venting ("back-pressure porosity") do not occur.

2. *Thermal expansion techniques.* With thermal expansion techniques, the mold is usually heated to about 700°C, in order to gain maximum mold expansion. A higher mold temperature should not be used or breakdown of the calcium sulfate binder can occur in the presence of carbon, thereby liberating sulfur dioxide. The carbon may be present as graphite added to the original investment powder as a reducing agent or may simply be carbon residue from burnout of the wax pattern. The reaction, which involves reduction of the calcium sulfate binder, takes place in two stages:

$$CaSO_4 + 4C \rightarrow CaS + 4CO$$
$$3CaSO_4 + CaS \rightarrow 4CaO + 4SO_2$$

The sulfur dioxide formed by the second reaction causes sulfide formation on the gold-alloy casting, resulting in discoloration and embrittlement of the alloy.

Investments for thermal expansion techniques may contain either cristobalite or quartz as the refractory; occasionally a mixture of both is used. Cristobalite investments have the advantage that thermal expansion is fairly constant over the temperature range 400° to 700°C, but have the disadvantage that the large expansion at 250°C, resulting from the $\alpha \rightarrow \beta$ inversion of cristobalite, can cause mold cracking if heating is not carefully controlled (Fig 5-15, curve A).

Quartz has a lower thermal expansion than cristobalite (see Fig 5-10), so most quartz investments for use in thermal expansion techniques contain additives to increase their thermal expansion. The expansion on heating is more gradual, so control of heating rate is not as important, but maximum expansion is available only in the temperature range 600° to 700°C (Fig 5-15, curve B).

At a burnout temperature of 700°C, residual carbon is oxidized rapidly, so venting of the mold cavity is not a problem.

3. *The effect of a wet liner.* In thermal expansion techniques, if a wet ring liner is used, not only the setting expansion but also the subsequent thermal expansion can be affected. Once the investment has set, the extra water it absorbed from the liner has the same effect as if it had been added when mixing (ie, an increased W/P ratio). Therefore, the thermal expansion may be reduced.

The same considerations apply to denture investments. The investment cast forms part of the final mold, and its expansion is the major factor determining the accuracy of the casting. It sets in contact with a duplicating impression, usually an aqueous gel, which, like a wet ring liner, makes free water available to the setting investment with the same effects as those already described.

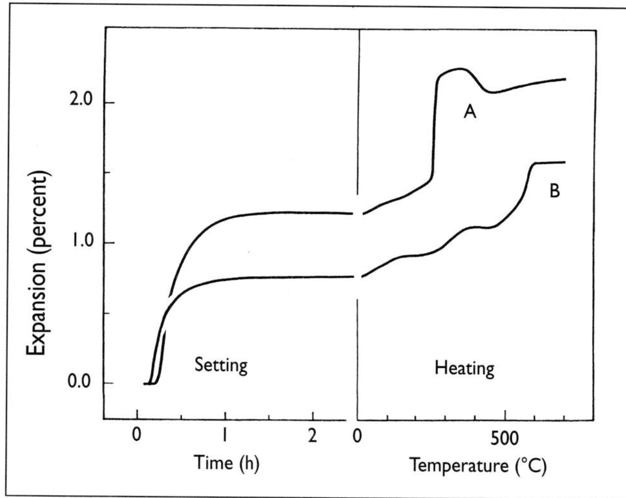

Fig 5-15 Setting and thermal expansion of two typical investments of the thermal expansion type (curve A: Kerr Cristobalite Inlay, W/P = 0.38; curve B: Ransom and Randolph Gray, W/P = 0.25). With both materials the specimens were surrounded by a wet ring liner while setting and were then heated to 700°C. The former material is an inlay investment based on cristobalite. The latter material is described as a universal investment but is most commonly used for casting dentures and is based on quartz, with the addition of sodium chloride to increase its thermal expansion.

Control of expansion

1. *Composition.* The manufacturer adjusts investment expansion by choice of refractory and binder and sometimes by the use of suitable additives.
2. *W/P ratio.* Decreasing the W/P ratio increases both setting expansion (in air or water) and thermal expansion. The W/P ratio must be carefully controlled for reproducible mold expansion. Changes in expansion can most easily be effected by changing the W/P ratio (Fig 5-16).

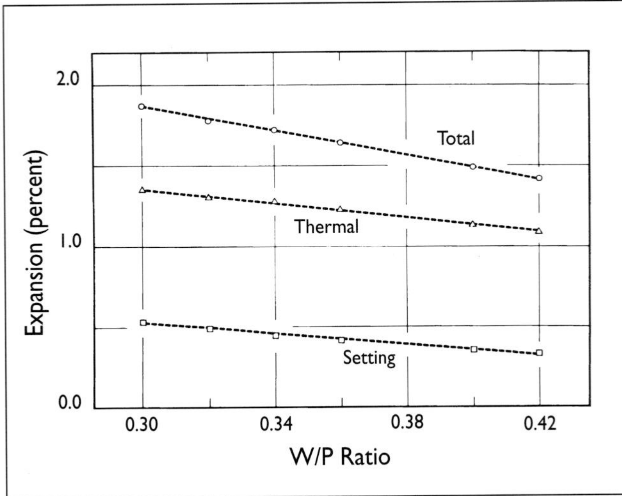

Fig 5-16 The effect of changing the W/P ratio on the setting, thermal, and total expansions of a typical investment of the thermal expansion type, set against a dry ceramic liner without vacuum investing, and then heated to 700°C.

3. *Period of exposure to water.* In hygroscopic expansion techniques, additional control can be obtained by varying the length of time the setting investment is exposed to an aqueous environment. This may be achieved by reducing the time for which the setting investment is immersed in a water bath, or by adding controlled amounts of water to the top of the investment mix in the ring instead of immersing it. In the latter case, if only a small volume of water is added, it will be completely absorbed by the investment before setting is complete, and subsequent expansion will be reduced. Varying the amount of added water varies the setting expansion proportionally.

Strength

The mold must be strong enough to withstand stresses at ambient temperatures (eg, during removal of the sprue former) and when heated to the recommended mold temperature for casting (eg, during rapid entry of molten alloy). Strength properties of investments are usually determined by testing in compression. Inlay investments have wet compressive strengths mostly in the range of 2 to 6 MPa. Because of the need to make a working cast, denture investments have higher compressive strengths when set, mostly in the range 9 to 14 MPa. In both investment types, changes in the compressive strength on heating to the recommended casting temperature vary according to the presence of additives to control investment thermal expansion. Unless it is known whether an additive is present in an investment, and if so what it is, it is impossible to predict strength at the casting temperature from measurements made at ordinary ambient temperatures. Little information is available on the compressive strength of gypsum-bonded investments at the casting temperature (hot strength). In one study on a limited number of materials (Earnshaw, 1969), it was found that the hot strength of four investments without additives was in the range 1.8 to 9.4 MPa; for three investments containing boric acid in the range was 6.3 to 13.3 MPa; and for three investments containing sodium chloride it was 3.1 to 5.2 MPa.

Casting accuracy

In all casting procedures, after the molten metal or alloy has filled the mold, a volumetric contraction occurs in the liquid and then in the solid casting as it cools. In addition, with almost all metals and alloys there is a volumetric contraction during solidification.

In dental casting, thermal contraction of the liquid alloy, and its solidification contraction, do not affect the dimensions of the casting because, under the influence of the casting force, continued feeding of liquid alloy occurs from the excess in the sprue and button. Interruption to the flow of liquid during solidification, which may be caused by premature freezing of an incorrectly designed sprue, will not cause an overall contraction of the casting, but will lead to localized shrinkage porosity.

Therefore, thermal contraction of the solidified casting, as it cools from solidus to ambient temperature, remains as the sole cause of the observed casting shrinkage. Although this is a volumetric contraction, in dental technology dimensional changes are usually studied on a linear basis. It is assumed that these changes occur isotropically—an assumption that is frequently unjustified.

The fact that the observed casting shrinkage is thermal contraction of the solid alloy can be confirmed, at least for pure gold, by comparing measured values for its linear casting shrinkage with a value calculated from its coefficient of linear thermal expansion (α) and the temperature difference between its freezing temperature and ambient.

Table 5-5 Measured values for the linear casting shrinkage of pure gold

Reference	Specimens (mm)	Linear casting shrinkage (%)*
Hollenback and Skinner (1946)	Cylindrical rod (5.6 × 25)	1.67 ± 0.02 (8)
Earnshaw (1960)	Cylindrical rod (6.3 × 60)	1.74 ± 0.03 (6)
Nakai et al (1980)	Rectangular prism (3 × 5 × 20)	1.73 ± 0.04 (9)

*Values are shown as mean and standard deviation, and (in parentheses) number of tests.

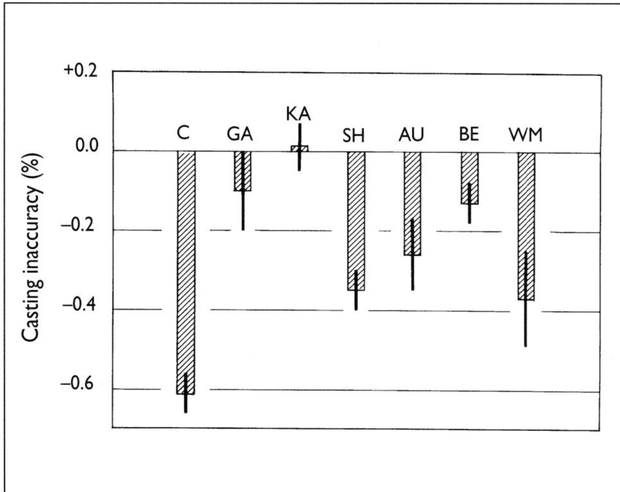

Fig 5-17 The effect of different prewetted ring liners on the relative inaccuracy of gold-alloy full-crown castings. The castings were made with a cristobalite inlay investment of the thermal expansion type used with vacuum investing. C = control castings made without a liner; GA, KA, and SH = castings made with asbestos liners; and AU, BE, and WM = castings made with cellulose liners. The height of each bar shows the mean of at least 10 castings, while the narrow superimposed bar shows the standard deviation.

Results of direct measurements of the linear casting shrinkage of gold are shown in Table 5-5. A theoretical value can be calculated as follows:

$$\alpha_{(20°–900°C)} = 16.7 \times 10^{-6}/K$$
$$\text{Melting temperature} = 1{,}064°C$$

If 20°C is taken as an average ambient temperature, the solidified gold cools through 1,044 K. Total linear contraction per unit length is given by $1{,}044 \times 16.7 \times 10^{-6} = 0.0174$, which converts to 1.74%.

Alloying gold will alter the value for α and for solidus temperature. Calculations similar to that given previously have been made on a group of 12 high noble-metal casting alloys, and the calculated linear casting shrinkages varied from 1.65% to 1.80% (Finger and Jørgensen, 1980). Thus an average value of 1.7% would apply to gold and high-gold alloys.

It is conventionally assumed that compensation for this casting shrinkage is provided by mold expansion. Calculations of available compensation, however, must be based on measurements of investment expansion made under conditions that reproduce those obtaining in the casting ring (Earnshaw, 1988).

Another factor that must be considered is the effect of the ring liner on investment expansion. Absorbent liners (asbestos and cellulose) vary in thickness, water uptake, and compressibility when wet. In thermal expansion techniques, some may not have sufficient compressibility to accommodate all of the increased setting expansion provided by the availability of extra water, so that restriction of expansion could occur in a diametral direction in the ring (Morey and Earnshaw, 1992). Thus they affect to a varying degree the available mold expansion. Ceramic liners also vary in thickness and compressibility, and if vacuum investing is used, they vary in the amount of water they absorb from the investment mix. Again they affect mold expansion in the ring to a varying degree (Earnshaw and Morey, 1992).

The choice of casting-ring liner can thus affect, often to a significant extent, the dimensional accuracy of the casting. Figure 5-17 shows the relative inaccuracy produced in full-crown castings made in a high-gold alloy with a gypsum-bonded cristobalite investment of the thermal expansion type, used with vacuum investing. The only variation in technique was the casting-ring liner used. All the liners were water absorbent, and all were prewetted under controlled conditions. Three were asbestos, and three cellulose.

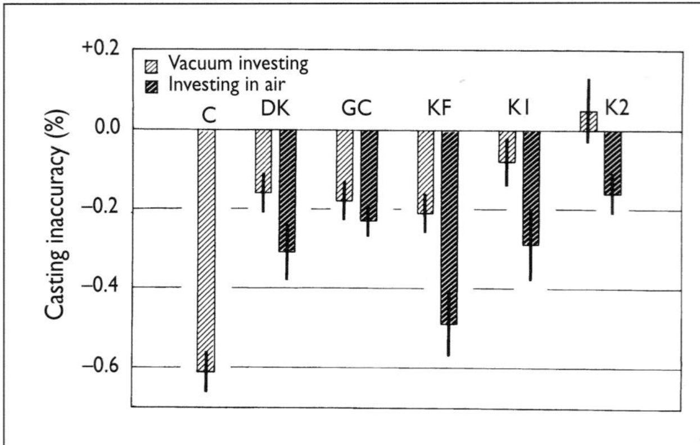

Fig 5-18 The effect of different dry ceramic ring liners on the relative inaccuracy of gold-alloy full-crown castings. Conditions were the same as in Fig 18-11, except that castings were made with and without vacuum investing. C = control castings made without a liner; DK, GC, and KF = castings made with ceramic liners supplied for dental use; and K1 and K2 = castings made with liners cut from commercial insulating material of the same type, supplied in sheets nominally 1 mm and 2 mm thick.

Figure 5-18 shows the results of similar experiments made with five different dry ceramic liners used with and without vacuum investing. These two graphs show the great variation in casting inaccuracy produced when the same investment is used with different casting-ring liners. This variation in inaccuracy is often not predictable; in these experiments, only when the ceramic liners were used with vacuum investing was there any correlation between measured liner properties and casting inaccuracy.

Although with gypsum-bonded investments mold expansion is the major factor affecting relative casting inaccuracy, mold strength at the casting temperature must also be considered. The average value of 1.7% for alloy thermal contraction represents the inherent casting shrinkage of the alloy—the shrinkage that would occur in a casting that was free to contract without constraint. Under practical conditions the casting is enclosed in a mold, and in all but the simplest castings its shape allows some interlocking between investment and mold. In the early stages of cooling the mold has a lower rate of thermal contraction than the casting; if the investment has a high hot strength, alloy thermal contraction will be opposed by the mold. The degree of constraint will depend on the casting shape and is usually directional. At temperatures near its solidus the alloy is weak and plastic, and mold constraint can cause anisotropic thermal contraction. When the alloy has cooled enough to attain rigidity, a strong mold can cause plastic deformation by hot-working the alloy. Both factors cause anisotropic contraction and distortion of the casting.

A constant pattern of distortion of gold-alloy mesio-occluso-distal inlays has been reported (Teteruck and Mumford, 1966) which can be attributed to directional restraint of alloy shrinkage by the mold (Earnshaw, 1969). The gypsum-bonded investment used in Teteruck and Mumford's experiments had a compressive strength at 700°C in the range of 4 to 6 MPa.

Therefore, although with gypsum-bonded investments the total investment expansion that occurs in the casting ring is the major factor affecting the casting inaccuracy, the hot strength of the mold must be considered. For the casting to reproduce accurately the size and shape of the original pattern, the investment expansion must compensate fully for the thermal contraction of the solid alloy, the ring and ring liner must allow the potential expansion of the investment to be achieved isotropically and the investment at the burnout temperature must not be so strong that it restricts the shrinkage of the alloy in any direction. On the other hand, it should not be so weak that it may fracture during casting. A safe minimum compressive strength at 700°C is 1.8 MPa, and this allows substantially isotropic alloy contraction (Morey and Earnshaw, 1995).

Storage of gypsum products

When hemihydrate powders are exposed to the atmosphere, water vapor is adsorbed; the extent to which this occurs depends on the prevailing water vapor pressure (Torrance and Darvell, 1990). If sufficient water is adsorbed to form a liquid film, and if this becomes thick enough to function as a solvent, the setting reaction begins on the surface of the powder particles, causing deterioration of the material. Gypsum crystals are formed which act as nucleation centers when the powder is mixed with water, and accelerate the setting rate. But if exposure of the powder continues, surface hydration will form a layer of gypsum on each particle, hindering the access of water to the hemihydrate, and the subsequent setting rate is retarded. If exposure continues over a long period, eventually the material will not set properly, because insufficient unreacted hemihydrate remains to form a coherent set mass. This is equally likely to occur in gypsum-bonded investments, and will have the same effects.

A long-standing recommendation to store gypsum products at relative humidities not greater than 70% (Farmer and Skinner, 1942) appears to be satisfactory only at temperatures of 25°C or lower, but of uncertain validity at higher temperatures (Torrance and Darvell, 1990). To avoid deterioration, especially at high temperatures and high relative humidities, bulk gypsum products should be stored in closed bins, in a cool dry area of the laboratory. "Topping up" of bins should not be done over old stock. Packaging of small quantities of powder, in waterproof containers, is a preferable method of storage in the laboratory. Many die stones and gypsum-bonded investments are now supplied by their manufacturers packaged in this way.

Glossary

acicular (of a crystal) Slender, needle-like.

apparent density (of a powder) The mass of a sample divided by the volume it occupies, measured at a specified degree of compaction. The measured volume includes all interstitial spaces and porosities, so powders with a poor packing ability show a low apparent density.

calcination Prolonged heating of a substance at some temperature below its melting temperature.

crystal habit (crystalline form) The external geometrical shape of a crystal.

crystal structure The regular three-dimensional arrangement of atoms within a crystal. This internal atomic arrangement is characteristic of a particular crystalline solid, but may or may not be the same as the external shape of individual crystals.

inversion A temperature-dependent change from one polymorphic form to another. **Rapid (high-low) inversions** involve only an alteration in bond angles within the crystal structure (shear or displacive transformation). This change requires only a small activation energy (excess energy required for the change to occur), so it occurs rapidly on heating to the critical temperature and is rapidly reversible on cooling. An example is the $\alpha \rightarrow \beta$ inversion of quartz or cristobalite. **Slow inversions** involve breaking of interatomic bonds and atomic diffusion to form a new crystal structure (reconstructive transformation). In a ceramic material in which a significant amount of the interatomic bonding is covalent, such as crystalline silica (Jastrzebski, 1976; Sosman, 1965), such a transformation involves a high activation energy, so prolonged high-temperature heating is needed for complete conversion. Because the transformation is so sluggish, the new high-temperature phase is retained during cooling to ambient temperature, where in most materials the rate of atomic diffusion is extremely slow. The high-temperature form therefore persists indefinitely as a metastable phase. An example is the quartz → cristobalite inversion.

isotropic Occurring equally in all directions. (Antonym: **anisotropic.**)

nucleation center In an aqueous solution, a region where spontaneous orderly deposition of ions or molecules forms nuclei that continue to grow, and so begin the process of crystallization. Normally this process involves heterogeneous nucleation, where nucleation centers are provided by the deposition of ions or molecules on existing solid surfaces, such as solid particles (seeds) already present in the solution.

nuclei poisoning The inactivation of nuclei of crystallization by the deposition of foreign material on their surfaces.

polymorphism The existence of an element or chemical compound in more than two different crystalline forms.

pseudomorph A crystalline material whose crystal habit differs from the normal shape that would be dictated by its crystal structure.

pseudoplasticity The behavior of non-Newtonian fluids in which the rate of shear increases more than in proportion to the shearing stress (shear-thinning liquids). Thick mixes of plaster or stone are typical examples; they appear to be very viscous when at rest but flow readily when subjected to a shear stress (eg, by stirring or vibration).

refractory A heat-resisting material (noun); capable of resisting high temperatures (adj.)

relative surface area (of a powder) The total surface area of a given mass.

specular (of reflections) Mirror-like.

spherulite A spherical aggregation of needle-shaped crystals radiating out from a common center.

water/powder (W/P) ratio The mixing proportions of plaster or stone, expressed as a decimal fraction. If 100 g of plaster is to be mixed with 50 g of water, the W/P ratio is 0.50.

water requirement The amount of water that must be added to a given mass of plaster or stone to produce a mix of suitable viscosity.

Discussion questions

1. How many different applications do gypsum products have in dentistry, as well as other fields?

2. Why are storage conditions and shelf life important considerations in the use of gypsum products? Why do these present special problems for the dental services of large organizations such as the armed forces?

3. Why is it essential to follow directions to achieve the higher strengths possible with improved die stones?

4. What are the main methods of reducing bubbles in gypsum casts and molds?

Questions and answers

1. **What differences in chemical composition are there in the powders of plaster, stone, and high-strength stone?** The major constituent is the same in all products—calcium sulfate hemihydrate. Minor differences in composition exist between stones and high-strength stones because of the presence of accelerators, retarders, and coloring matter.

2. **What physical differences are there in the powders of plaster, stone, and high-strength stone? How are these differences related to the methods of manufacture of the powders?** Plaster is produced by the dry calcination of ground gypsum (calcium sulfate dihydrate). Partial loss of water of crystallization is not accompanied by a change in shape or size of the individual particles, which are therefore irregular and porous, giving the powder a relatively low apparent density. Stone and high-strength stone are produced by wet calcination, which allows formation of dense regular crystals of hemihydrate, producing powders that have a higher apparent density than plaster. Careful grinding increases the apparent density still further.

3. **Give typical W/P ratios for plaster, stone, and high-strength stone. Why are these different? For each type, assuming that the setting reaction goes to completion, what percentage of the mass of the set material would consist of free water?** Typical W/P ratios: Plaster, 0.50; stone, 0.30; high-strength stone, 0.22. Lower W/P ratios can be used with stone and high-strength stone, because the apparent densities of their powders are higher, so less water is needed to make a workable mix. Uncombined water in set mass: for plaster, 100 g powder + 50 g water = 150 g set mass. Only 18.6 g water combines chemically. Therefore, after the setting reaction is complete, uncombined water is 31.4 g in 150 g, approximately 20%. Similarly, for stone, uncombined water is approximately 9%; for high-strength stone, approximately 4%.

4. **What chemical and physical changes accompany the setting of gypsum products?** Chemical change: Hydration of calcium sulfate hemihydrate to form the dihydrate (gypsum) $2CaSO_4 \cdot {}^1\!/_2H_2O + 3H_2O \rightarrow 2CaSO_2 \cdot 2H_2O$
Physical changes: The mix is first a viscous liquid, then a plastic mass, and then a rigid solid, friable at first but increasing in strength until the reaction has ceased.

5. **What is the difference between the microstructures of gypsum casts made from plaster and stone? What is the cause of this difference, and what is its effect on strength properties?** Set plaster has a higher proportion of inherent microporosity than set stone. The microporosity is caused by (*a*) residual unreacted water and (*b*) setting expansion. Both of these factors are greater in the case of plaster. Thus, set plaster is less dense and weaker than set stone.

6. **What is meant by the setting time of gypsum products? What is the practical significance of (*a*) the loss of surface gloss, (*b*) the Gillmore initial set, and (*c*) the Vicat initial set?** Setting is a continuous process. In practice, any figure given for setting time is arbitrary, unless it refers to the time when the setting reaction ceases. (*a*) Loss of surface gloss gives an indication of the time when the mix will not pour or flow under vibration. (*b*) and (*c*) Both the Gillmore and Vicat initial sets give an indication of the time when the solid material can be handled safely.

7. **Explain how the manufacturer of a dental gypsum product adjusts its rate of setting.** By the empirical addition of accelerators or retarders to the raw hemihydrate powder.

8. **For a given gypsum product, what is the effect of increasing the W/P ratio on the rate of setting? Explain this effect.** The setting rate is reduced, because increasing the W/P ratio increases the relative amount of aqueous phase present in the mix. Therefore, the physical changes associated with setting occur more slowly because interaction of growing gypsum crystals takes place later.

9. **Theoretically, the setting of gypsum products should be accompanied by a volumetric contraction. Why is a setting expansion observed in practice?** There is a decrease in the volume of the actual solid. However, the gypsum crystals formed are usually long and thin, and crystal growth creates microscopic voids that cause an increase in the total volume of the mass.

10. **Why do gypsum products show a greater setting expansion in water than in air?** When setting occurs in water, there is a continuous aqueous phase present and crystal growth is relatively unimpeded. When setting occurs in air, the water content of the mix decreases as the reaction proceeds. Residual liquid in the mix is drawn into voids created between growing gypsum crystals, over which it forms a film. Surface tension forces crowd the growing crystals together and restrain further expansion.

11. **What is the practical significance of the setting expansion of dental gypsum products?** It affects the dimensional accuracy of the ultimate dental restoration.

12. **Give typical values for the linear setting expansion in air of impression plaster, plaster, stone, and high-strength stone.** Impression plaster, 0.15%; plaster, 0.30%; stone, 0.15%; high-strength stone, 0.10%.

13. **Explain how the manufacturer of a gypsum product controls its setting expansion.** By the empirical addition of a blend of a suitable accelerator and retarder, both of which reduce setting expansion.

14. **What practical limits are placed on the extent of this control?** Accelerators and retarders also reduce the strength properties of the set material, so when strength is an important consideration the concentration that can be used is relatively low.

15. **For a given gypsum product, what is the effect of increasing the W/P ratio on setting expansion? Explain this effect.** Setting expansion is reduced, because the relative amount of aqueous phase is increased and interaction of growing gypsum crystals is less effective.

16. **What is the practical significance of the tensile strength and the compressive strength of dental gypsum products?** Tensile strength is an indication of resistance to fracture; compressive strength is an indication of surface hardness.

17. **For a given gypsum product, what is the effect of increasing the W/P ratio on tensile strength and compressive strength? Explain the effect.** It reduces both. With a higher W/P ratio there is more residual water remaining after setting is complete, and this causes increased microporosity which reduces strength properties.

18. **What is the effect of drying cast gypsum on its tensile strength and its compressive strength? Explain the effect.** Drying approximately doubles both tensile and compressive strengths, since the presence of free water in the cast material weakens it.

19. **What constituents are likely to be present in a gypsum-bonded investment powder? Give the function of each.** Calcium sulfate hemihydrate acts as a binder. Silica (quartz, or cristobalite, or a mixture of both) offsets the contraction of the binder that occurs on heating and often provides a positive thermal expansion. Modifiers may be present in small concentrations to adjust the rate of setting, to give a reducing atmosphere when the mold is heated, or to give an increased thermal expansion.

20. **Within normal limits, what effect does increasing the proportion of refractory filler in an investment have on *(a)* rate of setting, *(b)* setting expansion in air, *(c)* setting expansion in water, *(d)* thermal expansion, and *(e)* compressive strength?** *(a)* Rate of setting decreases; *(b)* setting expansion in air increases; *(c)* setting expansion in water increases; *(d)* thermal expansion increases; *(e)* compressive strength decreases.

21. **How does the investment set?** When the investment powder is mixed with water, the silica is unaffected. The calcium sulfate hemihydrate reacts with water to precipitate gypsum crystals, which bind the silica particles together.

22. **What is the practical significance of microscopic porosity formed in the investment mass during setting?** The porosity is continuous and provides venting of the mold cavity when the molten alloy is cast.

23. **What are the requirements for the particle size of an investment powder? Give reasons.** The powder should have a uniform fine particle size (not more than 75 µm). A uniform particle size ensures adequate venting of the mold cavity, because the silica particles show least-dense packing. A fine particle size produces a smooth casting; surface roughness of the casting can interfere with its fit.

24. **Why is the particle size of the refractory filler more important than that of the binder?** The particles of refractory filler remain unchanged during setting, and have a major effect on the smoothness of the mold surface. The particles of binder are dissolved during setting, and gypsum crystals are precipitated that are much smaller than the refractory particles.

25. **Which do you consider to be the most important property of an investment? Why?** Expansion, provided by a summation of setting and thermal expansions is most important. Mold expansion is used to offset the casting shrinkage of the alloy and thus produce an accurate casting.

26. **What is a hygroscopic expansion technique?** A casting technique in which most of the mold expansion is gained by the increased setting expansion that occurs when the setting investment is exposed to additional water. The need for thermal expansion of the mold is small.

27. **What is a thermal expansion technique?** A casting technique in which thermal expansion contributes greatly to mold expansion. In most thermal expansion techniques, setting expansion also plays an important part.

28. **In hygroscopic expansion techniques, why is prolonged heating of the mold at the burnout temperature necessary?** At the relatively low burnout temperatures used, oxidation of carbon remaining from the wax pattern is slow. Most of it must be removed to allow adequate mold venting.

29. **How can the user of a dental investment discover whether it contains cristobalite or quartz as a refractory? What is the practical importance of this information?** The refractory can be identified by studying the investment's thermal expansion curve, which should be provided by the manufacturer. Cristobalite investments show a large isothermal expansion at about 250°C. Quartz investments show a smaller isothermal expansion at about 570°C. The type of refractory filler in the investment affects the heating rate to be used and sometimes the burnout temperature.

30. **Why is control of the heating rate more important with a cristobalite investment than with a quartz investment?** Cristobalite investments undergo a large isothermal expansion at a relatively low temperature (250°C). If a large temperature gradient, resulting from rapid heating, exists within the mold at this temperature, nonuniform expansion can cause cracking. This can be prevented by following a slow heating rate below 300°C. The problem does not arise with quartz investments, which have a more gradual thermal expansion.

31. **Why is an accurate furnace pyrometer more important with a quartz investment than with a cristobalite investment?** With quartz investments, the required thermal expansion is available only over restricted temperature ranges (hygroscopic expansion techniques, 350°C to 480°C; thermal expansion techniques, 600°C to 700°C). With cristobalite investments, the thermal expansion is reasonably constant over a wide temperature range (400° to 700°C).

32. **Why should gypsum-bonded investments not be heated above 700°C?** At temperatures above 700°C the calcium sulfate binder decomposes in the presence of carbon, liberating corrosive gases that can adversely affect the casting.

33. **In thermal expansion techniques, what is the effect of a wet liner on the investment's setting expansion?** It increases it.

34. **What is the effect of increasing the W/P ratio on (a) the investment's setting expansion in air, (b) its setting expansion in water, (c) its thermal expansion.** (a) Setting expansion in air decreases; (b) setting expansion in water decreases; and (c) thermal expansion decreases.

35. **In hygroscopic expansion techniques, how can mold expansion be controlled by the user?** By varying the W/P ratio, or by varying the length of time additional water is available to the setting investment. In the latter case this may be achieved by delaying the immersion of the investment, or by adding controlled amounts of excess water to the setting investment instead of immersing it.

36. **In thermal expansion techniques, how can mold expansion be controlled by the user?** By varying the W/P ratio.

37. **What is the practical significance of the compressive strength of the investment at the casting temperature?** At the casting temperature, the investment mold may be strong enough to restrain the thermal contraction of the solidified casting as it cools. The effect will vary in different directions, depending on the amount of interlocking of casting and mold. This can cause distortion of the casting shape.

    An investment with a low hot strength is more likely to allow uniform thermal contraction of the alloy and give an undistorted casting. A safe lower limit for compressive strength at the casting temperature is 1.8 MPa.

38. **How should gypsum products be stored in a dental laboratory? How can incorrect storage conditions affect these materials?** They should be stored in airtight containers, in a cool dry region of the laboratory. When hemihydrate powders are exposed to the atmosphere, particularly when the water vapor pressure is high, the particles adsorb water from the air. This can react with the hemihydrate to form gypsum crystals. Initially this increases the setting rate of the material, but if deterioration proceeds further, the setting rate is retarded, and eventually the strength properties of the set material are adversely affected.

Suggested reading

Andrews H. The production, properties and uses of calcium sulphate plasters. London: Building Research Congress, Division 2, Part F, 135, 1951.

Asgar K. Casting alloys in dentistry. In Dickson G, Cassel JM, (eds.) Dental Materials Research. Washington, D.C.: National Bureau of Standards, SP 354, 63, 1972.

Asgar K, Mahler DB, Peyton FA. Hygroscopic technique for inlay casting using controlled water additions. J Prosthet Dent 5:711, 1955.

Barnard G. Recent developments in using ceramic fibres in reducing atmospheres. Metals Australasia 13:10, 1981.

Beretka J, Crook DN, King GA, Middleton LW. Applications of by-product gypsum in the plaster industry. Melbourne: Eighth Australian Chemical Engineering Conference, August 1980.

Bergman B, Bergman M, Olsson S. Alginate impression materials, dimensional stability and surface detail sharpness following treatment with disinfectant solutions. Swed Dent J 9:255, 1985.

Bever, MB, ed. Encyclopedia of Materials Science and Engineering. Elmsford, NY: Pergamon Press, 1986; 1098.

Buchanan AS, Worner HK. Changes in the composition and setting characteristics of plaster of Paris on exposure to high humidity atmosphere. J Dent Res 24:65, 1945.

Combe EC. Recent developments in model and die materials. In von Fraunhofer JA, ed. Scientific Aspects of Dental Materials. London: Butterworths, 1974:402–415.

Collins PF. Dental Investment Composition and Process. U.S. Patent: 2,006,733, 1935.

Collins PF. Dental Investment Composition and Process. U.S. Patent: 2,247,571, 1941a.

Collins PF. Dental Investment Composition and Process. U.S. Patent: 2,247,572, 1941b.

Collins PF. Dental Investment Composition and Process. U.S. Patent: 2,247,573, 1941c.

Combe EC, Smith DC. Studies on the preparation of calcium sulphate hemihydrate by an autoclave process. J Appl Chem 18:307, 1968.

Combe EC, Smith DC. The effects of some organic acids and salts on the setting of gypsum plaster. II. Tartrates. J Appl Chem 15:367, 1965.

Combe EC, Smith DC. The effects of some organic acids and slats on the setting of gypsum plaster. III. Citrates. J Appl Chem 16:73, 1966.

Craig, RG, ed. Restorative Dental Materials. 9th ed. St Louis: CV Mosby; 1993; 349.

Donovan T, Chee WWL. Preliminary investigation of a disinfected gypsum die stone. Int J Prosthodont 2:245, 1989.

Dootz, ER, Craig RG, Peyton FA. Influence of investments and duplicating procedures on the accuracy of partial denture castings. J Prosthet Dent 15:679, 1965.

Earnshaw R. Further measurements of the casting shrinkage of dental cobalt-chromium alloys. Br Dent J 109:238, 1960.

Earnshaw R. The effect of restrictive stress on the setting expansion of gypsum-bonded investments. Aust Dent J 9:169, 1964.

Earnshaw R. The effect of restrictive stress on the hygroscopic setting expansion of gypsum-bonded investments. Aust Dent J 14:22, 1969.

Earnshaw R. The compressive strength of gypsum-bonded investments at high temperatures. Aust Dent J 14:264, 1969.

Earnshaw R. Effects of additives on the thermal expansion of cast gypsum. J Dent Res 55:518, 1976.

Earnshaw R. The effect of casting ring liners on the potential expansion of a gypsum-bonded investment. J Dent Res 67:1366, 1988.

Earnshaw R, Marks BI. The measurement of setting time of gypsum products. Aust Dent J 9:17, 1964.

Earnshaw R, Morey EF. The fit of gold-alloy full-crown castings made with ceramic casting ring liners. J Dent Res 71:1865, 1992.

Earnshaw R, Mori T. Contraction of cast gypsum between 200°C and 500°C. J Dent Res 64:658, 1985.

Eberl JJ, Ingram AR. Process for making high-strength plaster of Paris. Ind Eng Chem 41:106, 1949.

Fairhurst CW. Compressive properties of dental gypsum. J Dent Res 39:812, 1960.

Farmer GJ, Skinner EW. Effect of relative humidity on the setting time of plaster of Paris. Northwestern Univ Bull 43:12, 1942.

Finger W, Jørgensen, KD. An improved dental casting investment. Scand J Dent Res 88:278, 1980.

Finger W, Jørgensen KD, Ono T. Strength properties of some gypsum-bonded investments. Scand J Dent Res 88:155, 1980.

Fusayama T. Factors and technique of precision casting. J Prosthet Dent 9:468, 486, 1959.

Fusayama T. Synthetic study on precision casting. Bull Tokyo Med Dent Univ 11:165, 1964.

Gay P. Some crystallographic studies in the system $CaSO_4$ — $CaSO_4{\cdot}2H_2O$. I. The polymorphism of anhydrous $CaSO_4$. Mineral Mag 35:347, 1965.

Gay P. Some crystallographic studies in the system $CaSO_4$ — $CaSO_4{\cdot}2H_2O$. II. The hydrous forms. Mineral Mag 35:354, 1965.

Gibson CS, Johnson RN. Investigations of the setting of plaster of Paris. J Soc Chem Ind (Transactions) 51:25, 1932.

Greener EH, Harcourt JK, Lautenschlager EP. Materials Science in Dentistry. Baltimore: Williams & Wilkins, 1972;276.

Gregg SJ. The Surface Chemistry of Solids. 2nd ed. London: Chapman and Hall; 1965; 232.

Gutt WH, Smith MA. The α form of calcium sulphate. Trans Br Ceram Soc 66:337, 1967.

Haddon CL. Gypsum plaster products. Chem Ind 22:190, 1944.

Haddon CL, Cafferata BJ. Improvements in the manufacture of plaster of Paris. British Patent 563, 019, 1944.

Harcourt JK, Lautenschlager EP. Accelerated and retarded dental plaster setting investigated by X-ray diffraction. J Dent Res 49:502, 1970.

Hoggatt GA. Method of producing gypsum plaster. U.S. Patent: 2,616,789, 1952.

Hollenback GM. A brief history of the cast restoration. J South Calif State Dent Assoc 30:8, 1962.

Hollenback GM, Skinner EW. Shrinkage during casting of gold and gold alloys. J Am Dent Assoc 33:1391, 1946.

International Standards Organization. International Standard 6873, Dental Gypsum Products. Geneva, 1983; 1.

International Standards Organization. International Standard 7490, Dental Gypsum-bonded Casting Investments for Gold Alloys. Geneva, 1990;1.

Ivanovski S, Savage NW, Brockhurst PJ, Bird P. Disinfection of dental stone casts: antimicrobial effects and physical property alterations. Dent Mater 11:19, 1995.

Jastrzebski ZD. The Nature and Properties of Engineering Materials. 2nd ed. New York: John Wiley & Sons; 1976; 59.

Johnson GH, Drennon DG, Powell GL. Accuracy of elastomeric impressions disinfected by immersion. J Am Dent Assoc 116:525, 1988.

Jørgensen KD, Posner AS. Study of the setting of plaster. J Dent Res 38:491, 1959.

Khalil AA, Hussein AT, Gad GM. On the thermochemistry of gypsum. J Appl Chem Biotechnol 21:314, 1971.

Kingery WD, Bower HK, Uhlmann DR. Introduction to Ceramics. New York: John Wiley & Sons; 81–87, 1976.

Koslowski T, Ludwig U. Retardation of gypsum plasters with citric acid: mechanism and properties. In Kuntze RA, ed. The Chemistry and Technology of Gypsum ASTM STP861. Philadelphia: American Society for Testing and Materials; 1984; 97–104.

Lager GA, Armbruster T, Rotella FJ, Jorgensen JD, Hinks DG. A crystallographic study of the low-temperature dehydration products of gypsum. Am Mineral 69:910, 1984.

Lautenschlager EP, Corbin F. Investigation on the expansion of dental stone. J Dent Res 48:206, 1969.

Lautenschlager EP, Harcourt JK, Ploszaj LC. Setting reactions of gypsum materials investigated by X-ray diffraction. J Dent Res 48:43, 1969.

Mahler DB, Ady AB. An explanation for the hygroscopic setting expansion of dental gypsum products. J Dent Res 39:578, 1960.

Matsuya S, Yamane M. Decomposition of gypsum-bonded investments. J Dent Res 60:1418, 1981.

McGill S, Narea EM, Suchak AJ, Stanford JW. The effect of disinfecting solutions on alginate and gypsum materials. J Dent Res 67:281, 1988.

Moore TE. Method of making dental castings and composition employed in said method. U.S. Patent: 1,924,874, 1933.

Morey EF, Earnshaw R. The fit of gold-alloy full-crown castings made with pre-wetted casting ring liners. J Dent Res 71:1858, 1992.

Morey EF, Earnshaw R. The effect of potential investment expansion and hot strength on the fit of full-crown castings made with a gypsum-bonded investment. Dent Mater 11:312, 1995.

Mori T. The effect of boric acid on the thermal behavior of cast gypsum. Dent Mater J 1:73, 1982.

Mori T. Transformation of $CaSO_4$(III) to $CaSO_4$(II) in gypsum-bonded investments. J Dent Res 64:658, 1985.

Mori T. Thermal behavior of the gypsum binder in dental casting investments. J Dent Res 65:877, 1986.

Mori T, Yamane M. Fractography of cast gypsum. Aust Dent J 27:30, 1982.

Nakai A, Nakamura K, Seki S-I, Kakuta K, Kawashima J-I. Measurement of casting shrinkage with U-type tungsten die. J Jap Dent Apparat Mat 21:122, 1980.

Neiman R. Investment. U.S. Patent 2,247,395, 1941. U.S. Patent: 2,313,085, 1943a.

Neiman R, Ernst RC, Steinbock EA. Investment composition. U.S. Patent: 2,313,086, 1943b.

O'Brien WJ, Nielsen JP. Decomposition of gypsum investment in the presence of carbon. J Dent Res 38:541, 1959.

Offutt JS, Lambe CM. Plasters and gypsum cements for the ceramic industry. Am Ceram Soc Bull 26:29, 1947.

Ohno H, Nakano S, Miyakawa O, Watanabe K, Shiokawa N. Effects of phase transformations of silicas and calcium sulfates on the compressive strength of gypsum-bonded investments at high temperatures. J Dent Res 61:1077, 1982.

Olsson S, Bergman B, Bergman M. Agar impression materials, dimensional stability and surface detail sharpness following treatment with disinfectant solutions. Swed Dent J 11:169, 1987.

Phillips RW. Skinner's Science of Dental Materials. 9th ed. Philadelphia: WB Saunders; 1991; 80–82.

Phillips RW. Skinner's Science of Dental Materials. 9th ed. Philadelphia: WB Saunders; 1991; 393–406.

Pomés CD, Slack GL, Wise MW. Surface roughness of dental castings. J Am Dent Assoc 41:545, 1950.

Priest G, Horner, JA Fibrous ceramic aluminium silicate as an alternative to asbestos liners. J Prosthet Dent 44:51, 1980.

Randel WS, Dailey MC. High strength calcined gypsum and process of manufacture of same. U.S. Patent: 1,901,051, 1933.

Ridge MJ. Acceleration of the set of gypsum plaster. Aust J Appl Sci 10:218, 1959.

Ridge MJ. Mechanism of setting of gypsum plaster. Rev Pure Appl Chem 10:243, 1960.

Ridge MJ. Factors determining the water requirement of gypsum plaster. J Appl Chem 11:287, 1961.

Ridge MJ. The hydration of calcium sulphate hemilhydrate. Proc Royal Austral Chem Inst 39:55, 1972.

Ridge MJ, Beretka J. Calcium sulphate hemihydrate and its hydration. Rev Pure Appl Chem 19:17, 1969.

Russell JJ. The effect of moisture content on the compressive strength of small cubes of some cast gypsum plasters. Zement-Kalk-Gips 13:345, 1960.

Schutt RW. Bactericidal effect of a disinfectant dental stone on irreversible hydrocolloid impressions and stone casts. J Prosthet Dent 62:605, 1989.

Selby A. The Relationship Between the Viscosity of the Mix and the Tensile Strength of Cast Gypsum. Sydney: University of Sydney, 1979. Thesis.

Sodeau WH, Gibson CS. The use of plaster of Paris as an impression material. Br Dent J 48:70, 1927.

Sosman RB. The Phases of Silica. New Brunswick: Rutgers University Press; 1965; 32, 36–42.

Souder W, Paffenbarger GC. Physical Properties of Dental Materials. Washington, D.C.: National Bureau of Standards, C433, 1942; 80–92.

Suffert LW, Mahler DB. Reproducibility of gold castings made by present day dental casting technics. J Am Dent Assoc 50:1, 1955.

Sweeney WT, Taylor DB. Dimensional changes in dental stone and plaster. J Dent Res 29:749, 1950.

Taylor NO, Paffenbarger GC, Sweeney WT. Dental inlay casting investments; physical properties and a specification. J Am Dent Assoc 17:2266, 1930.

Teteruck WR, Mumford G. The fit of certain dental casting alloys using different investing materials and techniques. J Prosthet Dent 16:910, 1966.

Torrance A, Darvell BW. Effect of humidity on calcium sulphate hemihydrate. Aust Dent J 35:230, 1990.

Weinstein LJ. Composition for dental moulds. U.S. Patent: 1,708,436, 1929.

Weiser HB, Milligan WD, Eckholm WC. The mechanism of dehydration of calcium sulfate hemihydrate. J Am Chem Soc 58:1261, 1936.

Whyte MP, Brockhurst PJ. The effect of steam sterilisation on the properties of set dental gypsum models. Aust Dent J 39:262, 1994.

Worner HK. Dental plasters. Part I. Aust J Dent 41:128, 1996.

Yli-Urpo A, Øilo G, Syverud M. The effect of asbest-alternatives on the accuracy of cast veneer crowns. Swed Dent J 6:127, 1982.

Chapter 6

Polymers and Polymerization: Denture Base Polymers

Polymers have a major role in most areas of dentistry. Their distinctive properties allow a range of clinical applications not possible with other types of materials. The most widely used impression materials (alginates, polyethers, polysulfides, and silicones) are polymers. A polymeric matrix with a particulate ceramic filler is the most commonly used anterior esthetic restorative material. Additional applications include artificial teeth, cements, dies, temporary crowns, endodontic fillings, tissue conditioners, and pit and fissure sealants. However, the primary use of polymers in terms of quantity is in the construction of complete dentures and the tissue-bearing portions of partial dentures. This chapter introduces concepts related to polymer composition and properties and concludes with a discussion of those polymers currently used in the construction of complete and partial dentures, liners, and tissue conditioners.

Polymers and polymerization

Composition

A polymer is a molecule that is made up of many units (*poly* = many; *mer* = unit). The oligomer is a short polymer composed of two, three, or four mer units. A mer is the simplest repeating chemical unit of which the polymer is composed, and is often the basis for naming the material. Thus, polystyrene is a polymer composed of styrene units.

Monomers (*mono* = single) are the molecules that unite to form a polymer, and the process by which this occurs is termed *polymerization*. If monomers of two or more different types are joined, copolymers are formed. Copolymers may be either random (mers do not appear in specific order), or block (large numbers of one type of mer appear arranged in sequence). Atoms along the length of any polymer are joined through strong, primary covalent bonds.

Molecular weight

The *degree of polymerization* is defined as the total number of mers in a polymer molecule. The *molecular weight* of a polymer molecule is the sum of the molecular weights of the mers of which it is made. Typical polymer molecules may be composed of thousands to millions of mers. Often, a distribution of molecular sizes is present in a material, and the reported molecular weight is the average molecular weight. The particular distribution is the result of conditions present during polymerization. Variations in conditions have a pronounced effect on the properties of the final material.

Spatial structure

There are three basic spatial structures of polymers: linear, branched, and cross-linked, shown in Fig 6-1. Linear and branched molecules are discrete but are

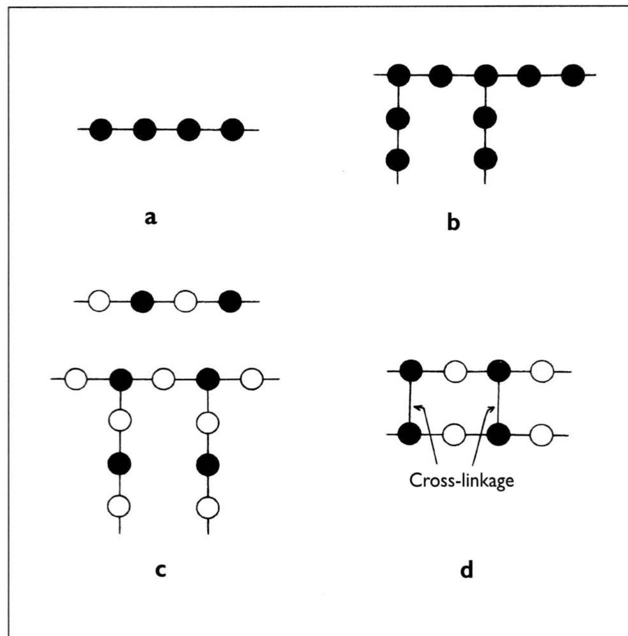

Fig 6-1 Polymer chains. (a) A linear chain; (b) a branched chain; (c) copolymer chains, linear *(upper)* and branched *(lower)*; (d) cross-linking chains.

bonded to one another through weak, physical bonds. Upon heating, the weak bonds break and the ability of the chains to then slide past one another results in a softened material. Upon cooling, the bonds reform and hardening occurs. Materials that are able to undergo this process are termed *thermoplastic*. Examples include polystyrene, polyvinyl acrylics, and poly(methyl methacrylate) (PMMA).

Cross-linking results in the formation of a network structure of covalently bonded atoms; primary linkages occur between chains, and the polymer actually becomes a single giant macromolecule. The spatial structure that allows chain sliding upon heating is not present in cross-linked materials. Cross-linked polymers therefore do not undergo softening upon heating and are termed *thermosets*. Typical examples are silicones, *cis*-polyisoprene, bisphenol A-diacrylate, and cross-linked poly(methyl methacrylate).

Polymerization

Most polymerization reactions are of two types: *addition polymerization*, in which no by-product is formed, and *condensation polymerization*, in which a low molecular weight by-product such as water or alcohol is formed. Materials that set by addition polymerization include poly(methyl methacrylate), used in the construction of dentures, and Bis-GMA, a common component of the matrix of composite resins. Materials that set by the condensation mechanism include polysulfide rubber and some silicone rubber impression materials.

The three stages in the free-radical addition polymerization reaction are described in the following subsections. They may be accelerated by heat, light, or small amounts of peroxides.

Initiation

The initiation step involves the production of free radicals which will encourage a polymer chain to begin growing (Fig 6-2). Free-radical molecules have chemical groups with unshared electrons. In chemically activated systems, free radicals are generally produced by the reaction of an organic peroxide initiator and an amine accelerator. In light-activated systems, the scission of camphoroquinone results in the production of two molecules with one unshared electron each. Whatever the means of production, the free radicals attack the double bonds of available monomer molecules, resulting in the shift of the unshared electron to the end of the monomer and the formation of activated monomer molecules.

Propagation

Activated monomers attack the double bonds of additional available monomers, resulting in the rapid addition of monomer molecules to the free radical. This second stage, propagation, continues as the chain grows in length.

Termination

Termination of the growing free radical may occur by several mechanisms and can result in the formation of branches and cross-links.

Small amounts of inhibitors, such as hydroquinone, may be added to the monomer to increase storage life. Hydroquinones react with free radicals, thereby decreasing the rate of initiation.

Properties

Many factors affect the properties of polymers, including the chemical composition of the chain, its degree of polymerization, and the number of branches and/or

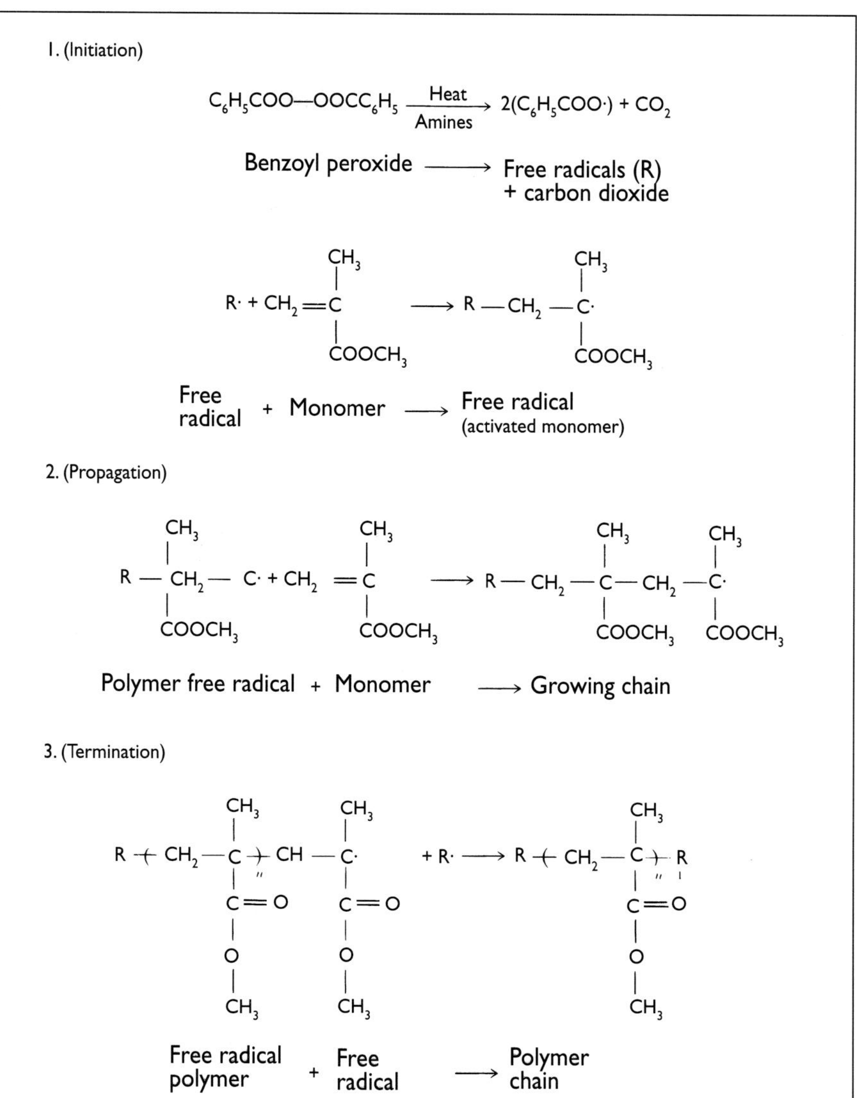

Fig 6-2 Three stages of addition polymerization of methyl methacrylate.

cross-links between polymer chains (Fig 6-3). In general, longer chains and a higher molecular weight result in the polymer's increased strength, hardness, stiffness, and resistance to creep along with increased brittleness. Composite resins, for example, have a highly cross-linked matrix, in which a large number of strong covalent linkages between chains transforms the molecules into a rigid, very high-molecular-weight material. The resulting increased strength and stiffness contribute to the ability of this material to withstand occlusal stresses during function.

In contrast, elastomeric impression materials are composed primarily of individual coiled chains with just a few cross-links. This type of molecular structure

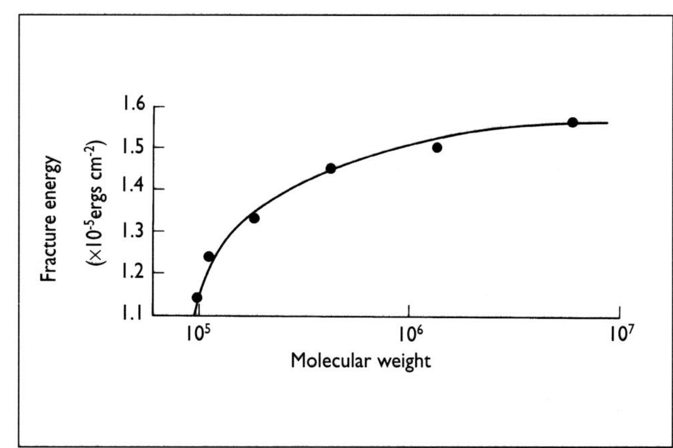

Fig 6-3 Relation between strength and polymer molecular weight. (From Mark, 1962. Reprinted with permission.)

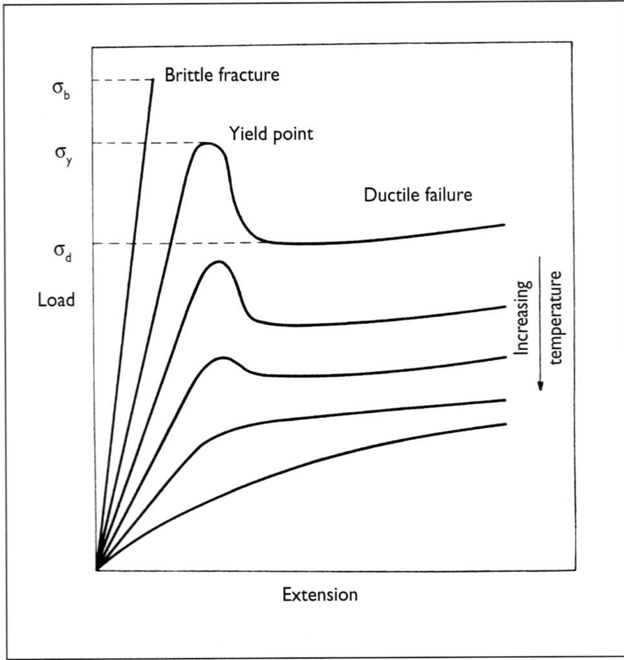

Fig 6-4 Effect of temperature on the tensile properties of a polymer. The temperature below which brittle failure occurs is called the glass-transition temperature. (From Berry and Bueche, 1962. Reprinted with permission.)

permits the large-scale uncoiling and recoiling of chains that gives these materials high flexibility.

The amount of *crystallinity* present in a polymer affects properties. Materials that are highly crystalline have atoms with a very regular arrangement in space and are stronger, stiffer, and absorb less water than do noncrystalline materials. Few dental polymers are crystalline. Most are *amorphous*, meaning that the atoms of which they are composed have irregular arrangements in space. Amorphous polymers are often called "glassy" polymers.

Small *plasticizer* molecules, when added to a stiff uncross-linked polymer, reduce its rigidity. When small molecules surround large ones, the large molecules are able to move more easily. A plasticizer therefore lowers the *glass-transition temperature* (T_g) of the polymer, so a material that is normally rigid at a particular temperature may become more flexible. The glass-transition temperature is the temperature at which a polymer ceases to be glassy and brittle and becomes rubber-like. The temperature of a polymer, as shown in Fig 6-4, has a strong effect on its strength properties.

Finally, during polymerization a volumetric decrease occurs resulting in shrinkage (up to 21% for unfilled acrylic resins, 6% for denture resins, 1% to 3% for composite resins) and the production of internal stresses. A change in shape, often called *warpage*, may occur when the polymer is reheated. Additionally, polymers have varying abilities to absorb water. A small amount of expansion may occur during this process.

Denture base polymers

This section concerns itself with selection and use of polymers used as denture bases, liners, and tissue conditioners, as well as problems associated with them. A classification is shown in Fig 6-5. The polymeric denture base can consist of either a simple stiff base on which the teeth are arranged, or a sandwich of stiff base and a resilient liner to provide greater retention and comfort. When the tissue underlying a loose denture is traumatized due to the constant motion of the hard plastic over the mucosa, a viscoelastic gel known as a *tissue conditioner* can be molded onto the fitting surface of the denture in situ so the tissue can heal and an accurate impression of the untraumatized fitting surface can be taken prior to making a new, better-fitting denture.

Advances in denture design have been mediated by the materials available at the time. In the 1800s the art of hand carving ivory and wooden denture bases resulted in dentures retained by mechanical devices such as springs. Goodyear's invention of vulcanized rubber, vulcanite, in 1839 provided not only a thermoplastic material that could be molded accurately, but also one that did not biodegrade and was strong enough to withstand masticatory forces for many years. Vulcanite's intrinsic dark color and opacity meant that the translucency and reflectivity of living mucosa was impossible to mimic.

With the commercial availability of man-made polymers in the early 1930s came an opportunity to apply some of the optically brilliant polymers to dentistry. It was the need for custom fit that delayed their use, however, since polymerization of the free monomer, with its inherent massive volume shrinkage, did not lend itself easily to the vulcanizing techniques used at the time. It was the adoption of the dough technique first described in the mid-thirties that made the use of acrylics in dentistry possible. In the dough

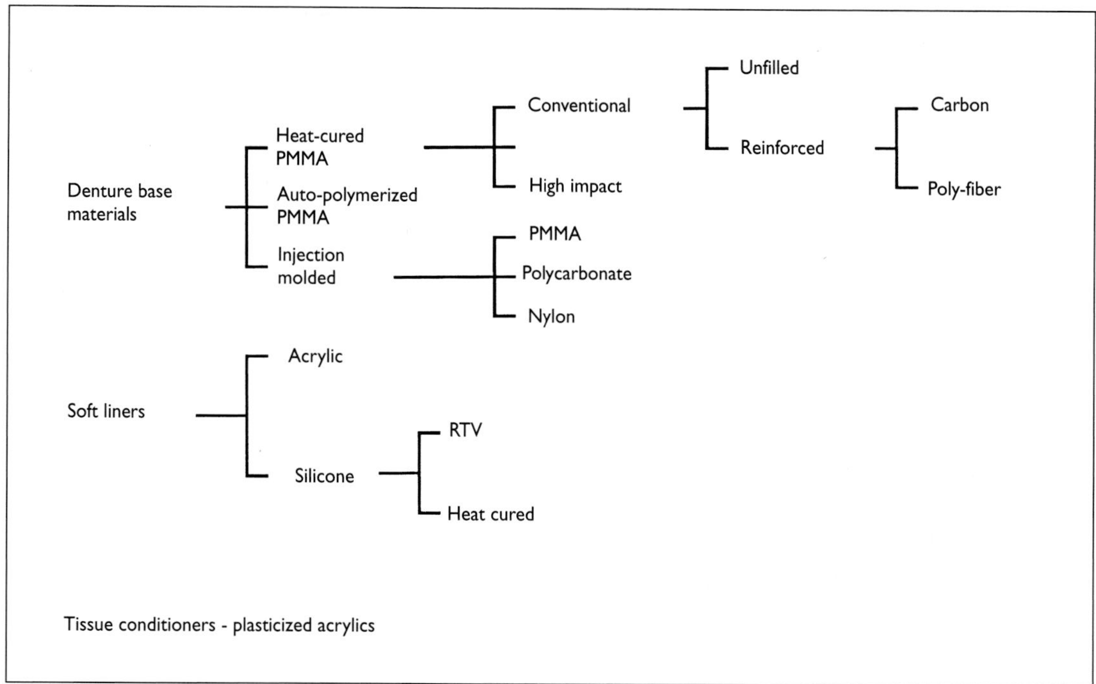

Fig 6-5 A classification of denture bases, liners, and tissue conditioners.

technique, a liquid component (monomer) is mixed with a powder component (polymer). The monomer wets the polymer to a dough-like consistency, which is packed into the mold prior to polymerization. Adoption of the new denture bases was rapid in America. However, in Europe, change was forced upon the profession by rubber shortages during World War II. By the end of the war the use of vulcanite for dentures had almost ceased. After the war, resins developed for aircraft production and the burgeoning plastics industry were offered for use as denture base materials, but the simplicity of the dough technique and the lifelike results have sustained acrylics as the market leader to the present day. Table 6-1 gives a comparison of current denture base materials.

Composition and manufacture

Heat-cured acrylic

The bulk of denture base acrylic is supplied these days in the form of a free-running powder and a liquid. Originally the powder was produced by grinding blocks of poly(methyl methacrylate). However, it was soon found that smoother, more consistent doughs resulted from the use of a spherical bead polymer. By suspending monomer liquid in water with the aid of either a surfactant or water-soluble polymer, the rate of polymerization can be well controlled by the cooling action of the surrounding water. The additives required to make the beads dough easily are fortunately very soluble in monomer globules and relatively insoluble in water. The globules can be thermally polymerized without a catalyst; however, benzoyl peroxide is usually added, partly to act as a catalyst in the polymerization of the beads, and partly so the beads become the source of the peroxy free radical during the polymerization of the dough in the dental flask (Fig 6-6).

To assist dough formation a plasticizer is also incorporated into the bead polymer. For many years this was an external plasticizer, that is, one that resided between the polymer chains rather than being chemically attached to them. Any inert, nontoxic organic molecule will suffice; dibutylphthalate was used for many years. Today, internal plasticizers are used instead, consisting either of methacrylate monomers with larger side groups than methyl methacrylate or acrylates. They locally soften the bead and allow the monomer to diffuse more rapidly into the bead during the dough stage. Pigment can be added to the bead either during polymerization or after, by ball milling. By this method, the manufacturer produces a PMMA

Table 6-1 A comparison of denture base materials

Material	Advantages	Disadvantages	Ideal properties
Heat cured	Good appearance High glass-transition temperature Ease of fabrication Low capital costs Good surface finish	Free-monomer content or formaldehyde can cause sensitization Low impact strength Flexural strength low enough to penalize poor denture design Fatigue life too short Radiolucency	Good appearance High flexural strength High impact resistance High stiffness Long fatigue life High craze resistance High creep resistance High radiopacity
Heat cured, rubber reinforced	Improved impact strength	Reduced stiffness	Low free-monomer content Good adhesion with teeth and liners
Heat cured, fiber reinforced	High stiffness Very high impact strength Good fatigue life Polypropylene fibers: Good translucency Good surface finish	Carbon and Kevlar fibers: Poor color Poor surface	Low solubility Low water uptake Dimensional stability Dimensional accuracy
Auto cured	Easy to deflask Dimensional accuracy Capable of higher flexural strength than heat cured	No cheaper over long term Increased creep Increased free-monomer content Color instability Reduced stiffness Tooth adhesion failure	
Injection molded	Dimensional accuracy Low free-monomer content Polycarbonate and nylon Good impact strength	High capital costs Difficult mold design problems Less craze resistance Less creep resistance	
Light activated	No methacrylate monomer Decreased polymerization shrinkage Possible improved fit compared to conventional material Requires little equipment Time savings	Decreased elastic modulus	

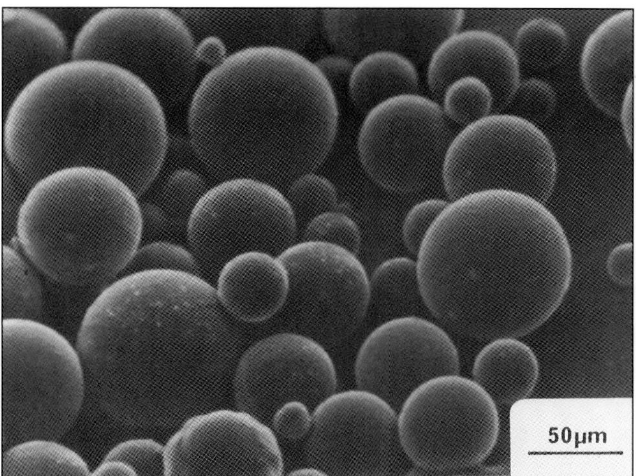

Fig 6-6 Scanning electron micrograph of poly(methyl methacrylate) beads.

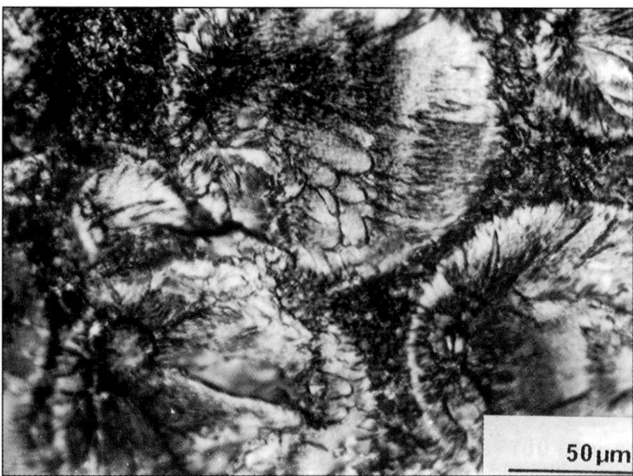

Fig 6-7 The fracture surface of heat-cured denture base acrylic resin showing that the bead structure remains and that cracks pass through, rather than around, beads during fracture.

bead mixture having a fairly wide molecular weight distribution with an average molecular weight on the order of 1 million. The all-important doughing characteristics of the bead are governed by particle size distribution, molecular weight distribution, and plasticizer content. The highest molecular weight distributions and lowest plasticizer content are favored, because they result in better physical and mechanical properties in the cured denture base.

The monomer used to form the dough is largely the same as that used to make the methyl methacrylate beads. Methyl methacrylate quickly diffuses into the polymer beads on contact, causing them to swell, and extracting some low-molecular-weight polymer into the monomer trapped in the interstices between the beads. As the beads swell, entanglements occur between the juxtaposed beads, and the bead/monomer mixture becomes a cohesive gel. The beads never dissolve completely (Fig 6-7), although the monomer infiltrates well into the core of each bead. In the swollen state, benzoyl peroxide can diffuse from the bead into the interstices, where later it will initiate the curing of the dough. In addition, cross-linking agent molecules, capable of diffusing into the beads, are present in the monomer phase.

The cross-linking agent confers two useful properties on the cured gel. It reduces the denture base's solubility to organic solvents, and it reduces the tendency of the denture base to craze (form pre-cracks) under stress. However, cross-linking agents also are very important from a practical point of view because they help to keep the denture-making apparatus simple. For a monomer to be converted to a solid polymer, the polymer chain produced must achieve a certain minimal length. Polymers having molecular weights below 5,000 are liquid and viscous; resilient polymers need to achieve a minimum molecular weight of about 150,000. Without a cross-linking agent the flask would have to be airtight and the monomer flushed with nitrogen to achieve the molecular weight required without being inhibited by air. Free-monomer levels would then be unacceptably high, and the denture would have a lower stiffness level and a greater tendency to creep. The cross-linking agent accelerates the increase in the curing system's molecular weight and combats the effects of oxgen inhibition. However, excessive levels of cross-linking agent in the monomer result in denture bases that are brittle. The most common cross-linking agents are dimethacrylates, either ethylene glycol dimethacrylate or 1,4 butylene glycol dimethacrylate.

High-impact acrylic

High-impact acrylic denture base is also made by the heat-cured dough method; impact resistance arises from the incorporation of a rubber phase into the beads during their suspension polymerization. Certain rubbers will dissolve in methyl methacrylate monomer, notably copolymers of butadiene with styrene and/or methyl methacrylate. The rubber remains soluble in the monomer globule until the polymer content of the globule becomes too high and the rubber begins to

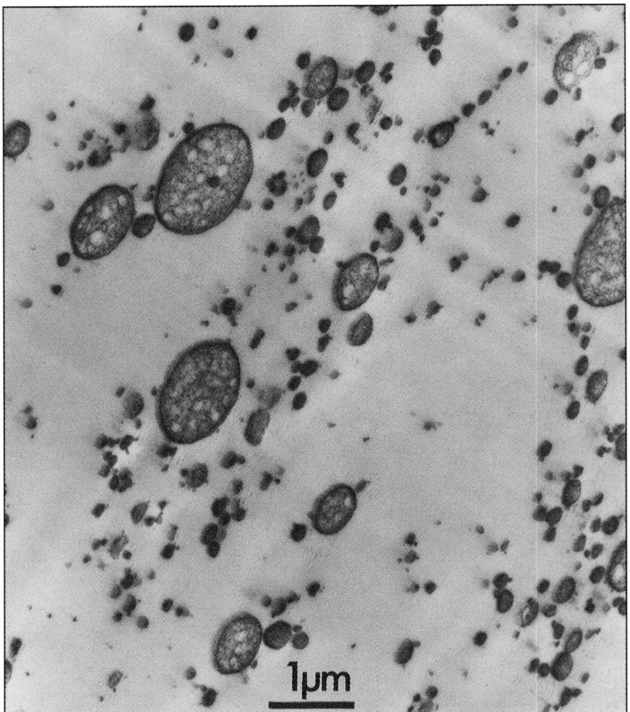

Fig 6-8 Electron micrograph of high-impact denture base showing the size and shape of the polystyrene-butadiene rubber inversion phase.

precipitate out. The nature of this precipitation is complicated by the fact that some of the growing chains of PMMA may have become grafted to the butadiene rubber. This results in what is known as a *phase inversion*, resulting in dispersion throughout the bead of tiny islands of rubber containing small inclusions of rubber/PMMA graft copolymer (Fig 6-8). Why these inclusions improve the impact strength of the cured denture base will be discussed later. There are, however, many patents that describe the formation of the beads, and dentistry uses examples that are either beads with uniformly distributed rubber inclusions, or beads that have a core of rubber-included polymer covered by an outer shell of conventional polymer to give a more conventional dough formation. Beads that have no shell often gel very quickly and may entrap air as a result. The monomer used to get high-impact beads differs from conventional monomers in that it contains either very little or no cross-linking agent. Fortunately, the inclusion of rubber does have a craze-inhibiting effect, as will be explained later.

Autopolymerizing denture base

The autopolymerizing, or pour-type, denture base is chemically similar to the heat-cured denture base except that a reducing agent is added to the monomer. The reducing agent is usually a tertiary aromatic amine, although barbituric acid derivatives also have been used. The reducing agent reacts with the benzoyl peroxide at room temperature to produce peroxy-free radicals, which initiate the polymerization of the monomer in the denture base. There is wide variation among manufacturers in the molecular weights of the polymers in the beads. Some have average molecular weights as low as 190,000. Cross-linker concentrations vary greatly in the monomer liquid, from 0% to 9%; interestingly, excess cross-linker is associated with high creep. The size, molecular weight, and plasticizer content are balanced to give a high penetration of monomer into the bead without too early an increase in viscosity of the mix to allow pouring of the acrylic into the mold and good wetting of the plastic teeth. This compromise is difficult to achieve and often results in high residual free-monomer contents and low cross-link densities. Manufacturers' attempts to achieve the best compromise result in the wide ranges of molecular weights and cross-linker concentrations found in materials, which inevitably result in large differences in physical and mechanical properties between the various products, especially where creep is concerned.

Injection-molded plastic

Injection-molded plastics have the advantage of consistent molecular weight, but the disadvantage of capital equipment costs, low craze resistance, and difficulties associated with attachment of teeth to the denture base. The plastics still offered for use as injection-molded denture base acrylic are polycarbonate and nylon. They represent a very small fraction of the market, although they offer a real alternative to metal dentures for patients sensitized to conventional methacrylate or to nickel or cobalt.

Acrylic. Acrylic is supplied as granules of low-molecular-weight (MW = 150,000) linear PMMA, with narrow molecular weight range and only a small amount of residual free-monomer. Note there is no cross-linking, as this would increase the melt viscosity during molding. Plasticization is low and often results in stiffnesses slightly in excess of conventional heat-cured denture base, despite the low molecular weight.

Polycarbonate. This tough plastic is supplied as granules but is not suited to injection into damp molds. It has a high melt viscosity and may depolymerize explosively if overheated in the presence of water. Again, absence of cross-linking results in poor solvent resistance and craze resistance. The high melt viscosity exacerbates problems of tooth attachment.

Nylon or polyamides. This is a family of condensation polymers that result from the reaction of a diacid with a diamine to give a variety of polyamides whose physical and mechanical properties depend on the linking groups between the acid or amine groups. The first dental use of nylon was not a success because of the excessive water absorption of the type chosen, which resulted in excessive creep and some biodegradation. More recent work on glass-reinforced nylons with much lower water absorptions (eg, nylon 66) has produced more encouraging results. These nylons are either filled with specially coated glass beads or chopped glass fibers. The glass fibers increase the stiffness of the nylon to about that of a conventional heat-cured denture base from a stiffness of half that when only glass-bead reinforcement is used. Glass-fiber reinforcement should be used with care, and patients should be warned not to abrade the fitting surface so as to avoid exposing irritation-causing fibers.

Light-activated materials

In recent years, a light-activated system has come on the market and is now used for many prosthetic applications. This material consists of a urethane dimethacrylate matrix with an acrylic copolymer and has a microfine silica filler. It is supplied in premixed sheet or rope form. A baseplate is made by adapting the material to a cast and polymerizing in a light chamber at 400 to 500 nm. Teeth are added to the base with additional material followed by a second light exposure. The system eliminates the need for flasks, wax, boil-out tanks, packing presses, and heat-processing units required for the construction of conventional dentures. The manufacturer claims a significant time savings in both the dental office and the laboratory.

Fabrication and its effect on physical and mechanical properties

When fabricating a denture base from polymers—by whatever means—certain physical and mechanical properties of the final polymer are important. The cured polymer should be stiff enough to hold the teeth in occlusion during mastication and to minimize uneven loading of the mucosa underlying the denture. The polymer should not creep under masticatory loads if good occlusion is to be maintained. The polymer must have sufficient strength and resilience to withstand not only normal masticatory forces, but sudden high stress caused by impact forces. The material should not deteriorate in the aqueous environment of the mouth, and crazes should not form due to attack by solvents present in food, drinks, or medicaments. The cured polymer should be biologically inert and slow to foul when in contact with oral flora.

During fabrication of a denture the physical and mechanical properties mentioned here can be influenced by cure conditions and choice of materials. Each cure cycle or fabrication technique is a compromise that attempts to optimize the properties thought important for a given application. For an allergic patient, low free-monomer content may be thought more important than stiffness. For a patient requiring a soft lining, stiffness is very important if the reduced cross-sectional area of the denture is not to cause stability or loading problems.

Heat-cured denture base

In the discussion of heat-cured denture base acrylic in the previous section, the mechanism of doughing was described. When manipulating the dough prior to packing, the operator is aware of various stages of gelation: the initial melting of the beads with the monomer, the sandy stage, the formation of first entanglements as the outer layers of the bead swell, and, when the dough is pulled, the formation of stringy threads that can be drawn out as low-molecular-weight components dissolve into and thicken the interstitial monomer. In the last stage, the dough becomes elastic as monomer penetration reaches the core of the beads, plasticizing them and lowering their glass-transition temperature from an initial 125°C to well below room temperature; the beads have become rubber. Curing the dough before the monomer has diffused to the core of the beads may result in reduced flexural strength and a tendency for cracks to propagate along lines of weakness between the cross-linked interstitial phase and the linear, more pliable beads. Allowing the monomer and cross-linker to diffuse to the center of the beads results in a more homogeneous distribution of stress, and the formation of a tough, three-dimensional network within the existing amorphous bead polymer to form what is known as an *interpenetrating polymer network* (IPN) (see Fig 6-7).

The curing cycle is designed to raise the temperature to a point at which (*1*) sufficient benzoyl peroxy radicals are produced to overcome the scavenging effect of oxygen, and (*2*) polymer chains form by free-radical addition polymerization. Too rapid a rise in temperature produces large numbers of radicals—a radical avalanche—and, as a result, many growing polymer chains. These chains collide either with other radicals, or even with polymer chains, producing an increase in branching and cross-linking of the interstitial polymer. This in turn reduces toughness. The polymerization reaction itself is exothermic; if the rate of reaction is too high, heat builds up in the dough until the boiling point of the monomer is exceeded. Porosity of the final denture base results, with a subsequent loss of strength and esthetics and an increase in the possibility of fouling.

Slow cures result in much tougher denture bases, producing fewer cross-links and branches, and having a higher overall molecular weight between cross-links because fewer polymer chains grew at any one time. Free-monomer content is often lower also, because the steadier rise in internal viscosity of the curing polymer allows the monomer easier access to the growing free radicals. The cross-linker is more completely polymerized in heat-cured systems; this results in significantly lower creep values due to removal of the plasticizing effect of unreacted pendant cross-linker groups.

The shrinkage that occurs when a liquid monomer is converted to a solid polymer can be largely compensated for by keeping the curing dough under compression. There are, however, hybrid systems that deliberately start the polymerization of the dough on one side of the mold, while forcing uncured dough into the mold on the opposite side. As curing progresses across the mold, the mold space is kept filled, with a resulting improvement in dimensional accuracy. The advantage of this system is that there is less tendency to raise the bite by overpacking the mold with dough, which can occur with conventional flasks.

Heat-cured systems have one great advantage over autopolymerized and injection-molding methods: an increased rate of monomer diffusion at the higher temperature. This is most beneficial when acrylic teeth are used, for it leads to better wetting of the teeth by the dough and the formation of chemical welds between the teeth and denture base. Conversely, an increased temperature of cure can also result in the annealing of stresses that build up in the structure due to polymerization shrinkage. If this stress is not released, it can act as the foci for crazes or distortions caused by overzealous cleaning regimes.

Autopolymerizing acrylic

The pour technique for dentures, originally developed during the 1960s, has lost much of its popularity because of problems that stem from incorrect processing. In this technique, the acrylic is mixed to a liquid consistency, then poured into a sprued mold that consists largely of reversible hydrocolloid. The fitting surface of the mold consists of the plaster model itself; the acrylic teeth occupy their positions in the agar mold in the same way they do in a conventional plaster mold.

The pour-type mold itself has design weaknesses. The gelatinous agar cannot grip the teeth as easily as the rock-hard plaster, and hence there is a greater tendency for the teeth to be displaced during the pouring of the acrylic. Prior to being placed in the mold, the teeth themselves have been part of the wax-up; any wax remaining on the teeth will prevent the monomer from wetting their surfaces. This problem is far less common when solution and diffusion of the wax can occur at the elevated temperatures of the heat-curing process.

The use of a hydroflask to produce an increased atmospheric pressure around the mold has two main advantages: (*1*) Most important, porosity caused by monomer boiling is prevented by the simple expedient of raising its boiling point; and (*2*) air included during mixing is compressed, raising the density of the cured resin and improving its transverse strength. However, the technician can do little to reduce free-monomer content to achieve high toughness, because this is built into the formulation when the manufacturer chooses the powder/liquid ratio, the cross-linker content, and the accelerator/catalyst ratio. In general, the creep of these products is greater than that of heat-cured acrylics.

Injection molding

The technician has little leeway when using injection-molded plastics. The mold should be dry to prevent the generation of steam during molding. Patience is required to ensure the melt has reached the right temperature and cools sufficiently after molding. Inadequate spruing will lead to underfilled molds, as can underheating the melt; overheating the melt can cause explosions, especially when polycarbonate is injected into moist molds.

Injection moldings rely almost totally on mechanical forces to retain the teeth. Low melt temperatures will cause strong forces to be put on the teeth during the injection phase and may dislodge some molars, even from plaster molds.

Depolymerization or oxidation from overheating the melt can result in porosity, loss of strength, color changes, and increased fouling.

Light-activated materials

Light-activated materials compare well to conventional heat-cured materials in terms of impact strength and hardness, but have a considerably lower elastic modulus. A denture constructed of light-cured material would therefore be expected to deform elastically to a greater extent than a heat-cured denture under the forces of mastication. However, transverse strength—a measure of the load required to fracture a thin strip of material in the transverse direction—is just slightly lower than that of the conventional material.

As a consequence of the higher-molecular-weight oligomers used in light-cured systems, polymerization shrinkage is smaller, about 3%, rather than the 6% shrinkage found in conventional systems. One study showed that denture bases processed by visible light fit better than conventional or quick heat-cured resins. Ideally, a total lack of polymerization shrinkage would allow the best fit.

Since light-activated materials contain no methyl methacrylate monomer, they may be considered for use in those patients who have demonstrated a sensitivity. The formulation of light-activated denture bases contains a copolymer of urethane dimethacrylate and an acrylic resin along with silica fillers. Blue light is used to polymerize thin sheets of the plastic raw material in a light chamber.

Future improvements in polymeric denture bases

The properties of polymeric denture bases that are closest to being offered as improved features of commercial products are radiopacity, impact strength, and stiffness.

Radiopacity in denture bases would be a desirable attribute. Denture wearers, be they motorists, members of the security forces, or athletes, can endure serious complications from relatively minor traumatic incidents if their denture fractures and a portion of it either is ingested into the lungs or intestines or, in more serious incidents, is driven through the skull into the brain pan. Fragments of radiolucent denture base are difficult to find even when sophisticated ultrasound techniques are used, and their presence is often suspected only after a secondary infection sets in.

The use of radiopaque salts and fillers often reduces esthetic properties and strength, and organometallic components have often proved too toxic for use. Bromine-containing organics can give good esthetics but often lack the heat stability necessary for heat processing or have to be added in such high quantities that the bulky bromine groups overplasticize the resulting acrylic denture base, causing creep, water adsorption, and stiffness problems. However, by phase-separating a bromo-polymer additive within the bead phase, it has been shown that sufficiently high glass-transition temperatures of 110°C and stiffnesses of 2.0 GPa (290,000 psi) can be achieved, while at the same time preserving esthetic properties and achieving high levels of radiopacity.

High-impact denture base materials can be prepared using inversion-phase separated polymer beads. However, a 50% improvement in impact strength (2.1 J/m) could be achieved, in combination with good esthetics and radiopacity, by the formation of a three-phase bead consisting of (*1*) PMMA, (*2*) styrene/butadiene rubber, and (*3*) the poly(2,3-dibromopropyl methacrylate) mentioned earlier. Processing conditions must be well controlled.

The availability and quality of high-modulus fibers is improving quickly, as is the variety of materials from which the fibers are made. Early experiments with glass fibers resulted in failure because of the irritant nature of the fibers that protruded from the finished surfaces. Carbon fibers had no such irritancy effects and greatly increased impact strength and flexural stiffness of the denture base for little material expense. However, the carbon fibers are black, so their use must be restricted to the lingual aspects of a denture. Kevlar fibers (poly-*p*-phenylene terephthalamide) have stiffnesses of 90 GPa (13 million psi), are straw-colored, and are not easy to pack. They can, however, greatly enhance the mechanical properties of the denture. As with carbon fibers, they are disappointing esthetically and need to be restricted to lingual aspects of the denture, although they can be extended to the midline of the teeth without being noticeable. This is an advan-

Table 6-2 A comparison of soft liners and tissue conditioners

Material	Advantages	Disadvantages	Ideal properties
Soft liners			
Acrylic	High peel strength to acrylic denture base High rupture strength Some can be polished if cooled Reasonable resistance to damage by denture cleansers	Poor resilience Loses plasticizer in time Some buckle in water	High resiliency Unaffected by aqueous environment and cleansers Good bond to denture base Good abrasion resistance
Silicone (RTV)	Resiliency	Low tear strength Low bond strength to dentures Attacked by cleansers Buckle in water Poor abrasion resistance	Biocompatible Antifouling properties Good dimensional stability
Silicone heat cured	Resiliency Adequate bond strength to acrylic More resistant to aqueous environment and cleansers than RTV	Low tear strength Poor abrasion resistance	
Tissue conditioners	Rheological and viscoelastic properties almost ideal Can be applied chairside Dentures fit well Can record freeway space	Low cohesive strength Affected by cleansers Alcohol can sting inflamed mucosa	Flow under constant force Resilient at high rates of deformation Remain viscous for several days Have a high tack to aid retention to denture base

tage, for if this were done with carbon fibers it would create a black shadow beneath the teeth in the plastic gum work.

Incorporation of the fibers into dentures produces conventional dentures that can withstand uncommonly rigorous treatment. When the fibers are combined with Bis-GMA, the flexural strength is such that they do not break in the conventional three-point flexural test apparatus, yet they have Young's moduli of 30 GPa (4 million psi), a figure comparable with ceramics. Lingual bars for partial dentures could be made using such materials, and, perhaps, with some changes in partial denture design, much less obtrusive polymeric partial dentures could be fabricated with only the clasps being made of metal.

Permanent soft lining materials

Permanent soft lining materials are resilient polymers used to replace the fitting surface of a hard plastic denture, either because the patient cannot tolerate a hard fitting surface or to improve retention of the denture. Because the lining is soft, its dimensional stability is important, as are its durability and resistance to fouling. However, because by definition soft lining materials are above their glass-transition temperature when in the mouth, such physical phenomena as water absorption, osmotic presence of soluble components, and biodegradability play a greater role in the clinical success of a liner than they do in the glassy polymers used as denture bases.

Acrylics and silicones are the two main families of polymers used commercially as soft liners, though other rubbers have been used in limited clinical experiments. Table 6-2 gives a comparison of soft lining materials.

Acrylic soft liners

The acrylics consist of either highly plasticized intrinsically glassy polymers or soft acrylics that have a natural glass-transition temperature at least 25°C less than that of the mouth. The plasticizer used to soften the acrylic can either be unbound to the acrylic and hence free to diffuse out during use, resulting in a loss of resilience, or it can be reacted into the cured matrix of the acrylic. The latter method is preferred because it should increase the clinical life of the soft liner; unfortunately, in practice, such acrylics are hard to formulate.

The reactive plasticizer often has a much lower rate of polymerization than the acrylic monomer. The result is a form of phase separation that leads to an uneven uptake of water by the soft liner. Water accumulates in the plasticizer-rich phase, and soluble impurities in the polymer create an osmotic pressure that causes it to swell and distort. Therefore, although such internally plasticized acrylics have been produced commercially, they have often been withdrawn after distortion problems have been noted in practice, often due to insufficient curing of very finely balanced formulations.

The plasticized acrylics are based on copolymer beads consisting mainly of ethyl methacrylate; both *n*- and isobutyl methacrylate can be used, as can 2-ethoxyethyl methacrylate. However, the latter monomer is used mainly in the liquid component. The beads are copolymerized with acrylates, which, in general, have much lower glass-transition temperatures than their methacrylate homologues, but unfortunately have very unpleasant odors. So that the beads are free flowing, the bead polymers have glass-transition temperatures slightly above room temperature. The monomer usually contains the plasticizer, which is a large phthalate ester. The monomer must swell sufficiently for the plasticizer to enter the beads. The plasticizer is then trapped inside the beads as the monomer polymerizes and the mean free path between the polymer chains decreases. The monomer can be methyl methacrylate, although its T_g, even when plasticized, is rather high; *n*- or isobutyl methacrylate is preferred because it has a much lower T_g when polymerized. Some manufacturers use isobutyl methacrylate to produce a balance of properties such that in ice water the liner can be polished like denture base acrylic, while the liner remains resilient in the mouth.

Water can, of course, be used as the plasticizer if the liner is hydrophilic. This was the principle behind the hydroxyethyl methacrylate soft liners. However, the water is not present when the denture is fabricated, and its uptake leads to a swelling of the liner, which must be compensated for. Water-swollen liners also allow ions into their matrices, which can subsequently crystallize and thus harden the lining as well as cause osmotic pressure effects, as in the polymerizable plasticizers.

Silicone soft liners

The silicones used as soft liners can be divided into two types: room-temperature vulcanizing (RTV) and heat curing. The resilience of silicones makes them at first seem to be the ideal soft lining materials. However, silicones have poor tear strength, no intrinsic adhesion to acrylic denture base, and, if not properly cured, a tendency to osmotic pressure effects. The RTV silicones' greatest drawback is their lack of adhesion, which is especially a problem around the edges of the attachment between acrylic and silicone. Heat-cured silicones have in their formulation a siloxane methacrylate that can polymerize into the curing denture base and into the heat-cured addition silicone. The RTV silicones use a condensation cross-linking system based on organo-tin derivatives such as those used in impression rubbers. Their degree of cross-linking is lower and their serviceability is low as a result, with frequent reports in the literature of swelling and buckling during use and excessive sensitivity to denture cleansers. The rupture strength of some RTV silicones is known to deteriorate considerably when exposed to water for long periods. The heat-cured silicones achieve a greater degree of cross-linking and have much longer clinical lifetimes.

Temporary soft liners and functional impression materials

Temporary soft liners, or tissue conditioners, need only survive in the mouth for a few weeks—although some are so well formulated as to remain resilient and in place for many months. However, it is their viscoelastic properties that are important, specifically their ability to flow under masticatory and linguistic forces, spreading the load on the mucosa evenly. When first mixed they flow easily, recording such voids as mean freespace. They soon become highly viscous, however, and thereafter only respond to persistent forces, such as changes in the shape of the mucosa beneath the denture. In this way swollen mucosa traumatized by ill-fitting dentures can recover while the denture, with its tissue conditioner lining, adapts to any lack of fit driven by masticatory forces.

The materials used for the temporary soft liners were many when the technique was first developed, and included many nontoxic, putty-like materials, such as plasticine and chewing gum. Modern materials are exclusively acrylic gels. An acrylic gel can be made by mixing swellable acrylic beads with alcohol. Poly(methyl methacrylate) is unsuitable for this purpose, although poly(ethyl methacrylate) or its copolymers with acrylates have proved most popular. To maintain the softness of the gel in the mouth, plasticizer is added to the alcohol which diffuses into the polymer beads and lowers their glass-transition temperature to well below that of the mouth. The beads are made of low-molecular-weight polymer and have a high tack when swollen. This has the advantage of increasing the cohesive strength of the gel and causing it to be well retained by the denture base acrylic.

There is no polymerization or curing reaction involved in the setting of the gel, just the entanglement of outer polymer chains of juxtaposed beads. The rate of gelling is increased by lowering the molecular weight of the bead, reducing its size, or increasing the amount of acrylate in its copolymers. The alcohol content of the liquid also can be used to control the rate of gelling, as can the size of the plasticizer molecule; the more alcohol used, the faster the rate of gelling. However, because the alcohol diffuses out of the gel and is only partially replaced by water, high-alcohol-content gels tend to harden much faster than others. Practitioners should be aware of the alcohol content of these products, first because they sting when initially inserted, and second because they give false positive results if the patient is given a breathalyzer test.

Glossary

addition polymerization A polymerization process involving free radicals in which no by-product is formed as the chain grows.

condensation polymerization A polymerization process in which a by-product, such as water or alcohol, is formed as the chain grows.

copolymer A polymer consisting of two or more types of mers or units joined together.

crazing Minute surface cracks on polymers; precursors to crack growth and subsequent failure of the material.

cross-linking agent A monomer having two or more groups per molecule capable of polymerization. When polymerized, each active group is capable of incorporation in a growing polymer chain, causing either a loop in the chain or a cross-link between two chains.

degree of polymerization The total number of mers in one polymer molecule.

denture base Materials used to contact the oral tissues and support artificial teeth.

glass-transition temperature (T_g) (softening temperature) The temperature at which the polymer ceases to be a glass (ie, fractures in a brittle manner) and becomes a rubber or leather (ie, tends to permanently deform under a load too small to cause fracture).

glassy polymer An amorphous polymer that behaves as a brittle solid.

hydrophilic liner A soft liner that is readily wet by water.

interpenetrating polymer network (IPN) A combination of two polymers in network form, at least one of which is synthesized and/or polymerized in the immediate presence of the other. An IPN can be distinguished from simple polymer blends, blocks, and grafts in two ways: (*1*) An IPN swells but does not dissolve in solvents; and (*2*) creep and flow are suppressed.

molecular weight The sum of the molecular weights of the mers of which the polymer is made.

oligomer A polymer made up of two, three, or four monomer units.

phase inversion The inversion of the internal and external phases in an emulsion, eg, the change of an oil-in-water emulsion to a water-in-oil emulsion.

plasticizer A small molecule that, when added to a polymer, lowers its glass-transition temperature and increases the rate at which solvents penetrate the polymer.

polymer A molecule made up of thousands or millions of repeating units. Polymers may be linear, branched, or cross-linked.

polymerization The process by which monomers unite to form a polymer.

soft liner A soft polymer used as a thin layer on the tissue-bearing surface of a denture.

thermoplastic A polymer that softens upon heating and rehardens upon cooling.

thermoset A polymer that is not able to undergo softening upon heating.

tissue conditioner A soft liner used to treat traumatized mucosa.

Discussion questions

1. Why is higher impact strength an important advantage for denture base materials?
2. How does the heat-curing rate affect the porosity and strength of acrylic denture bases?
3. Although cross-linking can improve mechanical properties, how can it lead to problems in the bonding between acrylic teeth and the denture base?
4. Why do acrylic polymers still dominate the denture base market?

Questions and answers

1. **What are the main types of denture base materials used?**

   Heat- and cold-cured acrylic resins
   Rubber- and fiber-reinforced acrylic
   Polycarbonate injection molded
   Nylon injection molded
   Dimethacrylate light-activated

2. **What are the ideal properties of a denture base material?**

   Good appearance
   High flexural strength
   High impact resistance
   High stiffness
   Long fatigue life
   High craze resistance
   High creep resistance
   High radiopacity
   Low free-monomer content
   Good adhesion with teeth and liners
   Low solubility
   Low water uptake
   Dimensional stability
   Dimensional accuracy

3. **What are the advantages and disadvantages of heat-cured acrylic denture base materials?**

   Advantages:

   Good appearance
   High glass-transition temperature
   Ease of fabrication
   Low capital costs
   Good surface finish

   Disadvantages:

   Free-monomer content or formaldehyde can cause sensitization
   Low impact strength
   Flexural strength low enough to penalize poor denture design
   Fatigue life too short
   Radiolucency

4. What are the advantages and disadvantages of auto-cured denture base materials?

Advantages:
Easy to deflask
Dimensionally accurate
Can have higher flexural strength than heat-cured materials

Disadvantages:
No cheaper over the long term
Increased creep
Increased free-monomer content
Color instability
Reduced stiffness
Tooth adhesion failure

5. What are the advantages and disadvantages of rubber-reinforced denture base materials?

Advantage:
Improved impact strength

Disadvantage:
Reduced stiffness

6. What are the advantages and disadvantages of fiber-reinforced denture base materials?

Advantages:
High stiffness
Very good impact strength
Good fatigue life
Polypropylene fibers: good translucency and good surface finish

Disadvantage:
Carbon and Kevlar fibers: poor color and poor surface

7. What are the advantages and disadvantages of injection-molded denture bases?

Advantages:
Dimensional accuracy
Low free-monomer content
Good impact strength

Disadvantages:
High capital costs
Difficult mold design problems
Less craze resistance
Less creep resistance

8. What are the advantages and disadvantages of light-activated denture base materials?

Advantages:
No methyl methacrylate monomer
Reduced polymerization shrinkage
Time savings
Possible better fit than conventional denture base materials
Processing procedure requiring little equipment

Disadvantage:
Somewhat increased elastic deformation during mastication

9. What are the materials currently being used as soft liners?

Acrylic, silicone (RTV), and heat-cured silicone.

10. What are the advantages and disadvantages of RTV silicones?

Advantage:
Resilient

Disadvantages:
Low tear strength
Low bond strength to dentures
Attacked by cleansers
Buckle in water
Poor abrasion resistance

11. What are the advantages and disadvantages of heat-cured silicones?

Advantages:
Resiliency
Adequate bond strength to acrylic
More resistant to aqueous environment and cleansers than RTV

Disadvantages:
Low tear strength
Poor abrasion resistance

12. What are the advantages and disadvantages of acrylic soft liners?

Advantages
High peel strength to acrylic denture base
High rupture strength
Some can be polished if cooled
Reasonable resistance to damage by denture cleansers

Disadvantages:
Poor resilience
Loses plasticizer in time
Some buckle in water

13. What are the ideal properties of tissue conditioners?

Flow under constant force
Resiliency at high rates of deformation
Remain viscous for several days
Have high tack to aid retention to denture base

Recommended reading

Anderson GC, Schulte JK, Arnold TG. Dimensional stability of injection and conventional processing of denture base acrylic resin. J Prosthet Dent 60(3):394–398,1988.

Bafile M, Graser GN, Myers ML, Li EKH. Porosity of denture resin cured by microwave energy. J Prosthet Dent 66:269–274, 1991.

Berry JP, Bueche AM. Ultimate strength of polymers. In P Weiss (ed). Adhesion and Cohesion. Amsterdam: Elsevier, 1962;20.

Davy KWM, Causton BE. Radio-opaque denture base: a new acrylic copolymer. J Dent 10:253–264, 1982.

Eichold WA, Woefel JB. Denture base acrylic resins: Friend or foe? Compend Cont Edu Dent 11:720–725, 1990.

Goll G, Smith DE, Plein JB. The effect of denture cleansers on temporary soft liners. J Prosthet Dent 50:466–472, 1983.

Khan Z, von Fraunhofer JA, Razavi R. The staining characteristics, transverse strength, and microhardness of a visible light-cured denture base material. J Prosthet Dent 57:384–386, 1987.

Mack PJ. Denture soft linings: Materials available. Aust Dent J 34:517–521, 1989.

Mark FF. Future trends for improvement of cohesive and adhesive strength of polymers. In P Weiss (ed). Adhesion and Cohesion. Amsterdam: Elsevier, 1962;241.

MacGregor AR, Graham J, Stafford GD, Huggett B. Recent experience with denture polymers. J Dent 12:146–157, 1984.

Qudah S, Harrison A, Huggett R. Soft lining materials in prosthetic dentistry: A review. Int J Prosthodont 3:477–483, 1990.

Ruyter IE. Methacrylate-based polymeric dental materials: conversion and related properties. Acta Odontol Scand 40:359–376, 1982.

Ruyter IE, Svendsen SA. Flexural properties of denture base polymers. J Prosthet Dent 43:95–104, 1980.

Schmidt WF, Smith DE. A six-year retrospective study of Molloplast-B-lined dentures. Part 1. Patient response. J Prosthet Dent 50(3):308–313, 1983.

Smith LT, Powers JM. Relative fit of new denture resins polymerized by heat, light and microwave energy. Am J Dent 5(3):140–142, 1992.

Smith LT, Powers JM, Ladd D. Mechanical properties of new denture resins polymerized by visible light, heat and microwave energy. Int J Prosthodont 5:315–320, 1992.

Takamata T, Setcos JC. Resin denture bases: Review of accuracy and methods of polymerization. Int J Prosthodont 2:555–562, 1989.

Wright PS. Soft lining materials: their status and prospects. J Dent 4:247–256, 1976.

Chapter 7

Polymeric Restorative Materials: Composites and Sealants

The first material developed for use as a direct esthetic restorative was silicate cement. Introduced in the late 1800s, the cement was prepared from an alumina-silica glass and a phosphoric acid liquid. Highly soluble in oral fluids, silicate deteriorated rapidly, yet remained the favored material until the early 1950s. Dissolution, discoloration, loss of translucency, and lack of adequate mechanical properties contributed to its eventual replacement. Its main advantage was the slow release of fluoride from the glass phase.

Self-curing unfilled acrylic resins were introduced around 1945 as a substitute for silicate cement and were in moderate use in the 1950s. These materials were related to denture base resins and were much less soluble and more color stable than silicates. They were easy to use, polishable, and had good initial esthetics. Their main problems were high shrinkage upon polymerization, large thermal dimensional change, eventual discoloration, and a high wear rate.

Composite resins, a combination of hard, inorganic filler particles bonded to soft dimethacrylate polymer, were introduced in the 1960s. As a consequence of the bonded filler phase, these materials had much better mechanical properties than did unfilled resins, approaching the properties of dentin and enamel. Originally intended for use in anterior Class III, IV, and V restorations where esthetics are important, improvements have included light curing, bonding to tooth structure, and reduced wear. Continued development has led to their use in conservative posterior restorations.

Classification

A composite is a material composed of two or more distinct phases. Composite resins for dental use were formulated to combine the esthetics and ease of use of a polymerizable resin base with the improved properties to be gained from the addition of a ceramic filler. Composite resins are often classified according to the size of the ceramic filler particle (Fig 7-1).

Fine-particle composites contain ground glass or quartz particles 0.5 to 3.0 µm in diameter, which occupy 60% to 77% of the composite by volume. Since the filler has a density greater than that of the polymer matrix, the fraction of the filler by weight is higher, about 70% to 90%. Particles present may be of uniform diameter or may have a distribution of diameters, in which case smaller particles fit in the spaces between larger particles, and packing is more efficient.

Microfine composites contain spherical colloidal silica particles 0.01 to 0.12 µm in diameter. Colloidal silica is produced by vapor-phase hydrolysis of silicon compounds resulting in an average surface area of 200 m^2/g, which greatly increases the viscosity of the polymer matrix upon incorporation. Filler loading in these composites is therefore limited to about 20% to 55% by volume or 35% to 60% by weight, and low-molecular-weight organic diluents of low viscosity are often added to give the composite a workable clinical consistency. Filler content may be increased and properties improved by grinding a polymerized microfine composite into particles 10 to 20 µm in diameter and sub-

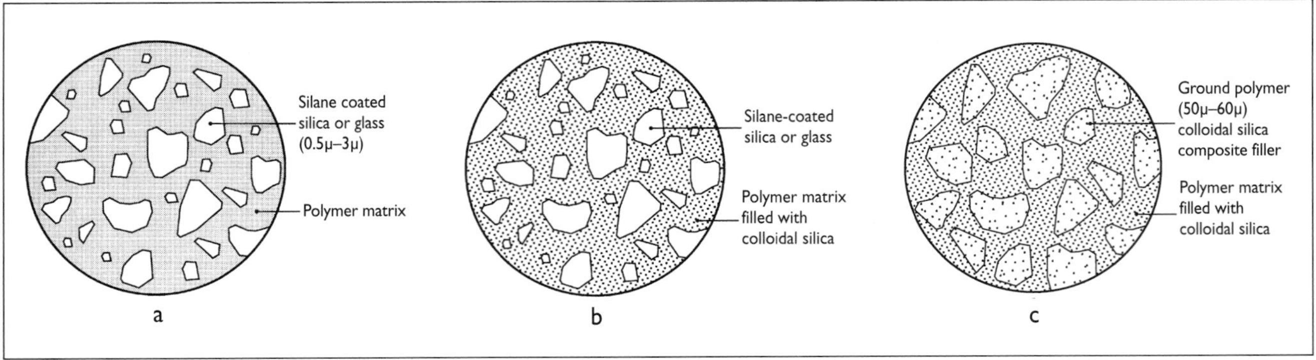

Fig 7-1 The microstructure of composite materials: (a) fine particle; (b) hybrid or blend; (c) microfill.

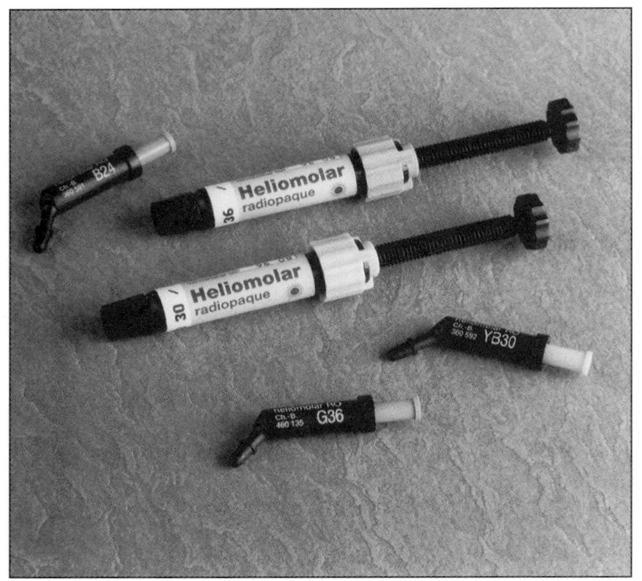

Fig 7-2 A heavily filled microfine light-cured composite restorative material that is syringe injected.

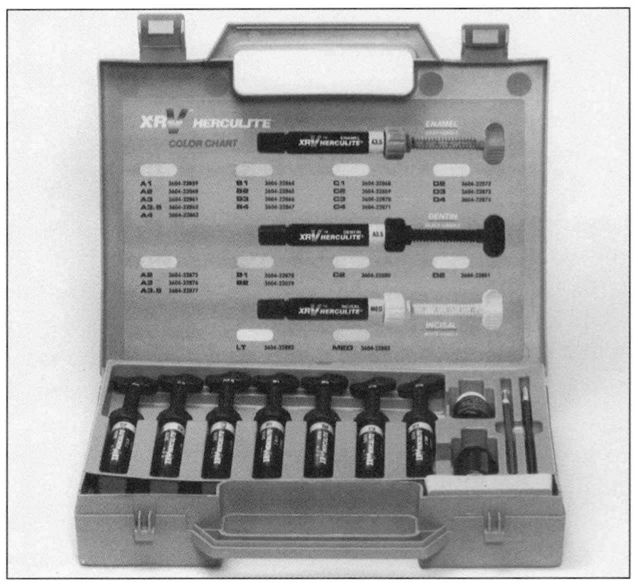

Fig 7-3 A well-established hybrid composite.

sequently using these reinforced particles as filler along with colloidal silica. Heavily filled microfine composites have a filler content of 32% to 66% by volume or about 40% to 80% by weight (Fig 7-2).

Hybrids (or blends) have a combination of colloidal and fine particles as filler. The colloidal particles fill the matrix between fine particles, resulting in a filler content of around 60% to 65% by volume. Hybrids (such as the one in Fig 7-3) currently dominate the market, followed by microfine materials.

Macrofills, the earliest composites, contain relatively large quartz particles ranging in size from 15 to 35 μm (Fig 7-4). Although these materials showed greatly improved properties relative to unfilled resins, large particles did not permit adequate polishability, resulting in rough surfaces and the retention of plaque. With the introduction in recent years of polishable small-particle materials, the use of macrofills has greatly declined.

Composition and reaction

Filler composition

Filler particles are of inorganic composition. In addition to quartz, fine-sized particles may be composed of barium or lithium aluminum silicate glasses;

borosilicate glass; or barium, strontium, or zinc glasses. Particles in microfine composites are colloidal silica.

Composites may be made radiopaque by incorporating elements of high atomic weight, such as barium, strontium, zirconium, or ytterbium, into the filler particle.

Organic matrix

The organic polymer matrix in currently available composites is most commonly an aromatic or urethane diacrylate oligomer such as bisphenol A-glycidyl methacrylate (Bis-GMA) or urethane-dimethacrylate (UDMA), represented by the simplified formula given here. R may be any of a number of organic groups, such as methyl-, hydroxyl-, phenyl-, carboxyl-, and amide-.

$$CH_2 = \underset{\displaystyle CH_3}{\underset{|}{C}} - R - \underset{\displaystyle CH_3}{\underset{|}{C}} = CH_2$$

The oligomers have in common reactive double bonds at each end of the molecule which are able to undergo addition polymerization in the presence of free radicals. The oligomer molecules are highly viscous and require the addition of low-molecular-weight diluent monomers, usually triethylene glycol dimethacrylate (TEGMA), so a clinically workable consistency may be maintained upon the incorporation of the filler.

Coupling agents

A bond between filler particle and matrix in the set composite is achieved by use of an organic silicon compound, or silane coupling agent. The silane molecule has reactive groups at both its ends and is coated on the filler particle surface by the manufacturer before mixing with the oligomer. During polymerization, double bonds on the silane molecule also react with the polymer matrix. A bond between filler and matrix allows the distribution of stresses generated under function. The net result is a material with strength properties greater than those of the particulate filler or the matrix separately. Bonding also enhances the retention of the filler particle during abrasive action at the composite surface. As a result, hard filler particles, in addition to soft matrix, are present to engage in abrasive wear with opposing enamel, for example, greatly improving the wear resistance of the material.

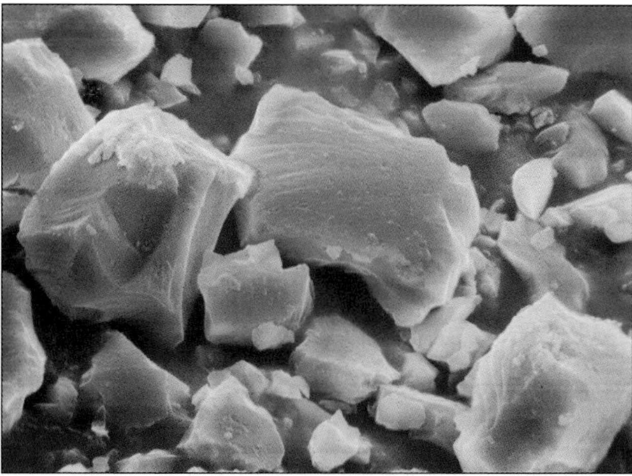

Fig 7-4 Scanning electron micrograph (SEM) of large quartz filler particles. (Original magnification × 2,000.)

Initiators and accelerators

Polymerization of composites may be achieved by chemical means (self-cure) or by visible light activation. Dual cure is a combination of light and chemical curing. In chemically activated systems, an organic peroxide initiator (or catalyst), upon reacting with a tertiary amine accelerator, produces free radicals that attack the double bonds of oligomer molecules and begin the process of addition polymerization.

Initiation of polymerization in light-activated systems depends upon the scission of the initiator molecule, often camphoroquinone, by visible light of appropriate wavelength. In the presence of an aliphatic amine accelerator, free radicals are produced and polymerization begins. For both systems, the following general reaction occurs:

Dimethacrylate	+	Initiator (peroxide or diketone + blue light)	+	Accelerator (amine)

+ Silane-treated particles → Dental composite

Since dimethacrylate oligomers as well as dimethacrylate diluent monomers have reactive double bonds at each end of the molecules, polymerization results in a highly cross-linked polymer.

Other ingredients

Inorganic oxide pigments are added to composites in small amounts to provide a range of standard shades. Most often, four shades, ranging from yellow to gray, are supplied. In response to consumer interest, manufacturers now offer an extended range of 16 or 25 shades, as well as shade selections from the Bioform and Vita ceramic shade guides. Most manufacturers offer modifiers such as highly pigmented tints for mixing with standard shades, as well as opaquers and glazes.

Polymerization inhibitors and stabilizers are added to the composite in order to lengthen shelf life.

Composite product systems

Composites are packaged as a two-paste system supplied in two jars, or as a single-paste system supplied in a syringe or in compules. An enamel acid etchant, along with an enamel and dentin bonding agent, also is usually supplied by the manufacturer.

In a *two-paste system* chemically cured composites are supplied as two pastes because the initiator and the accelerator must be kept separate until mixing. Each jar contains dimethacrylate and filler; one jar also contains the peroxide initiator, and the other contains the amine accelerator. A few composites are offered as two-paste, dual-curing systems. Setting begins after the catalyst and base are mixed and can be accelerated by light curing.

In a *single-paste system* light-activated composites are supplied as single pastes in opaque, disposable syringes or in color-coded compules for use with a syringe (see Fig 7-2). Light-activated composites are currently the most widely used systems available.

Commercially available curing units transmit light from a halogen lamp to the tooth surface by way of a curved quartz rod, a liquid-filled transmission tube, or a bundle of flexible quartz fibers attached to a fiber-optic handpiece. Ultraviolet light is generally filtered out at the light source.

Photosensitive initiator molecules in composite resins require blue light in the wavelength range of 468 to 480 nm to effect scission and initiate polymerization. Peak output wavelength of available curing units varies from 460 to 700 nm, with most units having peaks between 420 and 560 nm (Fig 7-5).

As with ultraviolet light used in early curing units, blue light has the potential to cause retinal damage. Fig 7-6 shows a curing light for composite materials. Protective eyewear during operation of curing units is also available and recommended.

Properties

Setting time

Composite systems that are chemically activated have setting times ranging from 3 to 5 minutes from the start of mixing. The setting time is determined at the time of manufacture by control of the concentrations of initiator and accelerator. However, studies show that even after a curing time of 24 hours, polymerization is not complete and 25% to 45% of double bonds remain unreacted.

The setting time of light-initiated materials and the depth of cure depend on the intensity and penetration of the light beam. Polymerization is approximately 75% complete at 10 minutes after exposure to blue light, and curing continues for a period of at least 24 hours. At 24 hours, up to 30% of double bonds still remain unreacted.

Polymerization shrinkage

The occurrence of shrinkage during polymerization creates stresses (~18 MPa) at the tooth/composite interface that may exceed the strength of any bond between composite and enamel or dentin. Bond failure

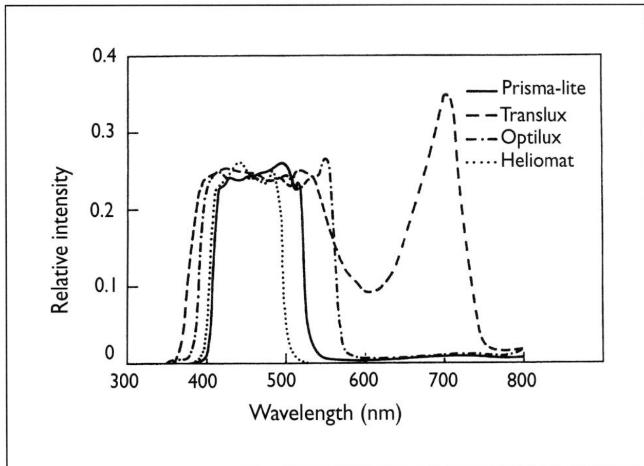

Fig 7-5 Spectra of four major dental curing lights: Prisma-lite (L.D. Caulk); Translux (Kulzer, Inc.); Optilux (Demetron Research Corp.); Heliomat (Vivadent USA, Inc.).

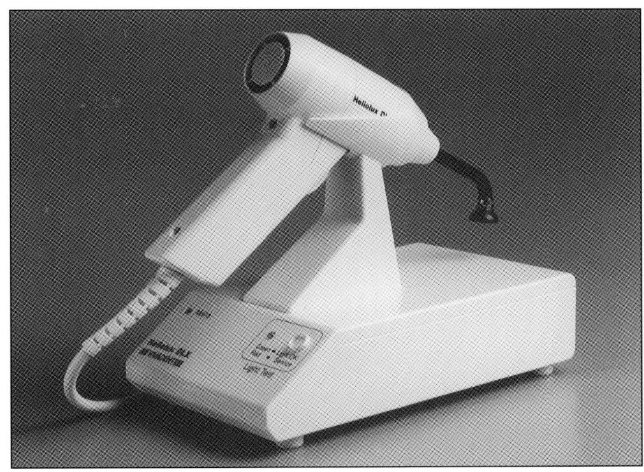

Fig 7-6 Blue curing light.

Table 7-1 Average properties of composite resins

Property	Microfine	Hybrid	Fine	Macrofill
Inorganic filler content (vol %)	20–55	60–65	60–77	50–65
Thermal conductivity	Insulator	Insulator	Insulator	Insulator
Coefficient of thermal expansion (/°C × 10^{-6})	50–68	20–40	19–38	17–35
Hardness (Knoop)	22–36	50–60	50–80	55
Water sorption (mg/cm^2)	1.2–2.2	0.5–0.7	0.3–0.6	0.3–0.7
Compressive strength (MPa) (psi × 10^3)	170–475 24.7–68.9	300–475 43.5–68.9	240–400 34.8–58.0	210–300 30.5–43.5
Tensile strength (MPa) (psi × 10^3)	25–50 3.6–7.3	50–90 7.3–13.1	35–90 5.1–13.1	35–65 5.1–9.4
Young's modulus (GPa) (psi × 10^6)	3–7 0.44–1.0	7–14 1.0–2.0	9–20 1.3–2.9	7–15 1.0–2.2
Polymerization shrinkage (%)	2–4	1.5–4	1.0–1.7	1.0–1.7

at the interface allows an influx of oral fluids and greatly contributes to the possibility of marginal staining, secondary caries, and postoperative sensitivity. In addition, stresses at the tooth/composite interface may exceed the tensile strength of enamel perpendicular to the enamel rods, resulting in fractures through the enamel along the interface.

Shrinkage is a direct function of the volume fraction of polymer matrix in the composite, and thus occurs to a larger degree in microfine composites than in fine-particle composites or hybrids. Microfine composites typically show setting contractions of 2% to 4% as compared to lower values of 1.0% to 1.7% for fine-particle composites, as given in Table 7-1.

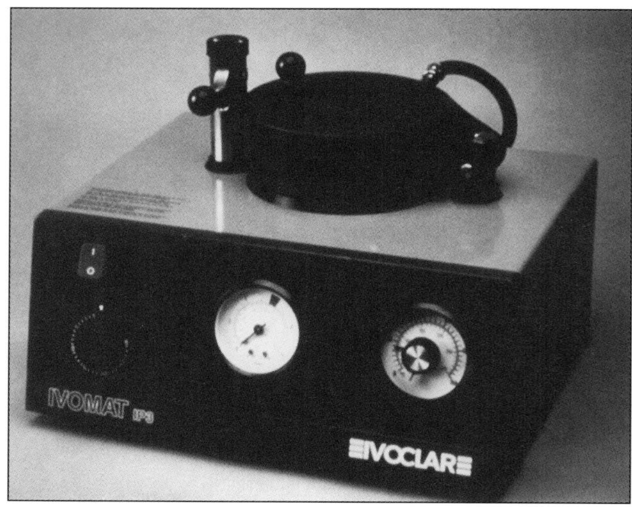

Fig 7-7 Composite inlay heat-processing unit.

The shrinkage problem can be partially overcome in two ways. First, incremental addition and polymerization of thin layers of a light-initiated material will result in decreased total setting contraction as opposed to bulk curing a single thick layer. However, although this method does result in lower stresses at the tooth/composite interface, studies show that marginal gaps may occur nonetheless.

A second approach involves the preparation of a composite inlay either directly in the mouth or indirectly as a laboratory procedure. In the latter procedure the inlay is heat processed (Fig 7-7), allowing the degree of polymerization to approach 100%, and cemented in the mouth with a thin layer of resin cement. The bulk of the composite resin cement layer needed is small, producing a very small amount of shrinkage and low interfacial stresses. Long-term studies are still underway, and composite inlays produced in this way are expected to show improved durability and increased wear resistance due to enhanced physical properties.

Thermal properties

The organic polymer matrix has low thermal conductivity, and composites therefore provide good thermal insulation for the dental pulp. Thermal conductivities of all composites closely match those of enamel and dentin and are much lower than that of dental amalgam.

As a consequence of the weak physical bonds by which individual polymer molecules are held together, polymers have a marked tendency to expand and contract in response to temperature changes. In contrast, the highly inorganic content of tooth structure is affected to a much smaller degree. Dimensional changes in the composite resulting from thermal cycling in the mouth produce further strain on the bond at the tooth/composite interface, increasing the possibility of marginal percolation. This effect occurs to a larger extent with resin-rich microfine composites than with fine-particle materials or hybrids.

Water sorption and solubility

The polymer matrix is able to absorb water, which is accompanied by some swelling of the composite, but this is not sufficient to counteract polymerization shrinkage. The uptake of water by composites has been correlated with decreases in surface hardness and wear resistance. As a result of their larger volume fraction of matrix, microfine composites have higher water sorption values and therefore a greater potential for discoloration by water-soluble stains.

Solubility of composite resins ranges from 1.5% to 2.0% of the original material weight. The major detected leachable components in water include residual oligomer or monomer, and, therefore, incomplete polymerization of the composite results in markedly increased solubility. Additional leachable molecules include degradation products of various composite components and may include formaldehyde, benzoic acid, and methacrylic acid. The largest part of the dissolution occurs within the first few hours of placement.

Elements from filler particles dissolve in water to varying degrees and are detected in quantities as high as 180 µmol/g. Boron and silicon are the main elements, but barium, strontium, and lead, other additives to glass particles, also leach out. The presence of silicon in solution may indicate degradation of the surface treatment of the filler.

Alcohol is a solvent of Bis-GMA and acidulated fluoride gels increase the rate of dissolution of filler particles. Therefore, alcohol-free rinses and neutral fluoride products should be used.

Table 7-2 **Mechanical properties of enamel and dentin**

	Compressive strength (MPa)	Tensile strength (MPa)	Young's modulus (GPa)	Hardness number (Knoop, Vickers)
Enamel	384	10.3	84.1	343 (408)
Dentin	297	51.7	18.5	68 (60)

Color stability

Darkening and a color shift to yellow or gray has often been noted in self-curing systems and has been attributed to the presence of the tertiary amine accelerator, which produces colored products upon oxidation. Photo-initiated systems do not contain a tertiary amine and have shown considerably improved color stability over long periods of time.

Under accelerated aging conditions in a weathering chamber, erosion of the resin matrix and exposure of filler particles of microfilled composites resulted in a lightening of the color of the material. Color stability of microfine composites, however, was affected by erosion only to a small degree.

Radiopacity

A degree of radiopacity slightly exceeding that of enamel may be useful in diagnosis. Radiopacity may be conferred by incorporating elements of high atomic number, such as barium, strontium, and zirconium, into the filler. The relative number of these atoms is still small, however, and the materials are much less radiopaque than is amalgam. Many composites currently available have some degree of radiopacity, and several for posterior use have radiopacities greater than that of enamel.

Mechanical properties

The higher compressive and tensile strengths of fine-particle and hybrid composites reflect the higher volume fraction of the high-strength filler component. Note that for all materials compressive strengths are several times higher than tensile strengths, reflecting the somewhat brittle behavior of composites. Composites probably fail under tensile loading. More highly filled composites have tensile strengths near that of dentin, and compressive strengths similar to or higher than that of dentin (Table 7-2). Some highly filled composites have compressive strengths greater than that of enamel.

The elastic (Young's) modulus is a measure of a material's stiffness. A material with low elastic modulus deflects under stress. As a group, composites have elastic moduli that are only a fraction that of enamel. Fine-particle materials, however, have moduli in the neighborhood of dentin's. Under high loads, such as occur in posterior teeth during mastication, deflection of the restoration strains the tooth/composite bond. Deflection additionally places considerable tensile stresses on adjacent cusps.

The lower filler content of microfine composites results in elastic moduli of one quarter to one half that of the more highly filled fine-particle composites, and are therefore recommended for cervical (Class V) restorations since deflection could reduce stresses at the tooth/composite interface.

Microindentation hardness of composites is directly related to volume fraction of the hard, inorganic filler component. Hardness is also related to the degree of polymerization. In laboratory experiments, composites that underwent a secondary heat treatment to increase the degree of polymerization showed higher Knoop hardness values than did composites that were light cured only.

As a group, the hardness of composites is a fraction of that of enamel but is similar to or higher than that of dentin.

Wear

Wear in composites is a complex phenomenon that depends on several intrinsic and extrinsic factors. The large amount of data collected for various available composites is confusing, at least in part because measuring techniques have not been standardized. In vivo

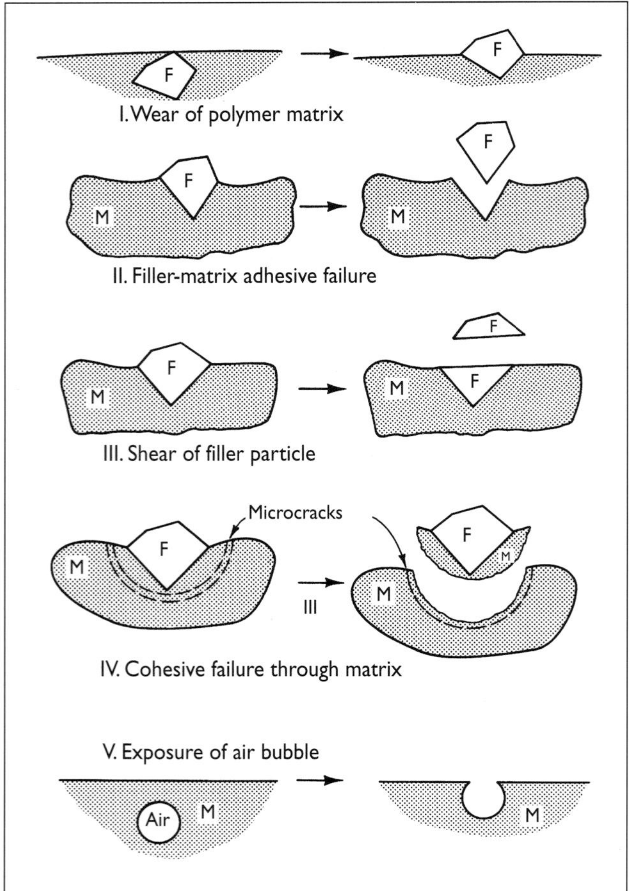

Fig 7-8 Several possible wear mechanisms for dental composites. (From O'Brien and Yee, 1979.)

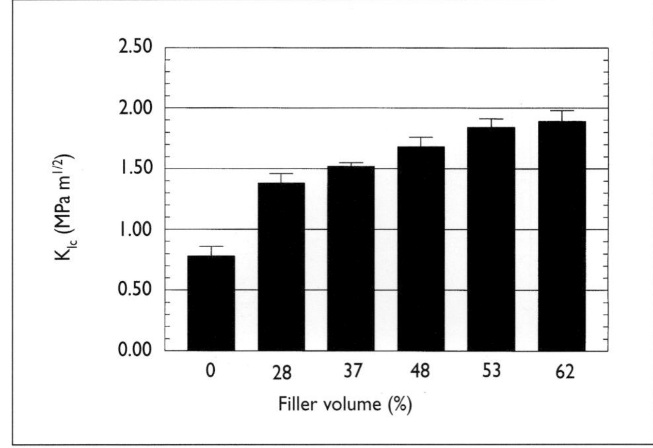

Fig 7-9 The effect of filler volume fraction on fracture toughness, K_{IC}. (Courtesy of J. Ferracane.)

wear has not been shown to correlate well with any single material property. In addition, the appearance of wear patterns in restorations of long duration is complicated by the presence of erosion, a degradative uniform loss of material across the composite surface; several wear mechanisms are shown in Fig 7-8. Nevertheless, a number of factors that contribute to wear have been identified.

1. *Filler content, particle size, and hardness.* Increased filler volume results in decreased wear. Laboratory studies demonstrate a greater loss of material volume during abrasive action for microfine as compared to more highly filled fine-particle composites. A higher filler volume results in a higher fracture toughness, as shown in Fig 7-9.

   Keeping volume fraction constant, wear resistance is increased by decreasing the size of the filler particle. Large, hard particles transmit considerable stress to the matrix, possibly resulting in microcracking and subsequent loss of material (Fig 7-10). By contrast, a reduced load per particle results when a large number of small particles is present per unit volume.

   It has been reported that wear of composites with filler particles smaller than 1.0 µm occurs at a constant rate with time. Wear of composites with particles larger than 1.0 µm is greatest in the year after placement, declining thereafter.

   The incorporation of softer filler particles with hardness characteristics similar to that of enamel appears to result in decreased wear. It is thought that soft particles are more capable than hard particles of absorbing energy generated during the masticatory process, thereby transmitting lower stresses to the matrix. Scanning electron micrographs of a material with hard quartz particles and another with soft glass particles are shown in Figs 7-10 and 7-11. Note the difference in the shapes of the particles that project from the occlusal surface.

   Interestingly, the presence of filler particles with hardness values greater than that of enamel has been shown to increase the roughness of opposing enamel over time.
2. *Tooth position in the arch.* In general, the more distally located the restoration, the higher the rate of wear.

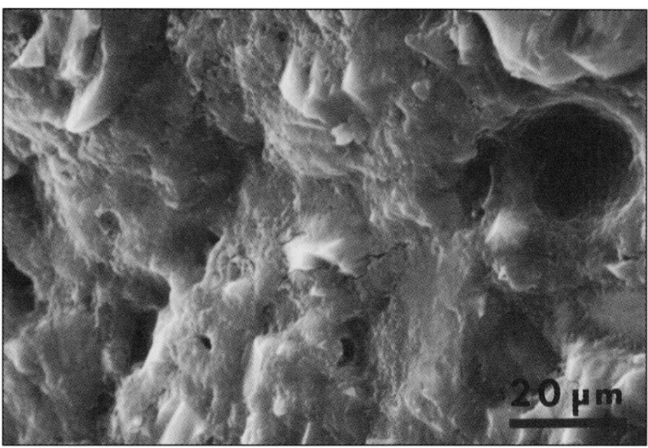

Fig 7-10 Worn surface of a composite restoration showing a protruding hard quartz filler particle with an adjacent microcrack. (SEM, original magnification × 1,000.) (From O'Brien and Yee, 1979.)

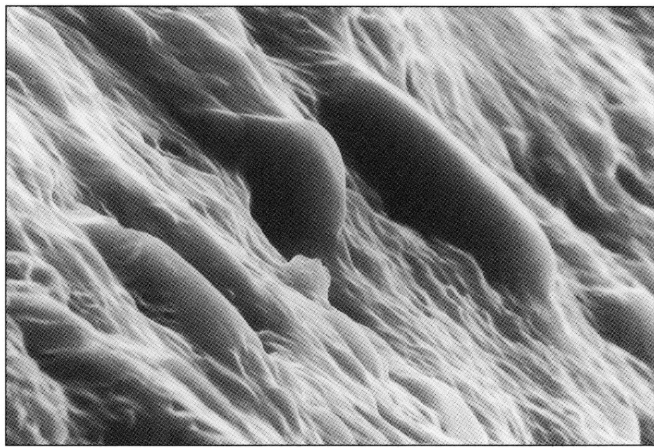

Fig 7-11 Worn surface of a composite with a soft glass filler. (SEM, original magnification × 2,500.)

3. *Porosity.* Internal porosity, particularly in stress-bearing areas, increases wear. It has been proposed that porosities concentrate stresses in the matrix, and under loading, contribute to the formation of microcracks. In addition, voids, produced during the spatulation process or during incorporation of filler during manufacture, are air-filled. An air-inhibited layer of incompletely polymerized matrix may exist at the void surface. Light-initiated systems requiring no spatulation have demonstrated higher wear resistance than self-curing systems.
4. *Degree of polymerization.* Strength properties of polymers are directly related to molecular size. During polymerization, molecular size increases enormously. The enhanced wear resistance found in some studies of heat-processed composite inlays is thought to be related to their higher degree of polymerization.
5. *Coupling agent.* The absence of a silane coupling agent at the matrix/filler interface reduces wear resistance by about half.
6. *Method of finishing.* Wear resistance decreases with the use of carbide or diamond finishing burs. Their use is thought to weaken the surface through the formation of microcracks or to degrade the matrix through the generation of heat. It has been reported that treatment of the surface after occlusal adjustment and subsequent curing with a low-viscosity unfilled resin decreases wear by about 50%.

Wear resistance of composites developed for posterior use has improved steadily over recent years.

Depth of cure

Polymerization in both chemically and light-activated composites is incomplete. Degrees of conversion are reported to be in the range of 60% to 75%. The number of unreacted double bonds at 24 hours is higher in light-activated than in chemically activated systems and results from a number of factors affecting depth of cure.

Light intensity at the surface and time of exposure are critical. The tip of the light source should be held within 3 to 4 mm of the surface in order to cure a light shade of material to a depth of 2.0 to 2.5 mm using a standard exposure time of 40 seconds. A longer exposure time will increase the degree of polymerization at all depths and is a necessity when using darker shades or more opaque materials. A reduction in thickness of the increment to be cured is a more reliable way of achieving polymerization than is an increase in exposure time. In addition, hardness of the top surface of a cured restoration is not a good indication of the extent of polymerization at the bottom surface.

Depth of cure is also influenced by the wavelength of light and the concentration of the activator-initiator system. The refractive indices of the resin and filler, as well as the size, shape, and number of filler particles, are important to the dispersion of the light beam. The small, highly numerous colloidal-sized particles of microfine composites scatter incident light very efficiently, necessitating a longer exposure time in order to obtain adequate polymerization.

Chemically activated systems are considered to have an infinite depth of cure.

Biocompatibility

Histological studies of the effect of residual monomer molecules on pulp tissue have shown a moderate degree of cytotoxicity, even in low concentrations. Recent in vivo biocompatibility studies, however, show that composite resins, whether completely or incompletely cured, cause little irritation to the pulp if an adequate marginal seal is present. It has been proposed that a significant degree of sensitivity after the placement of a restoration is a consequence of microbial invasion from the oral environment and not of toxicity of the material itself. A second possibility is that postoperative sensitivity may be a consequence of debonding between dentin and the composite at the cavity floor, causing a pumping action of dentinal fluid during chewing, possibly expressing irritants or bacterial toxins into dentinal tubules.

Until the precise mechanisms involved are understood, pulpal protection is recommended in deep parts of the cavity preparation.

Manipulation

Placement

Eugenol inhibits the polymerization of composite resins. Therefore, liners, bases, and interim restorations containing eugenol are not recommended. The use of cavity varnish is not recommended under composite restorations, as monomers present in the composite may solubilize and disrupt the integrity of the varnish film. Also, varnish will prevent bonding.

Following cavity preparation and prior to placement of the composite, a sealing procedure of some type is indicated. If any dentin bonding agent is to be used, the use of a rubber dam is indicated because moisture in exhaled air may interfere with bonding. The dentin is first conditioned according to the manufacturer's directions. Deep preparations may require the placement of a glass ionomer base over the dentin. Very deep cavities require pulpal protection in the form of a thin layer of a calcium hydroxide product on the dentin over the pulp.

Enamel is etched for 15 to 20 seconds using a 35% to 50% phosphoric acid solution or acid gel. High-viscosity gel etchants have the advantage of ease of control of the application to enamel walls. The preparation is thoroughly washed with water for at least 15 seconds to remove all residue. The surface is gently air-dried, at which point the enamel should have an opaque, white appearance. Any contamination by saliva after this step requires re-etching in order to clean the surface thoroughly.

A dentin bonding agent is applied to the clean enamel and dentin according to the manufacturer's directions. The bonding resin should be air-blown gently to ensure a thin film application. Dentin bonding agents work as well on enamel as do enamel bonding agents. While components of bonding systems should not be interchanged, any composite can be used with any bonding agent.

A transparent matrix band is sometimes applied for the purpose of contouring the restoration.

Two-paste system

To ensure uniform distribution of filler particles in the matrix, each paste should be stirred periodically with disposable plastic mixing sticks, taking care to avoid cross-contamination that will cause polymerization of the pastes in the jars. Less particle settling and an increase in shelf-life results if the pastes are refrigerated.

Equal amounts of the two pastes are dispensed onto a mixing pad with a disposable two-bladed plastic spatula. One blade of the spatula should be used to dispense one paste, and the other blade, the second paste. When needed, the two pastes are mixed thoroughly, requiring 20 to 30 seconds. Care should be taken to avoid the incorporation of air during mixing. Metal spatulas are not recommended for mixing, because filler particles are capable of abrading metal and small amounts of metal may be incorporated into the composite, resulting in discoloration.

Two-paste composites have a working time from the start of mixing of 1 to 1.5 minutes and a setting time of 3 to 5 minutes. The mixed material is inserted in one of two ways, depending upon the viscosity of the particular product. Viscous material is best placed with plastic instruments that do not adhere to the unset material. A small amount of bonding resin on the tip of the plastic instrument will prevent sticking. If the viscosity is low enough, the material may be injected into the cavity preparation from a syringe. A syringe placement tends to minimize the incorporation of voids into the restoration.

The cavity preparation is slightly overfilled. At 3.5 to 4 minutes after the start of mixing, the matrix band, if used, is removed. After an additional 2 to 6 minutes, the composite surface is sufficiently hard for finishing to begin.

Single-paste system

The shelf-life of composites supplied as single pastes and stored in a cool, dry environment is about one year.

The composite is best placed in small layers to minimize polymerization shrinkage. Shrinkage per layer placed is smaller if the tooth/composite bonding area per layer thickness is large. Each layer should be light cured for at least 40 seconds. After curing, a tacky, air-inhibited layer is present, through which the subsequent layer bonds.

Microfine composites require longer exposure times than do fine-particle composites because their colloidal-sized filler particles scatter blue light more efficiently.

Finishing

Composites are finished and polished in order to establish a functional occlusal relationship and a contour that is physiologically in harmony with supporting tissues. In addition, proper contour and high gloss give the restoration the appearance of a natural tooth structure. Early composites had large, hard quartz particles. Polishing preferentially removed the resin matrix, leaving filler particles exposed and giving the surface a dull appearance. In addition, quartz has a hardness about 2.5 times that of enamel and is difficult to polish compared to glasses, which have hardness characteristics similar to that of enamel.

Particles smaller than about 0.05 µm cannot be detected visually and allow polishing to a high luster. Fine-particle composites have no microfine particles, are considered to be only semi-polishable, and tend to have a rather opaque appearance. The colloidal-sized filler particles of microfine materials scatter light efficiently, giving these restorations a pleasing esthetic appearance. Hybrid composites are polishable, but are not as translucent as microfine composites.

Common prophylaxis pastes are very abrasive to composites and should not be used for polishing.

The composite surface may be contoured with a plastic matrix strip, but some gross reduction is often required. Finishing begins with coarse abrasives, such as 9- and 12-bladed finishing burs and fine diamonds, and progresses to 16- and 30-bladed finishing burs, ultrafine diamonds, and medium-grit abrasive points, discs, and strips. Polishing is accomplished with aluminum oxide polishing paste on a rubber cup at low speed.

A postocclusal adjustment cure of 40 seconds further hardens the surface. It is recommended that this step be followed by re-etching and the application and curing of a low-viscosity unfilled resin. The resin penetrates microcracks on the finished surface, further reducing wear.

Pitting has been observed on the surface of microfine-particle–reinforced composites after polishing. The pits are thought to occur at the junction of the new resin and the prepolymerized resin/filler, resulting in an increased susceptibility to chipping.

A properly placed anterior composite restoration has an expected clinical life of 7 to 10 years. Posterior restorations are generally serviceable for less than 5 years. The major reasons for replacing any composite include deterioration of esthetics, interfacial staining, wear, and secondary caries.

Material selection

A wide variety of composite resins is available for the clinician's use. The unique characteristics of composites make them desirable for a range of applications. Choosing the most suitable material requires matching a composite's desired properties under function to those of hard tissue. No one material is suited for all applications. Additionally, clinical performance data that may influence selection, such as long-term wear and serviceability of recently developed materials for posterior use, are still emerging.

The American Dental Association (ADA) classifies Class A materials as those intended for the restoration of occlusal surfaces, and Class B materials as those intended for other applications. Manufacturers are required to state the intended purpose of the product, describe the filler-particle size range, and list the major component of the resin matrix. At this point, ANSI/ADA Specification No. 27 for resin-based filling materials specifies minimum requirements for Class B materials only, and states that Class A materials should fulfill these requirements also. The acceptance of Class A materials must await further clinical evaluation programs beyond the limits of the current specifications.

For posterior use, hybrid composites with filler volumes of 60% to 65% appear to be most promising. These show Young's modulus values (7 to 14 GPa) similar to that of dentin, and Vickers hardness numbers (106 to 159) and compressive strengths (300 to 475 MPa) greater than that of dentin. As a group, these materials are most likely to withstand the higher stresses encountered during posterior function. A surface roughness (0.27 to 0.71 µm) matching or less than the average roughness of enamel-to-enamel occlusal contacts (0.64 µm) indicates that these materials are not likely to act as a destructive abrasive to opposing dentition.

For anterior use, both hybrid and microfine composites with filler volumes of 50% or higher appear to be satisfactory. These materials have Young's modulus values adequate to withstand the lower stresses present in anterior restorations under normal function (7 to 14 GPa). Their relatively low intrinsic roughness (0.11 to 0.34 µm) makes them suitable for anterior use. These materials are indicated for use in large Class III and V restorations and in Class IV restorations.

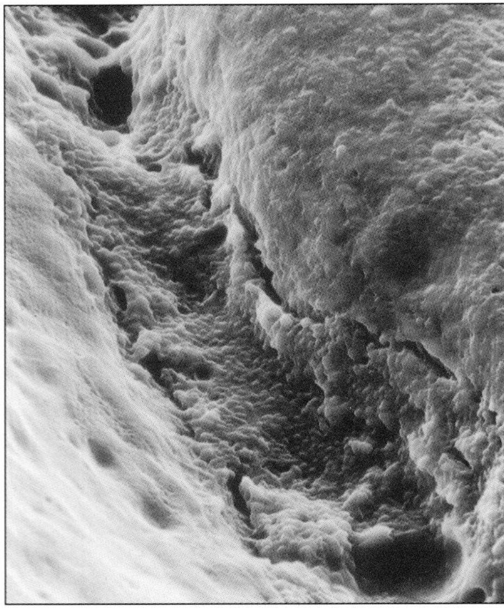

Fig 7-12 Ditching of a microfill composite margin. (Original magnification × 2,300.) (From Leinfelder K, 1979.)

Materials designated as microfine, with a mean particle size of 0.04 µm and volume fraction of 20% to 55%, are indicated in small Class III and V restorations because of their glossy appearance. These materials have low Young's modulus values (3 to 7 GPa), are susceptible to chipping, and are thus not indicated for larger, load-bearing applications. These materials also find application as veneers. None have radiopacities exceeding that of enamel. Another clinical characteristic of microfills is the occurrence of "ditching" from marginal fracture (Fig 7-12). This defect commonly occurs in areas under masticatory stress. In the case of anterior proximal restorations, this crevicing typically is found on the lingual aspect only. It apparently develops where the incisal edge of the mandible teeth contacts the lingual surface of the anterior teeth.

The traditional macrofills have largely been replaced. Though filler volume is moderately high, hard quartz particles impart a high intrinsic surface roughness (0.83 to 1.46 µm). In addition, quartz lacks radiopacity. Compressive strengths as a group fall slightly short of that of dentin (210 to 300 MPa), although these materials exhibit adequate longevity when used for posterior cores.

A third selection guideline, based on clinical judgment, is provided in Table 7-3.

Table 7-3 Clinical characteristics and selection of composite resins

	Filler size	Appearance	Polishability	Usage
Microfine	0.01–0.12 µm	Optical properties similar to enamel	Highly polishable	Non-stress-bearing esthetic restorations*
Hybrid	0.01–3.0 µm	Good gloss, luster, and smoothness	Polishable	Anterior and posterior restorations
Fine-particle	0.5–3.0 µm	Opaque appearance	Semi-polishable	Core buildups, conservative posterior restorations
Macrofill	15–35 µm	Dull, rough, and lusterless surface	Non-polishable	Core buildups

*Only heavily filled microfine materials may be used for posterior restorations.

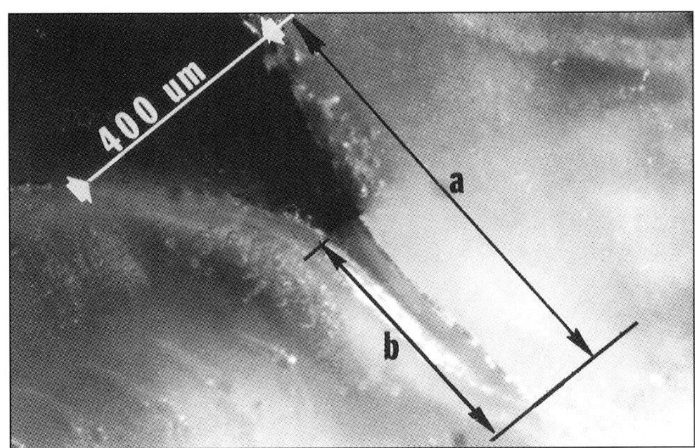

Fig 7-13 The penetration of a sealant into a fissure.

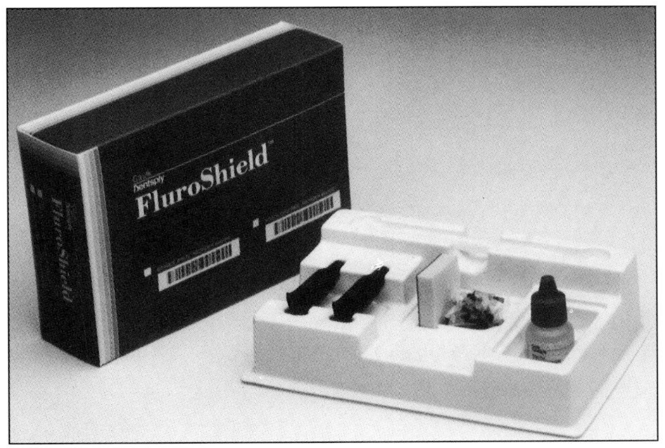

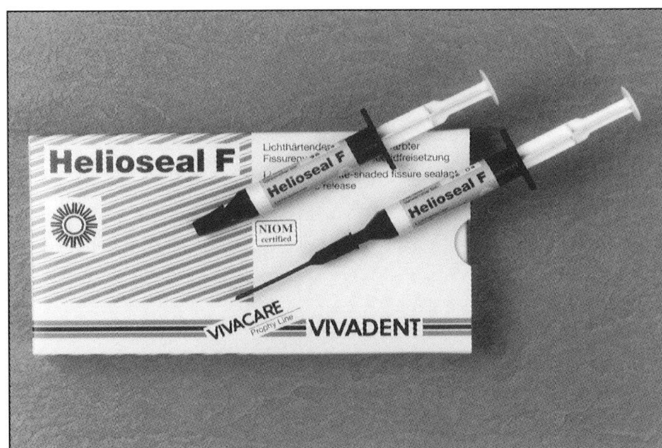

Fig 7-14 a and b Two commercial fluoride-containing sealants.

Pit and fissure sealants

These sealants are mainly fluid resins that are applied to posterior occlusal surfaces of caries-prone teeth to seal pits and fissures from bacterial action. The principal monomer used is Bis-GMA, which may be lightly filled with ceramic filler particles to improve wear resistance. Prior to application of the fluid monomer, the tooth enamel is etched with phosphoric acid. Upon application of the fluid resin, it penetrates into the pits and fissures by capillary action. There also is penetration into the microstructure of the etched enamel to form "tags" that lead to micromechanical action. Deep penetration is promoted by a high penetration coefficient (PC) which results from low viscosity, high surface tension, and low contact angle, that is, good wetting (Chapter 4). Figure 7-13 shows the penetration of a sealant into a fissure.

Sealants have been found to be effective in several studies. Long-term studies have shown around 50% decay reductions in sealed teeth compared with controls. About 90% of sealants are at least partially still present in 5-year studies. Also, partial loss or wear of a sealant does not prevent its preventive action in deep fissures. One disadvantage to using sealants is that they may trap food debris and bacteria that could lead to continued carious action. Studies have shown that although some food debris is usually trapped under sealants, the bacteria become dormant if they are isolated. Fluoride-containing sealants are also available. Figure 7-14 shows current fluoride-containing sealants.

Clinical decision scenarios for restorative materials

This section presents a formal approach to choosing restorative materials for specific situations. This approach is based on consideration of the advantages and disadvantages of each material and takes into account the different practitioner requirements, such as skill level, cost factors, and so on, as applicable.

Each scenario uses the following format:

1. A description of the situation
2. A list of the critical factors
3. A list of the advantages and disadvantages of each material prioritized using the following codes: *=of minor importance, **=important, ***=very important
4. An analysis of the situation and the decision reached

Situation Light-cured vs chemically cured composite materials for anterior Class III restorations

Description A patient is found to have a small interproximal carious lesion on the mesial surface of a permanent maxillary central incisor. He desires an esthetic restoration. The dentist has both visible light–cured composite material and chemically cured material in his armamentarium.

Critical factor Esthetics

	Light cure	Chemical cure
Advantages	*** 1. Good esthetics	*** 1. Good esthetics
	** 2. Better color stability	2. More complete cure
	3. Less porosity	3. Curing light not needed
	4. More working time	
Disadvantages	1. Less complete cure	1. More porosity
	2. Curing light needed	** 2. Poorer color stability
		3. Less working time

Analysis/Decision Although either material would be satisfactory, the greater color stability provides the determining factor in this instance and resulted in the selection for the light-cured material. The greater working time of light-cured material is convenient but not necessary to a dentist experienced in the use of the chemically cured material. The higher porosity of the chemically cured material—induced by the need to mix the paste and catalyst—as well as the activators and accelerators needed in the chemical cure, probably contribute to the lower color stability.

Situation Composite vs amalgam for cores

Description A patient comes to the office complaining of a broken tooth. Upon examination, the dentist finds that the lingual cusps of the lower right first permanent molar have fractured right at the gingival line. The tooth already has a large mesio-occlusodistal (MOD) amalgam in it, and the facial cusps are not sturdy. The patient is leaving for a winter vacation to Florida in 10 days and hopes to have the tooth repaired before then. The treatment plan is to prepare a pin-retained core buildup and then a full gold crown. The dentist has both amalgam and a composite core material available.

Critical factor Time

Advantages

	Amalgam	Composite
Advantages	1. Greater strength 2. Long clinical history	*** 1. Immediate set 2. Bonds to tooth 3. Can be prepared immediately
Disadvantages	*** 1. 24-hour set 2. No bond to tooth	1. Lesser strength

Analysis/Decision Although this may seem like an abbreviated list, these are essentially the main considerations. Even though the strength of the amalgam is thought to be greater in these applications, composites have served well if properly done. The deciding factor is often that the composite can be placed and prepared for the crown immediately, whereas it is recommended that the amalgam be allowed to set 24 hours before preparation. Thus, the composite may be done (and the tooth prepared) in one appointment. If amalgam had been the material of choice, a second appointment would have been necessary for the crown preparation. This, in fact, was the deciding factor that made the dentist choose the composite in this instance.

Glossary

acid-etch Selective etching of portions of the enamel rods with phosphoric acid, resulting in both high surface area and increased surface energy. Resin is able to flow into the enamel substructure and upon polymerization provides a mechanical bond to the enamel.

composite resin A material having two or more distinct components and with properties different from those of the individual components.

coupling agent A chemical attached to the filler surface for the purpose of creating a bond with the resin matrix upon polymerization. The presence of a coupling agent improves several properties of the composite, including strength and wear resistance.

cross-linked polymer A polymer with a three-dimensional network structure.

dimethacrylate A methacrylate monomer with reactive, or polymerizable, groups at each end.

fine-particle composite resins Composites containing fine-sized filler particles (0.5 to 3.0 µm). More polishable than macrofilled composites.

hybrid (blend) composite resins Composites containing colloidal silica (0.01 to 0.12 µm) in addition to fine-sized particles.

macrofilled composite resins First-generation composite resins that contain relatively large filler particles (15 to 35 µm).

microfine composite resins Composites containing colloidal silica as filler. Most polishable and translucent of the composite resins.

monomer A single molecule with double or triple bonds that are capable of uniting the monomers into oligomers or polymers.

oligomer A short polymer made up of two to four monomer units.

polymer A macromolecule formed by the linkage of monomers or oligomers.

polymerization The process by which a polymer is formed from monomers or oligomers.

Discussion questions

1. Why are these materials called "polymeric restorative materials" when they usually contain mostly ceramic phases?
2. How have composites overcome many of the problems of unfilled resin filling materials?
3. How are composite materials currently doing in replacing dental amalgam?
4. Although microfine composite materials have inferior mechanical properties, they continue to be widely used. Why?

Questions and answers

1. **What is the general composition of composite resin restorative materials?** Composite resins contain two major components: a polymer matrix and a ceramic filler. The polymer consists of a dimethacrylate oligomer (Bis-GMA or UDMA). Larger filler particles may be quartz or any of a number of glasses. The colloidal-size particles of microfine composites are silica. In addition, a silane coupling agent is attached to the filler surface to create a particle/matrix bond during polymerization.
2. **What are the applications for composite resin restorative materials?** Composite resins are commonly used for the restoration of Class III and Class V cavity preparations, for replacement of fractured incisal edges (Class IV), and for veneering of facial surfaces of natural teeth. Continued improvement has led to their use in selected, conservative posterior restorations. They are also used in the repair of porcelain and for the cosmetic recontour of anterior teeth.
3. **How long do composite restorations last?** Longevity of conventional composite resins varies. In general, composite restorations in anterior teeth provide adequate serviceability for up to 10 years. Class III restorations tend to last longer than those placed in cervical regions because they are exposed to less mechanical abrasion and stress due to tooth flexure. Posterior composite resins have a shorter service life, generally requiring replacement within 5 years. Reasons for replacement of any composite include deterioration of esthetics, wear, and recurrent decay.

4. **What are the disadvantages of macrofilled composite resins?** The large quartz filler particles of macrofilled composites produce a rough surface upon polishing, resulting in the retention of plaque. Quartz particles are hard enough that they are able to abrade opposing enamel. In addition, quartz lacks radiopacity. Macrofills also have poorer esthetics than microfills.

5. **What are the advantages of fine-particle composites?** Fine-sized particles (0.5 to 3.0 μm) permit maximal filler loading and improved polishability compared to macrofilled composites. Fine-particle composites have superior physical and mechanical properties compared to microfine composites, which have a lower filler content.

6. **What are the advantages of microfine composites?** Microfine composites contain colloidal silica (0.01 to 0.12 μm) as filler. Because the diameter of the particles is less than 0.05 μm, they cannot be detected visually, giving the composite a translucent quality and allowing polishing to a high luster.

7. **What is a "hybrid" or "blend" composite?** A hybrid composite contains colloidal silica in addition to larger filler particles. The colloidal silica is commonly added to improve certain handling characteristics, such as flow and packability. Hybrid composites can be used for both anterior and posterior restorations, because they combine the physical properties of fine-particle composites and the esthetics of microfills.

8. **What is polymerization shrinkage, and why is it a problem?** Polymerization of the polymer matrix after placement results in shrinkage of the matrix and places stresses on the bond at the tooth/composite interface. At present, the enamel/composite bond is more likely to withstand these stresses than is the dentin/composite bond. Loss of marginal integrity results in an influx of oral fluids and greatly increases the possibility of postplacement sensitivity and recurrent decay.

Recommended reading

Abdulrahman A-D, Wennberg A. Biocompatibility of dentin bonding agents. Endod Dent Traumatol 9:1–7, 1993.

Asmussen E. Factors affecting the quantity of remaining double bonds in restorative resin polymers. Scand J Dent Res 90:490–496, 1982.

Craig RG. Restorative Dental Materials. 9th ed. St. Louis: CV Mosby Co, 1993.

Eick JD, Robinson SJ, Byerley TJ, Chappelow CC. Adhesives and nonshrinking dental resins of the future. Quintessence Int 24:632–640, 1993.

Eliades G, Palaghias G, Vougiouklakis G. Surface reactions of adhesives on dentin. Dent Mater 6:208–216, 1990.

Farah JW, Powers JM. Anterior and posterior composites. The Dental Advisor 8(4):1–8, 1991.

McKinney JE, Wu W. Chemical softening and wear of dental composites. J Dent Res 64(11):1326–1331, 1985.

O'Brien WJ, Yee JJ. Microstructure of posterior restorations of composite resins after clinical wear. Oper Dent Vol 5(3):90–94, 1980.

Pearson GJ, Longman CM. Water sorption and solubility of resin-based materials following inadequate polymerization by a visible-light curing system. J Oral Rehabil 16:57–61, 1989.

Powers JM, Fan PL, Raptis CN. Color stability of new composite restorative materials under accelerated aging. J Dent Res 59(12):2071–2074, 1980.

Ruyter IE, Øysæd H. Composites for use in posterior teeth: Composition and conversion. J Biomed Mater Res 21:11–23, 1987.

Van Meerbeek B, Braem M, Lambrechts P, Vanherle G. Two-year clinical evaluation of two dentine-adhesive systems in cervical lesions. J Dent 21(4):195–202, 1993.

Van Meerbeek B, Lambrechts P, Inokoshi S, Braem M, Vanherle G. Factors affecting adhesion to mineralized tissues. Oper Dent Suppl 5:111–124, 1992.

Wendt SL Jr, Leinfelder KF. Clinical evaluation of a heat-treated resin composite inlay: 3-year results. Am J Dent 5:258–262, 1992.

Willems G, Lambrechts P, Braem M, Vanherle G. Composite resins in the 21st century. Quintessence Int 24:641–658, 1993.

Willems G, Lambrechts P, Braem M, Vanherle G. Three-year follow-up of five posterior composites; *in vivo* wear. J Dent 21:74–78, 1993.

Zidan O, Gomez-Marin O, Tsuchiya T. A comparative study of the effects of dentinal bonding agents and application techniques on marginal gaps in Class V cavities. J Dent Res 66(3):716–721, 1987.

Chapter 8

Abrasion, Polishing, and Bleaching

Abrasion is the process of wear on the surface of one material by another material by scratching, gouging, chiseling, tumbling, or other mechanical means. The material that causes the wear is called an *abrasive*; the material being abraded is called the *substrate*.

Polishing is the process of making a rough surface smooth to the touch and glossy (mostly specular reflection of incident light) (Fig 8-1a). Polishing is usually performed with very-small-particle–size (submicron-size) abrasives.

Grinding is the gross reduction of the surface of a substrate by the process of abrasion; it is usually performed with large-particle–size abrasives. The surface texture of the substrate after a grinding procedure is usually rough to the touch and gives a diffuse reflection to incident light (Fig 8-1b).

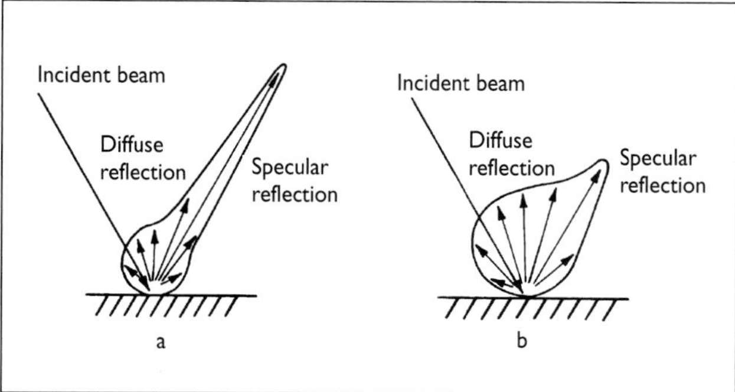

Fig 8-1 Schematic diagram of diffuse and specular reflection: (a) high gloss; (b) low gloss. (From O'Brien et al, 1984. Reprinted with permission.)

Abrasion

Many abrasives used in dentistry are particles that are bonded to a mandrel or disk for use in a rotary handpiece. Some abrasives are used as powders (or pastes) to be applied to the substrate using a cloth wheel, brush, or cup. The basic principles set forth in this chapter apply whether an abrasive is used in a bonded form or a powdered form.

Factors affecting rate of abrasion

1. *A large difference in hardness* between the abrasive and substrate (eg, tooth enamel, amalgam) allows the most efficient grinding to take place. Brinell and Knoop hardness values are functions of a material's resistance to indentation, whereas Mohs values indicate one material's resistance to scratching by another (Table 8-1).
2. *The particle size* of an abrasive may be expressed in micrometers. By convention, particles are classified as fine (0 to 10 µm), medium (10 to 100 µm), and coarse (100 to 500 µm), according to the average particle size of the sample. Larger abrasive particles will abrade a surface more rapidly than will smaller particles; however, they tend to leave coarser scratches in the abraded surface than do fine particles. Equivalent-sized scratches can be produced by different sizes of particles by varying the applied pressure (Fig 8-2a).
3. *The particle shape* also has an effect on rate of abrasion. Sharp, irregularly shaped particles will abrade

Table 8-1 Hardness of dental abrasives and substrates

Material	Hardness scale		
	Mohs	Brinell	Knoop
Abrasives			
Talc	1		
Gypsum	2		
Chalk	3		
Rouge	5–6		
Pumice	6	450	560
Tripoli	6–7		
Garnet	6.5–7	550	
Tin oxide	6–7		
Sand	7	650	800
Cuttle	7	650	800
Tool steel	—	800	
Zirconium silicate	7–7.5		
Tungsten carbide	9	1,200	2,100
Aluminum oxide	9	1,700	1,900
Silicon carbide	9–10	3,000	2,500
Boron carbide	9–10		2,800
Diamond	10	>3,000	7,000
Substrates			
Acrylic	2–3		25
Pure gold	2.5–3	30	
Hard gold alloys	3–4		
Amalgam	4–5	90	
Dentin	3–4		
Enamel	5–6	270	
Glass	5–6		
Composite	5–7		200
Porcelain	6–7	400	

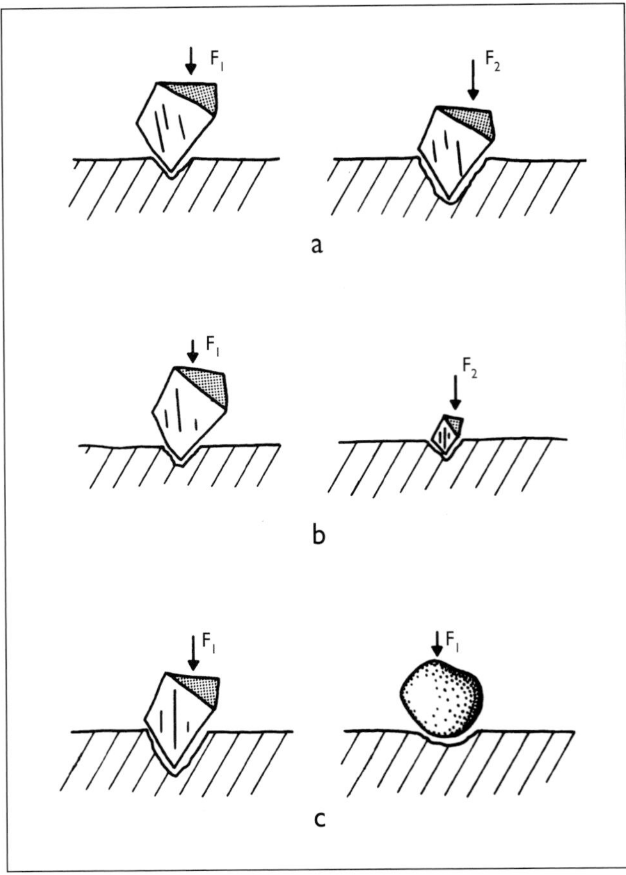

Fig 8-2 Factors affecting abrasion. (a) Large particle (*left*) produces similar scratches with lower applied force (F_1) than smaller particle (*right*). (b) Sharp particle (*left*) produces deeper abrasion than rounder particle (*right*) under applied force. (c) Deeper and wider scratches (*right*) are produced by increasing the applied force from F_1 to F_2.

a surface more rapidly than will more rounded particles having duller cutting angles. However, the former will produce deeper scratches than the latter (Fig 8-2b). The abrasion rate of an abrasive decreases during use; this is due partly to rounding of the particles and partly to contamination of the abrasive with some of the substrate material (debris).

4. *The greater the speed* at which the abrasive travels across the surface of the substrate, the greater the rate of abrasion. The greater friction at higher speeds, however, tends to create higher temperatures at the surface of the substrate.
5. *The greater the pressure* applied, the more rapid will be the abrasion for a given abrasive. Greater pressure produces deeper and wider scratches (Fig 8-2c) and creates higher temperatures (and patient discomfort).
6. *Lubricants* (eg, silicone grease, water spray, glycerol) are used during abrasion for two purposes: to reduce heat buildup, and to wash away debris to prevent clogging or "blinding" of the abrasive instrument. Too much lubrication can reduce the abrasion rate because it may prevent some of the abrasive from coming in contact with the substrate.

Polishing

In order to produce a smooth, lustrous surface by abrasion, successively smaller abrasive sizes must be used. Larger abrasive particles remove large amounts of material from the substrate, and smaller particles smooth out the roughness produced by the larger particles. Final polishing of a surface with a very fine abrasive produces a virtually scratch-free surface by creating a thin microcrystalline or amorphous layer on the surface of the substrate.

It is extremely important to remove all debris and abrasive particles from the surface of the substrate before using a finer abrasive during the polishing sequence. Even a single abrasive particle left on the substrate from a previous step will continue to scratch the surface during the subsequent polishing steps.

Appearance and feel of polished surfaces

A polished surface is important for esthetic and functional reasons. If the scratches produced by the abrasives are greater in width than the wavelength of visible light (ie, approximately 0.5 μm), the surface will appear to have a dull finish. If the scratches are less than about 0.5 μm in width, the surface will appear shiny. In addition, it has been found that the tongue can distinguish subtle differences in roughness; scratches more than 20 μm deep feel rough, whereas those less than 2 μm deep feel smooth.

Applications of abrasives

Dental prophylaxis pastes

Prophylaxis pastes should be chosen carefully and applied to remove exogenous stains without damaging the underlying tooth structure or adjacent restorative materials. The abrasive selected should be harder than the surface stain being removed and softer than the tooth surface, although this is not always practicable. If the tooth structure is excessively roughened during the procedure, it should be polished with a fine abrasive (such as zirconium silicate); otherwise, plaque and food substances will easily adhere to it.

The most common abrasives used in prophylaxis pastes are pumice, silica, zirconium silicate, and other silicates. They are usually supplied in various particle sizes (coarse, medium, fine), which produce different rates of abrasion and sizes of scratches. Sodium fluoride or stannous fluoride are incorporated into some prophylaxis pastes to help prevent dental caries.

Dentifrices

Dentifrice pastes are used for removing debris and minor stains from teeth and for polishing tooth surfaces. The most commonly used abrasives are dibasic calcium phosphate dihydrate, anhydrous dibasic calcium phosphate, tricalcium phosphate, calcium pyrophospate, and hydrated alumina.

Many dentifrices contain therapeutic agents, such as sodium fluoride, stannous fluoride, or sodium monofluorophosphate, to decrease the acid solubility of tooth enamel, decrease hypersensitivity, and interrupt the mechanisms of plaque attachment and calculus formation on tooth structure. Dentifrice pastes additionally may contain a humectant to reduce evaporation of water, a surface-active detergent, binders, flavoring and sweetening agents, and a preservative.

Abrasive values for dentifrice products have been reported as an abrasivity index (AI), which is a measure of the abrasion of dentin.

In selecting a dentifrice for a patient, the following factors should be considered: degree of staining, toothbrushing habits (force, stiffness of brush, method of brushing), presence of relatively soft restorative materials (eg, acrylic resin veneers, silicates), and the amount of exposed cementum and dentin.

Denture cleaners

Food debris, plaque, calculus, and stains may accumulate on denture base materials in the same way as natural teeth and are best removed on a regular basis by the patient. Daily soaking in a denture cleanser solution or brushing with or without a paste or powder is usually effective.

Chemical cleansers may contain sodium perborate, which releases peroxide. As peroxide decomposes, oxygen is released, resulting in effervescence. Effervescence, along with the oxidizing ability of peroxide, are assumed to be responsible for the cleaning action.

Dentures may also be soaked in a dilute solution of 5% sodium hypochlorite (1:3 water). Other chemical denture cleansers may contain dilute acids or enzymes.

Dentures should not be soaked in hot water, which may warp the denture base material.

Brushing may be needed to remove stains and stubborn deposits. Hard-bristle brushes or brushing with much force may abrade the plastic surface of the denture and should be avoided. Dentifrices are generally too abrasive for use with dentures, although some with gentle abrasives (sodium bicarbonate or acrylic resin) can be used. Organic solvents should be avoided, as they may cause crazing and eventual cracking of the denture material. Ultrasonic vibration has not been shown to adequately remove plaque from dentures.

Handpiece instruments

Handpiece instruments include stones, burs, rubber wheels, and disks. Bonded abrasives are available for dental use in various shapes, abrasive sizes, and hardnesses:

1. *Dental stones* are composed of abrasive particles that have been sintered together or bonded with an organic resin to form a cohesive mass. These stones are available in fine, medium, and coarse grades. The color of the stone is an indication of the particular abrasive used; green stones contain silicon carbide, and white stones contain aluminum oxide. Diamond stones generally have a higher cutting efficiency than silicon carbide or aluminum oxide.
2. *Dental excavating burs* have a cutting action on tooth structure that is similar to grinding and polishing. Low-speed burs are composed of either carbon tool steel or tungsten carbide. High-speed burs are almost exclusively composed of the harder tungsten carbide. Burs with eight blades can be used for gross reduction of tooth structure and removal of old restorations, and they produce a rather rough surface texture on the substrate. Burs with 12, 20, or 40 blades can be used for producing a smooth surface on tooth structure and restorations. Of significance is the relative hardness values of the burs and the substrates (see Table 8-1). Hard restorative materials (such as quartz-filled composite restorative materials and dental porcelain) will rapidly dull the sharp cutting edges of the high-speed tungsten carbide burs. Cutting efficiency and durability of the burs varies greatly among manufacturers and design types. Crosscut fissure burs have higher cutting efficiency than plain fissure burs, but they produce a rougher surface.
3. *Rubber wheels* are used for fine grinding of restorative materials (removing coarse scratches from rough grinding). They are made by molding fine abrasives (such as aluminum oxide, silicon carbide, and chromium oxide) in an elastomeric matrix.
4. *Disks and strips* are made by bonding abrasive particles onto a thin plastic backing. They generally wear out rapidly due to the loss of abrasive particles. They are particularly useful in finishing relatively flat surfaces. Abrasives commonly used on disks and strips are garnet, emery, aluminum oxide, and quartz (cuttle).

Techniques for polishing restorative materials

Dental amalgam

A polished surface is desirable on dental amalgam to retard the collection of plaque and help retard tarnish as well. Burnishing alone does not create as smooth a surface as does polishing. Although an amalgam restoration can be burnished immediately after carving, most brands should be left undisturbed for at least 24 hours before polishing in order to allow the amalgam to set completely. Polishing can then be performed with a rotary instrument (cup, brush, or felt) with a fine abrasive mixed with water or alcohol in a slurry or paste; flour of pumice (ground volcanic glass), extra-fine silex (various silicates, such as quartz or tripoli), or tin oxide may also be used for this purpose. Care must be taken to use sufficient water or alcohol to avoid frictional heating of the restoration, which could cause pulpal damage.

Fast-setting high-copper amalgams may be successfully polished 10 to 12 minutes following placement.

Gold alloys

Gold alloys are finished by using coarse, medium, and fine abrasives in sequence. Coarse scratches are removed with fine pumice or coarse abrasive rubber wheels; the surface is finished with a rubber wheel impregnated with a fine abrasive and finally polished with tripoli and rouge on rag wheels. Particular care must be taken to avoid overfinishing of contours and margins.

Acrylic resin denture bases and veneers

Gypsum material left on the denture base following processing and deflasking may be removed with a "shell blaster." Small blebs on the resin surface may be scraped off or removed with an acrylic finishing bur. Denture base material is comparatively soft and can be finished easily with a rag wheel and fine pumice followed by tripoli or tin oxide. Care must be taken not to alter the contour of the denture during finishing. Acrylic denture teeth are particularly easily abraded by pumice.

Composite resin restorations

Composite resin restorations present a unique polishing problem because they are composed of a relatively soft polymeric resin and a hard filler. Relief polishing may result due to unequal wear rates of the resin and filler, leaving "valleys" between the filler particles (Fig 8-3). This is very apparent in large-particle (conventional type) composite resins, which still look and feel rough after finishing with available dental abrasives (Fig 8-4). Although relief polishing still takes place during the finishing of microfilled composite resins, the valleys and filler particles are so small that the surface appears glossy (large specular component of reflection) and feels smooth (Fig 8-5). The new types of hybrid and small-particle composite resins also tend to appear shiny and smooth but cannot be polished as easily as the microfilled composite resins.

A typical sequence for polishing composite resins would be as follows: coarse grinding with a diamond stone or a green stone followed by a series of coarse to fine quartz or aluminum oxide abrasive disks or rubber wheels. Carbide burs with 12 or more blades have also been used to polish composite resins. Finishing instru-

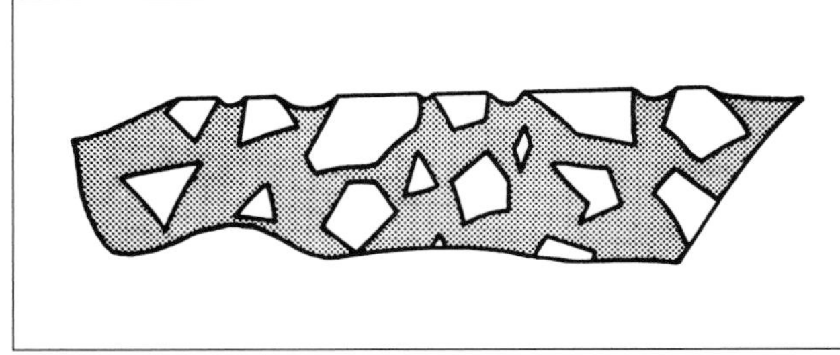

Fig 8-3 Uneven wear of composite surface producing valleys in the resin matrix between the hard filler particles.

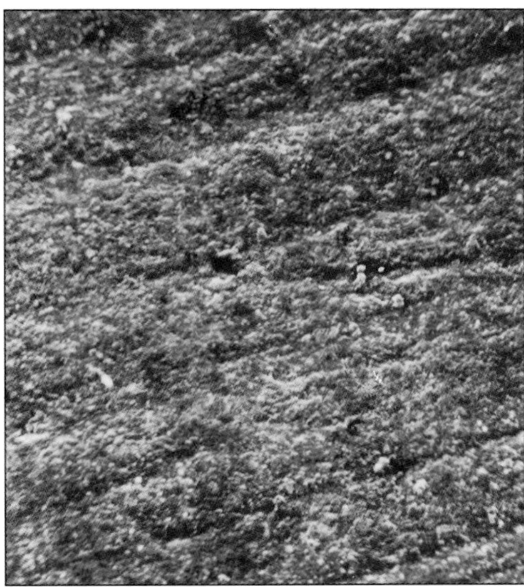

Fig 8-4 Scanning electron micrograph of a composite restorative material with conventional filler, finished with a 12-fluted bur. (From O'Brien et al, 1984. Reprinted with permission.)

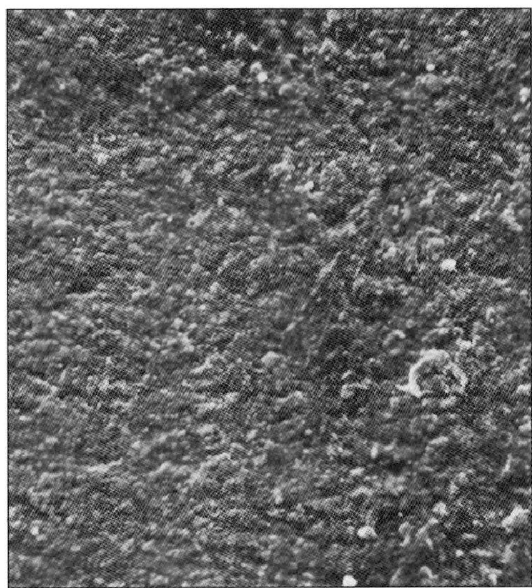

Fig 8-5 Scanning electron micrograph of a composite restorative material with smaller filler particles in the micron range, finished with the rubber-abrasive composite resin wheel. (From O'Brien et al, 1984. Reprinted with permission.)

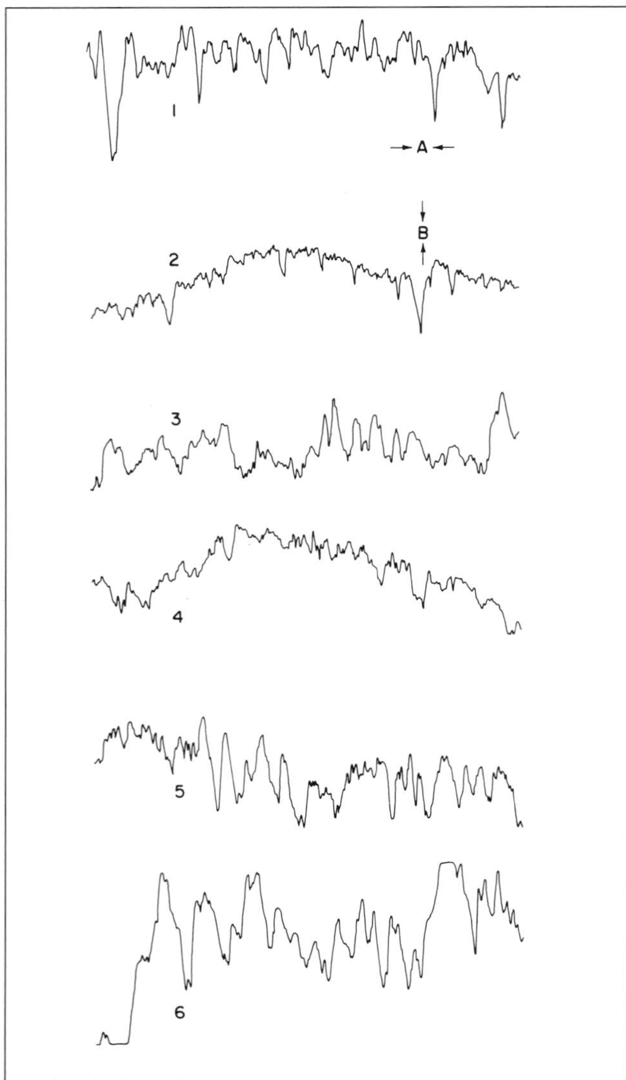

Fig 8-6 Roughness profiles of conventional composite resin surfaces finished with: (1) green to white stone; (2) SiC disks; (3) 12-fluted bur; (4) 40-fluted bur; (5) green to white stone to alumina paste; and (6)diamond stone. For scale: A = 50 µm; B = 2 µm. (From Tolley et al, 1978. Reprinted with permission.)

ments for composite resins are available commercially. The effects of several polishing sequences on the surface roughness of composite resins are shown in Fig 8-6, which are tracings from the surface analyzer shown in Fig 8-7.

Porcelain

The best way to obtain a smooth, glossy surface on dental porcelain is by glazing in a porcelain oven. After minor adjustments of the surface of a porcelain restoration, the porcelain can be polished using a series of coarse to fine abrasive rubber wheels (containing silicon carbide or aluminum oxide), followed by a fine-particle–size diamond paste applied on a felt wheel.

Bleaching

Bleaching has been used to whiten teeth since the 1800s, but with the introduction of home bleaching systems in 1989, its use has widened. In 1991, safety concerns led to a U.S. Food and Drug Administration ban, which has since been lifted while data are collected.

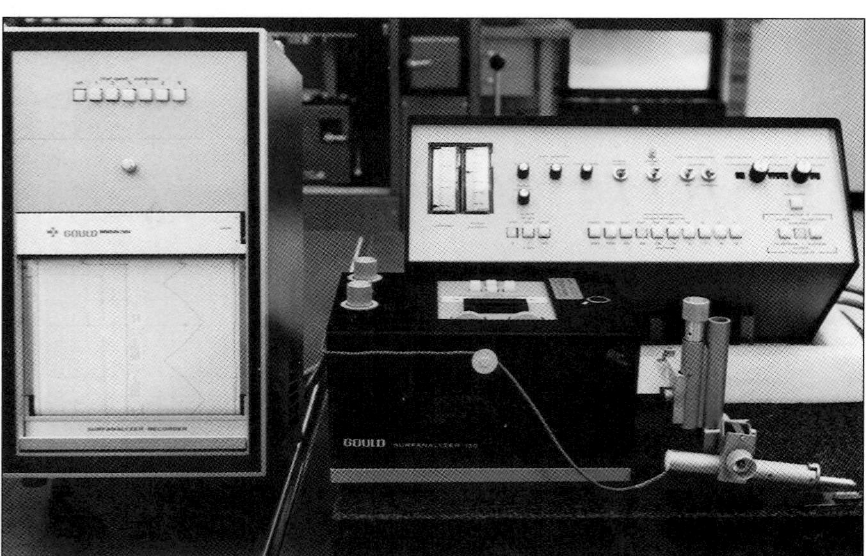

Fig 8-7 Surface analyzer using a diamond stylus to produce roughness profiles (Surfanalyzer, Gould, Inc.).

Dentist office systems usually employ 35% hydrogen peroxide with strong lights, which increase the bleaching effect, whereas home bleaching systems usually contain 10%–15% carbamide peroxide or 1%–10% hydrogen peroxide in a glycerine base. Dentist office treatments may also involve microabrasion to remove thin stained outer layers of enamel with hydrochloric acid and a fine abrasive.

The results of bleaching last about a year. Deep, dark stains are better handled with porcelain veneers. Side effects of bleaching include tooth hypersensitivity, soft tissue lesions, and sore throats and nausea from swallowing the bleach. Due to the possibility of tooth hypersensitivity, anesthesia should not be used during treatment, which would mask irritation of the pulp. About three office appointments are usually required for dark stains. Home bleaching techniques require that the bleaching gel be left in contact with the teeth for 3–4 hours per day in a tray. Considerable care is needed to protect the patient's eyes and to discontinue the treatment if painful. Although bleaching can be useful, many patients have an unrealistic view of the natural color of teeth and undergo unnecessary treatment.

Glossary

abrasion The mechanical process of wear of the surface of one material by another.

abrasive The material that causes the wear or abrasion of another material.

abrasivity index (AI) A method of rating the abrasiveness of dentifrices.

amorphous Without crystalline structure; having random arrangement of atoms in space.

blinding Clogging of an abrasive wheel with debris, causing reduction of abrasive action.

dental stones Grinding instruments composed of abrasive particles bound in a hard resin matrix or sintered together into a hard mass.

disks Grinding and polishing rotary instruments composed of abrasive particles cemented to a flexible plastic backing.

grit size Numerical grading of particle size. Larger numbers (eg, 600) denote fine particles, and smaller numbers (eg, 120) denote coarse particles.

mesh size Numerical grading of particle size (also called sieve sizes). Larger numbers (eg, 325) denote fine particles, and smaller numbers (eg, 100) denote coarse particles.

microcrystalline Composed of tiny (submicron) crystals.

micron 0.001 mm or 0.00004 inch.

rubber wheels Grinding and polishing instruments composed of abrasive particles in a flexible rubber matrix.

strips Instruments for grinding and polishing interproximal areas; composed of abrasive particles cemented to a flexible plastic backing.

substrate The material being abraded.

Discussion questions

1. Since many esthetic porcelain restorations are given a final thin layer of stain glaze for color matching, how could toothpaste cause an undesirable change in color?
2. How could polishing teeth reduce the need for bleaching?
3. Why is trying to obtain snow white teeth by bleaching unrealistic?
4. What are the dangers of bleaching teeth, and what are the current regulations regarding the use of these products?

Questions and answers

1. **What is an abrasive?** A material that causes wear of another material through mechanical means.
2. **Which factors affect the rate of abrasion?** Hardness, particle size and shape, speed and pressure, lubrication.
3. **Place the following in order of hardness: cuttle, rouge, silicon carbide, chalk, sand, diamond, aluminum oxide, and pumice.** Chalk, rouge, pumice, cuttle, sand, aluminum oxide, silicon carbide, diamond.
4. **Rouge is used to polish gold alloys. What effect do you think it would have on dental porcelain?** Little effect; it is too soft to be a good polishing agent for dental porcelain.
5. **Why is it important to obtain polished surfaces on dentition?** For esthetic and functional reasons (to retard plaque accumulation).
6. **During grinding and polishing, what would be the effect if coarse abrasive particles were present from a previous step during the final polishing step? How can this be avoided?** Coarse particles would leave scratches on the polished surface. Avoid contamination of the instruments used and have the patient rinse between the grinding and polishing steps.
7. **How sensitive is the tongue to scratches?** The tongue can distinguish between 20-μm and 2-μm scratch depths.
8. **What are some common abrasives found in**
   a. **prophylaxis pastes?** Pumice, sand, zirconium silicate, and chalk.
   b. **dentifrices?** Chalk, dibasic calcium phosphate dihydrate, anhydrous dibasic calcium phosphate, tricalcium phosphate, calcium pyrophosphate, and hydrated alumina.
   c. **stones, rubber wheels, and disks?** Aluminum oxide, silicon carbide, and sand.
9. **Which criteria would you use in selecting a dentifrice for a patient?** Degree of staining, toothbrushing habits, soft restorative materials present in the oral cavity, and amount of exposed cementum or dentin.
10. **When should you polish an amalgam restoration? Which materials would you use?** An amalgam restoration should be polished at least 24 hours after placing. Use flour of pumice, extra-fine silex, or tin oxide on a rotating cup, brush, or felt.
11. **Why are composite restorations difficult to polish? When would a rough surface on a composite restoration be desirable?** They are composed of two phases with greatly different hardnesses. A rough surface would be desirable if more composite material or surface glaze had to be added to a previously set composite restorative material.

Recommended reading

American Dental Association. Dentists' Desk Reference: Materials, Instruments and Equipment. 2nd ed. Chicago: ADA, 1983.

Ashmore H, et al. The measurement in vitro of dentine abrasion by toothpaste. Br Dent J 133:60, 1972.

Buehler Analyst. Sections 4 and 5. Evanston: Buchler Ltd, 1975; 111.

Council on Dental Therapeutics: Guidelines for the acceptance of peroxide-containing oral hygiene products. J Am Dent Assoc 125:1140, 1994.

Gerdin PO. Studies in dentifrices. IV. Size and shape of particles in commercial dentifrices. Svensk Tandlak T 64(7):447–461, 1971.

Grabenstetter RJ, et al. The measurement of the abrasion of human teeth by dentifrice abrasives: a test utilizing radioactive teeth. J Dent Res 37:1060–1069, 1958.

Haywood VB, et al. Effectiveness, side effects and long-term status of nightguard vital bleaching. J Am Dent Assoc 125:1219, 1994.

Hefferen JJ, et al. Abrasivity of dentifrice products. J Am Dent Assoc 81:1177, 1970.

Norton FH. Elements of Ceramics. 2nd ed. Reading, MA: Addison-Wesley, 1974; 260–268.

O'Brien WJ, et al. The surface roughness and gloss of composites. J Dent Res 63(5):685–688, 1984.

Phillips RW. Skinner's Science of Dental Materials. 7th ed. Philadelphia: WB Saunders Co, 1973; 623–640.

Powers JM, Roberts JC, Craig RG. Wear of filled and unfilled dental restorative resins. Wear 39:117–122, 1976.

Reder BS, Eames WB. The cutting rates and durability of diamond stones. J Dent Res (Abstr no 499) 55(B):186, 1976.

Stookey GK, Muhler JC. Laboratory studies concerning the enamel and dentin abrasion properties of common dentifrice polishing agents. J Dent Res 47(4):524–532, 1968.

Tolley LG, O'Brien WJ, Dennison JB. Surface finish of dental composite restorative materials. J Biomed Mater Res 12:233–240, 1978.

Whitehurst JF, Stookey GK, Muhler JC. Studies concerning the cleaning, polishing, and therapeutic properties of commercial prophylactic pastes. J Oral Therm Pharm 4(3):181–191, 1968.

Chapter 9

Impression Materials

Impression materials are used to make replicas of oral structures. All impression materials must be in a plastic or fluid state while the replica is being made. Physical change, chemical reaction, or polymerization convert these fluid materials into either elastic or nonelastic (ie, plastic or brittle) negative replicas of the soft and/or hard tissues of the mouth. A model or cast material (eg, high-strength stone) is poured into the impression and, upon setting, produces a positive impression of the tissues of interest. Nonelastic materials include impression plaster, impression compound, and zinc oxide–eugenol. Elastic materials in current use are agar hydrocolloid, alginate, polysulfide, condensation silicone, addition silicone, and polyether. These materials will be discussed separately. A classification key is shown in Fig 9-1.

The American Dental Association's (ADA's) Council on Dental Materials, Instruments, and Equipment is responsible for developing and disseminating specifications for dental materials, instruments, and equipment. The American National Standards Institute (ANSI) has made the Council the Administrative Secretariat of the American National Standards Commit-

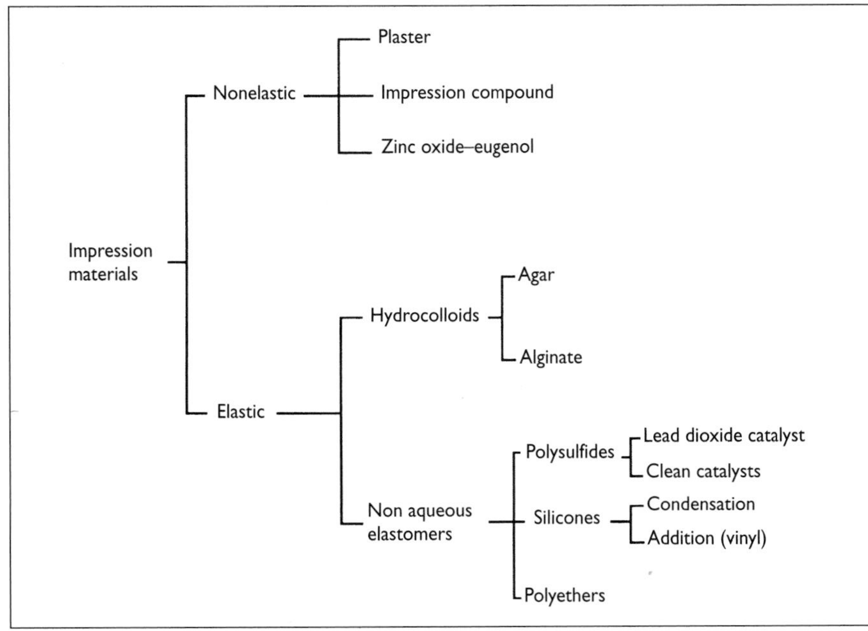

Fig 9-1 A classification key of impression materials.

Table 9-1 American Dental Association/American National Standards Institute specifications for dental impression materials

Material	ADA/ANSI Specification
Dental impression compound	3
Zinc oxide–eugenol impression paste	16
Dental agar impression material	11
Alginate impression material	18
Nonaqueous, elastomeric impression material	19
Dental duplicating material	20
Dental gypsum products	25

tee MD156 for Dental Materials, Instruments, and Equipment. Specifications relating to dental impression materials are listed in Table 9-1.

Nonelastic materials

Impression plaster

Plaster of Paris is seldom used as impression material now that elastomeric materials are available, but it can be used as a wash material for edentulous impressions. The main component of impression plaster is calcium sulfate hemihydrate, which reacts with water to form calcium sulfate dihydrate. Manufacturers incorporate additives to adjust the setting time and setting expansion. The water/powder (W/P) ratio recommended by the manufacturer should be measured out carefully. The powder should be sprinkled into the water, allowed to sit for 30 seconds to wet the powder, and then mixed for the minimum time necessary to obtain a homogeneous mix. Impression plaster is rigid and will break rather than bend. The plaster must be stored in an airtight container as it will absorb water from the air and its setting time will be adversely affected.

Dental impression compound (Types I and II)

There are two types of dental compound as defined by the American Dental Association. Type I is used for impression taking, and Type II is used for tray preparation. Although dental compound has fallen into disuse, it can be used for full crown impressions (Type I), impressions of partially or wholly edentulous jaws (Type I), and impression trays in which a final impression is taken with another material (Type II). Compound cannot be used to record undercuts since it is not elastic. Impression compound is available in either cakes or sticks in various colors from a number of manufacturers (JF Jelenko and Co., Kerr Corp., Mizzy, Inc., and Moyco Industries, Inc.).

Composition

Dental compound contains several ingredients. Natural resins, which comprise about 40% of the formulation, make the compound thermoplastic. Shellac is often used. Waxes (about 7%) also produce thermoplastic properties. Stearic acid (about 3%) acts as a lubricant and plasticizer. Fillers and inorganic pigments account for the remaining 50% of the formulation. Diatomaceous earth, soapstone, and talc are examples of commonly used fillers.

Thermal and mechanical properties

Dental compound is thermoplastic; it is used warm (45°C) and then cooled to mouth temperature (37°C), at which it is fairly rigid. The setting mechanism is therefore a reversible physical process rather than a chemical reaction. Dental compound is limited by its thermal properties. Type I materials have a flow of at least 85% at 45°C and less than 6% at 37°C. Type II materials flow about 70% at 45°C but less than 2% at 37°C. Both types become quite plastic with only an 8° rise in temperature. The thermal conductivity of dental impression compounds is very low. These materials do not conduct heat very well and therefore require heat soaking to attain a uniform temperature throughout the mass. When heated or cooled, they soften or harden quickly on the outside, but time is needed for the temperature to become uniform throughout the entire mass. If the impression is removed from the mouth before it has cooled completely, severe distortion may occur. Since these materials contain resins and waxes, they have high thermal expansion and contraction coefficients. Contraction from mouth temperature to room temperature may be as high as 0.3%. Therefore, the dimensions of the resulting impression could be significantly different than those of the mouth. Since compound has such a high viscosity, it is difficult to record details (Fig 9-2).

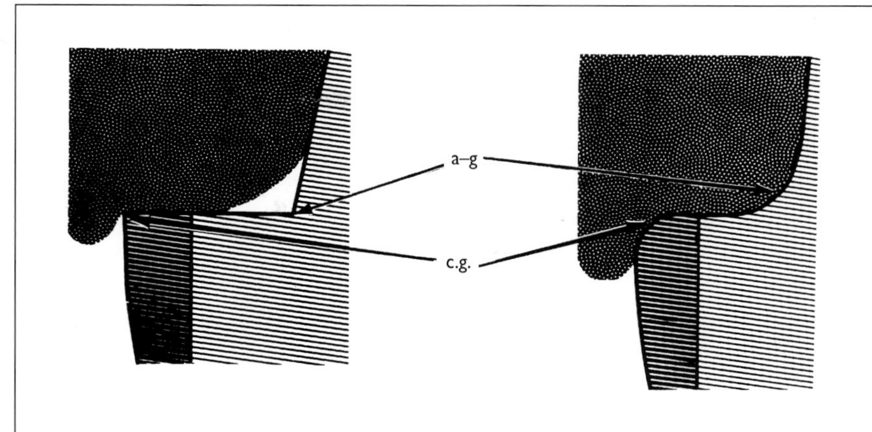

Fig 9-2 Problems in recording details with compound. The cavogingival region (c.g.) and axiogingival (a–g) line angles *(left)*. Better adaptation is obtained with rounded outlines *(right)*. (From Roydhouse, 1962. Reprinted with permission.)

Manipulation

The correct use of compound requires considerable judgment in handling. Compound is softened by heating over a flame or in a water bath. Care must be taken to prevent volatilizing ingredients over a direct flame. Kneading in water also may cause changes in composition and flow properties. The aim, therefore, is a thorough heating without excessive temperatures or long periods of storage in water. A room-temperature water spray is used to cool the impression in the mouth. Cooling must be continued until the entire mass is rigid to reduce plastic flow. Care must be taken to prevent overheating and burning of tissues. Also, cooling water should not be too cold, in order to prevent thermal shock.

To ease separation of the die stone, the impression should first be softened by immersion in warm water.

Advantages

Dental impression compound is compatible with die and model materials and is easily electroplated to form accurate and abrasion-resistant dies.

Disadvantages

The handling of dental impression compound is very technique sensitive. If it is not prepared properly, volatiles can be lost on heating, or low-molecular-weight ingredients can be lost during immersion in a water bath. Also, excessive wet kneading can incorporate water into the mix and change the flow properties of the compound. Due to a high coefficient of thermal expansion, the dimensions of the impression are not likely to be the same as the dimensions in the mouth. These materials are nonelastic and may distort on removal from the mouth. The casts should be poured within one hour.

Troubleshooting

1. *Distortion.* If the material is not completely cooled, the inner portions of the impression will still be soft when the impression is removed, resulting in distortion. Also, if water has been incorporated as the result of wet kneading, the material could have excessive flow at mouth temperature, producing distortion during removal from the mouth. If the tray used to carry the compound to the mouth is too flexible, distortion can result. It is important to select a tray that is strong and rigid. A delay in preparing the stone cast also may cause distortion. The cast should be poured as soon as possible after the impression has been removed from the mouth.
2. *Compound is too brittle or grainy.* Prolonged immersion in the water bath will cause low-molecular-weight components to leach out.

Disinfection

Dental impression compound can be disinfected by immersion in sodium hypochlorite, iodophors, or phenolic glutaraldehydes. The manufacturer's recommendations for proper disinfection should be followed.

Zinc oxide–eugenol

Zinc oxide–eugenol's main use is for full-mouth edentulous impressions with no or very minor undercuts for complete dentures. It can also be used as a wash impression with tray compound or an acrylic tray and for bite registration.

Composition

This material is commercially available as two pastes. One, called the base paste, contains zinc oxide (ZnO), oil, and hydrogenated rosin. The second paste, called the accelerator, contains about 12% to 15% eugenol, oils, rosin, and a filler such as talc or kaolin. These two pastes have contrasting colors so it can be determined when the pastes are thoroughly mixed. These materials are supplied as a soft- or hard-set type. Equal lengths of the two pastes, or properly proportioned amounts of the powder and liquid, are mixed with a stiff spatula on a special oil-resistant paper pad or on a glass slab. The mixed material is placed in a preliminary impression made from tray compound or tray acrylic. The setting time is shortened by increases in temperature and/or humidity. The set material does not adhere to set dental plaster or stone.

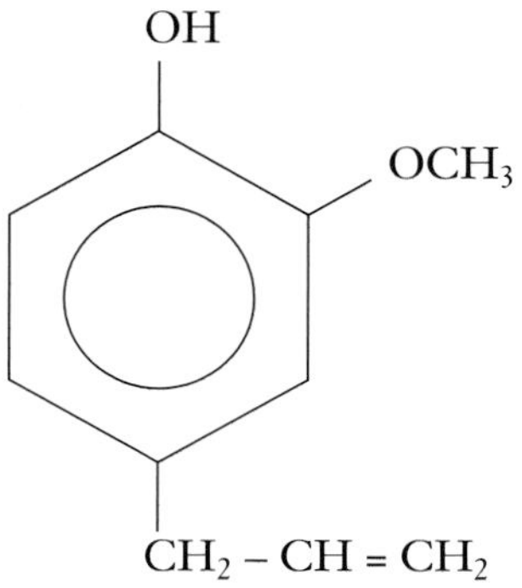

OH

OCH_3

$CH_2 - CH = CH_2$

eugenol

Zinc oxide, in the presence of moisture, reacts with eugenol to form zinc eugenolate, which acts as a matrix holding together the unreacted zinc oxide:

$$\underset{\text{(powder)}}{\text{ZnO (excess)}} + \underset{\text{(liquid)}}{\text{eugenol}} \xrightarrow{H_2O} \text{Zn eugenolate} + \underset{\text{(solid)}}{\text{ZnO (unreacted)}}$$

The setting reaction is accelerated by the presence of water, high humidity, and heat. A dimensional change of only about 0.1% shrinkage accompanies the setting.

Impression materials are classified as hard- and soft-set according to the American National Standards Institute, American Dental Association's specification. The hard-set material sets faster (in about 10 minutes, compared to 15 minutes for the soft-set material), although the hard- and soft-set materials both begin to set in about 5 minutes. The hard-set material is more fluid before setting than the soft-set material; after setting, it is harder and more brittle.

Noneugenol pastes contain carboxylic acids (eg, lauric or orthoethoxybenzoic acid) in place of eugenol to avoid the stinging and burning sensation experienced by some patients.

Mechanical properties

The hardness of zinc oxide–eugenol impression materials is determined using a Krebs penetrometer with a load of 100 g for 10 seconds. The hardness for Type I (hard-set) materials should be no greater than 0.5 mm and the hardness for Type II (soft-set) materials should be between 0.8 and 1.5 mm.

The shrinkage of these materials during the hardening process is approximately 0.1%. Subsequently, no additional dimensional change should occur.

Manipulation

These materials are usually mixed on a mixing pad with a spatula. Equal lengths of base and catalyst are extruded on the mixing pad. The components are mixed thoroughly with a stiff stainless steel spatula. Adequate mixing times are 45 to 60 seconds after which the mix should appear streak-free. The pastes have an initial set of 3 to 5 minutes, with the setting time decreasing as the temperature and/or humidity increases. The model or cast should only be made from gypsum-type plaster or stone. After the stone has set, the impression is immersed in warm water (60°C) to ease its removal from the cast.

The spatula may be cleaned by warming or by wiping with available solvents.

Advantages

The advantages of zinc oxide–eugenol include the accuracy of soft tissue impressions due to its low viscosity. The material is stable after setting, has good surface detail reproduction, and is inexpensive. It also adheres well to dental impression compound.

Disadvantages

The disadvantages of this material are messiness and a variable setting time due to temperature and humidity. Eugenol is irritating to soft tissues. This material is nonelastic and may fracture if undercuts are present.

Table 9-2 Properties of elastomeric impression materials*

	Agar	Alginate	Polysulfide	Condensation silicone	Addition silicone	Polyether
Elastic recovery (%)	98.8	97.3	96.9–94.5	99.6–98.2	99.9–99.0	99.0–98.3
Flexibility (%)	11	12	8.5–20.0	3.5–7.8	1.3–5.6	1.9–3.3
Flow (%)	—	—	0.4–1.9	<0.10	<0.05	<0.05
Reproduction limit (μm)	25	75	25	25	25	25
Shrinkage, 24 hours (%)	—	—	0.4–0.5	0.2–1.0	0.01–0.2	0.2–0.3
Tear strength (g/cm)	700	380–700	2,240–7,410	2,280–4,370	1,640–5,260	1,700-4,800

*See end-of-chapter glossary for definitions of terms.

Troubleshooting

1. *Inadequate working or setting time.* This could result from excessive humidity and/or temperature. An increase in either of these variables results in decreased working and setting time. It is important to select a material that provides the required setting time.
2. *Distortion.* If the tray warps on standing, the impression will also become distorted. It is important to select a stable tray material.
3. *Loss of detail.* If there is loss of detail, the impression material may not be compatible with the stone used to prepare the cast, and/or there may be adhesion between the impression and the stone.

Disinfection

Zinc oxide–eugenol impressions can be disinfected by immersion in 2% glutaraldehyde or 1:213 iodophor solutions at room temperature. The manufacturer's recommendations for proper disinfection should be followed.

Elastic materials

Agar (reversible) hydrocolloid

Agar hydrocolloids have been largely replaced by rubber impression materials but are still used for full-mouth impressions without deep undercuts, quadrant impressions without deep undercuts, and single impressions (less frequently). They can be used for crown-and-bridge impressions because of their high accuracy.

Composition

Agar hydrocolloids are available in both tray and syringe consistencies. They are supplied as a gel in plastic tubes and contain agar (12% to 15%) as a gelling agent, borax (0.2%) to improve strength, potassium sulfate (1% to 2%) to provide good surfaces on gypsum models or dies, alkylbenzoates (0.1%) as preservatives, and coloring and flavoring agents (traces) for ease of "reading" the impression and esthetics. The balance of the formulation (~85%) is water. The syringe consistency is prepared by increasing the water content and decreasing the agar content.

The material, supplied as a solid gel, can be converted to a sol (liquid) by heating; cooling a sol causes it to become a gel:

$$\underset{\text{(sol)}}{\text{agar hydrocoloid (hot)}} \underset{\substack{\text{heat to} \\ 100^\circ\text{C}}}{\overset{\substack{\text{cool to} \\ 43^\circ\text{C}}}{\rightleftarrows}} \underset{\text{(gel)}}{\text{agar hydrocolloid (cold)}}$$

The gel-to-sol and sol-to-gel transformations are dependent on time and temperature. The liquefaction and gelation temperatures are different (the latter being lower), and the effect is called *hysteresis*. A typical value of the gelation temperature is 43°C (109°F).

Mechanical properties

The mechanical properties of agar hydrocolloids are given in Table 9-2. They are highly elastic (98.8%) and sufficiently flexible (11%) to give accurate impressions of teeth with undercuts. They are stronger when stressed quickly; therefore, rapid removal is recommended.

Table 9-3 Dimensional change of hydrocolloid impressions

Storage conditions	Dimensional change	Causes
Air	Shrinkage	Evaporation of water from gel
H_2O	Expansion	Imbibition and absorption of water
100% relative humidity	Shrinkage	Syneresis
Inorganic salt solutions	Expansion or shrinkage	Depends on relationship of electrolyte in gel and in solution

Manipulation

Agar requires a special water bath with three chambers for heating, and water-cooled trays. The following sequence is used:

1. Heat in water at 100°C (212°F) for 8 to 12 minutes.
2. Store in water at 65°C (149°F).
3. Place in a tray (containing cooling coils) at 65°C (149°F).
4. Temper in 46°C (115°F) water for 2 minutes before taking the impression.
5. After seating the tray, cool it with water at no less than 13°C (55°F) until gelation occurs.
6. After the impression is removed from the mouth, wash it to remove saliva, which will interfere with the setting of the gypsum.
7. Shake off excess water and lightly blow off with air.
8. Disinfect the impression.
9. Pour mixed dental stone into the impression. If the impression is stored for a short time in 100% relative humidity, it should be washed as described in steps 6 and 7 to remove any exudate on the surface caused by *syneresis* (the exudation of water, accompanied by contraction) before pouring the model.
10. After the initial setting of the stone, store the gypsum model and impression in a humidor.

Agar impressions become less accurate during storage, and prompt pouring of gypsum casts is necessary. Table 9-3 lists the dimensional changes that occur upon storage under different conditions. If agar impressions must be stored, the minimum changes in dimensions are found upon storage in 100% relative humidity for no longer than one hour. However, the gel structure can absorb water, a process called *imbibition*, which is usually accompanied by expansion.

As the values in Table 9-4 indicate, agar materials have a long working time. Handling, however, offsets this convenience because of the need for storage tanks. Gelation, produced by circulating cool water through the special trays, also requires special equipment. Thermal shock produced by suddenly cooling the warm colloid may be painful to patients who have metallic restorations.

Contact with agar retards the setting of gypsum, resulting in dies and casts with poor surface finish. With older products, soaking the impression in a 2% potassium sulfate solution was necessary in order to achieve a smooth surface finish. Most agar products now contain potassium sulfate, which acts as an accelerator for the gypsum setting reaction, and soaking is no longer necessary.

Advantages

Agar impression materials are inexpensive, have no unpleasant odors, and are nontoxic and nonstaining. They do not require a custom tray or adhesives, and the components do not require mixing. These materials are hydrophilic and can be used in the presence of moisture, are able to displace blood and body fluids, and are easily poured in stone. The stone casts are easily removed from the hydrocolloid impressions.

Disadvantages

These materials require the use of expensive equipment, and the material must be prepared in advance. They tear easily, must be poured immediately, are dimensionally unstable, can only be used for single casts, and cannot be electroplated. The surface of stone casts will be weakened by compositions containing borax.

Table 9-4 Handling properties of elastomeric impression materials*

	Agar	Alginate	Polysulfide	Condensation silicone	Addition silicone	Polyether
Preparation	Boil, temper, store	Powder, water	2 pastes	2 pastes or paste-liquid	2 pastes	2 pastes
Handling	Complicated	Simple	Simple	Simple	Simple	Simple
Ease of use	Technique sensitive	Good	Fair	Fair	Good	Good
Patient reaction	Tedious, thermal shock	Pleasant, clean	Unpleasant, stains	Pleasant, clean	Pleasant	Unpleasant, clean
Ease of removal	Very easy	Very easy	Easy	Moderate	Moderate	Moderate to difficult
Working time (min)	7–15	2.5	5–7	3	2–4.5	2.5
Setting time (min)	5	3.5	8–12	6–8	3–7	4.5
Stability	1 h at 100% RH	Immediate pour	1 h	Immediate pour	1 w	1 w kept dry
Wetting and ease of pouring	Excellent	Excellent	Excellent	Fair	Fair to good	Good
Die material	Stone	Stone	Stone	Stone	Stone	Stone
Electroplating	No	No	Yes	Yes	Yes	Yes
Disinfection	Poor	Poor	Fair	Excellent	Excellent	Fair
Comparative cost	Low	Very low	Low	Moderate	High to very high	Very high

*See end-of-chapter glossary for definition of terms.

Troubleshooting

Sometimes problems of distorted impressions or loss of detail may be encountered when using agar hydrocolloids. The following are factors that could lead to distortion:

1. *Slow removal from the mouth.* To avoid permanent deformation, the impression should be removed with a quick jerk.
2. *Removal from the mouth before the gel reaches a temperature of 37°C (98.6°F) or less.* Above this temperature the impression material will still be plastic. The cooling rate of hydrocolloid is dependent on the temperature of water circulating through the tray.
3. *Cooling water that is too cold (<13°C).* Rapid cooling of the impression may cause a concentration of internal stresses that may be subsequently released.
4. *Application of force on the tray during gelation.* After the load is removed, relaxation of stresses will occur.
5. *Delay in pouring the cast.* Waiting any length of time to pour the cast will result in shrinkage of the impression owing to the loss of water.

If there is loss of detail, it may be caused by movement of the tray before gelation is complete. Failure to keep the impression stabilized will result in a multiple impression of the oral structures.

Disinfection

Agar hydrocolloids can be disinfected by immersion in sodium hypochlorite, iodophors, or phenolic glutaraldehydes. The manufacturer's recommendations for proper disinfection should be followed.

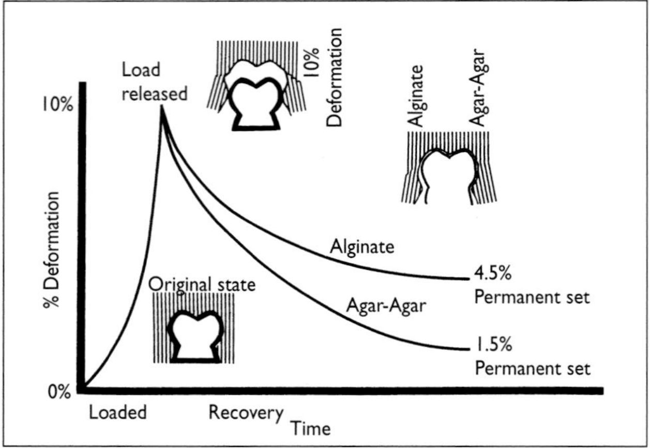

Fig 9-3 Illustration of agar hydrocolloids' greater accuracy due to their greater degree of recovery after deformation around undercuts. (From Roydhouse, 1962. Reprinted with permission.)

Alginate (irreversible) hydrocolloid

Alginates are the most widely used impression materials in dentistry. They are used for making impressions for partial dentures with clasps, preliminary impressions for complete dentures, and orthodontic and study models. They are not accurate enough for crown-and-bridge impressions.

Composition

Alginates are supplied as a powder containing sodium or potassium alginate (12% to 15%) and calcium sulfate dihydrate (8% to 12%) as reactants; sodium phosphate (2%) as a retarder; a reinforcing filler (70%), such as diatomaceous earth, to control the stiffness of the set gel; potassium sulfate or alkali zinc fluorides (~10%) to provide good surfaces on gypsum dies; and coloring and flavoring agents (traces) for esthetics. The sodium phosphate content is adjusted by the manufacturer to produce either regular- or fast-set alginates.

The powder is mixed with water to obtain a paste. Two main reactions occur when the powder reacts with water during setting. First, the sodium phosphate reacts with the calcium sulfate to provide adequate working time:

$$2\ Na_3PO_4 + 3\ CaSO_4 \rightarrow Ca_3(PO_4)_2 + 3\ Na_2SO_4$$

Second, after the sodium phosphate has reacted, the remaining calcium sulfate reacts with the sodium alginate to form an insoluble calcium alginate, which forms a gel with the water:

$$\underset{\text{(powder)}}{\text{Na alginate} + CaSO_4} \xrightarrow{H_2O} \underset{\text{(gel)}}{\text{Ca alginate} + Na_2SO_4}$$

To avoid the inhalation problems of alginate dust, some materials have been introduced in a dustless version in which the powder is coated with a glycol (Identic Dust Free, Cadco Dental Products, Inc.; Jeltrate Plus, L.D. Caulk).

Some products contain a chemical disinfectant in the alginate powder due to the concern for infection control (Coe Hydrophilic Gel, GC America, Inc.; Identic Dust Free, Cadco Dental Products, Inc.; Jeltrate Plus, L.D. Caulk). Two examples of these disinfectants are didecyl-dimethyl ammonium chloride and chlorhexidine acetate. When the quaternary ammonium compound is used, the detail reproduction and gypsum compatibility of the alginate improve. However, the impressions made from these materials should still be disinfected upon removal from the mouth.

Mechanical properties

Table 9-2 gives an elastic recovery value of 97.3% for alginates, which indicates less elasticity and therefore less accuracy than agar hydrocolloids and silicone and polyether impression materials. The compressive and tear strengths increase with increasing rates of deformation. The limit of reproduction is also lower, indicating that less fine detail will be obtained. Figure 9-3 compares the elasticity of alginates with the more accurate agar materials. Alginates have a higher permanent deformation upon stretching to pass over undercuts.

Manipulation

Although easy to use, care is required in handling alginate hydrocolloids. The powder, supplied in a can, should be shaken up for aeration and one scoop of powder is used for one measure of water. A powder scoop and a graduated cylinder for water are usually supplied with the product. With predispensed powder products, one packet of powder is used with the amount of water specified by the manufacturer. A lower W/P ratio increases strength, tear resistance, and consistency, and decreases working and setting times and flexibility. Cooling the water increases the working and setting times. Insufficient mixing results in a grainy mix and poor recording of detail. Adequate spatulation gives a smooth, creamy mix with a minimum of voids. One minute of thorough mixing for the regular-set material and 45 seconds for the fast-set material are generally recommended. Alginates have a relatively short working time of about 2.5 minutes (see Table 9-4) and set about 3.5 minutes after mixing. Alginates are as unstable as agar hydrocolloids because they are both gels and undergo shrinkage or expansion upon loss or gain of water. Storage in either air or water results in significant dimensional change; however, storage at 100% humidity results in the least dimensional change. Therefore, the cast should be poured soon after removal of the impression and cleaning (see Table 9-4). Alginates, like agar, retard the setting of the gypsum model and die materials when in contact. Potassium sulfate is added by the manufacturer to accelerate the setting of the gypsum and to obtain smooth model and die surfaces.

An alginate tray material can be combined with an agar syringe material to prepare impressions. These impressions take advantage of the agar hydrocolloid's detail reproduction and compatibility with gypsum qualities and at the same time minimize equipment needs. A simple heater can be used to prepare the syringe material, and the water-cooled trays are no longer necessary. The alginate is placed in a tray, the agar is syringed around the preparation, and then the alginate is seated on top of the agar. Care must be taken to select an agar-alginate impression pair with suitable bond strengths. It is best to select combinations recommended by the manufacturers. Best results are obtained when single-unit impressions are made by this technique.

Advantages

Alginate impression materials are inexpensive, easy to manipulate, pleasant tasting, able to displace blood and body fluids, hydrophilic, and easily poured in stone. They can be used with stock trays.

Disadvantages

Alginates tear easily, must be poured immediately after mouth removal, have limited detail reproduction, are dimensionally unstable, and can only be used for single casts. The gypsum compatibility varies with the brands of alginates and dental stones used. They are incompatible with many epoxy resin die materials.

Troubleshooting

Problems may sometimes be encountered when using alginate hydrocolloids. The following should serve as a guide for troubleshooting problems with these materials:

1. *Inadequate working or setting time*. The temperature of the mixing water may be too high. Generally, the temperature of the water should range between 18° and 24°C (65° and 75°F). If the mixture is incompletely spatulated, it may be inhomogeneous and may set prematurely. Under normal conditions, adequate spatulation requires 45 to 60 seconds. If the W/P ratio is too low as the result of incorrect dispensing, the setting time could be too fast. Improper storage of the alginate powder can result in deterioration of the material and shorter setting times.
2. *Distortion*. If the tray moves during gelation or if the impression is removed prematurely, the result will be a distorted impression. The amount and duration of compression should be considered. It is important, therefore, to remove the impression from the mouth rapidly. Since the weight of the tray can compress or distort the alginate, the impression should not be placed face down on the bench surface. If the impression is not poured immediately, distortion could occur.
3. *Tearing*. If the impression tears, it is possible that the impression was removed from the mouth before it was adequately set. Wait 2 to 3 minutes after loss of tackiness to remove the impression for development of adequate tear strength. Also, the rate of mouth removal may be a factor. Since the tear strength of alginate increases with the rate at which a stress is applied, it is desirable to rapidly remove the impression from the mouth. In addition, thin mixes are more prone to tearing than those with lower W/P ratios. The presence of undercuts also can produce tearing. Blocking out these areas will place less stress on the impression material during removal. It is also possible that there is not enough impression material; there should always be at least 3 mm of material between the tray and the oral tissues.
4. *Loss of detail*. If there is loss of detail, the impression may have been removed from the mouth prematurely. Multiple impressions of the oral structure will result if the material is still in the plastic state when removed.
5. *Consistency*. If the preset mix does not have the proper consistency (is either too thick or too thin), the W/P ratio is incorrect. Care must be taken to

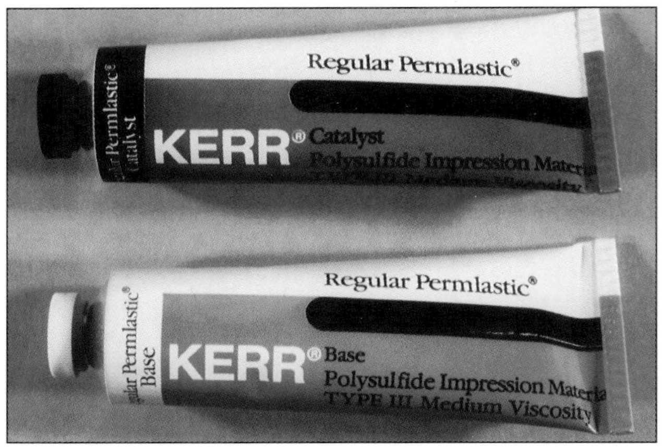

Fig 9-4 Polysulfide impression materials available as a two-paste system. The base is mixed with the catalyst paste.

fluff the powder before measuring and not to overfill the powder dispenser. Vigorous spatulation and mixing for the full recommended time is required to avoid consistency problems caused by inadequate mixing. If hot water is used, the mix may become grainy and prematurely thick.

6. *Dimensional change*. If dimensional change is a problem, a delay in pouring the die might be the cause. Such delays will result in a cast that is distorted as well as undersized, because alginate impressions lose water when stored in air.
7. *Porosity*. If the impression is porous, this could result from whipping air into the mix during spatulation. After the powder has been wetted by the water, the alginate should be mixed so as to squeeze the material between the spatula blade and the side of the rubber bowl.
8. *Poor stone surface*. If the set gypsum remains in contact with the alginate for too long a period of time, the quality of the stone surface will suffer.

Disinfection

Alginate hydrocolloids can be disinfected by immersion in sodium hypochlorite or iodophors. The manufacturer's recommendations for proper disinfection should be followed.

Polysulfide rubber (mercaptan)

Polysulfide rubbers are widely used for crown-and-bridge application, due to their high accuracy and relatively low cost. These materials are useful for multiple impressions when extra time is needed. The polysulfides are supplied in tubes of base paste and catalyst paste which are mixed together (Fig 9-4). Polysulfides are available in low, medium, and high viscosities.

Composition

The base paste contains the polysulfide polymer, fillers, and plasticizers. Low-molecular-weight (~4,000 MW) polysulfide polymer, having both terminal and pendant (near the center of the polymer) mercaptan groups (-SH), is used:

$$\begin{array}{c} C_2H_5 \\ | \\ HS - R_n - S - S - C - S - S - R_n - SH \\ | \\ SH \end{array}$$

mercaptan

The content of the reinforcing fillers (eg, zinc oxide, titanium dioxide, zinc sulfide, and silica) varies from 12% to 50% depending on the consistency (light, regular, or heavy). The fillers and plasticizers control the stiffness of the paste. The accelerator or catalyst paste contains lead dioxide (30%), hydrated copper oxide or organic peroxide, as a catalyst; sulfur (1% to 4%) as a promoter; and dibutyl phthalate or other nonreactive oils (17%) to form a paste. The balance of the catalyst paste is inorganic fillers used to adjust the consistency and reactivity. Those materials containing an organic peroxide may have decreased dimensional stability due to evaporation of the peroxide.

The lead dioxide catalyzes the condensation of the terminal and pendant -SH with -SH groups on other molecules, resulting in chain lengthening and cross-linking. In the process the material changes from a paste to a rubber. The reaction is accelerated by increases in temperature and by the presence of moisture.

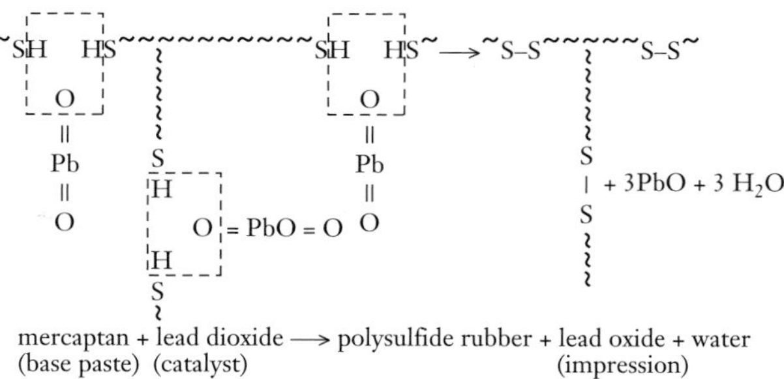

Note that this is a condensation polymerization with water as a by-product.

Mechanical properties

The values for the mechanical properties of these materials are summarized in Table 9-2. For elastic recovery, the polysulfides have values of about 96%, slightly lower than those for the other rubber impression materials (eg, silicone and polyether). Values for flow range from 0.4% to 1.9%, indicating a tendency to distort upon storage. The flow tends to be highest for the light-bodied and least for the heavy-bodied materials. Light-bodied polysulfides have flexibilities of about 16%; regular-bodied polysulfides have values of about 14%; and heavy-bodied polysulfides have values of about 10%. This is an advantage over the stiffer addition silicones and polyethers because removal from undercut areas is easier. Polysulfides have the highest tear strength of the rubber materials, which allows their use in deep subgingival areas where removal is difficult.

Manipulation

These materials are mixed on a mixing pad with a spatula. Equal lengths of base and catalyst are extruded on a disposable mixing pad. The components are mixed thoroughly with a stiff tapered spatula. The catalyst is dark and the base is white so thorough mixing is readily observed by lack of streaks in the mix. Adequate mixing times are 45 to 60 seconds. The working time is about 5 to 7 minutes (see Table 9-4), which is adequate considering the mixing times. Both working and setting times are shortened by higher temperatures and humidity. A value of 0.45% is given for shrinkage after 24 hours. Although this is less than that of the condensation silicones, the cast or die should be poured within 1 hour of taking the impression. Since polysulfides take longer to set than silicones, they require more chair time. They stain clothing permanently. They can be electroplated; some products can be silverplated, but copperplating is not recommended.

Advantages

Advantages of polysulfides include a long working time, good tear strength, good flow before setting, good reproduction of surface detail, high flexibility for easier removal around undercuts, and lower cost compared to silicones and polyethers.

Disadvantages

Disadvantages of these materials include the need to use custom-made rather than stock trays due to a greater chance of distortion, a bad odor, a tendency to run down the patient's throat due to lower viscosity, and the lead dioxide materials that stain clothing. Polysulfides must be poured within 1 hour and cannot be repoured.

Troubleshooting

Sometimes problems may be encountered when using polysulfide rubber impression materials:

1. *Inadequate working time.* This could result from excessive humidity and/or temperature. An increase in either of these variables results in decreased working and setting time. An improper base-to-catalyst ratio could also produce inadequate working time (too much catalyst will reduce working time).
2. *Distortion.* There are a number of causes of distortion, one of which is too much load. Because recovery after deformation is dependent upon the amount and duration of loading, the impression should not be placed face down on the laboratory bench. Improper mouth removal could also cause distortion of the impression; removal should be rapid because permanent deformation is a function of duration of stress. If a bubble is located just below the surface adjacent to a preparation (internal porosity), the impression may distort.
3. *Loss of detail.* Premature removal from the mouth may be a cause of this. Removal prior to sufficient polymerization or before the material is sufficiently elastic will result in inaccurate registration of detail. This may also be the result of incomplete mixing; failure to incorporate all the catalyst into the base will result in incomplete polymerization of portions of the surface. Movement of the tray prior to the time of removal could also cause loss of detail. The impression tray should be held firmly until the elastic stage is attained.
4. *Surface bubbles or voids.* These could be caused by the incorporation of air into the mix. The impression material should always be mixed carefully with only the flat surface of the blade. If the impression is partially polymerized prior to insertion in the mouth, voids may occur in the impression.

Disinfection

Polysulfide impressions can be disinfected by immersion in sodium hypochlorite, iodophors, complex phenolics, glutaraldehydes, or phenolic glutaraldehydes. The manufacturer's recommendations for proper disinfection should be followed.

Condensation silicone rubber

Condensation silicone rubber impression materials are used mainly for crown-and-bridge impressions. They are ideal for single-unit inlays. These materials are supplied either as two-paste or paste-liquid catalyst systems. Condensation silicones are available in low, medium, high, and very high (putty) viscosities.

Composition

The base paste usually contains a moderately high-molecular-weight poly(dimethylsiloxane) with terminal hydroxy groups (-OH), an orthoalkylsilicate for cross-linking, and inorganic filler. A paste will contain 30% to 40% filler, whereas a putty will contain as much as 75%. The catalyst paste or liquid usually contains a metal organic ester, such as tin octoate or dibutyl tin dilaurate, and an oily diluent. A thickening agent is used when making catalyst pastes. Sometimes a catalyst will contain both the orthoalkylsilicate and the metal organic ester:

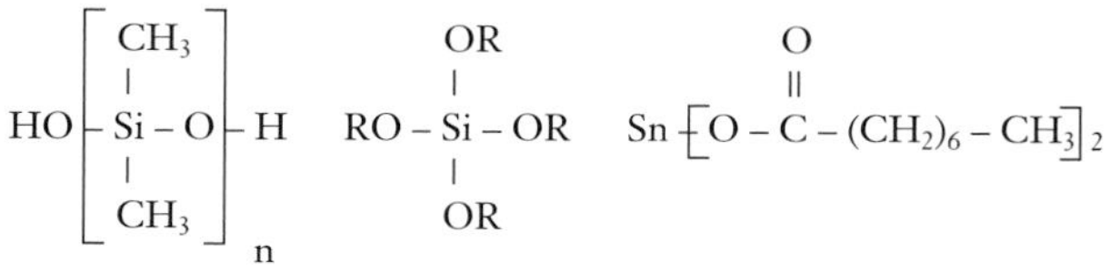

$$HO\left[\begin{matrix} CH_3 \\ | \\ Si-O \\ | \\ CH_3 \end{matrix}\right]_n H \qquad RO-\begin{matrix} OR \\ | \\ Si \\ | \\ OR \end{matrix}-OR \qquad Sn\left[O-\overset{\overset{O}{\|}}{C}-(CH_2)_6-CH_3\right]_2$$

hydroxy terminated poly(dimethylsiloxane) — orthoalkylsilicate — tin octoate

The metal organic ester catalyzes the reaction. One part of the polymerization involves chain extension by condensation of the terminal -OH group in a siloxane. The other part consists of cross-linking between chains by the orthoalkylsilicate molecules:

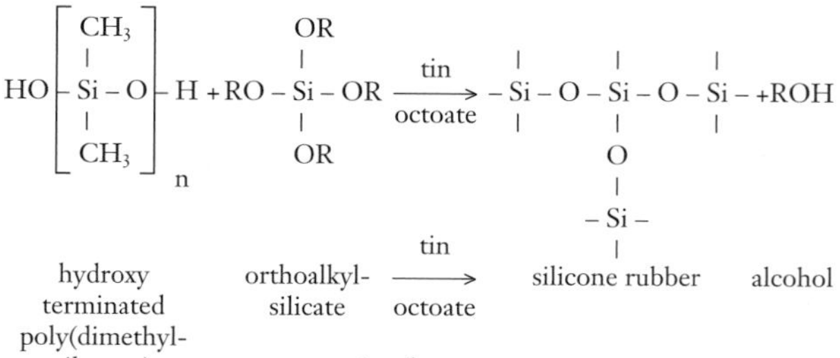

$$HO\left[\begin{matrix} CH_3 \\ | \\ Si-O \\ | \\ CH_3 \end{matrix}\right]_n H + RO-\begin{matrix} OR \\ | \\ Si \\ | \\ OR \end{matrix}-OR \xrightarrow[\text{octoate}]{\text{tin}} -\overset{|}{\underset{|}{Si}}-O-\overset{|}{\underset{\substack{| \\ O \\ | \\ -Si- \\ |}}{Si}}-O-\overset{|}{\underset{|}{Si}}- + ROH$$

hydroxy terminated poly(dimethylsiloxane) (base paste) — orthoalkylsilicate — tin octoate (catalyst paste or liquid) — silicone rubber (impression) — alcohol

Note that a volatile alcohol is formed as a by-product.

Mechanical properties

Accepted values for the mechanical properties of these materials are given in Table 9-2. An average value of 99% for elastic recovery is excellent. The flow of silicones is low; most values are less than 0.1%, indicating that less distortion is likely to be caused by light pressure on standing. The silicones are stiffer than polysulfides, as indicated by lower flexibility values in Table 9-2. The shrinkage in 24 hours ranges from 0.2% to 1.0%. About half the shrinkage takes place in the first hour, and it is greater than for polysulfides or polyethers. Polymerization and evaporation of the alcohol formed in the reaction are responsible for this high shrinkage. Accuracy is greatly improved by first taking an impression with a highly filled silicone putty and, after setting, taking a second impression with a light-bodied silicone. Thus, the final total shrinkage is lower.

Manipulation

The manipulation of condensation silicones is the same as for polysulfides, except that the silicone material may be supplied as a base paste plus a liquid catalyst. When it is supplied in this form, one drop per inch of extruded base paste is usually recommended. The setting time (6 to 8 minutes) is less than that of the polysulfides, which offers some advantage in chair time savings. Electroplating is possible. Because of the high polymerization shrinkage, the cast or die must be poured as soon as possible. Higher temperatures and humidity shorten the setting time.

Advantages

Condensation silicones are clean, pleasant materials for the patient. They are highly elastic, and the setting time can be controlled with the amount of accelerator. The use of a putty-wash system improves accuracy and eliminates the need for a custom tray.

Disadvantages

These materials tend to be inaccurate due to shrinkage on standing and should be poured within 1 hour. They are very hydrophobic, require a very dry field, and are difficult to pour in stone.

Troubleshooting

1. *Inadequate working time.* This could result from excessive humidity and/or temperature. Although not as critical as polysulfide rubber, the setting times of silicone impression materials are influenced by temperature and humidity. Increases in

these conditions tend to shorten both working and setting times. An improper base-to-catalyst ratio could also produce inadequate working time. Insufficient catalyst will result in prolonged setting times. Failure to polymerize in the predicted time may result from deterioration during storage.

2. *Distortion.* This may result from incorrect separation from impressed structures. Failure to remove the impression in a rapid, jerking motion may cause the impression to become permanently deformed. An impression can also become distorted if there is inadequate support of the impression after removal from the mouth. It may undergo permanent deformation if allowed to rest face down on the bench. Excessive delay in pouring the cast (30 minutes or more) also may result in dimensional changes. Possible shrinkage may result from continued polymerization and vaporization of volatiles in the silicone rubber. This shrinkage can be compensated for by use of the double impression technique. A preliminary impression is made with a very high (putty) viscosity material, providing space for the final impression, which is made with a low-viscosity material using the preliminary impression as the tray.
3. *Loss of detail.* Premature removal of the impression from the mouth could cause loss of detail. Failure to allow the impression material to set adequately will result in plastic deformation. Loss of detail also can be caused by incomplete mixing. Failure to adequately incorporate all the catalyst into the base will result in incomplete polymerization. Loss of detail can also result from movement of the tray after the impression has been seated. Failure to maintain the tray in a stable position will result in a blurred impression.

Disinfection

Condensation silicone impressions can be disinfected by immersion in sodium hypochlorite, iodophors, complex phenolics, glutaraldehydes, or phenolic glutaraldehydes. The manufacturer's recommendations for proper disinfection should be followed.

Addition (vinyl) silicones

Addition silicones represent an advance in accuracy over condensation silicones. This has been achieved by a change in polymerization reactions to an addition type and the elimination of an alcohol by-product that evaporates, causing shrinkage. These materials are available as two-paste systems in four viscosities and a range of colors, allowing monitoring of the degree of mixing. Due to their high accuracy, these materials are suitable for crown-and-bridge and partial denture impressions. They are rigid after setting and expensive, and therefore are not used for routine study models. Hydrophilic materials have been introduced that reportedly contain surfactants to improve the wetting characteristics compared to unmodified silicones. Monophase materials have been formulated with sufficient shear thinning to be used as both low-viscosity and high-viscosity materials.

Composition

These materials are based on silicone prepolymers with vinyl and hydrogen side groups, which can polymerize by addition polymerization. They are therefore called vinyl or addition silicones. The setting reaction is produced by mixing one paste containing the vinylpoly(dimethylsiloxane) prepolymer with a second paste that contains a siloxane prepolymer with hydrogen side groups. A platinum catalyst, chloroplatinic acid, is present in one of the pastes and starts the addition polymerization reaction as follows:

$$-\underset{\underset{CH_3}{|}}{\overset{\overset{CH_3}{|}}{Si}}-CH=CH_2 + H-\underset{|}{\overset{|}{Si}}-CH_3 \xrightarrow{H_2PtCl_6} CH_3-\underset{|}{\overset{|}{Si}}-CH_2-CH_2-\underset{|}{\overset{|}{Si}}-CH_3$$

vinyl terminated siloxane | silane | chloroplatinic acid | silicone rubber

Other reactions also occur that may release hydrogen gas that can on rare occasion produce porosity. Some manufacturers include hydrogen absorbers in their formulations to eliminate this problem. Since no volatile by-products are produced in the reaction, addition silicones have a much greater dimensional stability than condensation silicones. The pastes are available in light, medium, heavy, and putty viscosities. Some manufacturers include a retarder for extending the working and setting times.

Mechanical properties

The working and setting times of addition silicones are faster than polysulfides; a retarder is often supplied to extend the working time. They have excellent elasticity and show very low dimensional shrinkage

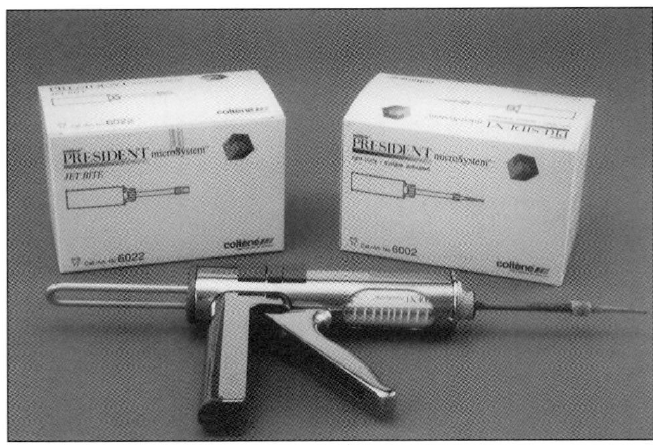

Fig 9-5 Automatic mixers, which provide quick, bubble-free mixes, are available with many addition silicone impression materials.

upon storage (see Table 9-2). Therefore, addition silicones can be safely poured up later or sent to a dental laboratory. Addition silicones do have greater rigidity, however, and therefore it is difficult to remove the impression around undercuts, as indicated in the lower flexibility value. The tear strength of addition silicones is similar to condensation silicones, but less than that of polysulfides.

Manipulation

Addition silicones are as pleasant to handle as condensation silicones. Because there is the possibility of hydrogen release upon setting, finely divided palladium is added to some products to absorb the hydrogen and prevent bubbles from forming on stone die surfaces. If a product does not contain a hydrogen absorber, an hour should pass before pouring dies, and the impression should stand overnight before epoxy dies are poured. Addition silicones can be electroplated with both copper and silver.

Automatic mixers that provide quick, bubble-free mixes are available with several products (Fig 9-5).

Advantages

Addition silicones are highly accurate and have high dimensional stability after setting. Recovery from deformation on removal is excellent. The material stays in the tray of reclined patients, does not stain clothing, has pleasant colors and scents, may be used with stock or custom trays, and can be copper- or silverplated. The materials may be poured 1 week after taking the impression, and multiple pours are possible.

Disadvantages

The disadvantages are that the material is expensive—twice the cost of polysulfides; is more rigid than condensation silicones and difficult to remove around undercuts; has a moderate tear strength, making removal from gingival retraction areas somewhat risky; and may release hydrogen gas on setting, producing bubbles on die surfaces if an absorber is not in the product. Hydrophobic materials are difficult to electroplate and to pour in stone. Also, sulfur in latex gloves and rubber dams can inhibit polymerization.

Troubleshooting

1. *Inadequate working time.* This can result from excessive temperature. As the temperature increases, the working and setting times decrease. If the impression material does not set, the catalyst may have been contaminated. The platinum-containing catalyst becomes inactive after contacting certain substances, such as tin or sulfur compounds. If addition silicones are combined with condensation silicones, the material will not set. Components from these two systems are not compatible and cannot be mixed together.
2. *Loss of detail.* This could occur if unmodified addition silicones are used. These hydrophobic materials cannot displace any moisture or hemorrhage that is not removed prior to placement of the impression material.
3. *Porosity.* The stone surface may appear porous if hydrogen gas is evolved. If this is the case, it is recommended the pouring of dies be delayed for at least 1 hour.
4. *Distortion.* This may occur if the polysiloxane adhesive does not provide adequate retention. Mechanical retention may be required in combination with the adhesive.

Disinfection

Addition silicone impressions can be disinfected by immersion in sodium hypochlorite, iodophors, complex phenolics, glutaraldehydes, or phenolic glutaraldehydes. The manufacturer's recommendations for proper disinfection should be followed.

Polyether rubber

Polyether rubbers are used for accurate impressions of a few prepared teeth without severe undercuts. Their high stiffness and short working time restricts their use to impressions of a few teeth. Polyethers are available in low-, medium-, and high-viscosity materials.

Composition

Polyethers are supplied as two-paste systems. The base paste contains low-molecular-weight polyether with ethylene-imine terminal groups:

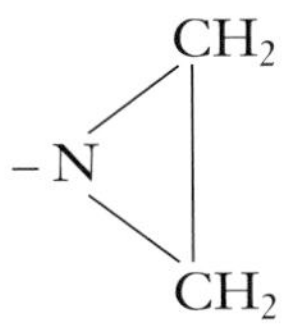

$$-N\begin{matrix} CH_2 \\ | \\ CH_2 \end{matrix}$$

along with fillers, such as colloidal silica, and plasticizers:

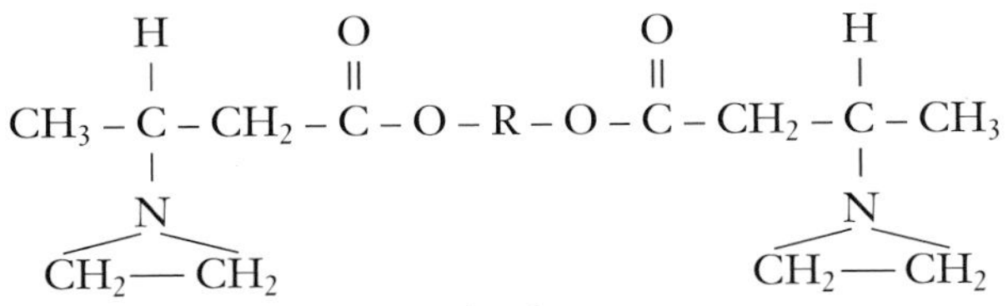

$$CH_3-\overset{\overset{H}{|}}{\underset{\underset{\underset{CH_2-CH_2}{N}}{|}}{C}}-CH_2-\overset{\overset{O}{\|}}{C}-O-R-O-\overset{\overset{O}{\|}}{C}-CH_2-\overset{\overset{H}{|}}{\underset{\underset{\underset{CH_2-CH_2}{N}}{|}}{C}}-CH_3$$

polyether

The catalyst paste contains an aromatic sulfonic acid ester plus a thickening agent to form a paste along with fillers:

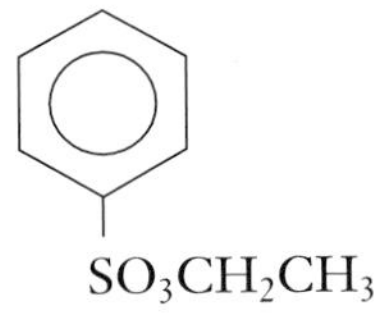

$$C_6H_5-SO_3CH_2CH_3$$

sulfonic ester

When the base paste is mixed with the catalyst paste, ionic polymerization occurs by ring opening of the ethylene-imine group and chain extension. The reaction converts the paste to a rubber as follows:

$$\underset{\text{(base paste)}}{\text{polyether}} + \underset{\text{(catalyst)}}{\text{sulfonic ester}} \rightarrow \underset{\text{(impression)}}{\text{polyether rubber}}$$

Mechanical properties

Polyethers are similar to addition silicones in properties. The early polyethers had short working and setting times and low flexibilities. Thinners were available to increase the working time and flexibility without any significant loss of other physical or mechanical properties. However, more recent formulations have a working time of 2.5 minutes and a setting time of 4.5 minutes. Shrinkage values of 0.3% in 24 hours place the polyethers at the upper end of the range for accuracy, but inferior to some addition silicones. Because this rubber absorbs water and changes dimensions, storage in water is not recommended. Elastic recovery values average 98.5%, between those for polysulfides and addition silicones (see Table 9-2). The flow of polyethers is very low and contributes to accuracy. The flexibility also is low (ie, the stiffness is high). This quality causes some problems on removal of the impression from the mouth or the die from the impression. More rubber between the tray and the impression area is recommended to relieve this problem. Polyethers have low tear strength values.

Manipulation

The manipulation of polyethers is similar to that of polysulfides and silicones. Equal lengths of base and catalyst paste are mixed vigorously and rapidly (30 to 45 seconds), because the working time is short. They are easy to mix. The impressions can be readily silver-plated to produce accurate dies. Precautions should be taken to mix the material thoroughly and to avoid contact of the catalyst with the skin or mucosa because tissue reactions have been observed.

A hand-held gun-type mixer that provides quick, bubble-free mixes is available for one product (Permadyne Garant, ESPE Premier Sales Co.). Also, an automatic mixing device (Pentamix, ESPE Premier Sales Co.) has been introduced for use with a polyether packaged in polybags (Impregum Penta).

Advantages

Advantages of polyethers include pleasant handling and ease of mixing. These materials are more accurate than polysulfide or condensation silicone impression materials. They have good surface detail reproduction and are easily poured in stone. If kept dry, they will be dimensionally stable for up to 1 week.

Disadvantages

Disadvantages of these materials include high cost, short working and setting times, and high stiffness after setting, which limit their use. Their bitter taste is objectionable to some patients. Storage of polyether impressions is critical, as they will distort if stored in water or high humidity. They cannot be left for long periods in disinfectant solutions

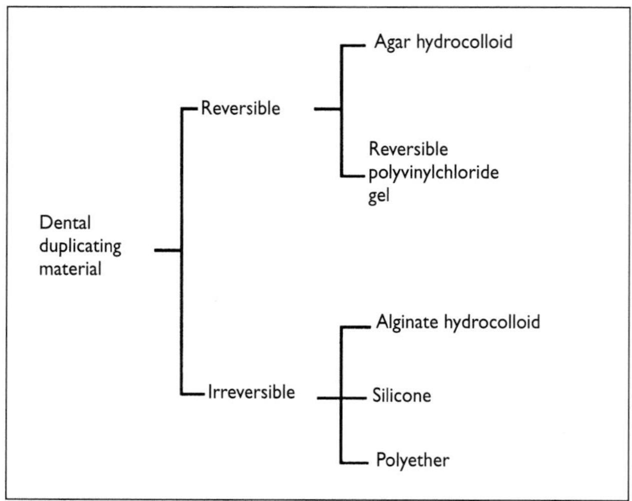

Fig 9-6 A classification key of dental duplicating materials.

Troubleshooting

1. *Inadequate working time.* This can result from excessive temperature. An increase in temperature will decrease the working and setting times. An improper base-to-catalyst ratio could also produce inadequate work time. Too much catalyst will decrease the working time.
2. *Tearing.* The rigidity of this material may result in tearing upon removal of the impression from the mouth or of the die from the impression. Tearing may occur if the rubber thickness is not adequate (at least 4 mm).
3. *Distortion.* The impression may distort due to moisture absorption and/or plasticizer extraction. These phenomena may result in dimensional change when impressions are stored in high-humidity environments or are exposed to water. The use of the thinner may increase the water absorption. Delay in impression placement may cause distortion. The onset of setting will result in the formation of elastic properties, which will cause deformation upon mouth removal.
4. *Loss of detail.* This can be caused by incomplete mixing. Failure to obtain a homogeneous mix will result in incomplete polymerization. If problems are encountered with multiple dies, it may be the result of gingival tearing and/or swelling. The rigidity and the relatively low tear strength of the polyethers may result in progressive deterioration at the gingival margin of the impression. The impression may absorb enough moisture from the gypsum that multiple pours could produce swelling.

Disinfection

Polyether impressions can be disinfected by immersion in sodium hypochlorite. The manufacturer's recommendations for proper disinfection should be followed.

Dental duplicating materials

Dental duplicating materials are used to prepare duplicate casts for prosthetic appliances and orthodontic models. These materials are used to make an impression of the original dental cast. Agar hydrocolloid duplicating materials are used most frequently. Their composition has a higher water content than agar hydrocolloid impression materials, and subsequently, a lower agar content. Therefore, the compressive strengths for duplicating materials is generally lower than those of impression materials. The advantages of the reversible materials include that they can be reused a number of times and may be stored in the liquid state for use as needed. The disadvantages include the fact that immediate pours are necessary, and degradation of the material will be accelerated by contamination. A classification key is shown in Fig 9-6.

Clinical decision scenarios for dental impression materials

This section presents one approach for choosing impression materials for specific situations. Each of the following scenarios uses the same format as that presented in Chapter 7:

1. The situation is described.
2. Critical factors are listed.
3. Advantages and disadvantages of each material are prioritized using the following codes: * = of minor importance, ** = important, and *** = very important.
4. The situation is analyzed, and the final decision is explained.

Situation Polysulfides vs addition silicones in a dental school clinic

Description In this scenario, the dentist is a dental school instructor who has been asked to determine which impression material will be used in the undergraduate crown-and-bridge clinics. There is a fixed budget that, typical of universities, dictates the use of inexpensive materials. The students are slow and unskilled at their stage of training, so a material allowing long working time is desirable. In addition, the students have not yet developed their gingival retraction techniques to the point that they have a wide sulcus into which to inject their syringe material. Because of this, a material with a high tear strength is desirable so the gingival area will not tear off from the main part of the impression and remain in the sulcus upon removal of the tray.

After review of the materials available, all are rejected except for the polysulfides (mercaptans) and the addition silicones (vinyl polysiloxanes).

The next steps in the selection process are to list the critical factors, list all the advantages and disadvantages of each material, and prioritize the advantages and disadvantages.

Critical factors Low cost, long working time, high tear strength

Advantages

Polysulfides

*** 1. Longer working time
*** 2. Lower cost
*** 3. Good tear resistance
* 4. High flexibility (easy to remove from undercuts)
*** 5. Good accuracy

Addition silicones

* 1. Good dimensional stability (can be mailed unpoured)
* 2. Short setting time
*** 3. Very accurate
* 4. Easy to mix and clean up
* 5. No disagreeable odor or taste
* 6. Rigid material

Disadvantages

Polysulfides:

* 1. Disagreeable odor and taste
* 2. Can stain clothing
* 3. Low dimensional stability (should be poured within 1 hour)
* 4. Longer setting time

Addition silicones:

*** 1. High cost
* 2. Low flexibility (harder to remove from undercuts)
*** 3. Shorter working time
*** 4. Lower tear resistance (may tear off in deep subgingival areas)
* 5. Some emit hydrogen gas (pouring must be delayed)

Analysis/Decision The lists include all the advantages and disadvantages obtainable from the available information, including some that were not mentioned in the discussion of the situation. Since the factors identified as important were low cost, high tear strength, and long working time, all advantages or disadvantages pertaining to these properties are marked ***, as is the property of good accuracy. This is essential in any impression material used for crown-and-bridge procedures. Because accuracy shows up as an advantage of both, it cancels out and is not a deciding factor.

In this example, the advantages the dentist is interested in all fall under the polysulfides, whereas the disadvantages fall under the addition silicones. This makes the choice easy—the polysulfides are selected.

The next step is to conduct a trial of the chosen material to see if this decision is well founded. For example, one half of the class takes impressions with the material chosen, and the other half uses the material previously used. If the polysulfide works well in the hands of students and is more inexpensive than the addition silicone, the trial confirms the decision.

Situation Polysulfides vs addition silicones in a busy practice

Description

In this scenario, the choice of impression materials is to be made by an experienced practitioner in a busy practice. She has been using agar hydrocolloid in water-cooled trays but has heard that the new elastomeric impression materials have become more dimensionally stable than they were originally. She is interested in trying either a polysulfide or an addition silicone. She has always obtained very good impressions with the agar hydrocolloid material but has never liked having to interrupt her busy schedule and pour the impressions right away. She feels that her time could be better used if a technician could set the dowel pins and pour the impression, but she has not felt that her practice is large enough to justify an in-office laboratory technician. She has likewise been unable to send the agar hydrocolloid impressions off to a laboratory for pouring because of the properties of the material.

The practitioner realizes that to use a polysulfide material, she should use custom trays due to the lack of dimensional stability of the material. But she does not like to take the dental assistant away from chairside for the time required to make a tray because she loses so much production by doing so. She would prefer a material with sufficient dimensional stability that it could be used in a disposable stock plastic tray. She is also looking for a material that will set much faster than the agar so she can decrease chair time for a crown impression.

Critical factors Low cost, short setting time, good dimensional stability

Advantages

Polysulfides

- * 1. Longer working time
- *** 2. Lower cost
- * 3. Good tear resistance
- * 4. High flexibility (easy to remove from undercuts)
- *** 5. Good accuracy

Addition silicones

- *** 1. Good dimensional stability (can be mailed unpoured)
- *** 2. Short setting time
- *** 3. Very accurate
- * 4. Easy to mix and clean up
- * 5. No disagreeable odor or taste
- * 6. Rigid material

Disadvantages

Polysulfides

- * 1. Disagreeable odor and taste
- * 2. Can stain clothing
- *** 3. Low dimensional stability (should be poured within 1 hour)
- *** 4. Longer setting time

Addition silicones

- *** 1. High cost
- * 2. Low flexibility (harder to remove from undercuts)
- ** 3. Shorter working time
- * 4. Lower tear resistance (may tear off in deep subgingival areas)
- * 5. Some emit hydrogen gas (pouring must be delayed)

Analysis/Decision

Here the decision is less obvious than in the previous example. The addition silicone seems to offer much of what the dentist desires, but it costs twice as much as the polysulfide. In this case, the decision might be in favor of the polysulfide due to the significant cost difference. After the trial period, however, the dentist confirmed her suspicion that the polysulfide was not stable enough to use stock trays. She also found that it took 15 to 30 minutes for either her or her assistant to fabricate the custom trays, and that use of "putty" material to line the stock tray greatly reduced the cost of the addition silicone. In addition, she found that placing dowel pins and pouring up the polysulfide took another 15 to 30 minutes of someone's time. The amount of time lost from chairside production more than offset the higher cost of the addition silicones, whose properties allowed her to use stock trays and to mail the impression off to her laboratory. Seeing this in her trial, the dentist reconsidered and changed to the addition silicone, which satisfied her needs.

Situation Polysulfides vs addition silicones for "triple tray"

Description This situation again addresses the choice between polysulfides and addition silicones, but this time due to a change in technique. In this scenario, the dentist has been using the polysulfides and is quite content but wishes to try a new impression technique that is gaining great favor among his peers. This method uses what is known as a "triple tray" and has the advantage for the single crown of obtaining the working impression, the opposing impression, and the bite relation all at the same time. This could significantly cut down the amount of time needed for each patient. The dentist finds, however, that the sides of the flimsy plastic trays sometimes spread apart when the dental arches impinge on them as the patient bites into position. The tray then attempts to spring back from this distortion when it is removed from the mouth. The recovery from the spreading requires that he use a material with sufficient rigidity that it can maintain its shape against this elastic recovery of the tray. If not, the tray recovery may distort the impression and result in a nonfitting crown.

Critical factors Low flexibility, good dimensional stability

Advantages

Polysulfides

- * 1. Longer working time
- * 2. Lower cost
- * 3. Good tear resistance
- *** 4. High flexibility (easy to remove from undercuts)
- *** 5. Good accuracy

Addition silicones

- *** 1. Good dimensional stability (can be mailed unpoured)
- * 2. Short setting time
- *** 3. Very accurate
- * 4. Easy to mix and clean up
- * 5. No disagreeable odor or taste
- *** 6. Rigid material

Disadvantages

Polysulfides

- * 1. Disagreeable odor and taste
- * 2. Can stain clothing
- *** 3. Low dimensional stability (should be poured within 1 hour)
- * 4. Longer setting time

Addition silicones

- * 1. High cost
- *** 2. Low flexibility (harder to remove from undercuts)
- * 3. Shorter working time
- * 4. Lower tear resistance (may tear off in deep subgingival areas)
- * 5. Some emit hydrogen gas (pouring must be delayed)

Analysis/Decision In this case, the trial period showed that the addition silicone was the only feasible choice. Here, the need for rigidity in the impression material for the triple tray is important enough that it becomes the deciding factor. Although other factors, such as accuracy, are important, unless the material is rigid enough to hold its shape, these other properties are meaningless.

Situation Polysulfides vs addition silicones for full-arch impression

Description In this situation, the dentist is a prosthodontist in an established specialty practice. He has a dental laboratory in his office and employs two dental laboratory technicians. He therefore has the capability of having custom trays made in his office and can have the impressions poured right away. Most of his patients have been referred from dentists who do the easier cases themselves. Consequently, his patients usually already have multiple crowns or bridges in different areas of the mouth. He feels that full-arch impressions are better because in the more extensive cases he needs the accuracy in bite relations that can only come from full-arch registration. He has heard that addition silicones are very accurate and that they have better dimensional stability than the material he has been using. This appeals to him for "pickup" impressions where a rigid material and better dimensional stability greatly enhance the probability of success. On the other hand, he is concerned that the stiffness of the addition silicone will make the removal of full-arch impressions from the mouth much more difficult. He is also concerned that the stiffness may pose a greater risk of inadvertently removing crowns or fixed partial dentures that his patients already have in other areas of the mouth.

Critical factors Good accuracy, high flexibility, good dimensional stability

Advantages

Polysulfides

* 1. Longer working time
* 2. Lower cost
* 3. Good tear resistance
*** 4. High flexibility (easy to remove from undercuts)
*** 5. Good accuracy

Addition silicones

*** 1. Good dimensional stability (can be mailed unpoured)
* 2. Short setting time
*** 3. Very accurate
* 4. Easy to mix and clean up
* 5. No disagreeable odor or taste
*** 6. Rigid material

Disadvantages

Polysulfides:

* 1. Disagreeable odor and taste
* 2. Can stain clothing
*** 3. Low dimensional stability (should be poured within 1 hour)
* 4. Longer setting time

Addition silicones:

* 1. High cost
*** 2. Low flexibility (harder to remove from undercuts)
* 3. Shorter working time
* 4. Lower tear resistance (may tear off in deep subgingival areas)
* 5. Some emit hydrogen gas (pouring must be delayed)

Analysis/Decision In this situation, some of the dentist's desires seem to conflict. The high flexibility listed under the advantages of polysulfides is offset by the rigidity listed as an advantage under addition silicones. He found that the rigidity was desirable for pickup impressions, but the flexibility was desirable for regular impressions. He decided to try the addition silicone and found that it did, indeed, give very accurate and dimensionally stable impressions. His pickup impressions were better than they had ever been. He also found that in normal situations the rigidity of the material made removal of the full-arch impressions much more difficult.

Some crowns and bridges on which he was not working came off in the impression material due to its rigidity. He found, however, that he could compensate for this rigidity by filling the impression tray only partially full in the areas where he only needed the occlusal registration and filling it full in the area of the preparations. After working with the material for a while, he decided to go back to the polysulfide for his normal working impressions. He had the necessary technicians in his office, so the disadvantages of needing custom trays and needing to pour the impressions right away were not a problem for him. In this case, he selected both materials, one for each use. It is not unusual to find that having more than one type of a given material may be advantageous.

Analysis/Decision (continued)

To this point some of the properties, such as taste and odor, have not been mentioned as critical factors. It is entirely possible that any one of these other properties could be significant to some situation and might become the deciding factor. A dentist who found the odor of the polysulfide completely unacceptable may rule out the material on this factor alone.

The discussion to this point demonstrates how the dentist making the choice between materials must carefully study all the information available on those materials. In addition, he or she must be able to interpret the significance of each bit of information. If, for example, the dentist does not realize that the dimensional stability will determine how long he or she can wait to pour the impression, the resulting choice could be incorrect.

Glossary

addition silicone A silicone polymer resulting from the free-radical polymerization of vinyl groups by platinum catalyst.

agar An ingredient in agar impression material. It is usually extracted from seaweed as a polysaccharide.

alginate Alginate impression material containing salts of alginic acid.

cast material Material used to form casts (models or dies) from impressions.

condensation (in polymerization) In a condensation polymerization (eg, to form silicone impression materials), two molecules unite and one small molecule (eg, H_2O, ROH) is released as a by-product.

~Si-OH + R-O-Si~ → ROH + ~Si-O-Si~

condensation silicone A silicone polymer resulting from the condensation of terminal -OH groups by orthoalkylsilicates and releasing alcohol as a by-product.

elastic recovery The amount of rebound after a cylinder of material is strained 10% for 30 seconds.

electroplate The process of depositing metal from solution onto the surface of an impression using an electric current.

eugenol Oil of cloves. As a derivative of phenol, eugenol reacts as an acid with zinc oxide.

flexibility The amount of strain produced when a sample is stressed between 100 and 1,000 g/cm^2. A flexible material shows a higher value of flexibility than a stiff material.

flow The amount of shortening of a cylinder when placed under a light load for 15 minutes.

gel A colloid system in which the solid (eg, agar) and liquid (eg, water) are continuous phases. A gel is usually flexible.

hydrocolloid A colloid system in which the liquid phase is water. Agar impression material is a hydrocolloid (agar + water).

hydrophilic material A material that has a strong affinity for water and is readily wet by water.

hydrophobic material A material that is resistant to wetting by water.

hysteresis The phenomenon of a gel's having a liquefaction temperature different from the solidification temperature of the sol.

imbibition The taking up of fluid by a colloidal system, resulting in swelling.

plasticizer A material that is added to increase flow.

polyether The polymer resulting from the ionic polymerization with ring opening of the ethylene-imine group and chain extension.

polysulfide The polymer resulting from the condensation of terminal mercaptan groups catalyzed by lead dioxide or other catalysts.

silicone rubber A polymer resulting from the formation of silicon-oxygen-silicon bonds (-Si-O-Si-). Silicone impression material is a silicone rubber.

sol A colloid system in which the solid phase is dispersed in the liquid phase. A sol usually has fluid properties.

stability Maximum time of storage of impressions after which acceptable casts can still be poured.

syneresis The exudation of a liquid film on the surface of a gel.

terminal group A chemical group at the end of a molecule (eg, -SH).

thermal conductivity The quantity of heat passing through a body 1 cm thick with a cross section of 1 cm^2 when the temperature difference between the hot and cold sides of the body is 1°C.

thermoplastic The property of softening on heating and hardening on cooling.

working time Duration from the start of mixing to the time when a test rod leaves a permanent indentation in the material upon withdrawal.

Discussion questions

1. Why are there so many impression materials in dentistry at the present time?
2. How could the movement of soft tissues during impression taking affect the accuracy of the final impression?
3. Since elastic impression materials are viscoelastic, wouldn't immediate pouring of a gypsum cast result in inaccuracy?
4. Why is it essential to sterilize an impression before sending it to a laboratory, and how is this done?
5. Why is the impression tray an important factor in obtaining a good impression?

Questions and answers

1. **What components are present in dental compound, and what is the purpose of each?** Natural resins and waxes provide thermoplastic properties. Stearic acid acts as a lubricant and plasticizer. Inorganic fillers and pigments give control of flow and color, respectively.
2. **What term describes the quality of dental compound that allows it to be repeatedly softened on heating and hardened on cooling?** Thermoplastic.
3. **What is the principal difference between the properties of impression and tray-type compounds?** Impression compound has a higher flow. Tray material, with a lower flow, does not record fine detail.
4. **What precautions should be taken when heating dental compound?** Avoid burning in a direct flame or heating in a water bath for long periods.
5. **What importance does low thermal conductivity have on the clinical handling of dental impression compound?** Low thermal conductivity requires time for thorough cooling to prevent distortion during removal.
6. **What factors affect the flow of impression compound?** The amounts of filler and water incorporated during kneading control the flow properties.
7. **What are the reactive ingredients in a zinc oxide–eugenol material?** Zinc oxide and eugenol.
8. **What is responsible for the setting of zinc oxide–eugenol impression paste?** ZnO + eugenol $\rightarrow$ Zn eugenolate, which forms a solid matrix holding unreacted ZnO.
9. **What factors affect the setting time of zinc oxide–eugenol?** Increases in temperature and/or humidity shorten the setting time.
10. **What are the functions of the various components in agar hydrocolloid?** Agar acts as a gelling agent. Borax improves strength. Potassium sulfate provides good surfaces on models or dies. Alkylbenzoates are preservatives.
11. **What is meant by hysteresis in agar hydrocolloid?** The liquefaction and gelation temperatures are different.
12. **What kinds of dimensional changes occur when an agar impression is stored in air, water, 100% relative humidity, or potassium sulfate solution?** Storage in air results in shrinkage; water, in expansion; 100% relative humidity, in shrinkage (synersis); and potassium sulfate solution, in shrinkage or expansion, depending on the ionic strength of the solution.
13. **What is the function of each of the components in alginate powder?** Sodium alginate and calcium sulfate are reactants to give calcium alginate. Sodium phosphate is a retarder; filler (eg, diatomaceous earth) controls stiffness; alkali zinc fluorides provide good surfaces on dies and models; and coloring and flavoring are for esthetics.

14. **What factors affect the setting time of alginates?** A low water/powder ratio and/or high temperature shorten the setting time.

15. **What reaction is responsible for providing the working time of alginate, and what other reaction is responsible for the setting of alginate?** $CaSO_4 + Na_3PO_4 \rightarrow Na_2SO_4 + Ca_3(PO_4)_2$ provides working time.
Na alginate + $CaSO_4 \rightarrow$ Ca alginate + Na_2SO_4, in the presence of water, provides setting time.

16. **Why are alginate impression materials called irreversible hydrocolloids?** Alginates do not revert to a sol on heating or by chemical means.

17. **What effect does the water/powder (W/P) ratio of alginates have on their properties?** A decreased W/P ratio increases strength, tear resistance, and consistency, but decreases working time, setting time, and flexibility.

18. **What effect does spatulation of alginates have on their properties?** Insufficient spatulation gives a grainy mix and poor recording of detail. Adequate spatulation yields a smooth, creamy mix with a minimum of voids.

19. **What effect does water temperature have on the working and setting times of alginates?** Decreased water temperature increases the working and setting times of alginates.

20. **How do the properties of alginate impression materials compare with those of agar impression materials?** Alginates and agars have similar properties.

21. **Describe the setting reactions for polysulfide, silicone, and polyether rubber impression materials.** Polysulfide cures by condensation of terminal mercaptan groups catalyzed by lead peroxide or other catalysts. Condensation silicones cure by condensation of terminal hydroxyl groups by orthoalkylsilicates to form polymer and alcohol. Addition silicones cure by free-radical polymerization with a platinum catalyst. Polyethers cure by ring opening of the ethylene-imine group.

22. **What effect do proportioning and temperature have on the working and setting time of the three rubber impression materials?**

	Proportioning	Increased temperature
Polysulfide	Decreases with increased amount of catalyst	Decreases
Silicone	Minimal	Decreases
Polyether	Decreases with increased amount of accelerator	Decreases

23. **What impression material may be used if you wish to use either a gypsum die, a silver-plated die, or a copperplated die?** Addition silicones.

24. **Compare the elastic recoveries of polysulfide, silicone, and polyether impression materials. How does elastic recovery affect clinical usage?** Addition silicone ≥ condensation silicone ≥ polyether > polysulfide. A large elastic recovery value indicates smaller distortion of the impression on removal.

25. **Compare the flexibilities of polysulfide, silicone, and polyether impression materials.** Polysulfide > condensation silicone ≥ addition silicone ≥ polyether.

26. **How would you disinfect your impression prior to sending it to the laboratory?** Follow the instructions given by the manufacturer for the impression material used, because the recommended procedure depends upon the material.

27. **List the advantages of each of the following recent advances in impression materials.**
    a. **Addition silicones with hydrophilic properties** Hydrophilic materials will wet the tooth surface more readily during impression-taking and are more readily wet by dental stone. Therefore, they are less likely to entrap air. Also, their wetting characteristics make them easier to electroplate.
    b. **Single-viscosity, or monophase, addition silicones** A single material can be used as both the low- and high-viscosity material for the syringe-tray impression technique.
    c. **Automatic mixers for addition silicones and polyethers** This method of mixing is quick and produces bubble-free mixes.

Recommended reading

Albers HF. Impressions: A Text for Selection of Materials and Techniques. Santa Rosa, CA: Alto Books, 1990.

American Dental Association. Clinical Products in Dentistry: A Desktop Reference. Chicago: ADA, 1993.

Anderson JN. Flow and elasticity in alginates. Dent Progr 1:63–74, 1960.

Anusavice KJ. Dental impression materials: Reactor response. Adv Dent Res 2:65–70, 1988.

Braden M. Characterization of the setting process in dental polysulfide rubbers. J Dent Res 45:1065–1071, 1966.

Braden M, Causton B, Clarke RL. A polyether impression rubber. J Dent Res 51:889–896, 1972.

Braden M, Elliot JC. Characterization of the setting process of silicone dental rubbers. J Dent Res 45:1016–1023, 1966.

Buchan S, Peggie RW. Role of ingredients in alginate impression compounds. J Dent Res 45:1120–1129, 1966.

Chee WW, Donovan TE. Polyvinyl siloxane impression materials: a review of properties and techniques. J Prosthet Dent 68:728–732, 1992.

Chong JA, Chong MP, Docking AR. The surface of gypsum cast in alginate impressions. Dent Pract 16:107–109, 1965.

Council on Dental Materials and Devices. Status report on polyether impression materials. J Am Dent Assoc 95:126–130, 1977.

Council on Dental Materials, Instruments, and Devices. Vinyl polysiloxane impression materials: a status report. J Am Dent Assoc 120:595–596, 598, 600, 1990.

Council on Dental Materials, Instruments, and Devices. Disinfection of impressions. J Am Dent Assoc 122(8):110, 1991.

Council on Dental Materials, Instruments, and Devices. Retarding the setting of vinyl polysiloxane impressions. J Am Dent Assoc 122(8):114, 1991.

Council on Dental Materials, Instruments, and Devices; Council on Dental Therapeutics; Council on Dental Research; Council on Dental Practice. Infection control recommendations for the dental office and the dental laboratory. J Am Dent Assoc 123(Supp):1–8, 1992.

Craig RG. A review of properties of rubber impression materials. J Mich Dent Assoc 59:254–261, 1977.

Craig RG. Evaluation of an automatic mixing system for an addition silicone impression material. J Am Dent Assoc 110:213–215, 1985.

Craig RG. Review of dental impression materials. Adv Dent Res 2:51–64, 1988.

Craig RG, O'Brien WJ, Powers JM. Dental Materials—Properties and Manipulation. 6th ed. St. Louis: Mosby, 1996.

Craig RG, Sun Z. Trends in elastomeric impression materials. Oper Dent 19:138–145, 1994.

Craig RG, Urquiola NJ, Liu CC. Comparison of commercial elastomeric impression materials. Oper Dent 15:94–104, 1990.

Farah JM, Powers JM (eds). Impressions and accessories. The Dental Advisor 9(4):1–8, 1992.

Fish SF, Braden M. Characterization of the setting process in alginate impression materials. J Dent Res 43:107–117, 1964.

Harris WT Jr. Water temperature and accuracy of alginate impressions. J Prosthet Dent 21:613–617, 1969.

Johnson GH, Craig RG. Accuracy and bond strength of combination agar/alginate hydrocolloid impression materials. J Prosthet Dent 55:1–6, 1986.

Kahn RL, Donovan TE, Chee WW. Interaction of gloves and rubber dam with a poly(vinyl siloxane) impression material: a screening test. Int J Prosthodont 2:342–346, 1989.

Kim K-N, Craig RG, Koran A III. Viscosity of monophase addition silicones as a function of shear rate. J Prosthet Dent 67:794–798, 1992.

Lautenschlager EP, Miyamoto P, Hilton R. Elastic recovery of polysulfide base impressions. J Dent Res 51:773–779, 1972.

MacPherson GW, Craig RG, Peyton FA. Mechanical properties of hydrocolloid and rubber impression materials. J Dent Res 46:714–721, 1967.

Marker VA. Dental impression materials. In T Okabe, S Takahashi (eds). Transactions International Congress on Dental Materials. Honolulu, HI, Nov 1–4, 1989; 114–138.

Merchant VA. Update on disinfection of impressions, prostheses, and casts. J Calif Dent Assoc 20:31–35, 1992.

McCabe JF, Wilson HJ. Addition curing silicone rubber impression materials: an appraisal of the physical properties. Br Dent J 145:17–20, 1978.

McLean JW. Physical properties influencing the accuracy of silicone and thiokol impression materials. Br Dent J 110:85–91, 1961.

Myers GE, Peyton FA. Clinical and physical studies of the silicone rubber impression materials. J Prosthet Dent 9:315–324, 1959.

Myers GE, Peyton FA. Physical properties of the zinc oxide-eugenol impression pastes. J Dent Res 40:39–48, 1961.

Myers GE, Stockman DG. Factors that affect the accuracy and dimensional stability of the mercaptan rubber base impression materials. J Prosthet Dent 10:525–535, 1960.

Naylor WP, Evans DB. An overview of impression materials and techniques for fixed prosthodontics. In JF Hardin (ed). Clark's Clinical Dentistry. Vol 4. Hagerstown, MD: Harper and Row, 1991.

Pratten DH, Craig RG. Wettability of a hydrophilic addition silicone impression material. J Prosthet Dent 61:197–202, 1989.

Pratten DH, Novetsky M. Detail reproduction of soft tissue: a comparison of impression materials. J Prosthet Dent 65:188-191, 1991.

Rosenblum MA, Asgar K, Leinfelder KF. Dental prosthetic materials. In JA Reese, TM Valega (eds). Restorative Dental Materials. Vol I. London: Quintessence Publ Co Ltd, 1985;158–168.

Roydhouse RH. Materials in Dentistry. Chicago: Year Book Medical Publishers, 1962.

Smith DC, Wilson HJ. Further studies on alginate impression materials. Dent Pract 15:380–382, 1965.

Stackhouse JA Jr. The accuracy of stone dies made from rubber impression materials. J Prosthet Dent 24:377–386, 1970.

Stackhouse JA Jr. Electrodeposition in dentistry. A review of the literature. J Prosthet Dent 44:259–263, 1980.

Stackhouse JA Jr. Impression materials and electrodeposits. Part I. Impression materials. J Prosthet Dent 45:44–48, 1981.

Stackhouse JA Jr. Impression materials and electrodeposits. Part II. Electrodeposits. J Prosthet Dent 45:146–151, 1981.

Stannard JG, Sadighi-Nouri M. Retarders for polyvinylsiloxane impression materials: evaluation and recommendations. J Prosthet Dent 55:7–10, 1986.

Wilson HJ. Some properties of alginate impression materials relevant to clinical practice. Br Dent J 121:463–467, 1966.

Wilson HJ. Elastomeric impression materials. I. The setting material. Br Dent J 121:277–283, 1966.

Wilson HJ, Smith DC. Alginate impression materials. Br Dent J 114:20–26, 1963.

Chapter 10

Waxes

Waxes have several applications in dentistry. They are used as patterns for inlays, crowns, pontics, and partial and full dentures. Waxes are very useful for bite registration and can be used to obtain impressions of edentulous areas. In addition, they have many applications for processing in all areas of restorative dentistry.

Composition

Waxes are organic polymers consisting of hydrocarbons and their derivatives (eg, esters and alcohols). The average molecular weight of a wax blend is about 400 to 4,000, which is low compared with structural acrylic polymers. Dental waxes are blends of ingredients, including natural (eg, paraffin, beeswax, carnauba, spermaceti, ceresin) and synthetic waxes, natural resins (eg, dammar), oils, fats (eg, stearic acid), gums (eg, gum arabic), and coloring agents.

Natural waxes are of mineral (petroleum oil), plant, insect, or animal origin. Paraffin wax is relatively soft with a low melting range (50° to 70°C). It is a mineral wax obtained from refined crude oil and used in inlay and modeling waxes. Beeswax is brittle with an intermediate melting range (60° to 70°C). It is an insect wax obtained from honeycombs and is added to many waxes because of its desirable flow properties at mouth temperature. Carnauba wax is a plant wax obtained from carnauba palm trees and is hard and tough with a high melting range (65° to 90°C). It is added to toughen paraffin wax and raise its melting range. Microcrystalline waxes have a high melting range (65° to 90°C) and are added to modify the softening and melting ranges of wax blends. They also serve to reduce stresses that occur on cooling. Microcrystalline waxes are obtained from petroleum.

Synthetic waxes have specific melting points and are blended with natural waxes. Low-molecular-weight polyethylene is an example of a synthetic wax. Natural waxes vary more depending on their sources and need to be monitored more for properties than synthetic waxes, which are more uniform in composition.

Classification

Dental waxes are classified according to their applications, into the categories of pattern, processing, and impression waxes (Fig 10-1).

Pattern waxes

Pattern waxes include inlay, casting, and base plate waxes. Inlay waxes (Kerr Manufacturing Co.) are used to make inlay, crown, and pontic replicas for the lost wax casting technique. Type I inlay waxes are hard and used for the direct-inlay technique. Type II inlay waxes are soft and used for preparing replicas on dies and

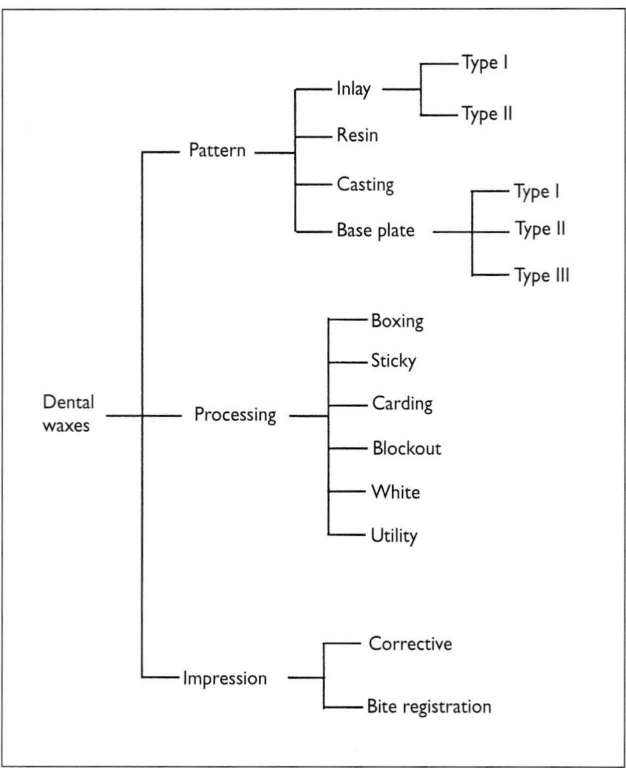

Fig 10-1 A classification of dental waxes.

models. In addition, inlay waxes are sometimes used for the attachment of miscellaneous parts.

Light-curing resin materials (eg, Triad VLC, Palavit GLC) are available for the fabrication of patterns for cast metal or ceramic restorations and precision attachments. The materials are provided as high- or low-viscosity pastes or liquids and are based on a diuethane methacrylate oligomer with a 40% to 55% resin filler.

Pattern resins are characterized by higher strength and resistance to flow than waxes, good dimensional stability, and burnout without residue. Full-crown patterns fabricated from pattern resins and inlay waxes have similar marginal discrepancies.

A pattern is fabricated by applying the resin in 3- to 5-mm layers and curing in a light chamber or by using a handheld light-curing unit. Resin is completely eliminated from the mold before casting by heating at 690°C for 45 minutes.

Casting waxes are used for thin sections of certain partial denture and crown-and-bridge patterns. They are particularly convenient in the preparation of copings or clasps requiring uniformly thin regions.

Base plate wax (Dentsply International, Inc.) is used in the construction of full denture patterns and for occlusion rims, although an occlusal rim wax is also available. Setup wax may be used instead of base plate wax to set denture teeth.

The American National Standards Institute/American Dental Association has established a specification that includes three types of base plate wax. Type I is a soft base plate wax for veneers and contours. Type II is a medium-hardness base plate wax designed for temperate climates for patterns to be tried in the mouth. Type III is the hardest base plate wax and is also for patterns to be tried in the mouth—but in tropical climates. The hardness is based upon the amount of flow the wax shows at 45°C (113°F).

Base plate wax is also used as a mold for the construction of temporary bridges and as a bite registration wax. It has some applications in orthodontics.

Processing waxes

Processing waxes include boxing, sticky, carding, blockout, white, and utility waxes. Boxing wax is used to form containers for pouring casts. It is also used to fabricate replacement pontics for temporary bridges. Sticky Wax (Kerr Manufacturing Co.) is used to join materials temporarily. Carding wax is used for attaching parts and in some soldering techniques. Blockout wax (Dura Block Out, Belle de St. Claire) is used to fill voids and undercuts for removable partial denture fabrication. White wax is used for making patterns to simulate a veneer facing. Utility wax (Modern Materials, Inc.) has miscellaneous applications for various laboratory procedures.

Impression waxes

Impression waxes (Bite Wax, Mizzy, Inc.) exhibit high flow and distort on withdrawal from undercuts. Waxes used for denture impressions are limited to use in edentulous regions of the mouth. Corrective waxes are used as wax washes to record detail and displace selected regions of soft tissue in edentulous impressions. Finally, bite waxes are used in certain prosthetic techniques; a typical use would be bite registration.

Properties

Waxes may consist of both crystalline and amorphous components, each with a distribution of molecular weights. Therefore, waxes melt over a range of 5° to 30°C (41° to 86°F) rather than at one temperature. Waxes have the highest coefficients of thermal expansion of any dental material. Resultant dimensional changes may produce poor-fitting castings if not balanced by compensating factors of mold expansion. The total wax shrinkage on cooling from liquid to solid at room temperature may be as great as 0.4% and consists of solidification shrinkages plus contraction on cooling to room temperature after solidification.

Flow is a measure of a wax's ability to deform under light forces and is analogous to creep. Flow increases with increasing temperature and force. At a temperature close to its softening range, a wax may flow under its own weight. In liquids, flow is measured by viscosity. In solids, flow is measured by the degree of plastic deformation over a fixed period of time. Type I direct-inlay technique waxes* need to flow well to reproduce details of the cavity preparation. However, when the wax is cooled to mouth temperature, flow must be minimized to reduce distortion when the pattern is removed.

Wax distortion

Waxes are partly elastic in behavior and tend to return to their original shape after deformation. A straight bar of wax bent into a horseshoe shape will slowly straighten out at room temperature (Fig 10-2). Residual stresses as a result of nonuniform heating also contribute to later distortion. There are four ways of minimizing pattern distortion. First of all, wax for the direct technique should be heated uniformly at 50°C (122°F) for 15 minutes before use. Next, the pattern should be invested quickly. The rigid walls of the set investment constrain the pattern and reduce distortion due to recovery and residual stresses. Also, the pattern should be stored at a low temperature if not invested right away.

Elastic recovery is slower at low temperatures; therefore, if immediate investing is impractical, storage in a refrigerator is preferred. If a pattern is refrigerated, however, it should be allowed to warm to room temperature before investing. Finally, it is essential that no wax residues are left in the mold after burnout in the lost wax process. Residues will result in poor castings because of inclusions or incomplete margins.

*American National Standards Institute/American Dental Association Specification no. 4 for dental-inlay casting wax.

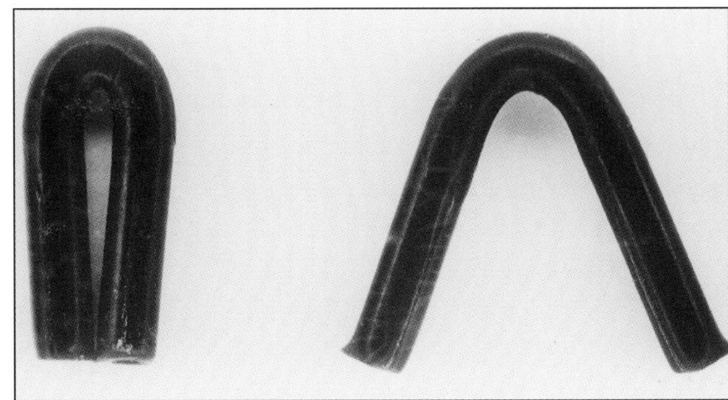

Fig 10-2 The rod on the right was originally bent to the shape of the rod on the left. After floating on room-temperature water for 24 hours, the rod opened as a result of the memory effect.

Commercial materials

Inlay waxes are supplied in geometric and anatomic forms as well as in bulk. Casting waxes are supplied in sheets and rods and in bulk. Preformed patterns are also available for partial denture applications. Bite waxes are supplied in a variety of forms and shapes. Base plate wax is supplied in sheet form.

Glossary

fats Substances similar to wax but characterized as being soft and greasy to the touch. An example of a fat used in dental waxes is stearic acid.

flow Continued deformation resulting from application of a static force.

gums Viscous substances from plant or animal sources that harden in air. Gums combine with water to form sticky, viscous liquids. An example of a gum is gum arabic.

natural resins Mixtures of high-molecular-weight organic substances obtained directly from plants or trees as exudates. An example of a natural resin used in dental waxes is dammar.

natural wax A hydrocarbon or hydrocarbon-derivative polymer with an approximate molecular weight of 400 to 4,000; of mineral, plant, insect, or animal origin.

pattern A form used to make a mold to be cast.

recovery Change in shape resulting from the release of internal stresses.

residual stress Internal stress independent of applied force.

synthetic wax A man-made wax synthesized from appropriate monomers.

Discussion questions

1. Waxes have the highest thermal expansion values of any dental material. What problems can result from this, especially in casting accuracy?
2. Which type of inlay wax (I or II) should be used for the indirect die technique? How do the different flow properties of the two types make them suitable for their application?
3. If a wax inlay pattern cannot be invested right away, it is recommended that it be stored in a refrigerator. Why and what phenomena will this storage affect?
4. Why are polymer cements recommended for use with CAD/CAM inlays with poor marginal fits?

Questions and answers

1. **List several common natural waxes used in dentistry.** Paraffin, beeswax, carnauba wax, spermaceti, ceresin.
2. **Why must natural waxes be carefully monitored for properties?** The properties of natural waxes vary with the conditions under which they are produced. For this reason, these waxes are not consistent in their properties. The properties of synthetic waxes are much more uniform, as the manufacturer may impose quality control procedures during their production.
3. **Name three types of pattern waxes and their applications.**
   a. Inlay wax: To form inlay, crown, or pontic replicas.
   b. Casting wax: Used for thin sections in certain partial denture and crown-and-bridge patterns.
   c. Base plate wax: Used in the construction of full denture patterns.
4. **Wax pattern contraction arises from two sources. What are they?** Solidification shrinkage and contraction on cooling to room temperature.
5. **List two means of increasing wax flow.** Increase temperature and apply force.
6. **Describe three steps to minimize wax pattern distortion.**
   a. Heat wax uniformly.
   b. Invest the pattern without delay.
   c. Store the uninvested pattern at a low temperature.
7. **Type I pattern wax must have two types of flow behavior. Why?** It must have high flow above mouth temperature to reproduce detail of cavity preparation, and it must have low flow at mouth temperature to reduce distortion when the pattern is removed.
8. **What is the memory or recovery effect in waxes, and what does it lead to?** Memory is the return of waxes to their original shapes over time. This produces distortion.
9. **Why is complete burnout of wax patterns critical in the lost wax casting technique?** Incomplete burnout leaves wax residue, which leads to poor castings from either inclusions or incomplete margins.

Recommended reading

American Dental Association. Dentists' Desk Reference: Materials, Instruments and Equipment. 2nd ed. Chicago: 1983.

Craig RG, ed. Restorative Dental Materials. 7th ed. St Louis: CV Mosby Co, 1985.

Phillips RW. Skinner's Science of Dental Materials. 8th ed. Philadelphia: WB Saunders Co, 1982.

Chapter 11

Dental Cements

Although dental cements are used only in small quantities, they are perhaps the most important materials in clinical dentistry because of their application as (*1*) luting agents to bond preformed restorations and orthodontic attachments in or on the tooth, (*2*) cavity liners and bases to protect the pulp and as foundation and anchor for restorations, and (*3*) restorative materials. This multiplicity of applications requires more than one type of cement because no one material has yet been developed that can fulfill the varying requirements.

Over the last two decades, the emphasis has been on materials for luting in view of the increase in crown-and-bridge prosthodontics. More recently, with the advent of glass-ionomer cements, interest in restorative applications has revived also. These different applications require different physical properties and appropriate clinical manipulative characteristics, and so, in response to the changing situation, new international standards are being developed (International Standards Organization [ISO]), as are various national standards (American National Standards Institute/American Dental Association [ANSI/ADA]) based on performance criteria rather than specific composition.

For acceptable performance in luting and restorative applications, the cement must have adequate resistance to dissolution in the oral environment. It must also develop an adequately strong bond through mechanical interlocking and adhesion. High strength in tension, shear, and compression is required, as is good fracture toughness to resist stresses at the restoration/tooth interface. Good manipulation properties, such as adequate working and setting times, are essential for successful use. The manipulation, including dispensation of the ingredients, should allow for some margin of error in practice. The material must be biologically acceptable.

Most cements are powder-liquid materials that may be dispensed and mixed manually or predispensed in capsules that are mixed mechanically. Some recent materials are composed of two pastes. Cements set by chemical reaction between the ingredients (often an acid-base reaction) or involve polymerization of a monomeric component.

In the early years of this century zinc oxide–phosphoric acid, zinc oxide–eugenol (clove oil 85%), and silicate glass–phosphoric acid cements were discovered. These zinc phosphate, zinc eugenate, and silicate cements were widely used until the 1970s when new cements began to be developed.

The introduction of new types of cements was prompted by the emphasis on improved biocompatibility and bonding to the tooth that began to develop 20 years ago. New information on pulpal histopathology resulting from particular clinical techniques and materials, as well as the demonstration of marginal leakage involving penetration of bacteria to the dentin interface and a reduction in retention of restorations, led to the realization that new materials possessing good wetting and bonding to enamel and dentin and low toxicity were needed.

These concepts were the basis of the development of cements based on polyacrylic acid: first the zinc polyacrylate (polycarboxylate) and later the glass-ionomer cements. The polycarboxylate cements have gradually become established as alternatives to zinc phosphate cement because of their minimal effects on pulp, similar strength and solubility characteristics, and adhesive properties. The glass-ionomer cements have developed more slowly, but their potential for luting and restorative applications is being more widely recognized by clinicians.

The advent of the acrylic resins led to the development of poly(methyl methacrylate) in the mid-1950s. These materials had limitations such as lack of adhesion, leakage, and toxicity that terminated their use for routine cementation. In the last decade, polymerizable Bis-GMA and other dimethacrylate monomer cements have become available in various forms for attachment of cast restorations and orthodontic brackets to enamel. More recently, similar systems containing (potentially) adhesive monomers have been marketed for crown-and-bridge cementation.

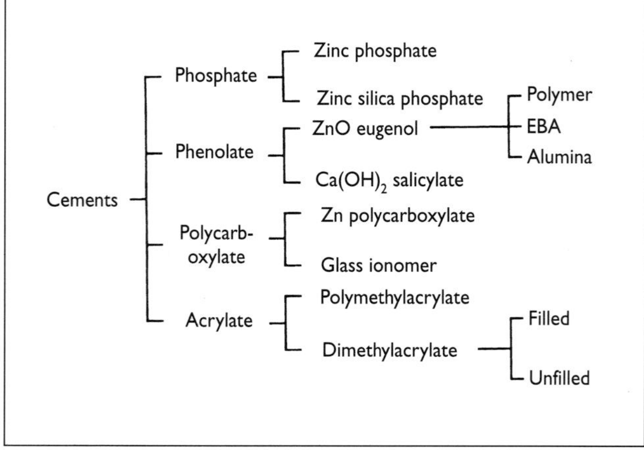

Fig 11-1 Classification of dental cements.

The cements based on the reaction between calcium hydroxide and a liquid salicylate also originated 25 years ago. They were primarily fluid, two-paste materials intended for the lining of deep cavities that had actual or potential exposure, thus providing an antibacterial sealing action to facilitate the formation of reparative dentin. The susceptibility to acid erosion of the original formulations, both through marginal leakage of restorations and exposure to phosphoric acid during acid-etch techniques, has resulted in more resistant compositions and, quite recently, to a light-cured, resin-based material.

As a result of the research of the last 10 years, there are cements of four basic types available, classified according to the matrix-forming species, as shown in Fig 11-1 and Table 11-1:

1. Phosphate bonded
2. Phenolate bonded
3. Polycarboxylate bonded
4. Polymethacrylate bonded

Table 11-1 Classification of dental cements

Matrix bond	Class of cement	Type
Phosphate	Zinc phosphate	Zinc phosphate Zinc phosphate fluoride Zinc phosphate copper oxide/salts Zinc phosphate silver salts
	Zinc silicophosphate	Zinc silicophosphate Zinc silicophosphate mercury salts
Phenolate	Zinc oxide–eugenol	Zinc oxide–eugenol Zinc oxide–eugenol polymer Zinc oxide–eugenol EBA/alumina
	Calcium hydroxide salicylate	Calcium hydroxide salicylate
Polycarboxylate	Zinc polycarboxylate	Zinc polycarboxylate Zinc polycarboxylate fluoride
	Glass ionomer	Calcium aluminum polyalkenoate Calcium aluminum polyalkenoate-polymethacrylate
Polymethacrylate	Acrylic	Poly(methyl methacrylate)
	Dimethacrylate	Dimethacrylate unfilled Dimethacrylate filled

Numerous brands of each type are available, and there is some overlap between properties. Since clinical and in vivo evaluation of cements is still very limited, the predictive value of laboratory data for assessment of clinical performance requires knowledgeable interpretation, not least since generalizations on specific types of cement cannot be made on the basis of the behavior of one or two brands. The applications of the different types of cements are given in Table 11-2. Examples of current widely used brands of cements are given in Tables 11-3 through 11-5. Typical properties of luting cements are given in Table 11-6.

Table 11-2 Selection of dental cements

Application	Cement type
Inlays, crown posts, multiretainers, fixed partial denture in or on:	Glass-ionomer cement
Nonvital teeth or with advanced pulpal recession and average retention	Zinc phosphate
Vital teeth with average retention, average pulp recession, thin dentin, especially for single units and small-span bridges	Zinc polycarboxylate
Multiretainer splints on vital teeth with above-average retention, minimal dentin thickness; hypersensitive patients	Zinc oxide–eugenol polymer
Temporary cementation	Zinc oxide–eugenol polymer Zinc polycarboxylate (thin mix)
Temporary cementation and stabilization of old, loose restorations; fixation of facings and acid-etched cast restorations	Dimethacrylate composite resin
Base/liner in:	
Cavity with remaining dentin more than about 0.5 mm	Glass-ionomer cement Zinc polycarboxylate Zinc phosphate (low-acid type)
Cavity with minimal dentin or exposure	Calcium hydroxide salicylate Zinc oxide–eugenol polymer

Table 11-3 "Permanent" luting cements

Product	Type	Manufacturer
Durelon	Zinc carboxylate	Premier/Premier-ESPE
Everbond	Glass ionomer	Kerr Manufacturing Co.
Fleck's Extraordinary	Zinc phosphate	Mizzy, Inc.
Fuji Type I	Glass ionomer	GC International Corp.
Fynal	Zinc oxide–eugenol	L.D. Caulk
Hy-Bond Polycarboxylate Cement	Zinc carboxylate	Shofu Dental Corp.
Hy-Bond Zinc Phosphate Cement	Zinc phosphate	Shofu Dental Corp.
Ketac-Cem	Glass ionomer	Premier/Premier-ESPE
Liv Cenera	Zinc carboxylate	GC International Corp.
Modern Tenacin	Zinc phosphate	L.D. Caulk
Opotow Alumina EBA	Zinc oxide–eugenol	Teledyne Getz
Tylok Plus	Zinc carboxylate	L.D. Caulk
Zinc Cement Improved	Zinc phosphate	Mission White Dental, Inc.

Table 11-4 "Maryland Bridge" composite restorative cements

Product	Type	Manufacturer
Comspan	2 pastes, translucent	L.D. Caulk
Conclude	2 pastes, opaque	3M Dental Products Div.
Den-Mat	2 pastes, translucent	Den-Mat Corp.
Duralingual	Primer, paste, opaque	Unitek Corp.
Epoxylite 9080	Powder/liquid, opaque	Lee Pharmaceuticals
Getz	2 pastes, opaque	Teledyne Getz
Resilute	2 pastes, translucent	Henry Schein, Inc.

Table 11-5 Temporary cements

Product	Type	Manufacturer
Flow-Temp	Zinc oxide–eugenol	Premier/Premier-ESPE
Freeginol	Eugenol free	GC International Corp.
Nogenol	Eugenol free	Coe Laboratories, Inc.
Temp-Bond	Zinc oxide–eugenol	Kerr Manufacturing Co.
Temporary Cement	Zinc oxide–eugenol	Buffalo Dental Mfg. Co.
ZOE 2200	Zinc oxide–eugenol	L.D. Caulk
Zone	Eugenol free	Cadco Dental Products

Table 11-6 Properties of dental luting cements

Material	Film thickness (mm)	Setting time (min)	Solubility (wt%)	Strength (MPa)		Modulus of elasticity (GPa)
				Compressive	Tensile	
Zinc phosphate	25–35	5–14	0.2 max	80–100	5–7	13
Zinc silicophosphate	30–40	5–7	1	140–170	8–13	—
Zinc oxide–eugenol						
Unmodified	25–35	2–10	1.5	2–25	1–2	—
Polymer reinforced	35–45	7–9	1	35–55	5–8	2–3
EBA-alumina	40–60	7–13	1	55–70	3–6	3–6
Zinc polycarboxylate	20–25	6–9	0.06	55–85	8–12	5–6
Glass ionomer	25–35	6–9	1	90–140	6–7	7–8
Polymer-based	20–60	3–7	0.05	70–200	25–40	4–6

Phosphate-based cements

Zinc phosphate cement

Applications

Because of their long history, these materials have the widest range of applications from the cementation (luting) of fixed cast alloy and porcelain restorations and orthodontic bands (Table 11-3) to their use as a cavity liner or base to protect pulp from mechanical, thermal, or electrical stimuli (Fig 11-2).

Composition and setting

The powder is mainly zinc oxide with up to 10% magnesium oxide and small amounts of pigments. It is fired at high temperature (>1,000°C) for several hours to reduce its reactivity. The liquid is an aqueous solution of phosphoric acid containing 45% to 64% H_3PO_4 and 30% to 55% water. The liquid also contains 2% to 3% aluminum and 0 to 9% zinc. Aluminum is essential to the cement-forming reaction, whereas the zinc is a moderator of the reaction between powder and liquid, allowing adequate working time and permitting a sufficient quantity of powder to be added for optimum properties in the cement.

Some zinc phosphate cements have modified compositions. One material, widely used as a cavity liner, has 8% aluminum and only 25% H_3PO_4 in the liquid and a powder that contains calcium hydroxide. Others may contain fluoride and have as much as 10% stannous fluoride.

The amorphous zinc phosphate formed binds together the unreacted zinc oxide and other components of the cement. The set cement consists of a cored structure of residual zinc oxide particles in a phosphate matrix:

zinc oxide + phosphoric acid → amorphous zinc phosphate

Manipulation

The measurement of components and the timing of mixing are essential to consistent success. The mixing slab must be thoroughly dried before use. The powder is added to the liquid in small portions to achieve the desired consistency. Dissipation of the heat of reaction by mixing over a large area on a cooled slab will allow a greater incorporation of powder in a given amount of liquid. The cement must be undisturbed until the end of the setting time. The cement liquid is kept stoppered to prevent changes in the water content. Cloudy liquid should be discarded. Increasing the powder/liquid ratio gives a more viscous mix, shorter setting time, higher strength, lower solubility, and less free acidity. Use of a chilled (5°C) thick glass slab slows down the initial reaction and allows incorporation of more powder, giving superior properties in the set cement.

Properties

The long persistence of zinc phosphates in clinical practice indicates that reasonable performance is obtained. Although the properties are far from ideal, they are usually regarded as a standard against which to compare newer cements (Table 11-6). The principal reasons for their satisfactory performance under routine conditions are that they can be easily manipulated and that they set sharply to a relatively strong mass from a fluid consistency.

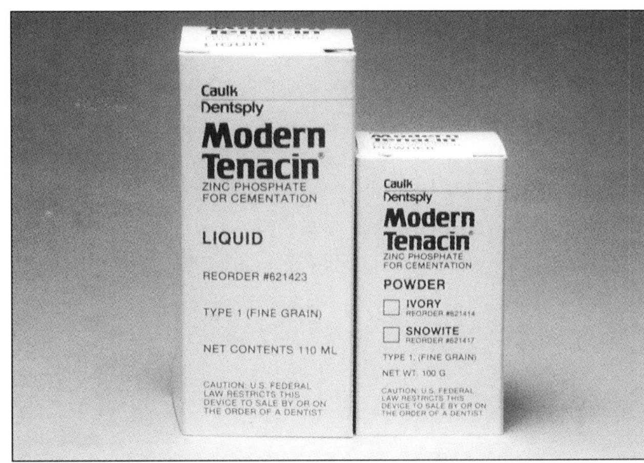

Fig 11-2 Zinc phosphate cements with a wide range of cementation applications.

For a given brand of material, the properties are a function of the powder/liquid ratio. For a given cementing consistency, the higher the powder/liquid ratio, the better the strength properties and the lower the solubility and free acidity.

At room temperature (21° to 23°C) the working time for most brands at luting consistency is 3 to 6 minutes; the setting time is 5 to 14 minutes. Extended working times and shorter setting times can be achieved by use of a cold mixing slab, which permits up to an approximate 50% increase in the amount of powder, improving both strength and resistance to dissolution.

The cement must have the ability to wet the tooth and restoration, flow into the irregularities on the surfaces it is joining, and fill in and seal the gaps between the restoration and the tooth. The minimum value of film thickness is a function of powder particle size, powder/liquid ratio, and mix viscosity. As measured by ISO and ANSI/ADA specifications, acceptable cements give film thicknesses of less than 25 µm. In practice, the cement fills in the inaccuracies between the restoration and the tooth and allows most castings to seat satisfactorily. Unless escapeways or vents are provided with full crowns, separation of powder and liquid may occur, with marginal defects in the cement film.

At the recommended powder/liquid ratio (2.5 to 3.5 g/mL), the compressive strength of the set zinc phosphate cement is 80 to 110 MPa (11,000 to 16,000 psi) after 24 hours. The minimum strength for adequate retention of restorations is about 60 MPa (8,500 psi). The strength is strongly and almost linearly dependent on powder/liquid ratio. The tensile strength is much lower than the compressive strength, 5 to 7 MPa (700 to 900 psi), and the cement shows brittle characteristics. The modulus of elasticity (stiffness) is about 13 GPa (1.8×10^6 psi).

According to the standard method, the solubility and disintegration in distilled water after 23 hours may range from 0.04% to 3.3% for inferior material. The standard limit is 0.2%. The fluoride-containing cements give a figure of about 0.7% to 1.0% because of the leaching of fluoride. The solubility in organic acid solutions, such as lactic or citric acid, is 20 to 30 times higher. These data are only a rough guide to solubility under oral conditions. The comparative evaluation of cement solubility under clinical conditions has shown significant loss but conflicting results. Dissolution contributes to marginal leakage around restorations and bacterial penetration. This may be facilitated by dimensional change. The cement has been found to contract about 0.5% linearly, giving rise to slits at the tooth/cement and cement/restoration interfaces.

Biologic effects

The freshly mixed zinc phosphate is highly acidic with a pH of between 1 and 2 after mixing. Even after setting 1 hour, the pH may still be below 4. After 24 hours, the pH is usually 6 to 7. Pain on cementing is due not only to the free acidity of the mix but also to osmotic movement of fluid through the dentinal tubules. Hydraulic pressure developed during seating of the restoration may also contribute to pulpal damage. Prolonged pulpal irritation, especially in deep cavities that necessitate some form of pulpal protection, may be associated with the extended duration of the set material's low pH. This is minimized by a high powder/liquid ratio and rapid setting. One material that has a low acid content and incorporates calcium hydroxide has little effect on pulp when used as a liner. Very thin mixes will also lead to etching of the enamel.

Advantages and disadvantages

The main advantages of zinc phosphate cements are that they can be mixed easily and that they set sharply to a relatively strong mass from a fluid consistency. Unless the mix is extremely thin (for instance, with a very low powder/liquid ratio), the set cement has a strength that is adequate for clinical service, so manipulation is less critical than with other cements.

However, zinc phosphates' distinct disadvantages include pulp irritation, lack of antibacterial action, brittleness, lack of adhesion, and solubility in oral fluids.

Modified zinc phosphate cements

Copper and silver cements

Black copper cements contain cupric oxide (CuO); red copper cements contain cuprous oxide (Cu_2O). Others may contain cuprous iodide or silicate. Since a much lower powder/liquid ratio is necessary to obtain satisfactory manipulation characteristics with these cements, the mix is highly acidic, resulting in much greater pulpal irritation. Their solubility is higher and their strength is lower than zinc phosphate cements. Their bacteriostatic or anticariogenic properties seem to be slight. Silver cements generally contain a few percent of a salt such as silver phosphate. Their advantages over zinc phosphate cement have not been substantiated.

Fluoride cements

Stannous fluoride (1% to 3%) is present in some orthodontic cements. These materials have a higher solubility and lower strength than zinc phosphate cement owing to dissolution of the fluoride-containing material. Fluoride uptake by enamel from such cements results in reduced enamel solubility and potentially anticariogenic effects.

Silicophosphate cements

These materials have been available for many years as a combination of zinc phosphate and silicate cements. The presence of the silicate glass provides a degree of translucency, improved strength, and fluoride release.

Applications

Their principal applications have been for the cementation of fixed restorations and orthodontic bands (Type I), as a temporary posterior filling material (Type II), and as a dual-purpose material (Type III).

Composition and setting

The powder in these materials consists of a blend of 10% to 20% zinc oxide (zinc phosphate cement powder) and silicate glass (silicate cement powder) mechanically mixed or fused and reground. The silicate glass usually contains 12% to 25% fluoride. Some materials have been labeled "germicidal" because of the presence of small amounts of mercury or silver compounds. The liquid is a concentrated orthophosphoric acid solution containing about 45% water and 2% to 5% aluminum and zinc salts.

The setting reaction has not been fully investigated, but may be represented as follows:

zinc oxide/aluminosilicate glass + phosphoric acid →
zinc aluminosilicate phosphate gel

The set cement consists of unreacted glass and zinc oxide particles bonded together by the alumino-silico-phosphate gel matrix.

Manipulation

The mixing is analogous to that for a phosphate cement; a nonabradable spatula and a cooled mixing slab should be used. The filling mix should be glossy, with puttylike consistency.

Properties

At cementing consistency, the setting time is 5 to 7 minutes; working time is about 4 minutes and may be increased by using a cold mixing slab.

These cements generally have shorter working times and a coarser grain size, leading to a higher film thickness than with zinc phosphate cements. One recent material is improved in these respects, and film thickness is adequate for cementation of cast gold and porcelain restorations.

The compressive strength of the set cement is in the range from 140 to 170 MPa (20,000 to 25,000 psi); the tensile strength is considerably lower at 7 MPa (1,000 psi) (Table 11-6). The toughness and abrasion resistance are higher than those of phosphate cements.

The solubility in distilled water after 7 days is about 1% by weight. Solubility in organic acids and in the mouth is less than for phosphate cements. Fluoride is leached out and may contribute to anticariogenic action. The durability in bonding orthodontic bands to teeth is greater, and less decalcification is observed.

The glass content gives considerably greater translucency than phosphate cements, making silicophosphate cements useful for cementation of porcelain restorations.

Biologic effects

Because of the acidity of the mix and the prolonged low pH (4 to 5) after setting, pulp protection is necessary on all vital teeth. Fluoride and other ions are leached out from the set cement by oral fluids, resulting in increased enamel fluoride and probable anticariogenic action.

Advantages and disadvantages

Silicophosphate cements have better strength, toughness, and abrasion resistance properties than zinc phosphate cements, and show considerable fluoride release, translucency, and, under clinical conditions, lower solubility and better bonding.

Disadvantages include an initial pH and total acidity that are greater than those for zinc phosphate cements. Pulpal sensitivity may be of longer duration, and pulpal protection is essential. Manipulation is more critical than with zinc phosphate cements.

Phenolate-based cements

There are three main types of cement under this classification:

1. The simple zinc oxide–eugenol combination that may contain setting accelerators
2. The reinforced zinc oxide–eugenol materials
3. The ortho-ethoxybenzoic acid (EBA) cements

Cements have also been formulated using other phenolic liquids, but these have seen little use except for those containing calcium hydroxide and a salicylate.

Zinc oxide–eugenol cements

Applications

The basic combination zinc oxide and eugenol finds its principal applications in the temporary cementation of restorations, in the temporary filling of teeth, and as a cavity liner in deep cavity preparations.

Composition and setting

The powder is essentially pure zinc oxide (United States Pharmacopeia [USP] or equivalent, arsenic free). Commercial materials may contain small amounts of fillers, such as silica. About 1% of zinc salts, such as acetate or sulfate, may be present to accelerate the setting. The liquid is purified eugenol or, in some commercial materials, oil of cloves (85% eugenol). One percent or less of alcohol or acetic acid may be present to accelerate setting together with small amounts of water, which is essential to the setting reaction.

A chemical reaction occurs between zinc oxide and eugenol, with the formation of zinc eugenolate (eugenate):

$$\text{zinc oxide} + \text{eugenol} \xrightarrow{\text{water}} \text{zinc eugenolate (eugenate)}$$

The precise mechanism is not fully understood, but the set mass contains residual zinc oxide particles bonded by a matrix of zinc eugenolate and some free eugenol. Water is essential to the reaction, which is accelerated also by zinc ions. The reaction is reversible because the zinc eugenolate is easily hydrolyzed by moisture to eugenol and zinc hydroxide. Thus, the cement disintegrates rapidly when exposed to oral conditions. The rate of reaction between the zinc oxide and the eugenol is dependent on the nature, source, reactivity, and moisture content of the zinc oxide and on the purity and moisture content of the eugenol.

Manipulation

The zinc oxide is slowly wetted by the eugenol; therefore, prolonged and vigorous spatulation is required, especially for a thick mix. A powder/liquid ratio of 3:1 or 4:1 must be used for maximum strength.

Properties

The working time is long because moisture is required for setting. Variable results are obtained with different samples of zinc oxide, depending on their mode of preparation and reactivity. For a given oxide, set time is controlled by moisture availability, accelerators, and the powder/liquid ratio. Mixes of cementing consistency set very slowly unless accelerators are used and/or a drop of water is added. Commercial materials set in the range of 2 to 10 minutes, resulting in adequate strengths at 10 minutes for amalgam restorations to be placed (Table 11-6).

The particle size of the zinc oxide and the viscosity of the mix govern the film thickness. Using a fluid mix gives values of about 40 µm.

Because of the weak nature of the binding agent, the compressive strength is low, in the range of 7 to 40 MPa (1,000 to 6,000 psi). The tensile strength is very low also.

The solubility is high, about 1.5% by weight in distilled water after 24 hours. Eugenol is extracted from the set cement by the hydrolytic decomposition of the zinc eugenolate/eugenate. The cement disintegrates rapidly when exposed to oral conditions.

Biologic effect

The presence of eugenol in the set cement under clinical conditions appears to lead to an anodyne and obtundent effect on the pulp in deep cavities. When exposed directly to oral conditions, the material maintains good sealing characteristics despite a volumetric shrinkage of 0.9% and a thermal expansion of 35×10^{-6}/°C. The sealing capacity and antibacterial action appear to facilitate pulpal healing; however, when in direct contact with connective tissue, the material is an irritant. Reparative dentin formation in exposed pulp is variable. Eugenol is a potential allergen.

Advantages and disadvantages

The main advantage of these materials is their bland and obtundent effect on the pulp tissues, together with their good sealing ability and resistance to marginal penetration.

Disadvantages include low strength and abrasion resistance, solubility, and disintegration in oral fluids, and little anticariogenic action.

Reinforced zinc oxide–eugenol cements

Applications

These materials have been used as cementing agents for restorations, cavity liners and base materials, and temporary filling materials.

Composition and setting

The powder consists of zinc oxide with 10% to 40% finely divided natural or synthetic resins (eg, colophony [pine resin], poly[methyl methacrylate], polystyrene, or polycarbonate) together with accelerators. The liquid is eugenol, which may also contain dissolved resins as mentioned earlier and accelerators such as acetic acid, as well as antimicrobial agents such as thymol or 8-hydroxyquinoline.

The setting reaction is similar to zinc oxide–eugenol cements. Acidic resins such as colophony (abietic acid) may react with the zinc oxide, strengthening the matrix.

Manipulation

More powder is required for a cementing mix than with other cements. The proper ratio must be adhered to for adequate strength properties. Measures are provided for some commercial materials. The mixing pad or slab should be thoroughly dry. The powder is mixed into the liquid in small portions with vigorous spatulation until the correct amount has been incorporated. Adequate time should be allowed for setting without disturbance of the cement. Both powder and liquid containers should be kept closed and stored under dry conditions.

Properties

These cements may have a long working time because moisture is needed for setting. Some commercial materials contain moisture and, therefore, have working and setting times in the same range as zinc phosphate cements, that is, 7 to 9 minutes under mouth conditions. Setting time is also lengthened by reducing the powder/liquid ratio.

At cementing consistency, values of film thickness from 35 to 75 µm have been obtained with commercial materials (Table 11-6). Clinical trials have shown satisfactory performance in seating castings for cements with the lowest values.

These materials have compressive strengths in the range from 35 to 55 MPa (5,000 to 8,000 psi). The tensile strength is 5 to 8 MPa (700 to 1,000 psi) (Table 11-6). The strength is adequate as a lining material and for luting single restorations and retainers with good retention form. The modulus of elasticity is 2 to 3 GPa (300,000 to 400,000 psi). The mechanical properties of these cements are reduced by immersion in water, which results in loss of eugenol, although this appears to be slower than with simple zinc oxide–eugenol materials. This tendency seems less pronounced with the polymer-reinforced materials.

Because of the presence of the resin, the solubility of these cements appears to be somewhat lower than that of zinc oxide–eugenol materials.

Biologic effects

Polymer-reinforced zinc oxide–eugenol cements have biologic effects similar to basic materials, although there is some variation in inflammatory reaction in connective tissue with the brand of material. There may be softening and discoloration of some resin restorative materials.

Advantages and disadvantages

The main advantages of these materials are the minimal biologic effects, good initial sealing properties, and adequate strength for final cementation of restorations.

The principal disadvantages are the lower strength, higher solubility, and higher disintegration compared to zinc phosphate cements; hydrolytic instability; and the softening and discoloration of some resin restorative materials.

EBA and other chelate cements

In order to further improve on the basic zinc oxide–eugenol system, many researchers have investigated mixtures of zinc and other oxides with various liquid chelating agents. The only system that has received extensive commercial exploitation for luting and lining is that containing ortho-ethoxybenzoic acid.*

Applications

These materials have been used for the cementation of inlays and crowns and bridges, for temporary fillings, and as a base or lining material.

Composition and setting

In EBA materials the powder is mainly zinc oxide containing 20% to 30% aluminum oxide or other mineral fillers. Polymeric reinforcing agents, such as poly(methyl methacrylate), may also be present. The liquid consists of 50% to 66% ethoxybenzoic acid with the remainder eugenol.

The setting mechanism has not been fully elucidated. It appears to involve chelate salt formation between the EBA, eugenol, and zinc oxide. The setting is accelerated by the same factors that are operative for zinc oxide–eugenol cements.

Manipulation

In general, the manipulation is similar to that of reinforced zinc oxide–eugenol cements. The cement mixes readily to a very fluid consistency even at a high powder/liquid ratio. In order to obtain optimal properties, it is important to use as high a powder/liquid ratio as possible; this is about 3.5 g/mL for cementation and 5 to 6 g/mL for liners or bases. Vigorous spatulation is required for about 2 minutes to incorporate all the required powder. The correct mix flows readily under pressure because of the long working time. Adequate setting time in the mouth should be allowed. Several days may be required to reach maximum strength.

*Noneugenol cements have also been developed in which fatty acids or low-odor phenolic derivatives are used to overcome the smell and taste of eugenol.

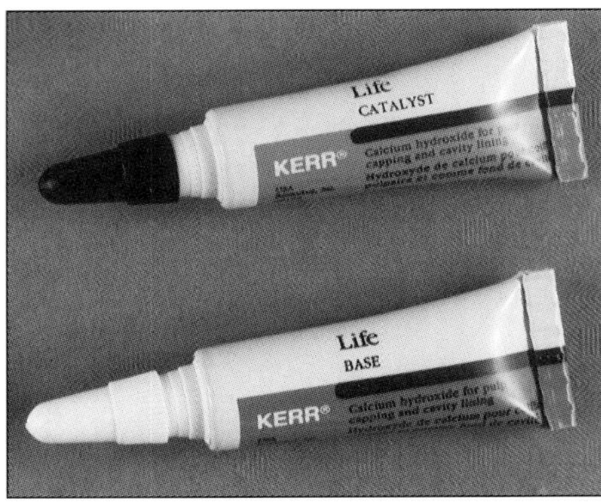

Fig 11-3 Calcium hydroxide cements used as pulp-capping materials to facilitate the formation of reparative dentin.

Properties

The working time at room temperature is long because of the dependence upon moisture. The setting time ranges between 7 and 13 minutes under oral conditions (Table 11-6).

The film thickness appears to be in the range of 40 to 70 µm for the different brands and seems adequate for permanent cementation of restorations at the lower level.

At cementing consistency, the compressive strength of these materials is in the range of 55 to 70 MPa (8,000 to 10,000 psi); higher values, similar to those of zinc phosphate cements, can be obtained by increasing the powder/liquid ratio. The tensile strength is considerably lower, about 3 to 6 MPa (500 to 900 psi). The modulus of elasticity is about 5 GPa (700,000 psi). The EBA cements show viscoelastic properties with very low strength and large plastic deformation at slow (0.1 mm/min) rates of deformation and at mouth temperature (37°C). This may explain why the retention values for crowns and orthodontic bands are considerably below those obtained using zinc phosphate cements.

The solubility is similar to that of the polymer-reinforced zinc oxide–eugenol materials in distilled water, although loss of eugenol also occurs. The resistance to solubility in organic acids appears to be greater than that of the zinc phosphate cements. When exposed to moisture, greater oral dissolution occurs than for other cements. However, a clinical survey by Silvey and Meyers (1978) of the performance of an EBA-alumina cement over 3 years showed only very slightly worse results than for zinc phosphate and polycarboxylate cements. Oral breakdown may thus depend on the precise brand and manipulation.

Biologic effects

The biologic properties of these materials appear to be similar to those of zinc oxide–eugenol materials.

Advantages and disadvantages

The principal advantages of EBA cements are their easy mixing, long working time, good flow characteristics, and low irritation to pulp. Strength and film thickness can be comparable to those of zinc phosphate cements (Table 11-6).

The main disadvantages are the critical proportioning, hydrolytic breakdown in oral fluids, liability to plastic deformation, and poorer retention than zinc phosphate cements. These materials seem best suited to luting of restorations with good fit and retention where there is no undue stress and as cavity bases.

Calcium hydroxide chelate cements

The value of calcium hydroxide as a pulp-capping material that facilitates the formation of reparative dentin has long been recognized. This action appears to be largely attributable to its alkaline pH and consequent antibacterial and protein-lyzing effect. Although a number of aqueous paste materials based on calcium hydroxide are available, their manipulation is not easy and the dried films tend to crack. In the early 1960s, phenolate-type cements based on the setting reaction between calcium hydroxide and other oxides and salicylate esters were introduced (Fig 11-3).

Applications

These materials are used as a liner in deep cavity preparations.

Composition and setting

These materials are usually formulated as two pastes: One paste contains calcium hydroxide, zinc oxide, and zinc salts in ethylene toluene sulphonamide; the other contains calcium sulfate, titanium dioxide, and calcium tungstate (a radiopacifying agent) in a liquid disalicylate ester of butane-1,3-diol. The calcium hydroxide is intended to be in excess to produce an alkaline pH that will effect an antibacterial and remineralization action. There is some variation among the materials in this respect. At least one material contains fluoride.

Calcium and zinc oxide react with the salicylate ester to form a chelate similar to the zinc oxide–eugenol reaction. Likewise the reaction is greatly accelerated by moisture and accelerators.

Manipulation
Equal lengths of the two pastes are mixed to a uniform color.

Properties
Working time may be 3 to 5 minutes, depending on the availability of moisture. In the mouth, setting is rapid, about 1 or 2 minutes.

The compressive strength at 7 minutes is about 6 MPa (900 psi), and the tensile strength 1.5 MPa (200 psi); at 1 hour the corresponding values are about 10 MPa (1,500 psi) and 1.5 MPa (200 psi); and at one day the values are 14 to 20 MPa (2,000 to 3,000 psi) and 1.7 to 2 MPa (250 to 300 psi). Thin films become resistant to 8 MPa (1,100 psi) penetration force in 90 seconds. At 37°C plastic flow without fracture occurs.

The solubility in 50% phosphoric acid during acid-etching procedures is significant. These cements seem to be subject to hydrolytic breakdown. When continued marginal leakage takes place, complete dissolution of linings of these materials can occur.

Biologic effects
These cements appear to exert a strong antibacterial action when free calcium hydroxide is available and to assist in remineralization of carious dentin. They facilitate the formation of dentin bridging when used for pulp capping on exposures. Their effect on exposed pulp is superior to that of zinc oxide–eugenol materials. These materials can also exert a pulp protective action by neutralizing and preventing the passage of acid and by acting as a barrier to the penetration of other agents such as methyl methacrylate.

Advantages and disadvantages
The advantages of these materials include their easy manipulation, rapid hardening in thin layers, good sealing characteristics, and beneficial effects on carious dentin and exposed pulps.

Their disadvantages are that they show low strength even when fully set, exhibit plastic deformation, are weakened by exposure to moisture, and will dissolve under acidic conditions and if marginal leakage occurs. The data on physical properties and clinical experience suggest that further improvements in these materials are required before they can be utilized as the sole liner in deep cavity preparations.

More recently polymerizable resin compositions containing calcium hydroxide have been introduced as alternatives to these materials.

Polycarboxylate (carboxylate)-based cements

Zinc polycarboxylate cements

The polycarboxylate cements were developed in the late 1960s as adhesive dental cements that would combine the strength properties of the phosphate system with the biologic acceptability of the zinc oxide–eugenol materials. These materials have gone through several stages of development since their inception, and progress is continuing.

Applications
Zinc polycarboxylates are used for the cementation of cast alloy and porcelain restorations and orthodontic bands, as cavity liners or base materials, and as temporary filling materials.

Composition and setting
The powder in these cements is zinc oxide with, in some cases, 1% to 5% of tin or magnesium oxide; 10% to 40% aluminum oxide or other reinforcing filler may be present in some brands. A few percent of stannous or other fluoride may be included also to improve mechanical properties and provide leachable fluoride. The liquid is approximately a 40% aqueous solution of polyacrylic acid or an acrylic acid copolymer with other organic acids, such as itaconic acid. The molecular weight of the polymer is generally in the range of 30,000 to 50,000, which accounts for the viscous nature of the solution. In some brands of the material the polyacrylic acid component is dried and added to the powder. In a brand that is encapsulated the liquid is a weak solution of NaH_2PO_4, which both reduces the viscosity of the polyacrylic acid and retards the setting of the cement. In still other brands water is simply added to the powdered ingredients.

The zinc oxide reacts with the polyacrylic acid, forming a cross-linked structure of zinc polyacrylate. The set cement consists of the residual zinc

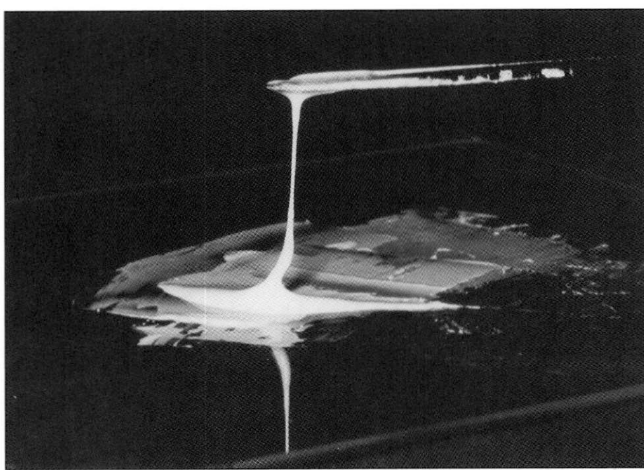

Fig 11-4 Typical consistency for water mix polycarboxylate and glass-ionomer cements. The mix is comparable to zinc phosphate cements.

oxide particles bonded together by this amorphous gel-like matrix:

zinc oxide + polyacrylic acid → zinc polyacrylate

Manipulation

The material should be carefully proportioned and the freshly dispensed components mixed rapidly in 30 to 40 seconds. The mix should be used while it is still glossy, before the onset of cobwebbing. The correct cementing mix is more viscous than a zinc phosphate mix, but because of its different rheology it flows adequately under pressure. The water mix materials are more fluid initially (Fig 11-4). The interior of restorations and tooth surfaces should be clean and free of saliva. The powder and liquid should be stored under cool conditions and kept stoppered. Prolonged or cold storage may cause the liquid to gel; to reverse this warm to 50°C. Loss of moisture from the liquid will lead to thickening.

Properties

The rate of setting is affected by the powder/liquid ratio, the reactivity of the zinc oxide, the particle size, the presence of additives, and the molecular weight and concentration of the polyacrylic acid. At luting consistency the recommended powder/liquid ratio for most materials is about 1.5:1 by weight. The working time is 2.5 to 3.5 minutes at room temperature, and the setting time is 6 to 9 minutes at 37°C; the water mix materials tend to give slightly longer setting times. As with other cements, working time can be substantially increased by mixing the material on a cold slab and by refrigerating the powder. The liquid should not be chilled, as this encourages gelation due to hydrogen bonding.

The freshly mixed cement shows shear thinning. Contrary to the subjective impression that the correct mix for a zinc polycarboxylate cement is much thicker than that of a luting zinc phosphate mix, under pressure they flow out to the same degree to a film thickness of 25 to 35 µm. In fact, the zinc phosphate mix tends to thicken more quickly than the zinc polycarboxylate mix. One of the most common errors made with the polycarboxylate cements is to make a mix that appears to be as fluid as a zinc phosphate mix; this will result in a low powder/liquid ratio with consequent poor properties in the cement. Measuring devices for these materials will ensure correct proportions.

At cementing consistency, the compressive strength of these materials is in the range of 55 to 85 MPa (8,000 to 12,000 psi), and the tensile strength is 8 to 12 MPa (1,100 to 1,700 psi) (Table 11-6). Strength increases with the powder/liquid ratio, reaching a maximum at about 2:1 by weight, and it is increased also by additives such as alumina and stannous fluoride. In general these cements have somewhat lower compressive strengths than zinc phosphate cements but are significantly stronger in tension. The cement gains strength rapidly after the initial setting period; the strength at 1 hour is about 80% of the 24-hour value. The modulus of elasticity is about 6 GPa (850,000 psi).

In distilled water, the solubility ranges from less than 0.1% to 0.6%. The latter high value relates particularly to cements that contain stannous fluoride. However, as in the zinc phosphate system, the solubility is appreciably higher in acids such as lactic and citric acid. In vivo solubility is similar to or less than that for zinc phosphate cements.

Bonding to clean enamel and dentin surfaces can occur through calcium complexation. In practice, adhesion to dentin may be limited because of debris and contamination. The material also sticks to clean stainless steel, amalgam, chrome-cobalt, and other alloys. Bond strength is related to the strength of the cement.

Biologic effects

The effect of zinc polycarboxylate cements on pulp is comparable to or less than that of zinc oxide–eugenol. The formation of reparative dentin in exposed pulp is variable. The generally good biocompatibility appears

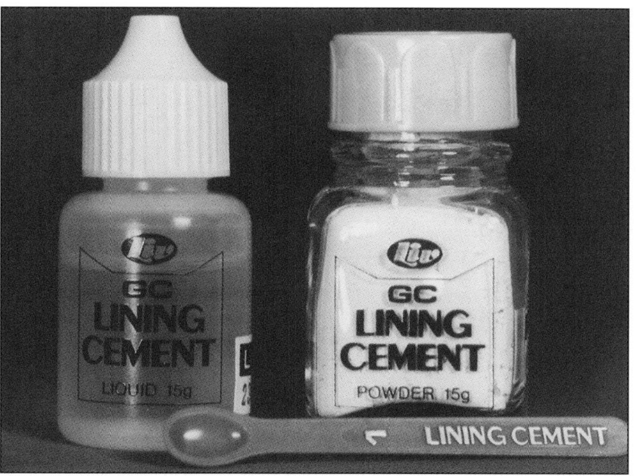

Fig 11-5 Glass-ionomer cavity preparation lining cements.

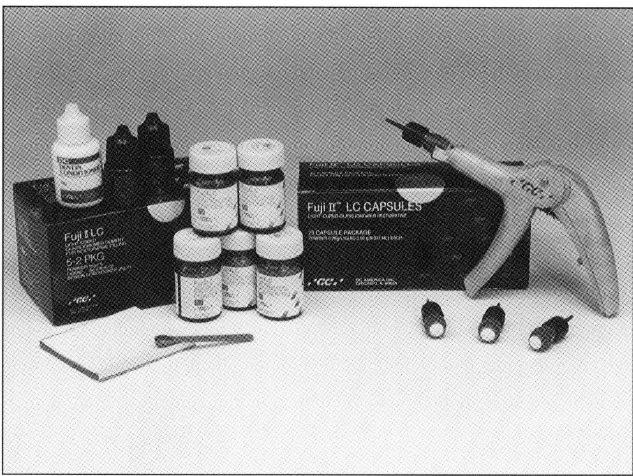

Fig 11-6 Glass-ionomer restorative materials.

to be primarily due to the low intrinsic toxicity and also to (*1*) the rapid rise of the cement pH toward neutrality; (*2*) localization of the polyacrylic acid and limitation of diffusion by its molecular size and ion binding to dentinal fluid and proteins; and (*3*) the minimal movement of fluid in the dentinal tubules in response to the cement. The presence of stannous fluoride does not appear to affect the mild response. The fluoride-containing cements release fluoride, which is taken up by neighboring enamel and which presumably will exert anticariogenic effects.

Advantages and disadvantages

The main advantages of these materials are the low irritancy, adhesion to tooth substance and alloys, easy manipulation, strength, solubility, and film thickness properties comparable to those of zinc phosphate cements.

The disadvantages are the need for accurate proportioning required for optimal properties and thus more critical manipulation, the lower compressive strength and greater viscoelasticity than zinc phosphate cements, the short working time of some materials, and the need for clean surfaces to utilize the adhesion potential.

Glass-ionomer cements

These materials were formulated in the 1970s by bringing together the silicate and polyacrylate systems. The use of an acid-reactive glass powder together with polyacrylic acid solution leads to a translucent, stronger cement that can be used for luting and filling materials.

Applications

Glass-ionomer cements are used for the cementation of cast-alloy and porcelain restorations and orthodontic bands, as cavity liners or base materials (Fig 11-5), and as restorative materials, especially for erosion lesions (Fig 11-6).

Composition and setting

The powder in these materials is finely ground calcium aluminum fluorosilicate glass with a particle size around 40 µm for the filling materials and less than 25 µm for the luting materials. One brand (Zionomer Liner, Den-Mat Corp.) also contains zinc oxide. Silver powder is fused into the glass in Ketac-Silver (Premier/Premier-ESPE) for improved physical properties. The liquid is a 50% aqueous solution of a polyacrylic-itaconic acid or other polycarboxylic acid copolymer that contains about 5% tartaric acid. Some other materials contain 10% to 20% added silver, silver alloy, or stainless steel. In some materials the solid copolymer is added to the powder, and the solution contains tartaric acid; in others, all the ingredients are in the powder, and the liquid is water.

On mixing, the polyacrylic and tartaric acids react with the glass, leaching calcium and aluminum ions from the surface, which cross-link the polyacid molecules into a gel. The tartaric acid serves to increase working time and gives a sharp setting by forming metal ion complexes. Differences in composition between brands affect the hardening rate and properties. Some recent evidence suggests that a polysilicate matrix may also form within the polygel over time.

In the new hybrid ionomer cements the acid-base setting reaction in these cements has been modified by the introduction of water-soluble polymers and polymerizable monomers into the composition. The use of copolymers of acrylic acid and methacrylate monomers in the liquid leads to materials that undergo the customary acid-base reaction on setting and can also be light-cured via the methacrylate groups. This gives improved lining and restorative materials with an immediate command set and thus higher early strength and water resistance. Some commercial materials contain a preponderance of polymeric components with minimal acid-base reaction.

The classification of these materials as glass-ionomer cements is controversial. Some light-cured restorative glass-ionomer cements are used with a dentin primer similar to dentin bonding composite resin systems and thus depend on surface infiltration for bonding in addition to chemical interaction. One hybrid ionomer cement (Vitremer Luting Cement, 3M Dental Products) is used for permanent cementation of crowns, orthodontic appliances, and core buildups.

Manipulation

The material should be carefully proportioned and the freshly dispensed components mixed rapidly in 30 to 40 seconds. Some brands are encapsulated, mechanically mixed, and injected. The powder/liquid ratio for luting is about 1.3:1 for the conventional types of glass-ionomer cement. This ratio appears to be critical with these cements to obtain optimal cementation properties. Best results are obtained by mixing the chilled powder with the liquid on a chilled slab. The correct cementing mix is fluid, similar to zinc phosphate. The lining mix is somewhat more viscous, depending on the brand. The restorative mix should have a puttylike consistency and a glossy surface. Tooth surfaces should be clean and free from saliva but not dehydrated. Restoration surfaces should be free from debris and contamination. The cement hardens slowly and should be protected from loss or gain of moisture when set clinically. Restoration margins or filling surfaces should be protected with a varnish or a light-curing sealant. This is less important with light-cured materials.

Properties

For the luting materials, the setting time is in the range of 6 to 9 minutes. The lining materials set in 4 to 5 minutes, and the restorative materials set in 3 to 4 minutes.

Materials that are light-cured set in approximately 30 seconds when exposed to a visible light source. The acid-base reaction continues slowly and properties further improve over time.

Film thickness is in the range of 25 to 35 µm, which is adequate to seat castings satisfactorily, although the flow properties are quite dependent on the powder/liquid ratio.

For the luting cements, the compression strength increases over 24 hours to 90 to 140 MPa (13,000 to 20,000 psi) depending on the brand. The tensile strength increases similarly to 6 to 8 MPa (900 to 1,100 psi). The compressive modulus of elasticity is about 7 GPa (900,000 psi). The lining materials have compressive and tensile strengths in the same range with some light-cured materials at the higher end of the range reaching 150 to 160 MPa (21,000 to 23,000 psi) in compression and 10 to 12 MPa (1,400 to 1,700 psi) in tension. The light-cured materials are significantly tougher with, in some brands, a lower modulus. The restorative materials range from 140 to 180 MPa (20,000 to 26,000 psi) in compression and 12 to 15 MPa (1,700 to 2,100 psi) in tension. The light-cured restorative materials may have strengths as high as 200 MPa in compression and 20 MPa in tension. Some silver-containing materials are in this range, and even higher strengths have been achieved in recent materials.

In general, with light-cured materials, properties are dependent on the depth of cure.

The solubility of the cements in water is about 1% for a luting material, and this is higher in lactic acid. Good resistance to dissolution is observed under oral conditions. Resistance to dissolution and disintegration is improved by varnish protection for conventional cements.

Erosion of clinical restorations of conventional cements by acid phosphate fluoride preventive-treatment solutions has been observed, making these solutions contraindicated.

Some studies show that light-cured glass-ionomer materials continue to absorb water over several months, with swelling and reductions in strength and stiffness. The clinical significance of this behavior is not yet clear.

Glass-ionomer cements exhibit bonding to enamel, dentin, and alloys in a similar manner to zinc polycarboxylates. In vitro and in vivo the adhesion is variable and is affected by surface conditions. Slight and variable marginal leakage has been observed. Bonding to dentin for conventional materials is not improved by pretreatment with polyacrylic acid solutions, whereas with light-mold materials it is dependent on the use of dentin primers.

Biologic effects

Pulpal response to the lining and restorative materials appears generally favorable. Variable behavior has been reported for the various luting materials with instances of postoperative sensitivity. This has been attributed to a prolonged initially low pH coupled with the effects of the toxic ions. This may be accentuated by mismanipulation and marginal leakage of bacteria. Leaching of fluoride and uptake by adjacent enamel occurs with these cements, and this continues for at least a year with potentially cariostatic effects. Antibacterial action has been attributed to low initial pH, leaching, release of silver and other ions, or a combination of these. Light-cured materials have been observed to show greater cytotoxicity.

Advantages and disadvantages

The advantages of glass-ionomer cement materials include easy mixing, high strength and stiffness, leachable fluoride, good resistance to acid dissolution, potentially adhesive characteristics, and translucency.

The disadvantages include initial slow setting and moisture sensitivity, variable adhesive characteristics, radiolucency, and possible pulpal sensitivity.

Polymer-based cements

The majority of the materials in this group are poly(methacrylates) of two types: (*1*) materials based on methyl methacrylate, and (*2*) materials based on aromatic dimethacrylates of the Bis-GMA type. The closely related cyanoacrylate monomers, notably ethyl and isobutyl, have found some limited use for the attachment of facings and for pin cementation. However, the hydrolytic stability and biologic effects in this situation are suspect and little use is made of them.

Acrylic resin cements

Applications

Acrylic resin cements are used for the cementation of restorations, facings, and temporary crowns.

Composition and setting

The powder in these materials is a finely divided methyl methacrylate polymer or copolymer containing benzoyl peroxide as the initiator. Mineral filler and pigments may also be present. The liquid is a methyl methacrylate monomer containing an amine accelerator.

The monomer dissolves and softens the polymer particles and concurrently polymerizes through the action of free radicals from the peroxide-amine interaction. The set mass consists of the new polymer matrix uniting the undissolved but swollen original polymer granules.

Manipulation

The liquid is added to the powder with minimal spatulation to avoid an incorporation. The mix must be used immediately because working time is short. Excess material must be removed at the final set hard stage and not when the material is rubbery, otherwise marginal deficiencies will be created.

Properties

The properties of these materials are comparable to those of the cold-curing acrylic resin filling materials. They are stronger and less soluble than other types of cement but display low rigidity and viscoelastic properties. They have no effective bond to tooth structure in the presence of moisture; thus they permit marginal leakage, although they may show better bonding than other cements to resin facings and polycarbonate crowns.

Biologic effects

As with acrylic resin filling materials, marked pulp reaction may occur and pulp protection is necessary.

Advantages and disadvantages

The advantages of these materials include relatively high strength and toughness and low solubility.

Disadvantages include a short working time, deleterious effects on pulp, and difficulty in removal of excess cement from margins.

Modified acrylic resin cements

Adhesive acrylic materials have been formulated by adding an adhesion promoter, 4-methyloxy ethyl trimelletic anhydride (4-META), to the methyl

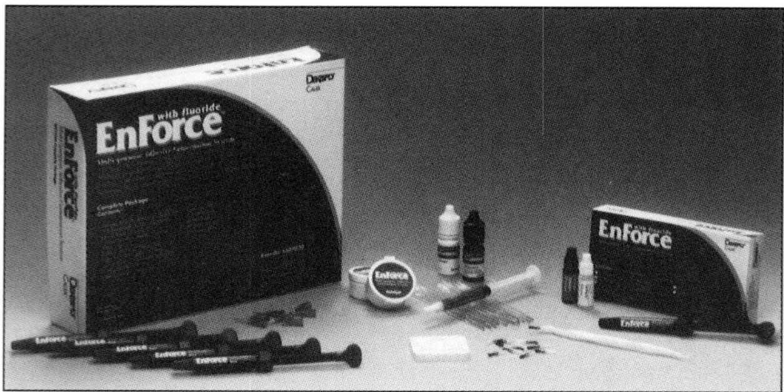

Fig 11-7 Dual-cure multipurpose resin cement.

methacrylate monomer as well as an additional polymerization initiator, tributyl boron, that is also believed to aid chemical bonding to dentin. Such materials have been developed as cements for metal crowns and bridges especially of base metal (Superbond, Parkell) and for bonding amalgam to dentin and composites (Amalgam bond, Parkell). In vitro tests have shown high bond strengths for the luting cement to oxidized, etched, or silica-coated casting alloy surfaces. Shear bond strength to amalgam is significantly less than the bond strength to dentin, which is comparable to other dentin bonding systems in the region of 20 MPa. Since these materials have only low (<10%) filler content the physical properties are typical of acrylic resins, that is, moderate strength with high deformation under load. Although the materials have been widely used for cementation of crowns and bridges, there is little clinical data on longevity, and the cements are said to be technique sensitive.

Dimethacrylate cements

Materials of more recent development are usually based on the Bis-GMA system: They are combinations of an aromatic dimethacrylate with other monomers containing various amounts of ceramic filler (Fig 11-7). They are basically similar to composite restorative materials. These materials have been supplied as two viscous liquids, two pastes, or as powder/liquid materials.

Applications

Dimethacrylate cements are used for the cementation of crowns, bridges, inlays, and veneers.

Composition and setting

A large number of brands are available that may be classified as (*1*) chemically (or auto-) cured; (*2*) visible light cured; and (*3*) chemically and light cured. The latter dual-cure cements are increasingly favored to achieve the rapid solidification associated with light cure while allowing for full polymerization of the cement in areas of the restoration that cannot be reached efficiently by light irradiation.

In the powder-liquid materials, the powder is generally a finely divided borosilicate or silica glass together with fine polymer powder and an organic peroxide initiator. The liquid is a mixture of Bis-GMA and/or other dimethacrylate monomers containing an amine promoter for polymerization. Some materials contain monomers with potentially adhesive groups, such as phosphate or carboxyl, similar to dentin bonding materials. The two-paste materials are of similar overall composition but with the monomers and fillers combined into two pastes. In light-cured and dual-cured materials, light-sensitive polymerization systems such as diketones (eg, camphorquinone) and amine promoters are present respectively in the two cement components in addition to the chemical-initiator systems.

On mixing the components, polymerization of the monomers occurs, leading to a highly cross-linked composite resin structure.

Manipulation

Correct proportioning of powder and liquid components using measures is important. Paste materials are usually proportioned 1:1 (equal lengths). Rapid, thorough mixing, minimizing air inclusion, until uniform is critical.

Properties

As with composite restorative resins, monomer conversion is incomplete, even under optimum cure conditions, and thus manipulation is critical to optimum physical properties. For light- and dual-cured materials, the maximum light exposure (eg, 60 seconds) is desirable. Maximum properties are generally reached about 10 minutes after polymerization; only small changes occur over the ensuing 24 hours.

Since polymerization systems vary and filler contents range between 20% and 80% for the various products, physical properties vary widely (Table 11-6) and the solubility of a specific material for a particular clinical application should be checked individually.

Compressive strengths have been reported to range between 100 and 200 MPa (14,000 and 28,000 psi), and diametral tensile strengths from 20 to 50 MPa (3,000 to 7,000 psi) with corresponding differences in microhardness. These values are considerably higher than traditional cements, and therefore high values can be obtained for retention of well-fitting crowns. However, optimum luting performance is very dependent on fluidity, seating capability, and film thickness. Many resin cements tend to show unacceptably high values for film thickness. Recently, to improve wetting of the tooth, preparation, and seating and to improve bond strength, some resin cements began being used with dentin bonding primers, thus increasing the clinical complexity of the system. Although these materials have been used widely in adhesive techniques, especially for ceramic restorations, there are comparatively few clinical reports of their longevity. Aside from failures induced by material and technique shortcomings during the critical clinical manipulation, studies indicate that resin cement bonds will most likely fail through cyclic fatigue stresses. Some studies on etched metal restorations cemented with chemically cured cements have indicated a median survival time of about 8 years.

Biologic effects

The materials themselves appear to pose few problems, although some patients experience objectionable odors. Cases of allergy among dental personnel have occurred, especially where reactive dentin bonding systems have been used. Skin contact should be avoided.

Pulpal pathology may be due to poor seating, polymerization contraction, and consequent microleakage. All systems show some microleakage that may contribute to tooth sensitivity and clinical failure. Microleakage appears to occur least with systems employing dentin bonding agents, but there are no long-term studies on this aspect.

Advantages and disadvantages

The advantages of these cements include high strength; low oral solubility; and high micromechanical (and possible chemical) bonding to prepared enamel, dentin alloys, and ceramic surfaces.

Disadvantages include the need for a meticulous and critical technique, more difficult sealing and higher film thickness than traditional cements, possible leakage and pulp sensitivity, and difficulty in removal of excess cement.

Selection and use of cements

None of the cements available is free from deficiencies in the required clinical characteristics, such as biocompatibility, ease of manipulation, satisfactory sealing, retentive properties, and long-term stability. A proportion of clinical failures is inevitable, but this can be minimized by proper selection and manipulation of the cement. The following factors should be kept under review:

1. Uniform and reproducible dispensing of the components
2. Rapid, thorough mixing on a cold slab
3. Moisture isolation where practical
4. An undisturbed setting
5. Careful removal of excess

Factors within the clinician's control, such as the design and execution of the preparation, adequate isolation, proper seating of the restoration, and finishing of the margins, are also important determinants of success as is the manipulation of the cement.

These considerations may influence cement selection and use but a governing factor is the biological state of the tooth tissue. Thus, as indicated in Table 11-2, the selection of particular cements for specific clinical situations is limited both by the preparation and the properties of the cement.

Clinical decision scenarios for dental cements

This section presents one approach for choosing dental cements for specific situations. Each of the following scenarios uses the same format as that presented in Chapter 7:

1. The situation is described.
2. Critical factors are listed.
3. Advantages and disadvantages of each material are prioritized using the following codes: * = of minor importance, ** = important, and *** = very important.
4. The situation is analyzed, and the final decision is explained.

Situation Zinc phosphate vs resin cement for crown cementation

Description A dentist has finished preparation of a full gold crown for a maxillary left permanent second molar and is ready to cement the crown. The preparation is normal, and the tooth is vital. There is no known pulpal pathology. In other words, this is a routine crown cementation. The dentist may choose from a resin cement and zinc phosphate cement.

Critical factors Ease of use, cost, effectiveness

Advantages

Zinc phosphate	Resin
*** 1. Low cost	*** 1. Bonds to tooth
2. Long clinical history	2. Fast setting time
3. High rigidity	3. Higher strength
4. Long working time	*** 4. Easy to use
*** 5. Easy to use	

Disadvantages

Zinc phosphate	Resin
*** 1. No bond to tooth	*** 1. High cost
2. Slow setting time	2. Short working time
3. Moisture sensitive during mixing	3. Film thickness ranges widely from brand to brand
	4. Difficult to remove excess

Analysis/Decision Comparing the properties of the two cements reveals they are balanced in advantages and disadvantages for this situation. The choice finally rests in the personal preference of the dentist. Since this dentist had more experience with zinc phosphate, she chose to use that material.

Situation Glass ionomers vs zinc phosphate cement for crown cementation

Description An older gentlemen with a history of periodontal surgery to correct bony defects has broken the cusps off a previously restored mandibular first molar. The patient's plaque control is only fair, and he is taking medications that could result in some degree of "dry mouth." He has had a slightly increased level of caries activity since the surgery and since beginning the medication. The dentist has elected to restore the tooth with a cast crown, which has now been returned from the laboratory and is ready for cementation. The dentist has both zinc phosphate and glass-ionomer luting cements available and must decide which to use.

Critical factors Caries resistance, good seal

Advantages

Zinc phosphate	Glass ionomer
*** 1. Good seal	*** 1. Good seal
** 2. Reasonable cost	*** 2. Fluoride release
** 3. Adequate strength	** 3. Adequate strength
** 4. Little sensitivity	** 4. Reasonable cost

Disadvantages

Zinc phosphate	Glass ionomer
*** 1. No fluoride release	** 1. Occasional sensitivity

Analysis/Decision Both cements have a good seal, but only the glass ionomer releases fluoride after cementation. Fluoride is generally accepted to reduce caries and seems to do so in individuals such as this patient. For this reason, the glass ionomer was selected. Careful attention to instructions allowed cementation without the sensitivity sometimes experienced with glass-ionomer cements. The dentist was satisfied that this was the treatment of choice.

Situation Glass ionomers vs zinc phosphate for bases under amalgam restorations

Description A patient has a mandibular molar that exhibits extensive carious destruction. Due to the patient's finances, a large, pin-retained amalgam restoration is selected. Following caries removal and preparation, it is determined that the cavity needs a base prior to placement of the amalgam restoration. The dentist has zinc phosphate and glass-ionomer cements available and must choose between them for a base material.

Critical factors Strength, modulus of elasticity

Advantages

Zinc phosphate	Glass ionomer
*** 1. Adequate modulus of elasticity	*** 1. Adequate modulus of elasticity
*** 2. Adequate strength	*** 2. Adequate strength
** 3. Ease of use	** 3. Fluoride release
** 4. No sensitivity	** 4. Ease of use

Disadvantages

Zinc phosphate	Glass ionomer
** 1. No fluoride release	** 1. Occasional sensitivity

Analysis/Decision Since the advantages and disadvantages were essentially balanced for this situation, neither cement had a clear advantage. The highly significant modulus of elasticity, essential for a good base, was roughly equivalent. In this case, the dentist chose glass ionomer because of the added advantage of fluoride release, which is thought to reduce recurrent decay. However, because that was not a problem with this patient, either cement would have been an acceptable choice.

Situation Zinc oxide–eugenol vs calcium hydroxide as liners under amalgam restorations

Description A patient in need of a slightly deep mesio-occlusodistal (MOD) amalgam on a mandibular left first molar was seen by the dentist. The patient reported that the last two amalgams the dentist placed had been quite sensitive for several weeks following placement. They had finally lost their sensitivity, but the patient felt they had hurt unusually long for new restorations. Upon preparation, the dentist decided that a base was indicated. He had both calcium hydroxide and zinc oxide–eugenol base materials available.

Critical factors Strength, modulus of elasticity

Advantages

Zinc oxide–eugenol	Calcium hydroxide
** 1. Ease of use	** 1. Ease of use
** 2. Decreases sensitivity	** 2. Stimulates secondary dentin
** 3. Low cost	** 3. Low cost

Disadvantages

Zinc oxide–eugenol	Calcium hydroxide
*** 1. Low strength	*** 1. Low strength
*** 2. Low modulus of elasticity	*** 2. Low modulus of elasticity

Analysis/Decision In this situation, again, there is no clear advantage for either base. Both have low strength and low modulus of elasticity, necessitating that they be applied as very thin layers. The zinc oxide–eugenol, however, does have the advantage of the anodyne eugenol, which is known to reduce tooth sensitivity. The calcium hydroxide, on the other hand, will stimulate the formation of secondary dentin and thus is good if the restoration is near the pulp. This was the case in the situation described, and the patient had a history of sensitive teeth following amalgam restorations. This advantage allowed the dentist to select the zinc oxide– eugenol as the liner of choice.

Situation Zinc oxide–eugenol vs calcium hydroxide as liners under amalgam restorations

Description A patient with a deep cavity on the maxillary right first premolar was seen by the dentist. Upon excavation of the caries, the remaining dentin was estimated to be very little by the dentist. In fact, she could see the pink outline of the pulp through the remaining dentin after caries removal. When questioned about sensitivity following placement of earlier amalgam restorations, the patient reported no unusual sensitivity. The dentist had zinc oxide–eugenol and calcium hydroxide from which to choose as a base.

Critical factors Strength, modulus of elasticity

Advantages

Zinc oxide–eugenol	Calcium hydroxide
** 1. Ease of use	** 1. Ease of use
** 2. Decreases sensitivity	** 2. Stimulates secondary dentin
** 3. Low cost	** 3. Low cost

Disadvantages

Zinc oxide–eugenol	Calcium hydroxide
*** 1. Low strength	*** 1. Low strength
*** 2. Low modulus of elasticity	*** 2. Low modulus of elasticity

Analysis/Decision In this situation, the advantages and disadvantages are identical to the last situation, but this time the cavity is very deep and near the pulp. In this case, the dentist chose the calcium hydroxide because of its ability to stimulate the formation of secondary dentin. It was hoped that this would help the tooth repair itself from the insult caused by the deep decay.

Situation All-purpose adhesives vs cavity varnish under amalgam restorations

Description A patient is seen and diagnosed as needing numerous amalgam restorations, some large. Upon preparation, the cavities turn out to be normal in size and depth. There is little remarkable about the patient or the restorations. The dentist has both cavity varnish and new all-purpose adhesives to use under the amalgam restorations. The all-purpose adhesives are reported by the manufacturer to bond the amalgam to the teeth, but the dentist knows that such claims are as yet probably exaggerated.

Critical factors Marginal leakage, bond to tooth, cost, time required for application

Advantages

Varnish	Adhesives
*** 1. Low cost	*** 1. Superior marginal seal
*** 2. Mediocre seal	*** 2. Bonds to tooth
*** 3. Easy placement	

Disadvantages

Varnish	Adhesives
*** 1. No bond to tooth	** 1. High cost
	*** 2. Complex placemnt

Analysis/Decision Since there is no evidence of excessively weakened cusps, the possible bonding of the new adhesives is not significant in this case. The superior seal makes them desirable, but their high cost and complex placement process complicates the choice. The dentist had been to a recent lecture on dental materials in which the speaker claimed the new materials should be a standard of practice, so he chose to place these materials. The patient reported a complete lack of postoperative sensitivity in the new restorations.

Situation Dentin adhesives vs glass-ionomer liners under composite restorations

Description A patient has several Class V toothbrush abrasion lesions on his maxillary and mandibular premolars. At first, they were no problem, but over the years they have become sensitive, and the patient wants the discomfort relieved. The lesions are not carious but are somewhat deep. The occlusal, mesial, and distal margins are on enamel, but the cervical margin is on cementum. The dentist decides against glass-ionomer restorations because she feels a better esthetic result can be obtained with a composite material. In addition, she feels the composite will better resist further toothbrush abrasion. She is uncertain whether to use a dentin bonding agent alone or a glass-ionomer lining cement under the cervical margin to prevent leakage. She has heard that composites often leak on margins that are on cementum.

Critical factors Marginal seal, bond strength

Advantages

Bonding agent only	Glass ionomer
** 1. Shorter procedure	*** 1. Better marginal seal
*** 2. Adequate bond strength	*** 2. Adequate bond strength
** 3. Lower cost	

Disadvantages

Bonding agent only	Glass ionomer
*** 1. Poorer marginal seal	** 1. Additional cost
	** 2. Additional procedure

Analysis/Decision Although there are more advantages for the bonding agent, the most significant advantage—better marginal seal—favors the glass-ionomer liner. It adds to the cost and the time to do the procedure, but it provides a significantly better seal. The better seal results in a superior restoration that justifies the extra cost and time. The glass-ionomer liner was selected.

Situation Glass ionomer vs amalgam for cores

Description A patient comes to the office complaining of a broken tooth. Upon examination the dentist finds that the lingual cusps of the mandibular right first permanent molar have fractured right at the gum line. The tooth already has a large MOD amalgam in it, and the facial cusps are none too sturdy. The treatment plan is to prepare a pin-retained core buildup and then a full gold crown. The dentist has both amalgam and a glass-ionomer core material available.

Critical factor Strength

Advantages

Amalgam	Glass ionomer
*** 1. High strength	1. Immediate set
2. Long clinical history	2. Fluoride release
	3. Bonds to tooth

Disadvantages

Amalgam	Glass ionomer
1. 24-hour set	*** 1. Low strength
2. No fluoride release	
3. No bond to tooth	

Analysis/Decision Despite the more numerous advantages for the glass ionomer, its low strength makes it unsuitable for a full buildup, and the amalgam was selected. Glass ionomers have been advertised for this use, but time has shown that they do not hold up well if they are the entire support for the crown. They are useful for filling in some small depressions in the preparation but not for the complete core.

Glossary

accelerator (promoter) Substance that facilitates decomposition of an initiator.

cored structure A material consisting of at least two phases, for example, as residual particles of a component embedded in a matrix of reaction product.

initiator Substance capable of decomposing into free radicals that initiate polymerization.

lute A cementlike material that also fills and seals gaps.

obtundent A material that reduces irritation or has a soothing effect on tissue.

rheology Science of the deformation and flow of matter.

setting time Time from the beginning of mixing of the cement to the development of a hard and rigid (usually brittle) state in the mouth.

working time Time available, measured from the beginning of mixing at room temperature, for clinical manipulation of a cement before viscosity becomes too great for seating of the restoration.

Discussion questions

1. Why is fluoride release so important in a cement?
2. What is the source of fluoride in a glass-ionomer cement?
3. What is the difference in function between a cement liner and a cement base?
4. Why are polymer cements recommended for use with CAD/CAM inlays with poor marginal fits?

Questions and answers

1. **What is the minimum compressive strength required of a dental cement for adequate retention of restorations?** About 55 MPa (8,000 psi).
2. **What is the structure of set zinc phosphate cement?** A cored structure of unreacted zinc oxide particles in an amorphous zinc phosphate matrix.
3. **How does the solubility of phosphate cements in citric or lactic acid compare with their solubility in water?** The solubility in organic acid solutions, such as citric or lactic acid, is 20 to 30 times higher than in water.
4. **What is the composition of silicophosphate cements?** The powder contains zinc oxide and silicate glass mechanically mixed or fused and reground. The liquid is a concentrated phosphoric acid solution containing about 45% water and 2% to 5% aluminum and zinc as phosphates.
5. **Are silicophosphate cements usually stronger than zinc phosphate cements? If so, by how much?** Silicophosphates have a compressive strength about 50% higher than that of zinc phosphate cements. Their tensile strength is about 25% higher.
6. **What agents accelerate the setting of zinc oxide–eugenol cements?** Water, zinc salts such as acetate and sulfate, and other acidic materials.
7. **Why do zinc oxide–eugenol cements have a high solubility?** The high solubility of zinc oxide–eugenol cements is due to hydrolytic breakdown of zinc eugenolate and the extraction of eugenol from the set cement.
8. **What materials can be added to zinc oxide–eugenol cements to improve their strength?** Mineral fillers, such as silica or alumina; natural resins, such as pine rosin; and synthetic polymers, such as poly(methyl methacrylate), polystyrene, or polycarbonate.
9. **What effects do zinc oxide–eugenol cements have on resin restorative materials?** Zinc oxide–eugenol cements inhibit the polymerization of resin restorative materials, resulting in softening and discoloration.
10. **How does the composition of EBA cements differ from that of zinc oxide–eugenol cements?** The powder of EBA cements contains more mineral filler, such as alumina, than does the powder of zinc oxide–eugenol cements, and in the liquid only about one third is eugenol; the remainder is ethoxybenzoic acid.

11. **What factors affect the setting reaction of polycarboxylate cements?** The powder/liquid ratio, the reactivity and particle size of the zinc oxide, the presence of additives, and the molecular weight and concentration of the polyacrylic acid.

12. **Give possible reasons for the minimal effect of polycarboxylate cements on pulp.** The mild effect of polycarboxylate cements on pulp may be due to the relatively high pH of the setting cement; localization of the polyacrylic acid molecules; and/or the minimal osmotic effects on fluid in the dentinal tubules.

13. **What are important considerations in manipulating polycarboxylate cements?** The components of the cement should be carefully proportioned and mixed on a cooled slab. All the powder may be added to the liquid at one time so the total mix time is no more than 30 to 40 seconds. The mix should be used while it is still glossy, before the onset of cobwebbing.

14. **What are the advantages of light curing glass-ionomer cements?** They set by both acid-base reaction and polymerization of monomer groups, giving higher early strength, improved physical properties, and water resistance.

15. **What are the major advantages of glass-ionomer cements?** High strength and stiffness, adhesion, translucency, leachable fluoride and potential cariostatic effect, and good resistance to dissolution in the mouth.

16. **Define the two types of polymer-based cement.** The two types of resin cement are acrylic resin cements, based on poly(methyl methacrylate) and methyl methacrylate monomer, and resin composite materials, based on a ceramic filler and a Bis-GMA dimethacrylate monomer.

17. **What are the principal disadvantages of polymer-based cement?** Short working time, viscous behavior of the mix, microleakage and pulpal irritation, and difficulty of removal of excess cement.

18. **What are adhesive resin cements?** These cements contain monomers with polar groups, such as phosphate or carboxyl, that improve wetting and are potentially adhesive to the tooth or restorative material surface. Adhesive cements may also utilize a dentin bonding primer system before application of the cement.

Recommended reading

Arfaci AH, Asgar K. Bond strength of selected cementing materials. Microfilmed Paper No. 549. Delivered at the Annual Meeting of the International Association for Dental Research, Dental Materials Group, Atlanta, GA, March 21–24, 1974.

Beagrie GS, Smith DC. Development of a germicidal polycarboxylate cement. J Can Dent Assoc 44:409, 1978.

Boyer DB, et al. Analysis of debond rates of resin-bonded prostheses. J Dent Res 72:1244–1248, 1993.

Brännström M, Nyborg H. Bacterial growth and pulpal changes under inlays cemented with zinc phosphate cement and Epoxylite CBA 9080. J Prosthet Dent 31:556, 1974.

Burgess JO, et al. A comparative study of three glass ionomer base materials. Am J Dent 6:137–141, 1993.

Burke FJT, McCaughey AD. Resin luting materials; their current status. Dent Update, April 1993; 109–115.

Causton BE. Primers and mineralizing solutions. In DC Smith, DF Williams (eds). Biocompatibility of Dental Materials. Vol 2. Boca Raton, FL: CRC Press, 1982; 125–144.

De Freitas JF. The long-term solubility of a stannous fluoride-zinc phosphate cement. Aust Dent J 18:167, 1973.

Dennison JD, Powers JM. A review of dental cements used for permanent retention of restorations. Part I. Composition and manipulation. J Mich Dent Assoc 56:116, April 1974.

Eames WB, Hendri K, Mohler HC. Pulpal response in rhesus monkeys to cementation agents and cleaners. J Am Dent Assoc 98:40, 1979.

Eames WB, O'Neal SJ, Miller CB. Cementation variables in the seating of castings. Microfilmed Paper No. 545. Delivered at the Annual Meeting of the International Association for Dental Research, Dental Materials Group, Atlanta, GA, March 21–24, 1974.

Eames WB, O'Neal SJ, Monteiro J, et al. Techniques to improve the seating of castings. J Am Dent Assoc 96:432, 1978.

Forss H. Release of fluoride and other elements from light-cured glass ionomers in neutral and acidic conditions. J Dent Res 72:1257–1262, 1993.

Glenn JF. Composition and properties of unfilled and composite resin restorative materials. In DC Smith, DF Williams (eds). Biocompatibility of Dental Materials. Vol 3. Boca Raton, FL: CRC Press, 1982; 97–130.

Grieve AR. A study of dental cements. Br Dent J 127:405–410, 1969.

Grieve AR, Jones JC. Marginal leakage associated with four inlay cementing materials. Br Dent J 151:331, 1981.

Griffith JR, Cannon RWS. Cementation—materials and techniques. Aust J Dent 19(2):92–99, April 1974.

Hatton PV, Brook JM. Characterization of the ultrastructure of glass ionomer (poly-alkenoate) cement. Br Dent J 173:275–277, 1993.

Hembree JH Jr, George TA, Hembree ME. Film thickness of cements beneath complete crowns. J Prosthet Dent 39:533, 1978.

Hoard RJ, Caputo AA, Contino RM, et al. Intracoronal pressure during crown cementation. J Prosthet Dent 40:520, 1978.

Hood JA, Childs WA, Evans DF. Bond strengths of glass ionomer and polycarboxylate cements to dentin. N Z Dent J 77:141, 1981.

Jarzynka W. Effect of fluorine contained in the phosphate cement "Fluostable" on tooth pulp. Czas Stomatol 31:1003, 1978.

Jendresen MD. New dental cements and fixed prosthodontics. J Prosthet Dent 30:684, 1973.

Johnson GH, Herbert AJ, Powers JM. Properties of glass ionomer luting cements. Microfilmed Paper No. 189. Delivered at the Annual Meeting of the American Association for Dental Research, Dental Materials Group, Cincinnati, OH, March 17–20, 1983.

Kent BE, Wilson AD. The properties of a glass ionomer cement. Br Dent J 135:322, 1973.
Kidd EAM, McLean JW. The cavity sealing ability of cemented cast gold restorations. Br Dent J 147:39, 1979.
Kohmura TT, Ida KA. A new type of hydraulic cement. J Dent Res 58:1461, 1979.
Markowitz K, et al. Biologic properties of eugenol and zinc oxide-eugenol. A clinically-oriented review. Oral Surg Oral Med Oral Pathol 73:729–737, 1992.
McComb D. Retention of castings with glass ionomer cement. J Prosthet Dent 48:285, 1982.
McLean JW. The clinical use of glass ionomer cements. Dent Clin North Am 36:693–711, 1992.
Miller RA, Bussell NE, Richetts CK, et al. Analysis of purification of eugenol. J Dent Res 58:1394, 1979.
Mitchem JC, Gronas DG. Clinical evaluation of cement solubility. J Prosthet Dent 40:453, 1978.
Mitchem JC, Gronas DG. Continued evaluation of the clinical solubility of luting cements. J Prosthet Dent 45:289, 1981.
Mount GO, Makinson OF. Clinical characteristics of a glass ionomer cement. Br Dent J 145:67, 1978.
Myers CL, Drake JT, Brantley WA. A comparison of properties of zinc phosphate cements mixed on room temperature and frozen slabs. J Prosthet Dent 40:409, 1978.
Norman RD, Swartz ML, Phillips RW, et al. A comparison of the intraoral disintegration of three dental cements. J Am Dent Assoc 78:777, 1969.
Øilo G. Adhesive bonding of dental luting cements: influence of surface treatments. Acta Odontol Scand 36:263, 1978.
Øilo G. Extent of slits at the interface between luting cements and enamel, dentin and alloy. Acta Odontol Scand 36:257, 1978.
Øilo G, Espevik S. Stress/strain behavior of some dental luting cements. Acta Odontol Scand 36:45, 1978.
Pameijer GH, Segal E, Richardson J. Pulpal response to a glass ionomer cement in primates. J Prosthet Dent 46:36, 1981.
Peacocke LE, Jones DW, Sutow E, et al. Direct tensile strength of glass ionomer, polycarboxylate and phosphate cements. Microfilmed Paper No. 1212. Delivered at the Annual Meeting of the International Association for Dental Research, Dental Materials Group, New Orleans, LA, March 29–April 1, 1979.
Peterson WG, Joos RW, Boyer LV, et al. Initial response of $Ca(OH)_2$ bases in simulated oral conditions. Microfilmed Paper No. 210. Delivered at the Annual Meeting of the International Association for Dental Research, Dental Materials Group, Washington, DC, March 16–19, 1978.
Powers JM, Dennison JD. A review of dental cements used for permanent retention of restorations. Part II. Properties and criteria for selection. J Mich Dent Assoc 56(7–8):218–225, 1974.
Reisbick MH. Working qualities of glass ionomer cements. J Prosthet Dent 46:525, 1981.
Rueggeberg FA, Caughman WF. The influence of light exposure on polymerization of dual-cure resin cements. Oper Dent 18:48–55, 1993.
Sivey RG, Myers GE. Clinical studies of dental cements. VII. A study of bridge retainers luted with three different cements. J Dent Res 57:703, 1978.
Smith DC. A review of the zinc polycarboxylate cements. J Can Dent Assoc 37:22, 1974.
Smith DC. Dental cements. Dent Clin North Am 15:3, 1971.
Smith DC. Past, present and future of dental cements. In RG Craig (ed). Dental Materials Review, Ann Arbor: University of Michigan Press, 1977; 52–77.
Smith DC. Dental cements. Current status and future prospects. Dent Clin North Am 27:763–792, 1983.
Smith DC. Composition and characteristics of dental cements. In DC Smith, DF Williams (eds). Biocompatibility of Dental Materials. Vol 2. Boca Raton, FL: CRC Press, 1982; 143–199.
Smith DC. Glass ionomer contents. In H Kawahara (ed). Implantology and Biomaterials in Stomatology. Tokyo: Ishikayn Publisher Inc, 1980; 26–54.
Smith DC. Dental cements. Adv Dent Res 2:131–141, 1988.
Smith DC. Dental cements. Curr Opin Dent 1:228-234, 1991.
Vougiouklakis G, Smith DC. The bonding of cervical restorative materials to dentin. J Oral Rehabil 9:231, 1982.
White SN, Yu Z, Kipmio V. Effect of seating force on film thickness of new adhesive luting agents. J Prosthet Dent 68:476–481, 1992.
White S, Yu Z. Compressive and diametral tensile strengths of current adhesive luting agents. J Prosthet Dent 69:568–572, 1993.
White S, Yu Z. Physical properties of fixed prosthodontic resin composite luting agents. Int J Prosthodont 6:384–389, 1993.
Williams JA, Billington RW, Pearson GJ. The comparative strengths of commercial glass-ionomer cements with and without metal additions. Br Dent J 172:279–282, 1993.
Wilson AD. The chemistry of dental cements. Chem Soc Rev 7:265, 1978.
Wilson AD, Paddon JM, Crisp S. The hydration of dental cements. J Dent Res 58:1065, 1979.
Wilson AD, Prosser HJ. Alumino silicate dental cements. In DC Smith, DF Williams (eds). Biocompatibility of Dental Materials. Vol 3. Boca Raton, FL: CRC Press, 1982; 42–77.
Wilson AD, McLean JW. Glass Ionomer Cements. Chicago: Quintessence, 1988.

Chapter 12

Structure and Properties of Metals and Alloys

A wide variety of metals is used in dentistry, as indicated in Table 12-1. Each has a melting or solidification temperature that is characteristic of that element. When elements are alloyed together to change their properties, this single melting temperature is changed to a range of temperatures over which the liquid is in equilibrium with solid crystals nucleated in the liquid metal.

Table 12-1 Metallic elements used in dentistry

Element	Unit cell	Melting temperature (°C)
Mercury	Rhombohedral	–39
Gallium	Orthorhombic	30
Indium	Tetragonal	156
Tin	Face-centered cubic	419
Aluminum	Face-centered cubic	660
Silver	Face-centered cubic	960
Gold	Face-centered cubic	1,063
Copper	Face-centered cubic	1,083
Manganese	Cubic	1,244
Beryllium	Hexagonal close pack	1,284
Nickel	Face-centered cubic	1,452
Cobalt	Body-centered cubic	1,493
Iron	Body-centered cubic	1,535
Palladium	Face-centered cubic	1,552
Titanium	Hexagonal close pack	1,668
Platinum	Face-centered cubic	1,769
Chromium	Body-centered cubic	1,875
Molybdenum	Body-centered cubic	2,610

The upper temperature for the liquid-solid alloy range is called the *liquidus temperature*, and the lower temperature limit is called the *solidus temperature*. When a liquid alloy melt is being cooled, the liquidus temperature is the temperature at which solid crystals start to nucleate. When a mixture of an alloy liquid and crystals is being heated, the liquidus temperature is the temperature at which the crystals dissolve away into liquid. The solidus temperature is the temperature at which the last liquid solidifies on cooling or the first liquid is formed on heating.

Complete melting is needed for casting and soldering and at least an additional 100°C superheat is needed for a fluid melt to cast. Note that a gas/air torch cannot be used to cast a metal with a liquidus temperature above 1,000°C because the flame does not get hot enough. Also, a reducing flame rich in gas should be used for casting or soldering, otherwise the liquid metal will be oxidized by the oxygen in air. Oxidation keeps the solder from wetting the surface and flowing. To provide a margin of safety against melting the castings in a dental bridge, the liquidus temperature of the solder should be at least 50°C lower than the solidus temperature of the casting alloy being soldered.

Unit cells of crystal lattices

Liquid metals nucleate crystals upon cooling (Fig 12-1). The atoms joining the crystals form a unique packing arrangement in space that is characteristic of that metal or alloy at equilibrium. The smallest division of the crystalline metal that defines the unique packing is called the *unit cell*. When the unit cell is repeated in space, the repeating atomic positions form the crystal lattice structure of a crystalline solid (Fig 12-2). The atoms at the corners of the unit cell are shared among the adjacent eight unit cells, as shown for the body-centered unit cell. Therefore, one eighth of the corner atom is associated with the cell; there are eight corner atoms, so they each contribute one atom to the unit cell. The body-centered atom is totally inside the unit cell and is not shared, so it contributes the second atom to the unit cell mass. Using the lattice parameters to calculate the volume of the cubic cell, the density of the metal can be calculated by dividing the mass of atoms in the unit cell by its volume. The lattice parameters for metals and alloys range between 2 Å and 10 Å for the different unit cells formed.

It has been observed that the position of the neighboring atoms surrounding every atom of a crystal lattice is identical in a pure crystalline metal. When the property of identical periodic points in space was explored mathematically, it was discovered that there are 14 unique ways to arrange points in space (Fig 12-3). These are called *space lattices*. A pure metal crystal lattice is similar to one of the space lattices except that each mathematical point is the site of an atom. Complex crystal lattices like amalgam alloy and enamel have the points of their space lattices replaced by the different atoms of the material or by groups of atoms. The unit cell of each crystalline material, no matter how complex, corresponds with one of these 14-space lattice unit cells (See Table 12-1).

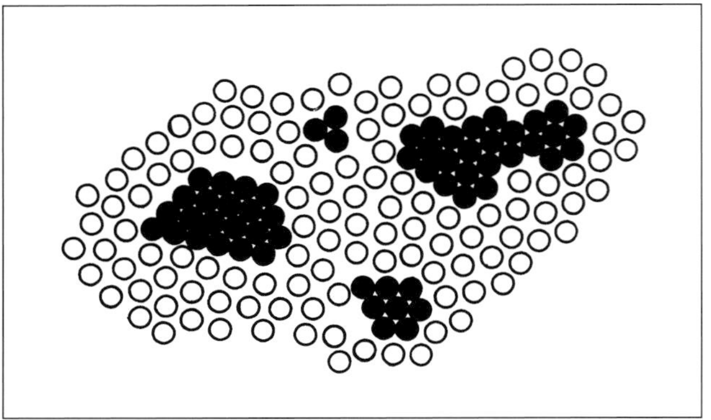

Fig 12-1 Formation of crystal nuclei in liquid metal. ○ = atoms in liquid state; ● = atoms in solid state.

Nucleation and polycrystalline grain structure

As the melt of metal is cooled, clusters of atoms come together from the liquid to form solid crystal nuclei. These nuclei will be stable and grow into crystallites or grains if the energy of the system is favorable, that is, the energy is lowered by the process. The energy is lowered by an atom bonding to the solid nuclei, thereby giving up its liquid-state kinetic energy of motion.

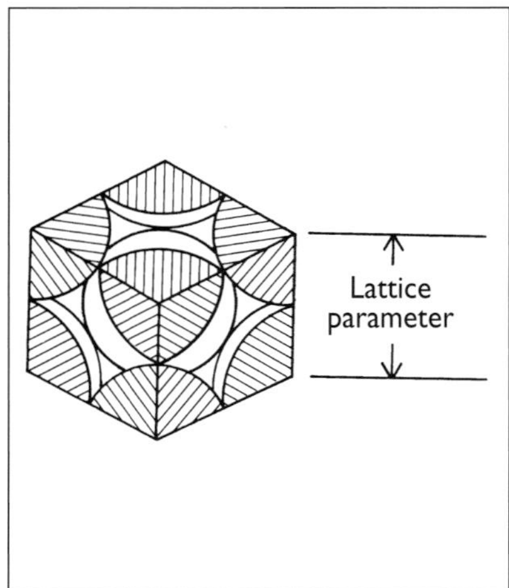

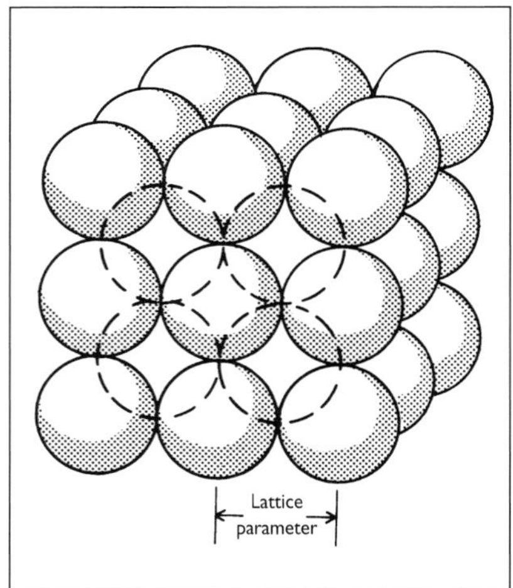

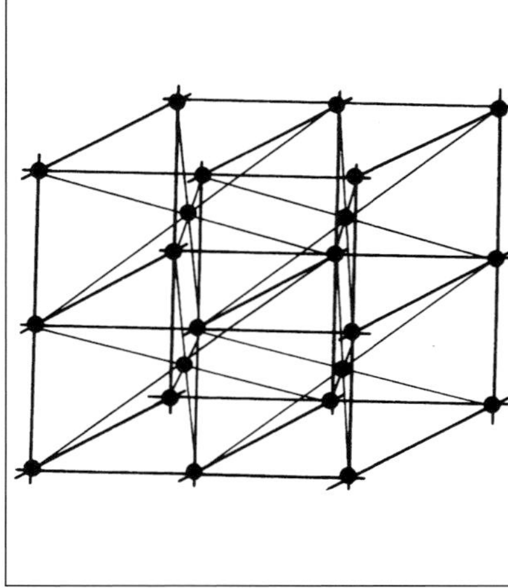

Fig 12-2 (a) The body-centered cubic unit cell is typical of the crystal lattice of pure iron at room temperature. The lattice parameter for iron is 2.87 Å. (b) A part of a body-centered cubic crystal lattice. It could extend in all directions. In this "hard sphere model," the atoms are visualized as hard spheres of a definite radius in contact. (c) The body-centered cubic space lattice can be visualized as a "point skeleton" of the body-centered cubic crystal lattice.

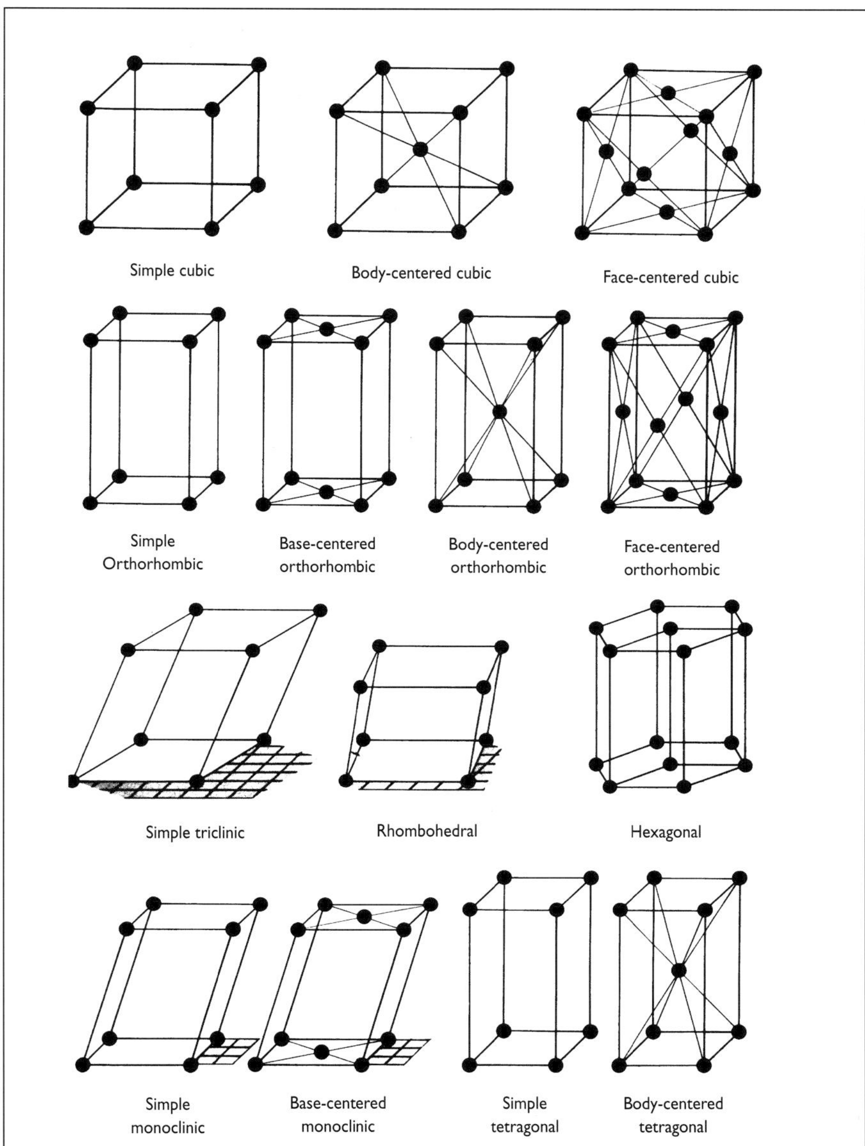

Fig 12-3 Unit cells of the 14-space lattice contain atoms arranged so that each one has identical surroundings. (From Mott, 1967. Reprinted with permission.)

However, when an atom bonds to the nuclei the energy can also be raised by the creation of more interfacial surface energy as a result of the increased surface area of the nuclei in contact with the liquid. The energy of the system is favorable for stable nuclei and growth when more energy is lost by bonding than is gained by increasing the interfacial surface area (ie, energy).

Nucleation can occur by two processes. The first, called *homogeneous nucleation*, is enhanced by rapid cooling so the nuclei are supercooled. The result for the system is that more energy is lost when an atom of the liquid bonds to the solid. With rapid cooling (quenching in water) more nuclei are formed per unit volume. These nuclei grow together to form the irregular polycrystalline grains or crystallites that fit together like a three-dimensional puzzle to form the bulk of the metal shape (Figs 12-4 and 12-5). The more nuclei that are formed by rapid cooling, the smaller the grain size or crystallite dimensions. Another means of decreasing the grain size (grain refining) is by adding to the melt a foreign solid particle or surface to which the atoms are attracted, such as a very fine high-melting metal or oxide powder. This process of seeding the nuclei is called *heterogeneous nucleation*.

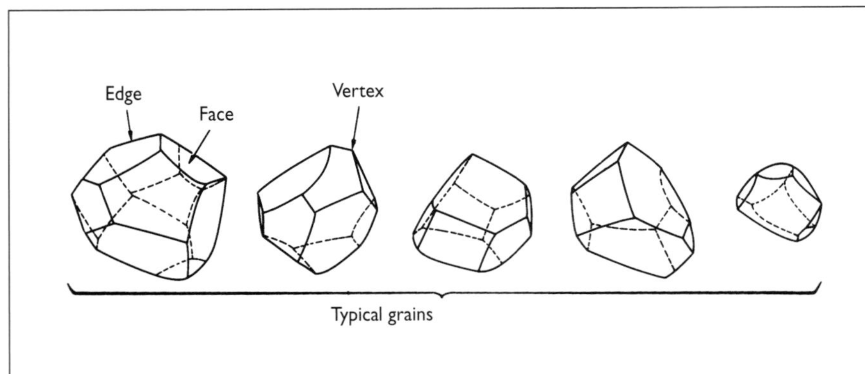

Fig 12-4 Irregular polygons called grains or crystallites. An average distance measured across the faces of the crystal grains is called the grain size. It may be less than 1,000 Å or more than 1 cm, depending on the number of nuclei present during solidification. (From Guy et al, 1971. Reprinted with permission.)

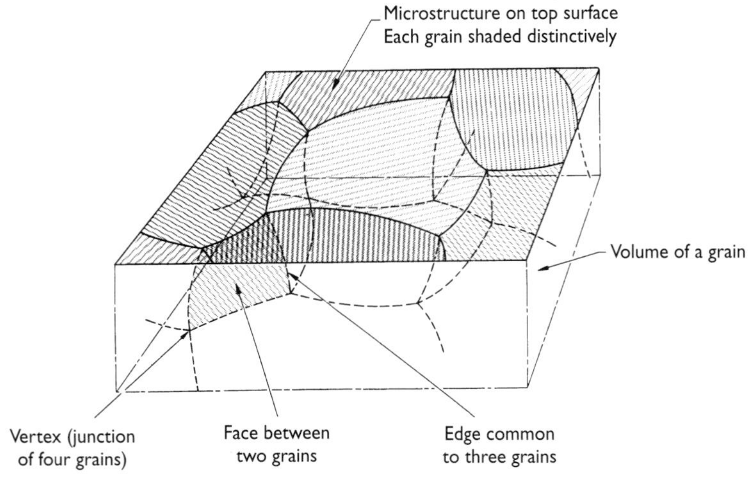

Fig 12-5 The grain structure of a metal is revealed by polishing the surface to a mirror finish and etching lightly in acid. To study the grain structure of metals used for dental appliances, a light or scanning electron microscope is needed for magnification because of the small grain sizes. (From Guy et al, 1971. Reprinted with permission.)

Grain size and properties

Decreasing the grain size can have a number of beneficial effects on the cast alloy structure of a crown or removable partial denture. The finer grain size can raise the yield stress, increase the ductility (percent elongation), and raise the ultimate strength. The change in these properties with grain size is related to the processes of plastic deformation and fracture, and to how the boundaries between grains relate to these processes. The size of metal grains in different metals may range from less than 1,000 Å to more than 1 cm. Grains contain large numbers of unit cells—even grains of only 1,000 Å across. The lattices of the grains are formed in random directions when they grow from the melt. A boundary is formed where the grains grow into contact, because the atoms in one grain's crystal lattice are not in position to mesh with the repeating atoms in the crystal lattices of adjacent grains. These grain boundaries are layers several atoms thick that are distorted from normal atomic positions in order to bridge the mismatch in the lattice orientations of adjacent grains.

Only metals with simple body-centered or face-centered cubic unit cells have enough densely packed planes of atoms in their lattices to allow plastic deformation at yield stress. These lattice types permit shearing of the densely packed planes of atoms like cards of a microscopic deck sliding over each other. However, the lattice of adjacent grain can be viewed as a second microscopic card deck at a different angle. To get the metal to deform, it is necessary to force the cards of one deck into other decks at an angle. But the more grains per unit volume, the more difficult it is to get the planes (cards) to slide because the dislocated slipping planes run against the grain boundaries sooner. Thus, a greater resistance to slippage is created by more grain boundaries, and higher yield stress results.

On the other hand, a material will fracture because a crack opens up on a grain boundary. This is more likely to occur in large-grain metals, when the planes cannot be slipped into the adjacent grains. Many smaller grains in various orientations can divide the plastic strain among the grains more easily with more oriented for slipping. Large grains must each accommodate a larger strain and will have fewer properly oriented to slip. The result is lower ductility and lower ultimate strength for large-grain metals, which open cracks more readily at grain boundaries because the plastic deformation cannot be accommodated. For these reasons, grain-refined or "micrograin" alloys produced by heterogeneous nucleation are advantageous for developing crown-and-bridge alloys with higher yield stress, better ductility, and improved ultimate strength.

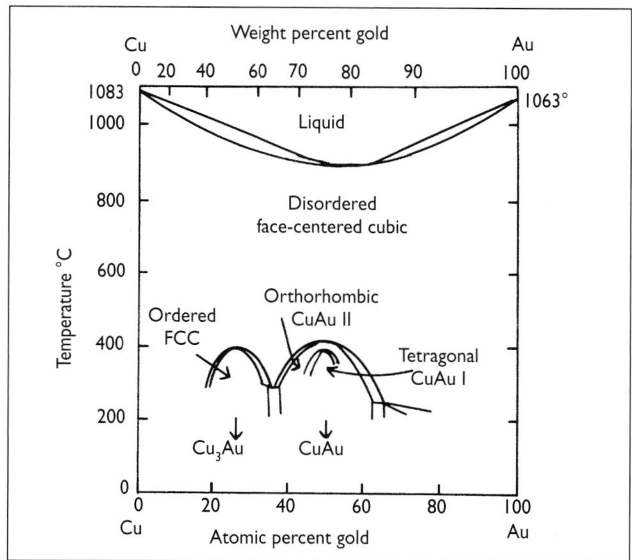

Fig 12-6 Copper-gold phase diagram. The disordered solid solution (softer) and ordered solid solutions (harder) are produced by heat treatment.

Alloy systems

Most pure metals are miscible in the liquid state when melted together. When two metals form a solution in the liquid state so their atoms mix randomly on the atomic scale, they are said to form an alloy. As the alloy liquid freezes, the atoms may remain randomly distributed on the unit-cell lattice sites in each crystal grain. This random distribution in the solid alloy is called a *solid solution*. But, if like atoms tend to prefer to bond among themselves, then as the nuclei form from the melt, the atoms of different elements may segregate in different grains. The grains of the two different metal elements are mixed together.

Different grains may be practically pure if their elements are insoluble in each other's lattices in the solid state. Or they can have a limited solubility in the other's crystal lattice if the elements exhibit partial solubility in one another. Metal atoms of two different metal elements are more likely to be soluble in each other's lattices if they (*1*) have the same atomic lattice type, (*2*) have similar atomic radii (ie, a difference of less than 10%), (*3*) have the same valence number, and (*4*) form bonds to other atoms of similar strength to those they form among themselves. On the other hand, if these rules are not followed and the unlike atoms have a strong affinity to each other, grains of an intermetallic compound may be formed at definite ratios of the alloying *elements* (eg, dental amalgam alloy Ag_3Sn).

The energetically stable (ie, at equilibrium) crystal lattice structures and their compositions for an alloy that is preferred by "nature" varies with temperature and ratio of the alloying elements that are melted together. It is not possible to calculate the equilibrium composition and structures and at what temperatures these change. They must be determined experimentally by measuring the temperatures at which the latent heat is liberated when alloy liquid solidifies or solid lattices transform to different crystal lattices. The type of crystal lattice is determined by X-ray diffraction from the crystal atomic planes. The angle and intensity of the X-ray beam reflections (ie, diffraction) are characteristic of the atomic composition, type of crystal lattice, and position of atoms in their unit cell. Thus, experimental detection of the temperature when heat is liberated indicates when an alloy is changing its structure, and X-ray scattering identifies what lattices are present. This information is portrayed in a phase diagram of the alloy system (Figs 12-6 and 12-7). The alloy system represents all possible ratios of the elements.

When two elements are alloyed, the system is called a *binary system*; when three elements are alloyed, the system is a *ternary system*, and so on. An alloy is named by listing its elements in descending order of percent composition. For example, Ag_3Sn is called silver-tin alloy. If more than two elements are involved, the number of phase changes and their representation becomes complex, but their description follows the same principle.

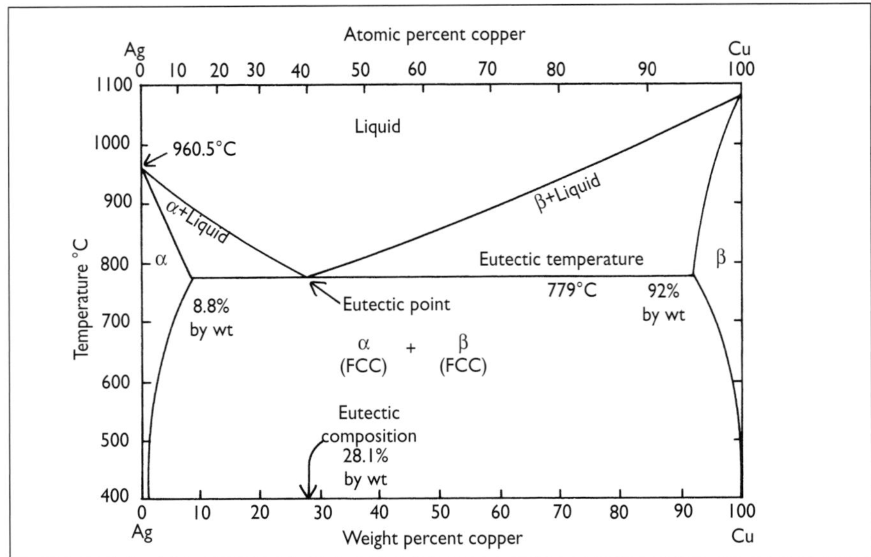

Fig 12-7 Silver-copper phase diagram showing a eutectic (lowest melting) point at 28.1% copper.

An *equilibrium phase* is defined as a homogeneous body of matter that is physically distinct and mechanically distinguishable. For a pure material like water, the vapor, liquid, and solid phases are physically distinct because there is a definite boundary between the regions when they exist together. Also, they are mechanically distinguishable in properties like hardness, compressibility, and elastic modulus. However, when the phase definition is applied to an alloy system, it is important to recognize that if two different types of unit cells nucleate from the melt—as, for example, at the eutectic (lowest melting) point in Fig 12-7—a two-phase region is formed. The two phases nucleate as separate grains. They are physically distinct, as indicated by grain boundaries that define their limits. Their mechanical properties differ, as can be measured by a microhardness tester impinging on individual grains. Note that two-phase alloys are not as corrosion resistant as like single-phase alloys, because microscopic galvanic corrosion cells are set up between the grains of the different phases. Also, porcelain bonding to multiphase alloys is considered potentially weaker because of composition differences of the grains.

Deformation in metals

There are three types of deformation that can occur in metals, which arise from different mechanisms. The simplest deformation, *elastic strain*, is the elastic stretching of lattice in which all the atoms are shifted from their equilibrium positions by a fraction of their atomic spacing. The strain is directly proportional to the applied stress (ie, force/area or force intensity) up to the proportional limit stress. When the stress is removed, the atoms return to equilibrium atomic spacing. Compared with most polymeric materials, metals generally have strong metallic bonds and resist elastic stretching. This stiffness or resistance to elastic strain is indicated by the high elastic modulus of metals. Stiffness is desirable for removable partial dentures, so forces can be transmitted by the framework across an arch to better distribute the load. It is desirable for the alloy of resin-bonded bridges to resist flexing of the bond.

Another type of deformation is *plastic deformation*, a permanent deformation that begins when the elastic limit stress or its approximation, yield stress, is reached. This mode of deformation requires that atoms be shifted to new atomic sites on the lattice. These lattice sites must be identical to the old sites and not far away, so the energy to shift atoms is not too great. Thus, ductility is associated with face-centered and body-centered cubic metal lattices, which have more identical sites and more closely packed planes, so atoms do not have to slide far to reach the new lattice sites. Intermetallic compounds are usually brittle because the atomic sites are specific to the different atoms of the compound and not interchangeable.

The mechanism of plastic deformation is called *dislocation motion* and produces the slipping of the closely packed planes over each other. A dislocation (Fig 12-8a, D_x) is the line of atoms that denotes the edge of an additional half-plane of atoms that appears to be wedged

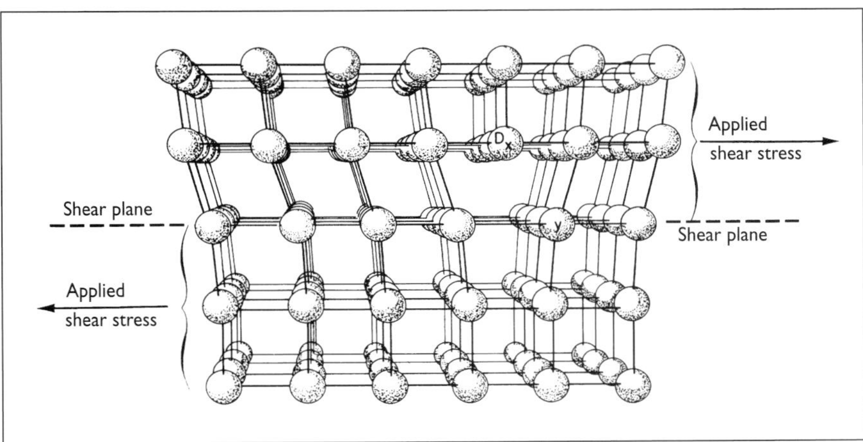

Fig 12-8a The distortion (strain) around a dislocation in a simple cubic crystal lattice. The size of the atoms has been reduced so the perspective can be seen. The row of atoms of the dislocation is D_x. (From Ziman, 1967. Reprinted with permission.)

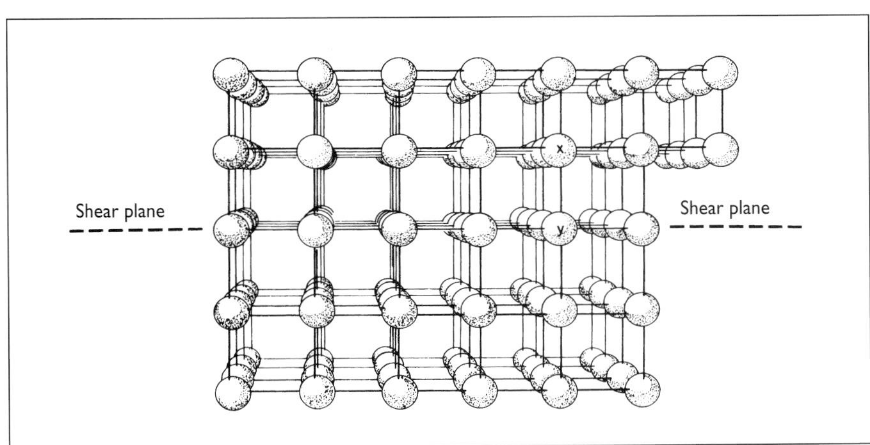

Fig 12-8b The crystal lattice as it would appear after the yield stress has been exceeded and the dislocation has moved through the lattice. The solid has been deformed to this new shape.

into the lattice. The lattice is distorted (strained) by the presence of the dislocation line of atoms. Dislocation motion shifts atoms from one lattice site to the next, rather than moving all the atoms of the plane at one time, which would take much more energy (Fig 12-8b).

It is important to understand that any process that impedes dislocation movement tends to harden a metal, raise its yield stress, and, often, lower its ductility. Some processes are reversible, allowing the hardness to be low when making an appliance, for example, after which the metal can be hardened to provide better service if necessary.

One process for hardening metal is called *cold working* or *work hardening*—any plastic deformation of metal by hammering, drawing, cold forging, cold rolling, or bending. These processes produce many dislocations in the metal that cannot slip through each other as easily as the lattice becomes more distorted. The yield stress can be raised more than 100% when a drawn orthodontic wire is compared to the as-cast metal. In dentistry, cold working occurs when gold foil is compacted, a denture clasp is bent, an inlay margin is burnished, or a deformed metal layer forms on a crown during finishing and polishing.

A second process for hardening a metal is *precipitation hardening*. In this process a second phase of finely dispersed clusters of atoms are precipitated from a metastable supersaturated solid solution by reheating an alloy that was quench-cooled to form the metastable supersaturated solid.

Heat treatment can also be used to harden gold-copper alloys by a slightly different process. In this case, because the gold-copper system forms a complete solid solution at all compositions, the atoms can be interchanged on the lattice sites. However, as the atoms are cooled, the copper and gold atoms tend to separate on alternating planes of the lattice in ordered arrangement. This ordering makes dislocation motion more difficult, raising the yield stress. These alloys are soft if quenched but hard if cooled slowly on the bench

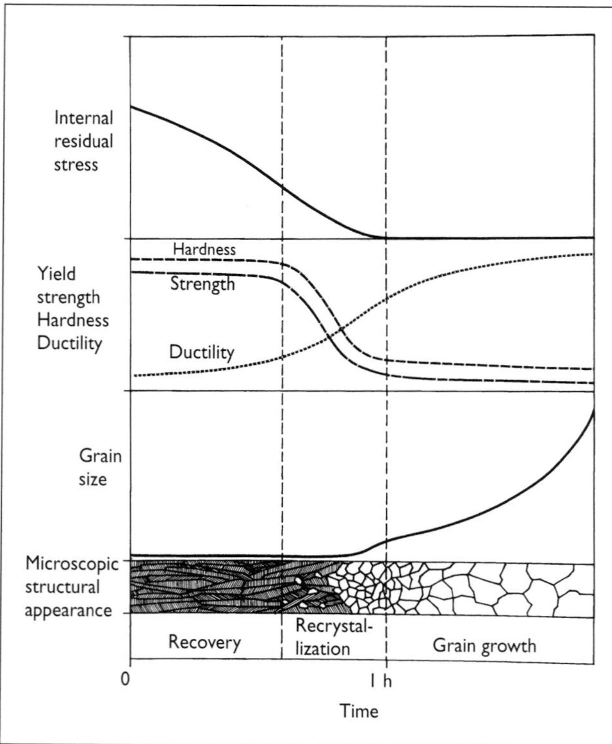

Fig 12-9 A microscopic view of the stages that a cold-worked metal, such as an orthodontic wire, goes through when subjected to prolonged heating. The higher the temperature and the greater the cold working, the more quickly the transitions occur. This figure shows recrystallization being completed in 1 hour, which means the temperature of heating was the recrystallization temperature as per the definition. The changes in properties can be compared with the structural changes. (From Jastrzebski, 1959. Reprinted with permission.)

top or held in the furnace at the ordering temperature range (350°C for 30 minutes).

Other heat treatments are used to homogenize the grains of an alloy that have developed composition gradients by rapid cooling and crystallization of the melt. When cooled rapidly, the grains of the alloy cannot maintain an equilibrium or uniform composition in the grain. The first part of the grain to cool will be richer than the average composition of the higher-melting-temperature element, and the last part of the grain to solidify is richer in the low-melting alloy component. This inhomogeneity, termed *coring*, tends to reduce corrosion resistance of the metal because of the galvanic cell created between the center of the grain and the grain boundary. Heating the solid at a temperature and for a duration that allows the atoms to reach equilibrium will improve corrosion resistance.

Diffusion in metals

Atoms of a crystalline solid vibrate about their fixed lattice positions. As they absorb heat with increasing temperature, they vibrate at greater amplitude. Also, a small fraction of the atom sites are vacant in a metal. As the temperature increases, an atom may momentarily experience an increase in vibrational energy, which will be sufficient to permit it to jump from one lattice site to another. As the temperature and time increase, more atoms will be able to jump or diffuse to new lattice sites. This random jumping during heat treatment allows the rearrangement of the crystal lattice. Atomic diffusion also permits rearrangement of cold-work metals and permanent deformation of metals at stress levels far below the yield stress if the stress lasts long enough. In general, these rearrangements by diffusion begin to occur at a significant rate as the temperature of metal exceeds one half of its absolute melting temperature. The rate of rearrangement accelerates rapidly as the metal or alloy approaches its solidus temperature.

There are several heat treatment processes for metals that utilize diffusion. Among them is an annealing heat treatment for residual stress release. It allows the dislocations and atomic vacancies to move and realign to lower the internal residual stress fields in a cold-worked metal at a relatively low temperature and short heating time.

If the temperature and heating times are extended for a cold-worked metal, the metal can experience "recrystallization," in which stress-free grains are crystallized out of the deformed grains. A recrystallization temperature is the temperature at which it would take 1 hour for the cold-worked metal to recrystallize. This temperature is between one third and one half of the absolute melting temperature for most metals (Fig 12-9). As the temperature and time are further extended, "grain growth" occurs, during which the stress-free grains grow larger at the expense of the disappearing small grains.

The residual stress heat treatment relaxes the internal stress, which may cause warpage over time. The chance of corrosion related to residual stress differences on the metal surface are reduced. Recrystallization heat treatment lowers the yield stress and increases the ductility. Grain growth further reduces yield stress and increases ductility yield stress. When soldering a cold-worked wire in which a high yield stress is desired (eg, a partial denture wire clasp or an orthodontic appliance), a low-melting solder and a short soldering time are desirable to minimize recrystallization and grain growth.

Glossary

alloy system An atomic mixture of metallic elements.

annealing A relatively low-temperature heat treatment for removing residual stress.

austenitic stainless steel An alloy of iron, often with nickel and chromium, whose normally high-temperature face-centered cubic phase exists at room temperature.

binary alloy An alloy composed of two elements.

binary phase diagram A map with temperature and composition as coordinates, which displays the regions where each stable phase exists.

brittle Exhibiting no permanent deformation before fracture (in common usage, exhibiting *very little* permanent deformation before fracture).

carbon steel An alloy of carbon and iron with less than 2% carbon present.

cold working Deforming a metal at temperatures that are low compared with its melting temperature.

crystal A solid with periodic arrangement of atoms in space, usually with atomic planes forming facets on the surface.

crystal lattice The periodic arrangement of atoms in three-dimensional space.

crystallite A crystal with irregularly shaped surfaces instead of facets.

crystallization The process of crystal and crystallite formation.

deformation The process of changing the shape of a metal by applied stresses.

dislocation A row of atoms displaced from their normal positions in the lattice.

dislocation motion The movement of a dislocation through a crystal under an applied stress.

ductile Capable of being permanently deformed.

eutectic alloy An alloy, easily melted with respect to its component elements, that can transform at one temperature from liquid to two phases separated as distinct grains in the solid metal.

eutectic composition The alloy composition at which the eutectic transformation occurs.

eutectic temperature The temperature at which the eutectic transformation occurs.

grain Another name for crystallite.

grain boundary The interface or junction of adjacent grains.

grain growth Enlargement of grains by heating.

hardening A process in which the yield stress and resistance to indentation are increased.

homogeneous Having uniform composition throughout.

homogenization The process of developing a uniform composition.

intermetallic compound An alloy phase with a composition usually near a definite fixed atomic ratio of the elements.

lattice parameters The distances between corners of the unit cell.

metastable phase An energy phase that is often produced when the atoms do not have time to reach an equilibrium lattice configuration because of rapid cooling; not the lowest energy phase.

nuclei The embryos of the crystallites formed from the liquid.

phase A homogeneous body of matter that is physically distinct and mechanically distinguishable.

polycrystalline Composed of many crystallites.

porosity A state in which there are voids in a solid.

recrystallization The process of forming new crystallites from existing crystallites by heating.

residual stress Internal stress remaining between parts of a solid after the applied stress is removed.

solid solution An alloy phase in which one alloying element enters the lattice of the other.

space lattice A pattern of points in space that satisfies the condition that each point is surrounded by the same arrangement of points.

ternary alloy An alloy composed of three elements.

ultimate strength The maximum stress a solid can support based on its original cross-section area.

unit cell The minimum grouping of atoms of an homogeneous crystalline solid that gives the geometric relationships, composition, and distance between the atoms in space.

yield stress The stress at which dislocation motion and permanent deformation and plastic flow begin.

Discussion questions

1. Gold and copper are completely soluble in each other in the liquid state. What is the connection between this mutual solubility and their lattice structure?
2. Which mechanical properties of a metal are affected if dislocation motion in the lattice is impeded?
3. How can you raise both the strength and ductility of gold castings by alloying and process control?
4. Why does overheating orthodontic wires lead to brittleness?

Questions and answers

1. **How does the melting of a pure metal differ from the melting of an alloy?** Pure metals have a melting temperature, whereas alloys usually exhibit a melting temperature range. Alloys of eutectic composition are an exception—they melt and solidify at a single temperature.
2. **What effect does incomplete melting have on dental castings and solder joints?** If a casting alloy is incompletely melted or not heated above its melting temperature range, it will not flow into all areas—especially not thin areas—of the investment mold of a wax pattern. An incomplete casting will result. In the case of soldering, the solder will not flow adequately, and voids may be left in the solder joint.
3. **What is the relationship between the density of a molten alloy and its crystalline solid? Is it the same, less, or greater? Why?** The density of a molten metal is less than that of its crystalline solid, because the atoms pack more closely together in a crystalline solid's crystal lattice than in the disordered liquid state.
4. **How can the density change from liquid to solid damage a dental casting?** If more molten liquid cannot flow from the casting button to take up the volume shrinkage in the casting as it solidifies, porosity will result.
5. **How many atoms are contained in a face-centered cubic unit cell?** Each corner atom is shared with eight other unit cells, so one eighth of each corner atom belongs to a unit cell. There are eight corner atoms, so together they contribute one atom to the unit cell. Each face-centered atom is shared between two unit cells, so one half of each face-centered atom belongs to each unit cell. The six face-centered atoms together contribute three atoms to the unit cell. The face-centered cubic unit cell thus contains four atoms.
6. **Outline how the density of a face-centered cubic metal can be calculated from knowledge of the composition of the unit cell, the atomic weight of the atoms present, the type of unit cell, and the lattice parameters for the unit cell. The density is equal to the mass divided by the volume of the unit cell.**

$$\text{Density} = \frac{\text{Number of atoms} \times \text{Atomic weight}}{(\text{Lattice parameter})^3}$$

7. **The following metals have the unit cell types listed. Which metals are capable of experiencing a large amount of ductility?**
   beryllium—hexagonal
   Ag_3Sn—orthorhombic
   copper—face-centered cubic
   iron—body-centered cubic
   gold—face-centered cubic

   Copper, iron, and gold.
8. **List several ways in which the yield stress of a metal or alloy may be increased.** Work hardening, hardening heat treatment, and a decrease in grain size.

9. **How can dislocation motion be impeded so as to raise the yield stress?**
   a. Increase the number of grain boundaries (ie, smaller grains).
   b. Increase the number of dislocations (ie, cold work).
   c. Treat with heat to create phase changes to lattices that are more resistant to dislocation motion.
10. **Is it better to have large crystallites or small ones in order to have a high yield stress and ultimate strength?** Small-grain metals have a higher yield stress and more uniform plastic deformation, which result in a higher ultimate strength.
11. **The grain boundaries of the crystallites at the surface of a metal can be made visible by polishing to a mirror finish with fine abrasives and etching the surface lightly with an acid.**
    a. **If 0.5 µm is the resolution of a light microscope, how small a crystal grain might one see?** The smallest grain visible would equal the resolution of the microscope, ideally 0.5 µm.
    b. **Why does acid etch the grain boundaries more than the interior of the grain? Why are different grains etched at different rates?** The atoms at the grain boundaries are not as chemically stable because they do not pack together as well as interior atoms of the grain. Different grains etch at different rates because their orientations present planes of atoms of different atomic densities to the polished surface. If the metal is multiphased, the different compositions of the grains will respond differently to the acid etch.
12. **What are the eutectic temperature and composition for the silver-copper system?** The eutectic temperature is 779°C, and the composition is 71.9% Ag and 28.1% Cu.
13. **At what temperatures does solidification begin and end for an alloy containing 40% by weight copper and 60% by weight silver?** It begins to solidify (liquidus temperature) at 833°C and is completely solidified (solidus temperature) at 779°C.
14. **The composition of an alloy can be specified by the weight percentages or the atomic percentages of its elements. Given the alloy Ag_3Sn, calculate the atomic percentage of silver and the weight percentage of silver if the gram atomic weight of silver is 107.9 and the gram atomic weight of tin is 118.7.** The atomic percentage of silver in Ag_3Sn is 75%: 3 Ag atoms ÷ (3 Ag + 1 Sn) = 0.75. The weight percentage of silver in Ag_3Sn is 73.2%:

    $$3(107.9) \div [3(107.9) + 1(118.7)] = 0.732.$$
15. **How do a crystal lattice and a space lattice differ?** A crystal lattice indicates the location and periodic spacing of atoms in a crystalline solid. A space lattice indicates the way in which mathematical points can be located in space so that every point has a similar grouping of points surrounding it. This requirement develops a repeat pattern of points that correlates with the periodic table of elements.
16. **Discuss how the yield strength and percentage elongation change during heating of a drawn wire with time.** During the recovery stage, the yield strength decreases only slightly, and the percentage elongation begins to increase. During recrystallization, the yield strength drops rapidly, and the percentage elongation increases rapidly. There is a further small increase in percentage elongation and decrease in yield strength with grain growth.
17. **If the recrystallization temperature of an iron wire is 450°C, how long would it take a drawn iron wire to recrystallize at that temperature? What fraction of the absolute melting temperature (ie, degrees Kelvin) of iron is 450°C?** By definition, it takes 1 hour for a metal to recrystallize at its recrystallization temperature; at a higher temperature it would take less time and at a lower temperature it would take more. The melting temperature of iron in degrees Kelvin is 1,535°C + 273°C (1,808 K). The recrystallization temperature in degrees Kelvin is 450°C + 273°C (723 K). The recrystallization temperature divided by the absolute melting temperature is 0.42.

Recommended reading

Greener EH, Harcourt JK, Lautenschlager EP. Materials Science in Dentistry. Baltimore: Williams & Wilkins Co, 1972.

Guy AG. Elements of Physical Metallurgy. Reading, MA: Addison-Wesley, 1959.

Guy AG, et al. Introduction to Materials Science. New York: McGraw Hill, Inc, 1971.

Jastrzebski ZD. Nature and Properties of Engineering Principles. New York: John Wiley & Sons, Inc, 1959.

Mott N. The solid state. Sci Am, Sept 1967; 80–90.

Reed-Hill RE. Physical Metallurgy Principles. 2nd ed. New York: Van Nostrand Reinhold Co, 1973.

Van Vlack LH. Materials Science for Engineers. Reading, MA: Addison-Wesley, 1970.

Wulff J, et al. The Structure and Properties of Materials. Vols 1–4. New York: John Wiley & Sons, Inc, 1965.

Ziman J. The thermal properties of materials. Sci Am, Sept 1967; 180–194.

Chapter 13

Dental Amalgams

Amalgam has been an accepted part of dental therapeutics for more than 150 years. It is still used for over 75% of direct posterior restorations today. The reasons for its popularity lie in its ease of manipulation, relatively low cost, and long clinical service life. Recently, some concern has arisen with reference to mercury from both a biological and an environmental viewpoint; however, it is presently believed that dental amalgam presents an acceptable risk-to-benefit ratio when properly used. An exception to this position has been taken in northern Europe where concerns have been raised regarding amalgam use in populations thought to be susceptible to mercury exposure, such as pregnant women and pedodontic patients.

Amalgam's primary application in dentistry is for the restoration of posterior teeth and, to some degree, for cores for crown-and-bridge buildups. Small Class V restorations, although formerly representing a major clinical use for amalgams, now are virtually always carried out using composite and hybrid glass-ionomer restorative materials. Posterior lesions are restored primarily by amalgam, although as a result of recent improvement in their clinical handling, composites have been employed successfully in small cavities.

Chemical composition and microstructure

A general classification of amalgam alloys is given in Fig 13-1 and Table 13-1. Contemporary amalgams are mainly classified as high-copper amalgams and have

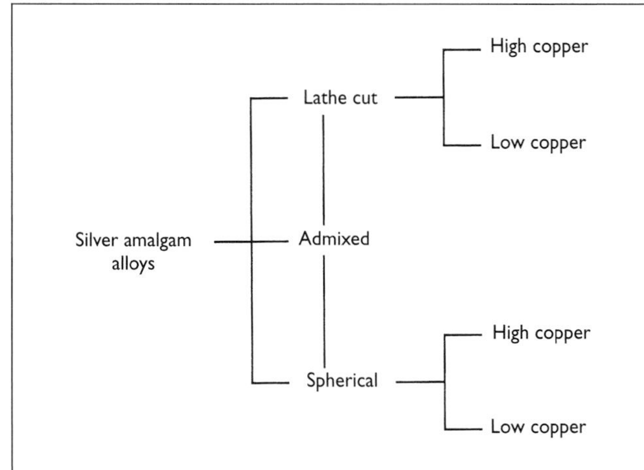

Fig 13-1 A general classification of types of amalgam alloys.

Table 13-1 Classification of amalgam alloys

Composition	Morphology	Example
Traditional	Lathe cut	Aristaloy
Traditional	Spherical	Spheraloy
High copper	Lathe cut (single composition)	Epoque 80
High copper	Spherical (single composition)	Tytin
High copper	Admixed (traditional + Ag-Cu eutectic)	Dispersalloy

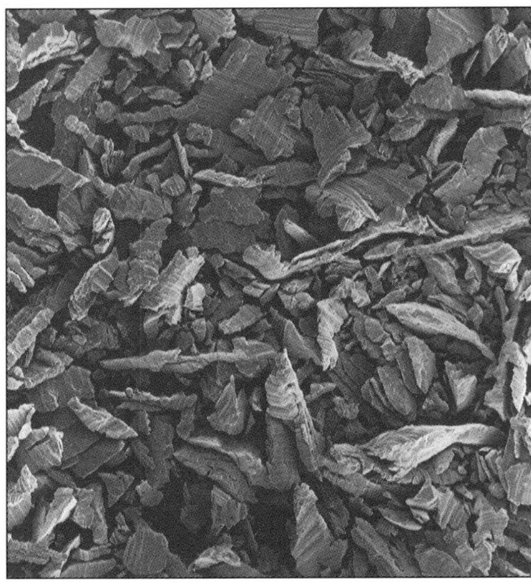

Fig 13-2 Traditional lathe-cut amalgam alloy. (Original magnification × 100.)

existed since the 1960s. Recently, in an attempt to circumvent the problems with mercury, a radically new composition has appeared containing a gallium-indium-tin liquid that completely replaces mercury. To understand the significance of these materials and how knowledge of the solid-state reactions occurring in amalgams has made superior clinical materials, it is first necessary to look at the so-called traditional amalgams.

Traditional amalgam alloys

Lathe cut

Until the 1960s, the chemical composition and microstructure of available amalgam alloys were essentially the same as those of the most successful systems investigated by G.V. Black (Black, 1895). Traditional alloys were delivered to the dentist as filings, which were lathe cut from a cast ingot. Milling and sifting produced the ultimate particle size distribution, as well as the final form of the amalgam alloy particles. Figure 13-2 illustrates a typical traditional alloy.

A commercial alloy evolved into a blend of different particle sizes rather than a unimodel system, in order to optimize packaging efficiency. The length of particles in a commercial lathe-cut alloy might range from 60 to 120 μm, their width from 10 to 70 μm, and their thickness from 10 to 35 μm. The particle size has become still smaller (<30 μm) due to the introduction of so-called spherical alloys, as discussed later. The traditional alloys contain 66% to 73% silver by weight; tin varies from 25% up to 29% by weight, and the amount of copper may be as high as 6% by weight. Zinc may be present up to 2% by weight. Up to 3% mercury by weight may also be present.

The structures of these traditional alloys are essentially phase mixtures of the gamma phase of the silver-tin system (Ag_3Sn) and the epsilon phase of the copper-tin system (Cu_3Sn). It has been shown that Ag_3Sn produces the best physical properties when reacting alloys of the silver-tin system with mercury (Gruber et al, 1967). Some of these traditional alloys are still available, but they represent only a minor component of the overall amalgam market.

Spherical

The spherical alloys were introduced on the market during the 1960s. Generally, their particle shape is created by means of an atomizing process whereby a spray of tiny drops is allowed to solidify in an inert gaseous (ie, argon) or liquid (ie, water) environment. Although all alloys produced in this way are classified as spherical, their particle shape might be irregular (Fig 13-3). Generally, the maximum particle size in a spherical alloy powder is 40 to 50 μm or less, although there usually is a particle size distribution. Spherical traditional amalgam lowered the necessary mercury/alloy ratios and dramatically reduced condensation pressures.

High-copper blended and single composition

During the late 1960s, alloys with a significantly different chemical composition were introduced on the market. All of these alloys could be characterized by their higher copper content. A list of current high-copper alloy products is given in Table 13-1.

The first alloy of this type (Dispersalloy, Johnson & Johnson Dental Care Co.) (Innes and Youdelis, 1963) was a mechanical mixture of two parts of a traditional lathe-cut alloy with one part of a spherical alloy (Fig 13-4). The chemical composition of the spherical particle was 72% silver by weight and 28% copper by weight; it corresponds to the eutectic composition of the silver-copper system. The overall composition of this alloy contained approximately 13% copper by weight. This was more than twice the maximum amount permitted in the American Dental Association's (ADA's) specifications for dental amalgam alloy at that time. Amalgams made from this alloy, however, were clinically superior to traditional amalgams with respect to marginal

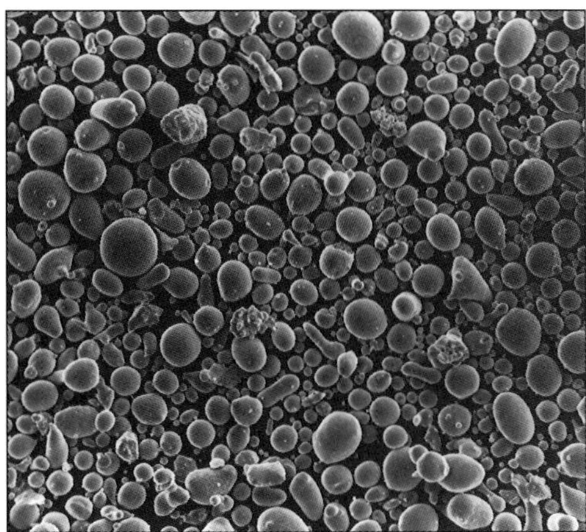

Fig 13-3 Spherical traditional alloy. (Original magnification × 500.)

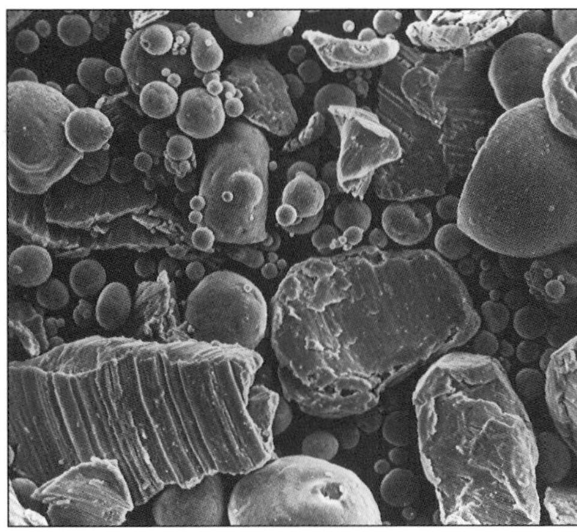

Fig 13-4 Blended high-copper amalgam alloy with spheres of silver-copper and lathe-cut particles of a traditional alloy. (Original magnification × 1,000.)

integrity (Mahler et al, 1970), and, consequently, other manufacturers developed similar compositions featuring some with a copper content greater than that found in traditional amalgam. At present, the copper content varies up to approximately 30% by weight in some commercial amalgam alloys (Table 13-2).

The structures of several high-copper alloys are similar to that of Dispersalloy. They can be classified as "blended" alloys in which the traditional and high-copper phases are mechanically blended. Other alloys are produced by melting together all components of a high-copper system and creating a single-composition spherical or lathe-cut alloy, rather than a mechanical mixture of two distinct powders. Depending on the number of components involved, these systems are also referred to as *ternary* or *quaternary alloys*, or as a *single-composition system*.

Some amalgam alloy producers, in an effort to improve clinical handling properties, supply "admixture" types of high-copper alloys. In these, the chemical compositions and physical forms of the basic powders (lathe or spherical) are varied. This system further differs from those using Dispersalloy in that both blended components are representative of copper-enriched alloys. Several typical classifications and compositions of high-copper systems are presented in Table 13-2. It is important to stress that all of these copper-enriched alloys contain >10% copper by weight in the form of either the silver-copper eutectic or the copper-tin system. The listing in Table 13-2 is a representative one but is by no means comprehensive. The dynamics of the current marketplace preclude a comprehensive listing as a great number of alloys appear and disappear worldwide in response to local demand.

Table 13-2 Typical compositions of amalgam alloys. Chemical composition (wt %)

Type*	Ag	Sn	Cu	An	Other
TL	70.9	25.8	2.4	1	—
TS	72	26	1.5	0.5	—
HCS	41–61	24–30.5	13–28.3	0–0.5	In 3.4
HCAd	62–69.7	15.1–18.6	12.0–22.7	0–0.9	In 10
HCL	43	29	25	0.3	Hg 2.7
GA	50	26	15	—	Pd9

*TL = traditional lathe cut; TS = traditional spherical; HCS = high-copper spherical; HCAd = high-copper admixed; HCL = high-copper lathe cut; GA = alloy for gallium amalgam.

Although amalgam alloys containing many other metals have been proposed or investigated on an experimental basis, at present only indium, palladium, and selenium have been utilized as commercial additives. Because of economic reasons, the alloys intended for mercury amalgamation and containing palladium feature a relatively low (<1%) concentration. Selenium has been added in an attempt to improve the biocompatibility of the amalgam (Sato and Kumei, 1982). Indium has been admixed in large concentrations (10% by weight) in metallic form to a high-copper amalgam in order to reduce the mercury vapor released in the mastication process (Powell et al, 1988; Youdelis, 1992).

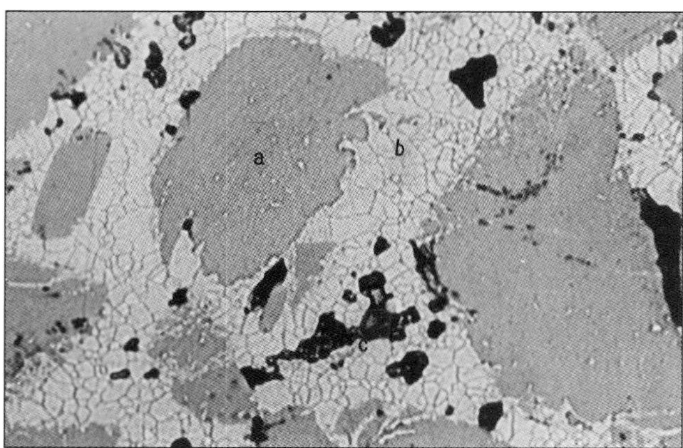

Fig 13-5 Microstructure of a traditional dental amalgam containing gamma 2 (c) and unreacted gamma (a) in a gamma 1 matrix (b).

Gallium alloys

Although called gallium alloys, these systems make use of the fact that the melting temperature of gallium can be suppressed below room temperature with the addition of appropriate amounts of indium and tin. This liquid can be then triturated with a silver-tin-copper alloy powder (spherical) in the same fashion as dental amalgam. Significant additions of palladium are added to the alloy powder in current commercial compositions to improve corrosion properties. A current composition marketed in Japan is known as Gallium alloy GF (Tokuriki Honton Co. Ltd.) comes as a powder and contains the following elements (by weight): silver, 50%; tin, 25.7%; copper, 15%; palladium, 9%; and traces, 0.3%. It is also available as a liquid containing gallium, Ga 65%; indium, 18.95%; tin, 16%; and traces, 0.5%.

Setting reactions and microstructure

Traditional amalgams

The amalgamation reaction of the traditional alloy with mercury (known as *trituration*) as well as its microstructure after setting are described on the basis of a reaction of Ag_3Sn (gamma) with mercury. Copper and/or zinc are not usually taken into account, but their presence has important effects. During hardening, new reaction products with mercury are formed at the cost of the original alloy particles. The main reaction products formed are the gamma 1 (silver-mercury) and gamma 2 (tin-mercury) phases. Formation of a network is completed before all the original reactant is consumed. This amalgamation reaction can be symbolized as follows:

$$Ag_3Sn + Hg \rightarrow Ag_2Hg_3 + Sn_7Hg + Ag_3Sn$$

$$\text{gamma} + \text{Hg} \rightarrow \text{gamma 1} + \text{gamma 2} + \text{gamma (remnant)}$$

After completion of the amalgamation reaction, the remnants of the high-melting-point silver-tin particles are embedded in a matrix of reaction products with mercury (Fig 13-5). In the majority of the traditional amalgams both the gamma 1 and gamma 2 phases form a continuous network. The formation of such an interconnecting structure is extremely important because the gamma 2 phase is prone to corrosion and should be considered the weak link in many traditional dental amalgams. The copper contained in the original alloy will react with tin during trituration to form the eta prime phase of Cu_6Sn_5. The presence of copper has long been associated with improving the physical properties of amalgam, particularly its flow or deformation under static load. This effect is magnified in high-copper amalgams. The presence of zinc appears to extend the working time and, hence, the plasticity of the traditional amalgam.

High-copper amalgams

All high-copper amalgams are characterized by the gamma 2 phase being either absent or substantially reduced, because tin preferentially reacts with copper rather than with mercury, preventing the formation of the tin-mercury reaction product. During amalgamation of blended-typed alloys, Cu_6Sn_5 is created from copper and tin. (The same process occurs in traditional amalgams, but to a lesser extent, as the copper concentration is less.) Because most of the reactive copper is present in the silver-copper spheres, the Cu_6Sn_5 phase is formed at the surface of these particles, creating a reaction zone that is easily identified in the microstructure (Fig 13-6). The mechanism to form Cu_6Sn_5 can be described by

$$6\,Cu + 5Sn \rightarrow Cu_6Sn_5$$

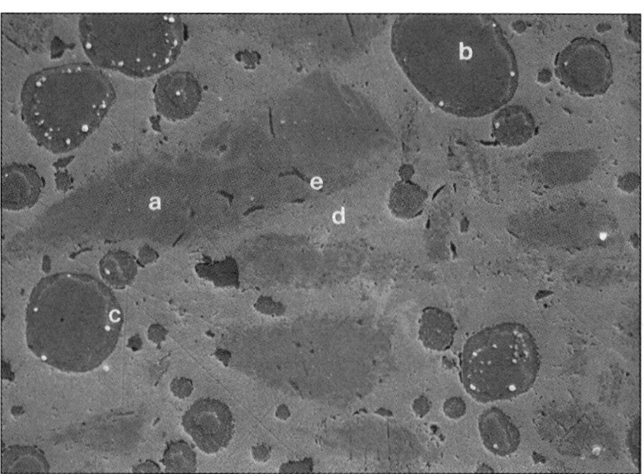

Fig 13-6 Scanning electron micrograph of Dispersalloy amalgam. (a) Ag_3Sn; (b) silver-copper eutectic; (c) eta prime phase (Cu_6Sn_5); (d) gamma 1 phase (Ag_2Hg_3); (e) epsilon phase (Cu_3Sn). (Original magnification × 1,000; courtesy of T. Okabe.)

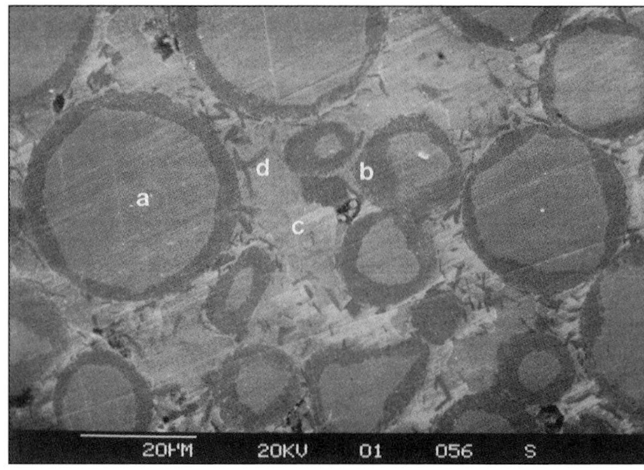

Fig 13-7 Scanning electron micrograph of gallium amalgam, (GF Alloy). (a) Unreacted alloy particle; (b) reaction zone (copper-gallium and palladium-gallium compounds); (c) matrix (silver-indium); (d) beta tin. (Original magnification × 1,000; courtesy of S-Y Lee.)

In single-composition systems, Cu_6Sn_5 also will be formed during amalgamation reactions. In this case, however, the reaction is thought to be

$$2Cu_3Sn + 3Sn \rightarrow Cu_6Sn_5$$

because the source of copper is the epsilon phase in single-composition alloys. It is obvious that in dental amalgam alloys where equivalent amounts of copper and Cu_3Sn are present, both types of reaction to form Cu_6Sn_5 may play equally important roles. It should be stressed here that some high-copper amalgams may initially contain the gamma 2 phase if the mercury content is higher than a certain critical percentage. In these amalgams, the elimination of gamma 2 may occur over a substantial time period as the reactions are diffusion controlled. In general, in lathe-cut and blended alloys the mercury/alloy ratios are ≥1.0, whereas in spherical alloy systems the mercury/alloy ratios are <1.0 and may be as low as 0.7. As mentioned earlier, the gamma 2 phase is considered the weak link in a traditional low-copper amalgam. However, in high-copper amalgams the gamma 2 phase is absent. In that case, attention should be focused on the least resistant phase in the multiphase structure associated with high-copper amalgams. Preferential corrosion of the Cu_6Sn_5 phase reportedly has been shown to be significant both in vivo (Marshall et al, 1980) and in vitro (Averette et al, 1978) studies.

Recently, evidence has been presented for the presence of an additional tin-mercury phase, delta 2 (Sarkar, 1994a), at the grain boundaries of the resulting gamma 1 network. This phase results from the lower tin concentration in the last mercury to solidify. Since it is located at grain boundaries, it will have significant influence in determining the structure-sensitive properties of amalgam. Since copper and tin will preferentially combine in dental amalgam, the higher copper concentrations will also reduce the formation of delta 2.

As mentioned earlier, admixing of indium metal has lowered the amount of mercury vapor released from amalgam. This phenomena has also been verified recently for amalgams prepared from a mercury-indium liquid in which the indium concentration was as high as 30% (Okabe et al, 1994). It is possible that through solid solution, indium may increase the stability of the gamma 1 phase (Sarkar, 1994b).

Gallium amalgams

The structure of gallium amalgams has been interpreted in terms of a reaction zone of $CuGa_2$ and $PdGa_5$ surrounding the unreacted alloy particles which are held together by a matrix of Ag_9In_4 in which islands of Ag_9Ga_3 and beta-tin can be found. The structure of set gallium amalgam (GF alloy) is shown in Fig 13-7.

Table 13-3 Physical properties of amalgam

Type*	Compressive strength (MPa) 30 min/1 hr/1 day	Tensile strength (MPa)	Knoop hardness	Creep (%)	Dimensional change (µm/cm)
TL	53, 89, 430	52	146	2.05	8
TS	170, 265, 444	55	174	0.21	0
HCS	122, 220, 486	63	173	0.07	–7
HCL	59, 97, 477	45	174	0.17	5
HCB	79, 123, 434	50	155	0.24	–7
GA	—, 343, 383	57	—	0.17	16

*TL = traditional lathe cut; TS = traditional spherical; HCS = high-copper spherical; HCL = high-copper lathe cut; HCB = high-copper blend; GA = alloy for gallium amalgam.

Physical properties

The physical properties of dental amalgam are usually compared to those specified in the American National Standards Institute/American Dental Association (ANSI/ADA) specifications for dental amalgam. These properties are (*1*) 1-hour compressive strength, (*2*) creep (or resistance to static load), and (*3*) dimensional change. The ANSI/ADA limits are (*1*) 1-hour compressive strength of at least 80 MPa (11,000 psi), (*2*) dental creep of no more than 3% and (*3*) dimensional change of ±20 µm/cm. The corresponding properties of several commercial alloys are given in Table 13-3. The rationale for these properties is that high early strength is important to withstand dental finishing procedures and occlusal stresses. Low creep is desirable for maintaining marginal integrity, and dimensional change must be controlled to prevent excessive marginal leakage.

Continual reaction occurs as a function of time. The 24-hour compressive strengths shown in Table 13-3 are adequate for most occlusal loadings. If the biting force is assumed to be 750 N (170 lb) and the contact area 2mm^2, the compressive stress offered to the amalgam would be on the order of 380 Mpa (55,000 psi). As can be seen from Table 13-3, this is similar to the compressive strengths of most set amalgams. Little additional hardening occurs beyond 24 hours, although additional phase changes are possible.

The amount of residual mercury is very important in the determination of mechanical properties. In general, the compressive strength will decrease 1% with each 1% increase in mercury above 60%. Low mercury/alloy ratios after condensation are therefore desired. In addition to the effects of residual mercury, compressive strength will also decrease 1% with each 1% of porosity. Adequate condensation of amalgam is, therefore, mandatory in achieving maximum strength.

It should also be emphasized that amalgam is a brittle material. Generally, the tensile strength of a brittle material is much less than its corresponding value in compression. As can be seen from Table 13-3, the tensile strength values are about one seventh of the compressive strength values. This means tensile failure is much more likely to occur than compressive failure. Tensile failure is particularly apt to occur in the margins where the amalgam may be unsupported or the mercury concentration is higher due to the condensation process. Obviously the last bit to condense will have the higher mercury concentration, because mercury expression occurs as the amalgam is packed. Because of the higher mercury concentration at the margin, this area may contain greater amounts of the delta 2 phase, contributing to weakness in this region. Tensile failure may also occur at the isthmus of mesio-occlusodistal (MOD) restorations with too little bulk at the step. Both traditional and high-copper amalgams display brittle behavior.

Creep and flow are both deformations produced by constant load. The creep of amalgam is important because amalgam at oral temperatures is at 0.9 T_m, where T_m is the melting temperature. At these temperatures, atomic diffusion occurs easily, and deformation under static load is possible. As can be seen from Table 13-3, the creep of higher-copper amalgam is at least an order of magnitude lower than the upper limit of 3% for traditional amalgams. This lower creep has been associated with the presence of Cu_6Sn_5 in the gamma 1 network and the decreased amount of available tin (Okabe et al, 1977). The lower creep of high-copper amalgams may also now be related to the absence of the delta 2 phase. The lower creep of higher-copper amalgam has been suggested as a possible reason for its demonstrably better marginal integrity.

The wear of amalgams is approximately the same magnitude as that of tooth enamel. The wear resistance of amalgams exceeds that of most posterior composite restorative materials; therefore, amalgams are much more likely than most composite restorative materials to maintain occlusal contacts.

The physical properties of gallium amalgam can be seen from Table 13-3 to be intermediate compared to traditional and high-copper amalgams.

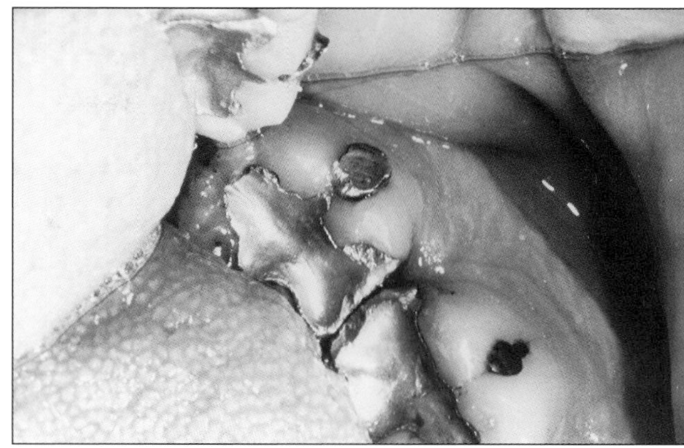

Fig 13-8 Marginal breakdown of traditional amalgam. (Original magnification × 2.5.)

Corrosion

Traditional amalgams are susceptible to corrosion, with chlorides attacking the gamma 2 phase. This phase has been shown to corrode according to:

$$8Sn_7Hg + 21O_2 + 42H_2O + 28Cl^- \rightarrow 14\ Sn_4(OH)_6Cl_2 + 8Hg$$

This process then leads to two deteriorating effects: (*1*) The corrosion of interconnected gamma 2 further weakens the amalgam, particularly the tensile strength; and (*2*) the mercury liberated by the corrosion process can react with the remaining unreacted gamma in the amalgam to produce additional reaction products (gamma 1 + gamma 2). The formation of these new reaction products could produce an additional dimensional change (mercuroscopic expansion), leading to unsupported amalgam at the margin, which can easily fracture in tension. The entire mechanism has been associated with the phenomenon of amalgam ditching (Fig 13-8), which was quite prevalent in the clinical use of traditional amalgam. The liberation of mercury as a corrosion by-product of amalgam has created additional concerns from a bicompatibility point of view.

The advent of high-copper amalgams eliminated or reduced the corrosion associated with gamma 2, because the formation of this phase was prevented or retarded and the formation of eta prime (Cu_6Sn_5) occurred instead. As will be discussed in the next section, this immediately led to an improvement in the marginal integrity of high-copper amalgams. However, the eta prime phase has also proven to be susceptible to corrosion in the oral cavity, with the following reaction possible:

$$4Cu_6Sn_5 + 19O_2 + 18H_2O + 12Cl^- \rightarrow 6\{CuCl_2 \cdot 3Cu(OH)_2\} + 20SnO$$

This reaction will not substantially affect the strength of the high-copper amalgam in the margin because the Cu_6Sn_5 is not an interconnected phase. However, corrosion of Cu_6Sn_5 has raised questions as to possible biocompatibility of the copper-containing corrosion products of high-copper amalgams.

The addition of <1% by weight of palladium to a commercial high-copper single-composition amalgam alloy and 5% by weight to an experimental dispersed-phase high-copper amalgam alloy has produced amalgams that appear to have superior corrosion behavior (Greener and Szurgot, 1982). Palladium may be soluble in gamma 1 with a resultant improvement in the corrosion behavior of that phase.

Recent studies have also shown that mercury is released during free corrosion of amalgam in vitro in various artificial salivas. Over the short term, this mercury burden was found to be in the range of 4 to 20 μg/day, or about the same value as the dietary intake; over longer periods, the mercury released from amalgams was considerably lower than dietary intake (Brune, 1986). The concentration of the dissolved mercury found in such in vitro tests may be unrealistically high compared with in vivo, because

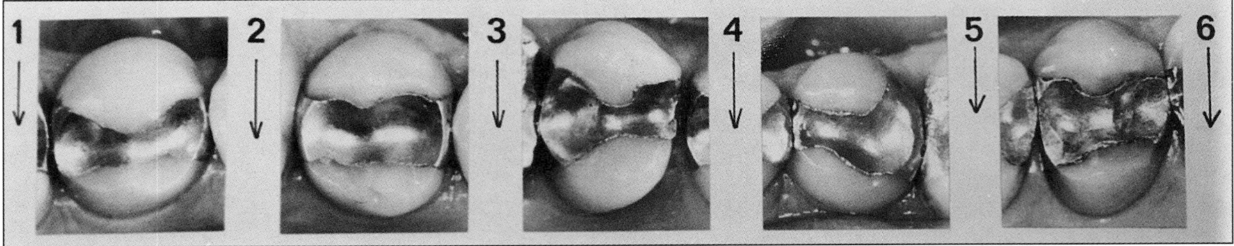

Fig 13-9 Categorical ranking scale for clinical evaluation of marginal breakdown. (Courtesy of H. Letzel and M.M.A. Vrijhoef.)

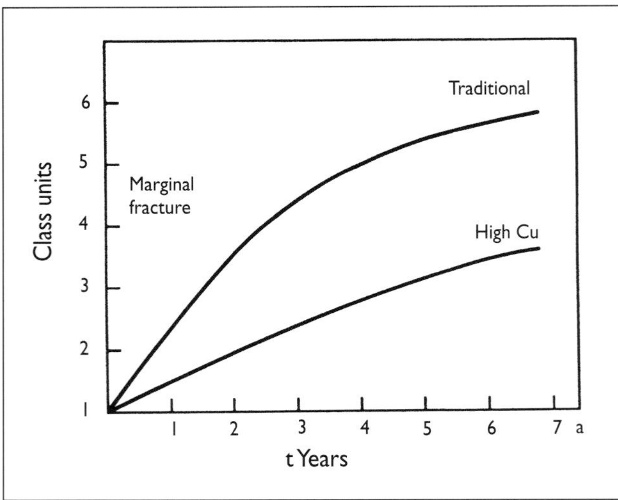

Fig 13-10 Idealized version of marginal fracture of traditional and high-copper amalgams as a function of time.

the natural buffering capacity of saliva, along with the attendant organic proteins, may appreciably lower corrosion kinetics. Porosity will have a significant effect on corrosion of both traditional and high-copper amalgams in effecting increases in surface area and surface energies.

Corrosion of gallium amalgams

In vitro corrosion studies have shown that gallium amalgams corrode at rates similar to those of traditional amalgams with the attendant release of cations of gallium, copper, tin, indium, and silver. This is understandable in terms of the high concentrations of beta-tin present in the matrix. In addition, substantial amounts of gallium were leached out into neutral and acidic saline solutions (Herø and Jørgensen, 1993).

Clinical performance

Amalgam is a successful clinical material when careful technique is applied to all parts of the restorative process, such as cavity preparation, mixing of the alloy and mercury (trituration), packing of the plastic amalgam mix into the preparation (condensation), and finishing. The most significant factor in amalgam behavior under oral conditions is the choice of amalgam alloy. Estimated median clinical lifetimes vary from values as low as 6 years for some traditional products available two decades ago up to median lifetimes exceeding 20 years for the best contemporary high-copper systems.

Unfortunately, only a few of the available commercial systems have been documented as to their long-term clinical function for two reasons: (*1*) The tradition of clinical research is a relatively young one, and (*2*) many of the high-copper systems have only recently been put on the market. Consequently, clinical reports are restricted to specific characteristics, such as marginal deterioration, surface roughening, and surface discoloration, all of which can be evaluated in the short term. Most clinical reports in the literature concern marginal fracture. Although these short-term phenomena give some indication as to the stability of dental amalgam restorations under oral conditions, it should be realized that they are not genuine parameters related to the ultimate lifetime.

The choice of the amalgam alloy is the most prominent factor in marginal deterioration. Marginal deterioration is measured in vivo by comparison of intraoral photographs with a graded scale of marginal failure (Fig 13-9). When treated with appropriate statistics, a quantitative measurement of marginal deterioration may be obtained. These techniques have also allowed for measurement of the kinetics of marginal breakdown (Fig 13-10).

High-copper amalgams tend to give less marginal fracture, although the best traditional systems available might be as good as, or even better than, the least effective high-copper amalgams. The admixing of up to 10% by weight indium did not adversely affect the marginal integrity or luster of a high-copper amalgam (Johnson et al, 1992). Other factors, such as cavity preparation, application of a cavity varnish, mode of packing, and type of finishing, reportedly may have an influence on marginal fracture in a statistical sense. However, their influence is moderate when compared with the differences due to alloy selection.

Several investigators have shown that the risk of marginal fracture increases with increasing cavity size (Mahler and Marantz, 1980). An investigation of the influence of the cavosurface angle (CSA) on marginal fracture indicated that a CSA of 90 degrees produced slightly less marginal fracture than a SCA of less than 90 degrees (Akerboom, 1985). This observation is consistent with published theoretical considerations (Jørgensen, 1965). Finishing the margins with tungsten carbide burs or chisels did not have any detectable influence; however, amalgam restorations with an applied layer of cavity varnish have been shown to have slightly more marginal fracture than those without it (Borgmeijer, 1985). It has also been shown that from the standpoint of marginal fracture, careful application of cotton rolls in combination with vacuum ejection was equivalent to restorations made using a rubber dam (Letzel et al, 1979). Similarly, different modes of packing or condensing (hand vs. four distinct commercial mechanically and air-driven vibrators) did not reveal any marginal deterioration differences (Letzel and Vrijhoef, 1982).

Commercial amalgamators are available for the mechanical trituration of the alloy and mercury (Fig 13-11). In the case of modern high-copper amalgams, different types of post-carving burnishing produce some differences in marginal fracture compared with the traditional polishing methods (carried out after one day). These differences are smaller than those between the distinct amalgam systems commercially available (Letzel and Vrijhoef, 1984).

Thus, the differences in marginal fracture due to operative variables are small compared with differences between amalgam systems and patients. The dentist may, therefore, seem to have only a small influence on the results of clinical reports found in the literature. However, caution must also be taken in extrapolating clinical literature results to the general practice situation because neither the dentists nor the patients in these published studies may be representative. In this regard, cross-sectional clinical performance data from general practices show a dramatic reduction in lifetimes as compared to controlled clinical trials in academic centers (Letzel et al, 1989). It is thus necessary to realize that the manufacturer makes the amalgam alloy, but the dentist makes the amalgam restoration. It is of ultimate importance to control the dentist factor, as well as the patient factor, in a general practice situation.

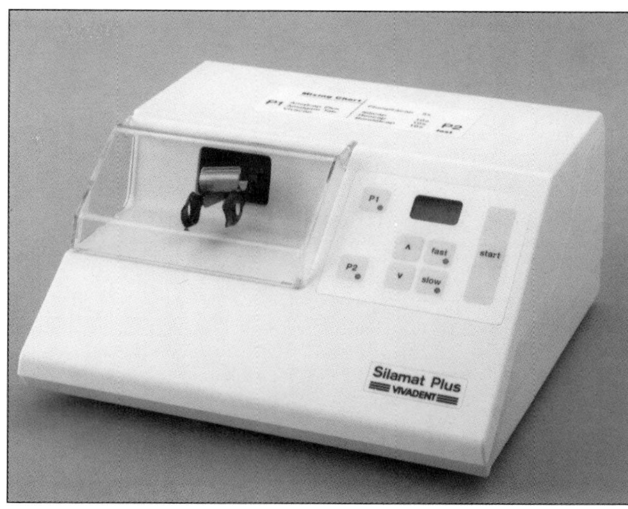

Fig 13-11 A programmable amalgamator available for the mechanical trituration of the alloy and mercury.

Clinical behavior of gallium amalgams

Changes in marginal integrity, surface texture, luster, and color were measured clinically over time periods of up to 2 years by several Japanese clinical groups (eg, Sakai et al, 1993). It was found that significant changes in luster and surface roughness occur within time periods as early as 4 months after placement, with occlusal changes being more severe than buccal changes. In light of the significant corrosion behavior associated with the presence of free tin and the selective attack of gallium in the current commercial formulation, this is probably not too surprising.

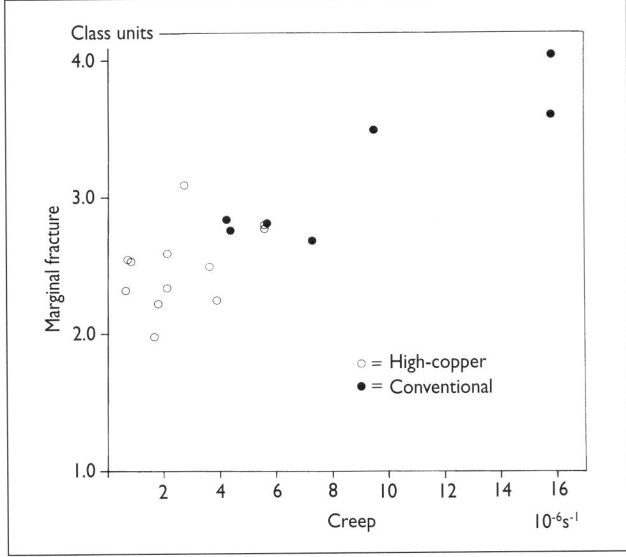

Fig 13-12 Correlation of marginal fracture and creep for traditional and high-copper amalgams. (After Vrijhoef and Letzel, 1986.)

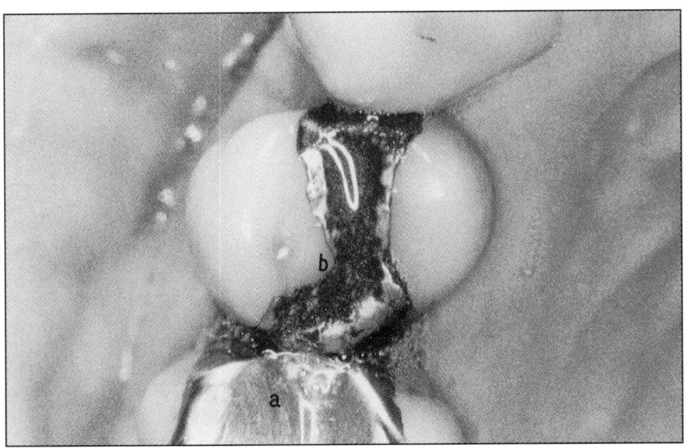

Fig 13-13 Corroding amalgam (b) in interproximal contact with gold casting alloy (a).

Correlations between laboratory properties and clinical data

Creep

In 1970, correlation between creep and the susceptibility of both traditional and high-copper amalgam restorations to marginal fracture was reported with a higher creep corresponding to more marginal breakdown (Mahler et al, 1970). This correlation between creep and marginal breakdown was subsequently verified in a large number of published studies. It attracted, and still attracts, much attention among researchers and in product advertisements. Frequently, statements can be found in contemporary literature expressing, either explicitly or implicitly, that a low-creep amalgam would solve the marginal fracture problem. But this statement is not necessarily true. Several investigators have shown that no correlation between creep and marginal deterioration is present for the gamma 2 free amalgams. However, there are indications of a positive correlation between creep and marginal fracture for the group of traditional amalgams containing gamma 2 (Fig 13-12). At this time, enough clinical/laboratory studies support this correlation to stress that caution is required not to overestimate creep as a selection criterion for the prediction of marginal fracture. General practitioners should not buy their alloy on the basis of creep data alone but rather as part of a complete picture in which clinical evidence from a controlled clinical study plays a substantial role.

Creep will also be affected by porosity. An increase in creep of 30% for a 1% increase in porosity was noted for traditional amalgams.

Corrosion

A well-known and frequently recognized phenomenon in the early life of an amalgam restoration is the "galvanic pain" due to galvanic action of amalgam restorations in combination with other metallic restorations in interproximal or occlusal contact (Fig 13-13). Clinical studies have found that this type of pain occurred only in a small percentage of cases and was generally not serious; it usually occurred in the first hours and in no instance did it last longer than a few weeks after the insertion of the material. It is also possible that the galvanic currents produced could have a harmful effect on the soft tissues or on the organism as a whole; however, the frequency of the occurrence of these effects is supposed to be low or absent.

Galvanic corrosion can adversely affect both the amalgam and the dissimilar metal in contact with it. For example, if the amalgam is in interproximal contact with a gold restoration the amalgam will corrode as the anode. It will suffer surface attack, lose luster, and become rough. Mercury, when produced as a corrosion product, will amalgamate with the gold alloy producing a color change as well as an embrittling effect.

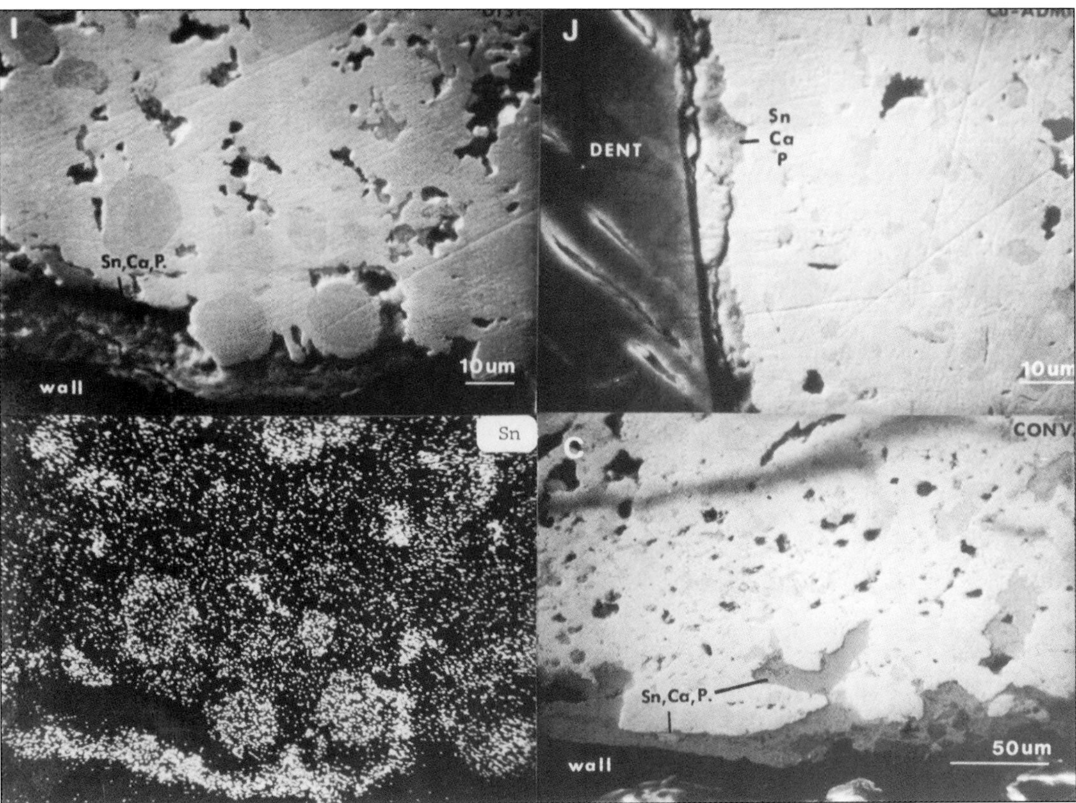

Fig 13-14 Scanning electron micrograph of Dispersalloy, high-copper admixed, and conventional amalgams, that have been retrieved from failed clinical restorations. Note buildup of tin, calcium, and phosphorous corrosion products at the cavodentinal wall. (After Marshall et al, 1980.)

Galvanic effects with dissimilar metals in occlusion are often greater, because occlusal forces at points of contact are usually great enough to rupture protective films of corrosion products that would form in the absence of contact. Thus, mixed metals in contact, either permanent or intermittent, should be avoided in clinical practice.

The loss of luster and the discoloration of the restoration's surface have been the subject of many clinical studies. They are the first indications as to the deteriorating surface of the amalgam restoration and the bulk of material underneath. A rough surface of the amalgam restoration is prone to the formation of plaque and can cause irritation to adjacent soft tissues. The aggressive attack of the oral cavity on amalgam is primarily due to the chloride ion contained in saliva. In addition to this attack, the silver in amalgam can tarnish due to action of the sulfide ion. This damage is confined to the surface layers and can easily be removed by polishing. Further, the sulfide ion concentration is controlled by such factors as the patient's diet and health.

Amalgam corrosion products coming out of the restoration also might have a positive effect. If these products precipitate in the interspace between the cavity wall and the restoration (Fig 13-14), less saliva can penetrate it and marginal leakage through percolation may be minimized. Sealing of the cavosurface margin takes place within the first several days. Both traditional and high-copper amalgams display this effect. The corrosion products at the cavosurface margin are phosphates, whereas the corrosion products seen within the bulk of the restoration are oxides and hydroxychlorides.

Sensitivity and amalgam bonding

Clinical experiences indicate that many of the modern high-copper spherical amalgams produce more postoperative sensitivity than other systems. It is speculated

Table 13-4 Estimated absorption of mercury (after USPHS report, 1993)

Source	Type	Absorption (ng/d)
WHO	Total	43,000
OSHA (air workplace)	Elemental	429,000
Amalgam	Elemental	1,240–29,000
Water	Inorganic	5
Food	Organic + organic	2,220–5,572
Saliva	Inorganic	180–1,400
Air (home)	Elemental	4,160
Air (ambient)	Elemental	32–96

that these materials, which universally contract upon setting, produce large gaps at the cavosurface margins that cannot be sealed by the resulting formation of corrosion products. In addition, the dynamic dimensional changes produced by thermal and mechanical stresses to the margin may potentiate this phenomenon. Obviously, an open margin is a preferred pathway for bacterial invasion. For these reasons, the sealing of amalgam cavity walls with a dentin adhesive or glass ionomer has recently become popular. Traditional dentin adhesives, newer amalgam/dentin adhesives, and hybrid glass ionomers have all shown the ability to reduce leakage and in some cases reduce caries when used under amalgams (Pashley et al, 1991; Manders et al, 1990). Bond strengths of amalgam to dentin with these systems range from a few MPa for traditional dentin adhesives and ionomers up to 10 MPa for the newer systems. A choice of system should not be made solely on the basis of strength values, however, as some of the systems that are lower in strength have been more effective in sealing the margin (CRA, 1994).

Biocompatibility

Dental amalgam has been clinically employed for over 150 years. Yet periodically, concern is expressed about its biocompatibility. Additionally, contemporary society has expressed great concern over the contribution of mercury to the total environmental burden of dental amalgam.

A recent report submitted to the U.S. Public Health Service (USPHS) summarizes the risk/benefit ratio involved in amalgam usage (USPHS, 1993). From a risk standpoint there is no doubt that the presence of amalgams will increase mercury levels in blood, urine, and tissue. The level of increase, however, is currently thought to be below that associated with clinical symptoms. Table 13-4, adapted from the USPHS report, summarizes what is currently known about mercury uptake from a wide variety of sources, and includes as benchmarks the World Health Organization (WHO) total mercury uptake and the Occupational Safety and Health Administration (OSHA) workplace limit. Values for mercury intake from amalgam are around one half to one tenth of these levels. Mercury uptake from amalgam is similar to that absorbed from food associated with normal saliva.

Biological testing procedures have revealed some interaction within cell cultures that has been associated either with unreacted mercury or with copper leached out during corrosion of high-copper amalgam systems. Implantation studies have demonstrated that traditional and high-copper amalgams are well tolerated by connective tissue and bone.

Inflammatory reactions and formation of secondary dentin have been noted, but proper use of lining materials in deep cavities should minimize possible pulpal and dentinal reactions.

Amalgam may also produce gingival reaction due to corrosion or to "tattoos" caused by the accidental subgingival condensation of amalgam. Utilization of amalgams of superior corrosion resistance is, in any case, indicated to minimize these effects.

Under normal service conditions, amalgam restorations are covered by a film of saliva. This both reduces the vapor pressure dramatically and largely reroutes the mercury from the respiratory to the esophageal tract. The esophageal route's tolerance to mercury is greater than that of the respiratory route.

Elevated sera mercury levels have been identified in populations of dental practitioners only after 20 years of clinical practice. However, these levels were far below those producing clinical toxicity, and the dentists were symptom free.

Properly handled dental amalgam should be regarded as safe for general use as a direct restorative material. This position has been accepted, based on available scientific evidence, by the leading regulatory, professional, and research organizations in the world (USPHS, 1993). An important step in the use of this material is the awareness of clinicians and support staff in the proper handling and disposal of mercury and dental amalgam.

Glossary

admixed alloy An amalgam alloy containing particles of different composition, that is, silver-tin particles and silver-copper particles.

alloy for dental amalgam A silver-tin alloy containing other metals, usually copper and zinc, that will be mixed with mercury to form dental amalgam.

amalgamation Reaction that occurs between mercury and an amalgam alloy.

beta (β)-tin An allotropic form of tin.

biocompatibility The ability of a material to provide successful service in a host while causing minimal response.

burnishing Smoothing the surface of a dental amalgam after initial carving by rubbing with a metal instrument having a broad surface.

condensation Packing dental amalgam into a prepared cavity.

corrosion Degradation due to the electrochemical process.

creep Permanent (plastic) deformation under constant load after the material has set.

delta 2 (-2) phase A tin-mercury compound that is a reaction product in dental amalgam.

dental amalgam An alloy that results when mercury is combined with a silver alloy and that is initially a plastic mass that hardens after placement in a prepared cavity.

epsilon (ε) phase A copper-tin compound (Cu_3Sn) that occurs in particles in traditional alloys.

eta prime (η′) phase A copper-tin compound (Cu_6Sn_5) that is a reaction product in dental amalgam.

eutectic composition An alloy or solution whose components are proportioned so the melting point is the lowest possible for those components. Upon cooling, the single liquid phase is transformed into two or more solid phases, the number of solid phases being equal to the number of components.

flow Permanent (plastic) deformation that occurs while the material is setting and in the process of developing its final strength.

gallium amalgam A product formed by the reaction of an alloy powder (silver-tin-copper) with a gallium-based liquid alloy (gallium-indium-tin).

galvanic action Electric potentials in the mouth caused by the contact of dissimilar metals in interproximal or occlusal contact.

gamma (γ) phase A silver-tin compound (Ag_3Sn) that forms a substantial part of the amalgam alloy and is also present in the resulting amalgam structure after reaction with mercury has occurred.

gamma 1 (γ_1) phase A silver-mercury compound (Ag_2Hg_3) that is a reaction product in dental amalgam.

gamma 2 (γ_2) phase A tin-mercury compound (Sn_7Hg) that is a reaction product in dental amalgam.

high-copper alloy Dental amalgam alloy with a relatively high copper content (10% by weight). This alloy is characterized by the corrosion-prone gamma 2 phase being either absent or substantially reduced.

ingot Cast rod of alloy.

lathe-cut alloy Amalgam alloy made by machining small, irregularly shaped chips from a large cast bar of alloy.

mercuroscopic expansion The expansion that occurs when mercury, released by the corrosion of the gamma 2 phase, reacts with the remaining amalgam alloy particles. This will produce an unsupported wedge at the margin of the restoration.

mercury alloy ratio The ratio of the amount of mercury to be mixed with an amount of amalgam alloy.

single-composition alloy Each alloy particle contains the same components in the same ratios.

spherical alloys An alloy whose particles are created by means of an atomization process whereby a spray of tiny drops is allowed to solidify in an inert gaseous or liquid environment.

traditional (or conventional) alloys An alloy composed of the following composition: 66% to 73% silver by weight, 25% to 29% tin by weight, 2% to 6% copper by weight, 0% to 2% zinc by weight, and 0% to 3% mercury by weight.

trituration Mixing dental amalgam alloy with mercury.

Discussion questions

1. Are dental amalgams a health hazard?
2. Why is dental amalgam so popular, even though it is not esthetic?
3. What are the advantages and disadvantages of using a bonding agent with amalgam restorations?
4. How does copper affect the set microstructure of amalgam?

Questions and answers

1. **How can the working time of amalgam be controlled?** It is best not to alter the trituration conditions because other properties may be degraded. Choose an amalgam that has the working time characteristics desired.
2. **Should a zinc-free amalgam be used?** Zinc in the presence of moisture decreases the performance of amalgams. Proper moisture control will give a zinc-containing amalgam better performance than a zinc-free system.
3. **Can some amalgams be finished the same day they are placed?** Yes, fast-setting alloys. Read the instructions for use.
4. **Why are spherical amalgams difficult to condense?** The small spherical-shaped particles tend to slip past one another. Less mercury, however, is required for plasticity. These amalgams also require less packing force to condense.
5. **Does creep predict marginal fracture?** Creep is a bad predictor for clinical marginal fracture in high-copper amalgams, but it has some value as a predictor for traditional systems. The best predictor, however, is proof from clinical trials.
6. **Why are seal/bond amalgam restorations of particular interest?** The primary reason for the sealing/bonding of amalgam restorations is the attempt to reduce postoperative sensitivity seen in teeth restored with some high-copper spherical amalgams.
7. **How safe are amalgams?** Except for allergic reactions affecting a small segment of the population, there is no credible scientific evidence that dental amalgam restorations cause disease in humans. Environmental concerns regarding mercury in amalgam can be addressed by proper office procedures for handling, dispensing, and waste management.

Recommended reading

Akerboom HBM. Amalgam restauraties nader bekeken. De caviteitspreparatie. PhD thesis. Amsterdam: Free University, 1985.

Averette DF, Hochman RF, Marek M. The effects of corrosion in vitro on the structure and properties of dental amalgam. J Dent Res 57 (Spec Issue A): 165, 1978.

Black GV. An investigation of the physical characters of the human teeth in relation to their diseases, and to practical dental operations, together with the physical characters of filling materials. III. Filling materials. Dent Cosmos 37:553–571, 1895.

Borgmeijer PJ. Amalgamrestauraties nader bekeken. De caviteits behandeling. PhD thesis. Amsterdam: Free University, 1985.

Brune D. Metal release from dental biomaterials. Biomater 7:163–175, 1986.

CRA Newsletter 18(2):3, 1994.

Greener EH, Szurgot K. Properties of Ag-Cu-Pd dispersed phase amalgam. J Dent Res 61:1192–1194, 1982.

Gruber R, Skinner EW, Greener EH. Some physical properties of silver-tin amalgams. J Dent Res 46:497, 1967.

Herø H, Jørgensen RB. Corrosion of gallium alloys. Trans Acad Dent Mat Abstr. B-23, 1993.

Innes DBK, Youdelis WV. Dispersion strengthened amalgams. J Can Dent Assoc 29:587–593, 1963.

Johnson GH, Bales DJ, Powell LV. Effect of admixed indium on the clinical success of amalgam restorations. Oper Dent 17:196–202, 1992.

Jørgensen KD. The mechanism of marginal fracture of amalgam fillings. Acta Odontol Scand 23:347–389, 1965.

Letzel H, Fick JM, Aardening CJMW, Van Leusen J, Vrijhoef MMA. Influence of rubber dam use on clinical behavior of amalgam restorations. J Dent Res 58:180, 1979.

Letzel H, Vrijhoef MMA. Condensation methods vs. the clinical behavior of amalgam restorations. J Dent Res 61:567, 1982.

Letzel H, Vrijhoef MMA. The influence of polishing on the marginal integrity of amalgam restorations. J Oral Rehabil 11:89–94, 1984.

Letzel H, Van Hof MA, Vrijhoef MMA, Marshall GW, Marshall SJ. Failure, survival and reasons for replacement of amalgam restorations. In KJ Anusavice (ed). Quality Evaluation of Dental Restorations. Chicago: Quintessence, 1989; 83–92.

Mahler DB, Marantz RL. Marginal fracture of amalgam: effect of type of tooth and restorations. J Dent Res 59:1497–1500, 1980.

Mahler DB, Terkla LG, Van Eysden J, Reisbick MH. Marginal fracture versus mechanical properties of amalgam. J Dent Res 49:1452–1457, 1970.

Manders CA, Garcia-Godoy F, Barnwell GM. Effect of Copal Varnish, ZOE or Glass Ionomer cement bases on the microleakage of amalgam restorations. Am J Dent 3:63–66, 1990.

Marshall GW, Jackson BL, Marshall SJ. Copper rich and conventional amalgam restorations after clinical use. J Am Dent Assoc 100:43–47, 1980.

Okabe T, Mitchell R, Wright AH, Fairhurst CW. Amalgamation reaction on high copper single composition alloys. J Dent Res 56 (Spec Issue A):79, 1977.

Okabe T, Yamashita T, Nakajima H, Berglund A, Zhao L, Ferracane JL. Mercury release from amalgams prepared with binary Hg-In liquid alloys. J Dent Res 73(Spec Issue), Abstr 27:105, 1994.

Pashley EL, Comer RW, Parry EE, Pashley DH. Amalgam buildups: shear strength and dentin sealing properties. Oper Dent 16:82–89, 1991.

Powell LV, Johnson GH, Bales DJ. Effect of admixed indium on mercury vapor release from dental amalgam. J Dent Res 68:1231–1233, 1989.

Sakai T, Kaga M, Oguchi H. Two year clinical observation of gallium alloy in pediatric patients. Trans Acad Dent Mat Abstr P-053, 1993.

Sarkar NK. Intergranular structure in dental amalgams. J Mat Sci (Mater Med) 5:171–175, 1994a.

Sarkar NK. Private communication, 1994b.

Sato A, Kumei Y. New selenium-containing silver amalgam. Bull Tokyo Med Dent Univ 29:19, 1982.

Dental Amalgams: A Scientific Review and Recommended Public Health Strategy for Research, Education and Regulation. Final Report of the Subcommittee on Risk Management of the Committee to Coordinate Environmental Health and Related Programs, January 1993. United States Public Health Service.

Vrijhoef MMA, Letzel H. Creep versus marginal fracture of amalgam restorations. J Oral Rehabil 13:299–303, 1986.

Youdelis W. Amalgam as Restorative Material: Is There Anything New? J Esthet Dent 4:61–63, 1992.

Chapter 14

Direct Gold Filling Materials

Direct gold has several properties that make it an excellent filling material. It is one of the most malleable of dental materials; thus, gold restorations can be directly inserted and adapted to the cavity wall. Although pure gold has a Brinell hardness number (BHN) of approximately 25, it can be work hardened to approximately the hardness of Type II casting gold, which ranges between 70 and 100 BHN. Direct gold filling material is ductile, that is, it can be drawn over the margins of the prepared area. It has been demonstrated with the aid of radioactive phosphorus that condensed direct gold fillings exhibit excellent marginal seal. In addition, direct gold filling material will not tarnish or corrode in the mouth.

In addition to its physical properties, direct gold filling material produces biophysical effects that make it attractive as a restorative material:

1. Gingival health and resultant periodontal support are excellent when tissues are in contact with gold restorative materials.
2. Health of the epithelial tissue is promoted and histologically appears comparable to tissue abutting sound enamel or glazed porcelain.
3. Records indicate that with the use of proper technique, pulp damage can be avoided.

There are four different types of direct filling gold (DFG) materials (Figs 14-1 and 14-2). These are: (*1*) foil and platinized (Williams-Ivoclar), beaten pure gold and platinized gold, respectively; (*2*) mat foil (Williams-Ivoclar), a combination of mat and pure gold foil; (*3*) mat and Electraloy RV (Williams-Ivoclar), electrolytically precipitated pure gold and calcium gold respectively; (*4*) EZ Gold (Williams-Ivoclar) and Stopfgold (Degussa), mixed-powder pure gold encased in foil and chemically precipitated pure gold, respectively. These substances are referred to as direct filling golds because they may be placed directly into a prepared cavity where "cold welding" takes place rather than having to be cast in a dental laboratory. Direct filling materials include amalgam, composites, and other metals (now under development) that the dentist can place directly into the prepared cavity.

Gold foil may be classified further as *cohesive* or *noncohesive*. Cohesive gold is essentially free of surface contaminants and is therefore inherently cohesive. Noncohesive gold is gold that has been subjected to a volatile agent, such as ammonia, which has been adsorbed onto the gold's surface. This keeps gold sheets from adhering to each other and also keeps other harmful gases or fumes, such as sulfur, from irreversibly contaminating the gold. Noncohesive gold filling materials are converted to a cohesive state by desorption, by either flame or hot plate. Pure, uncontaminated gold foil, when properly desorbed, is always cohesive. The use of ammonia to render gold noncohesive was previously said to make it *temporarily* noncohesive. Permanently noncohesive gold is no longer available; it was made by depositing an inorganic salt on the foil surface.

Indications

In general, direct gold restorations are indicated for patients with a low caries index. Further, direct gold should be used only in nonstress areas and areas that are relatively nonesthetic. Direct gold may be used to restore incipient carious lesions, cervical erosions, and developmental defects.

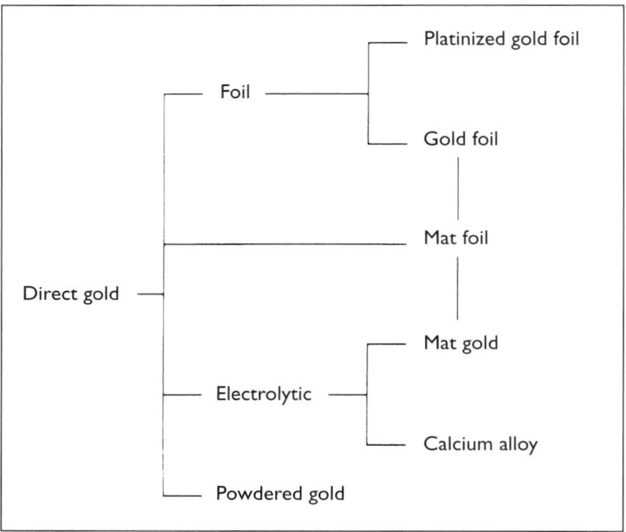

Fig 14-1 Classification of direct gold restorative materials.

Advantages

Direct gold is insoluble in oral fluids and will not readily tarnish or corrode, maintaining a high polish. Due to its high ductility, direct gold is capable of adapting perfectly to cavity walls. It may be welded in a cold state and has a thermal expansion similar to that of dentin. Oral tissue readily accepts the polished surface of direct gold restorations. Although the initial cost may seem high, the long-term cost of a direct gold restoration is relatively low compared with other restorative materials. Although there is a yellow hue in gold, this is harmonious with the color of tooth structure. In contrast to silver alloy filling materials, direct gold causes no tooth discoloration.

Disadvantages

Direct gold is difficult to manipulate, requiring patience and skill from the clinician. Due to its low surface hardness, it is unacceptable in areas of high shear stress. In addition, direct gold cannot be used in areas where displays of gold are objectionable. With some patients, the initial higher cost of a direct gold restoration may prohibit its use.

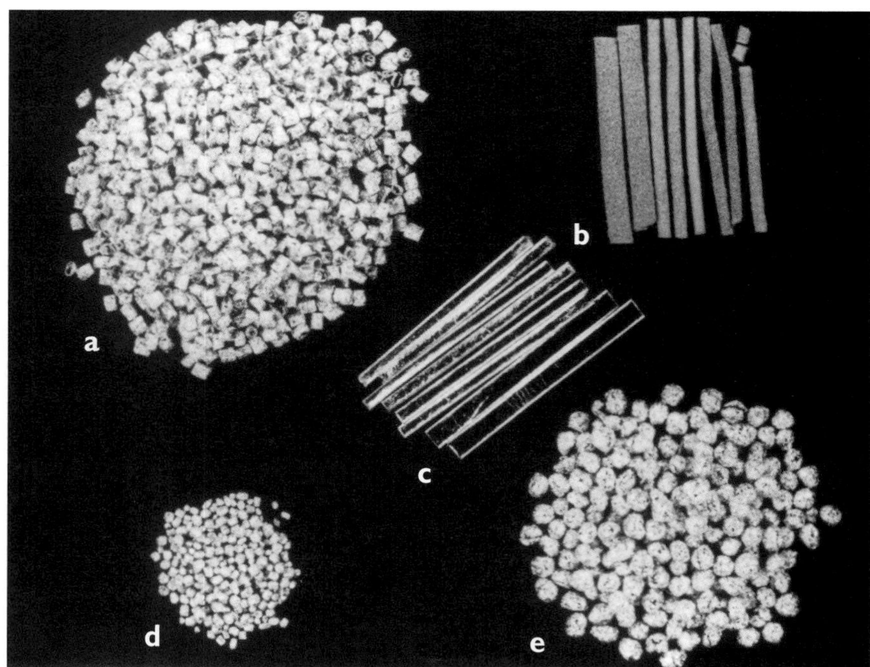

Fig 14-2 Equal weight of (a) machine-rolled cylinders, (b) mat gold, (c) Electraloy RV, (d) EZ Gold, and (e) hand-rolled pellets.

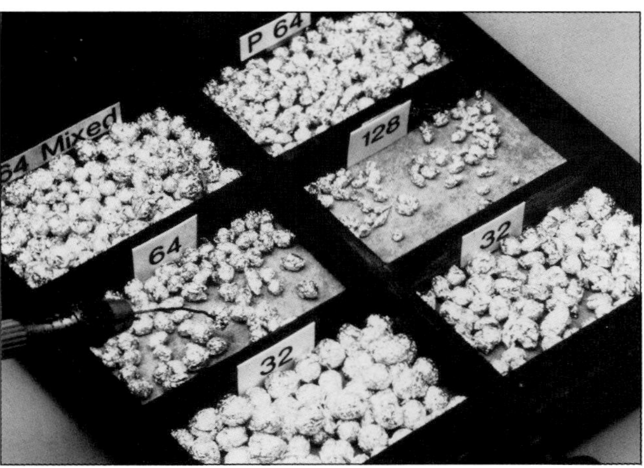

Fig 14-3 Gold foil box with labels for various sizes of foil pellets.

Types of gold filling materials

Gold foil

Manufacture

Sheets of 0.25-mm gold, 2.5 × 2.5 cm, are placed between layers of special paper measuring 12.5 × 12.5 cm and are held together with bands of parchment paper to form a *cutch*. The cutch is beaten by a mechanical 16-pound hammer for approximately 1.5 hours; it is moved into a different position after each blow. The beating increases the surface size of the sheets while making them thinner. The beating process is continued after quartering the gold sheets and interleaving and stacking them with a special plastic "skin" called a *shoder*. Parchment paper is again used for wrapping.

The second beating is done by hand with hammers until the gold reaches the edges of the parchment. The sheets are cut into 10 × 10-cm squares and passed through ammonia gas, which leaves the gold noncohesive. The thickness of foil is designated by a number; for example, one sheet of no. 4 foil weighs 4 grains. Each sheet is cut into portions of varying sizes for different applications. Cylinders and ropes are formed from the sheets and cut by machine to form pellets of varying sizes and weights. The dentist or dental assistant may also form hand-rolled pellets from no. 4 gold foil sheets from portions equal to ⅛, 1/16, 1/32, 1/64, and 1/128 of a sheet (Fig 14-3).

Table 14-1 Properties of direct gold filling materials (effects of condensation on hardness)*

Material	Knoop hardness number†	Measured density† (g/cc)
Gold foil		
Hand condensed	68.5 (12.8)	15.90 (0.41)
Electromallet	69.7 (16.0)	15.83 (0.42)
Combined	68.6 (15.7)	15.83 (0.44)
Mat gold		
Hand condensed	52.2 (16.8)	14.33 (1.04)
Electromallet	61.5 (18.2)	14.66 (0.48)
Combined	53.3 (22.2)	14.48 (1.05)
Mat foil		
Hand condensed	69.7 (15.3)	14.99 (0.48)
Electromallet	70.9 (12.4)	15.15 (0.17)
Combined	75.0 (9.6)	14.95 (0.52)
Powdered gold		
Hand condensed	55.2 (17.9)	14.40 (0.89)
Electromallet	63.7 (16.5)	14.50 (0.30)
Combined	57.6 (16.2)	14.93 (0.66)

*From Richter and Cantwell (1965).
†Parentheses indicate standard deviation.

Table 14-2 Properties of direct gold filling materials (effects of composition)*

Material	Theoretical density
Gold foil	19.32
Platinized gold foil	19.64
Mat gold	19.32
Mat foil	19.32
Powdered gold	19.32
Electraloy RV	19.30

*Measurements taken by permission from an unpublished study conducted by Clyde Ingersoll, Ivoclar Williams Co. (1994) in cooperation with the author.

Properties

Because of its softness and lack of mass, gold foil takes longer to build up than other direct gold filling materials (Tables 14-1 and 14-2). However, gold foil can be used throughout the cavity and is suitable as a surface material.

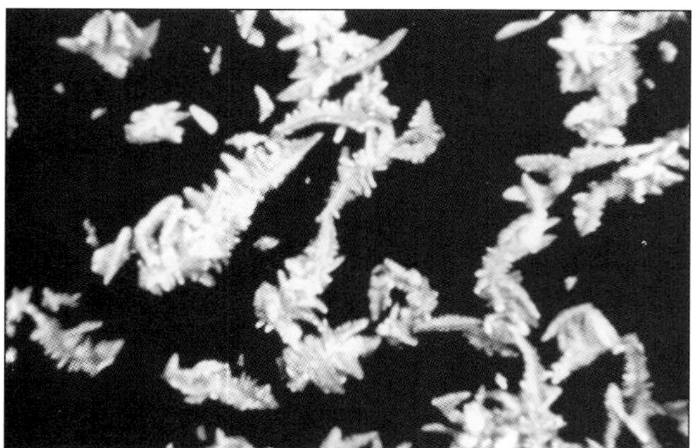

Fig 14-4 The dendritic structure of mat gold crystals.

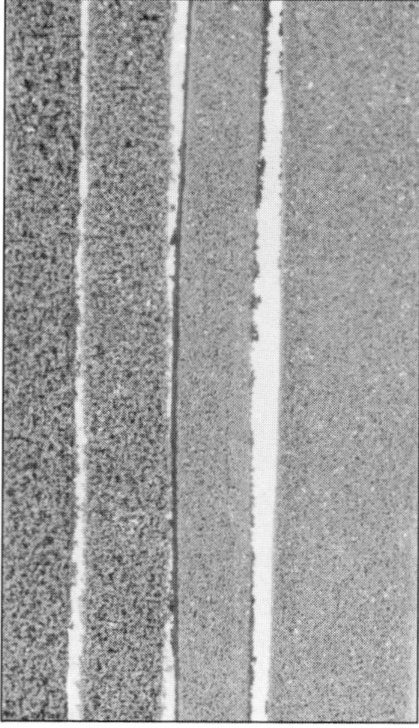

Fig 14-5 Low magnification photomicrograph of mat gold, showing both tops and bottoms of strips. Note that sintering has not proceeded to the extent of producing a solid mass.

Advantages and disadvantages

The advantages of gold foil include its ease of manipulation and workability, whereas its primary disadvantage is the fact that it requires considerable time to build up the restoration. Thus, it may be unsuitable for large lesions or preparations.

Platinized gold foil

Manufacture

Platinized gold foil is manufactured similarly to gold foil, except that a layer of platinum leaf is sandwiched between the two layers of gold foil before the hammering procedure. Platinum is 15% of the total volume of the alloy.

Properties

Platinum increases the hardness of the finished restoration (see Table 14-2). This alloy is generally used only in areas of excessive stress or wear, such as the incisal edge of anterior teeth, since it is difficult to manipulate. Platinized gold foil may also be used on the surface of a restoration because of its strength. In studies comparing the hardness values of all five types of gold filling materials, platinized gold foil was found to have a significantly higher Knoop hardness number (KHN) than other types of gold.

Advantages and disadvantages

Because of its hardness, platinized gold foil is excellent for heavy-access trauma areas and crown repairs. However, it is more difficult than other direct gold filling materials to condense and finish.

Electrolytic precipitate (mat gold)

Manufacture

The basic steps in manufacturing mat gold are as follows:

1. A gold bar anode and a thin gold cathode are used in an electrolytic bath. Ordinarily, gold from an electrolytic bath under good plating condition will deposit a dense shiny sheet of metal. In the mat process, however, the voltage (potential) is increased, and the gold atoms are attracted so rapidly to the cathode that they do not orient themselves into a dense solid metal surface. Instead, they form crystals in a helter-skelter pattern over the surface with large voids between them, creating the characteristic porosity of uncondensed gold mat (Fig 14-4).
2. The gold is removed from the electrical cathode, washed, and dried.
3. The gold is fragmented as crystals for sizing through a sonic (vibrating) sifter. Enclosed within the sifter are six screens, the largest on top and the smallest on the bottom. It takes a blend of various sizes of gold particles to form mat gold. (The average particle size for mat gold is 10 to 20 μm.)
4. The crystalline gold powder is shaped into strips about 3 to 6 mm wide by about 15 mm long and

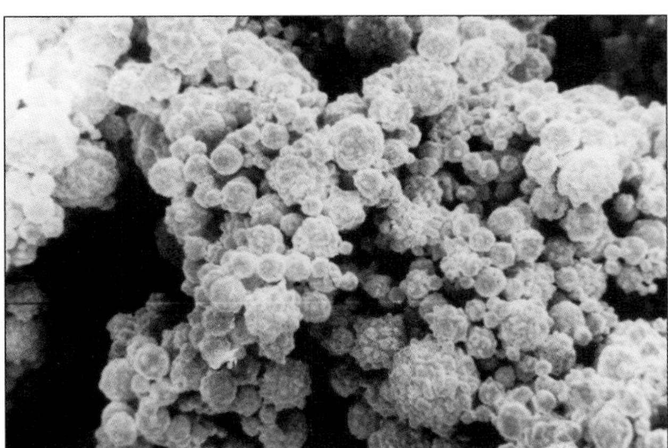

Fig 14-6 The blend of spherical gold particles in EZ Gold. (Original magnification × 4,000; courtesy of Ivoclar-Williams Co.)

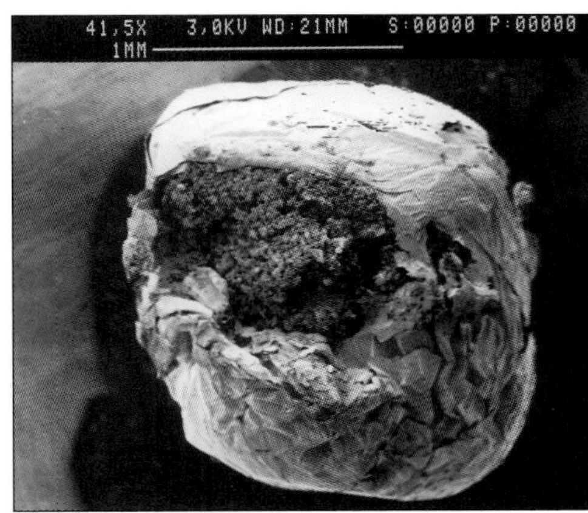

Fig 14-7 Scanning electron micrograph of EZ Gold showing gold leaf wrapping around spherical particles of gold pellets.

presintered before being transferred to heat-resistant trays for sintering (Fig 14-5).

5. The strips are sintered at a temperature well below the melting temperature of gold. Gold sinters very rapidly when near its melting temperature and exceedingly slowly at room temperature. A temperature is selected where proper sintering can be done in a reasonable time. Undersintering results in a product that can readily break up into powder. Oversintering results in too much joining of particles, which leaves the product harsh and hard to condense.

Properties

Mat gold has more mass than gold foil; thus it can be used internally in a restoration and is often used to rapidly fill the preparation. Due to the dendritic structure of the mat gold crystals (see Fig 14-4), condensation into a fully dense restoration is difficult; note the standard deviation of the measured density of mat gold in Table 14-1. There is also a greater tendency for porosity and surface pitting with mat gold.

Advantages and disadvantages

With its rapid filling properties, mat gold is especially suited for use as an internal filling material in a cavity preparation. One reason for this is mat gold's adaptability to the cavity walls and to the retentive portions of the restoration. One disadvantage of using mat gold, however, is that bridging and surface pits are difficult to prevent. Mat gold is no softer than other pure gold DFGs, and its undesirability is due only to its tendency for pits at the surface.

Mat foil

Mat foil is a combination of mat gold and gold foil, in which a layer of mat gold is sandwiched between layers of gold foil.

Properties

Mat foil, as shown in Table 14-1, has a hardness that is not significantly different from any of the other pure gold DFGs—as should be expected because they are all pure gold.

Advantages and disadvantages

Like mat gold, mat foil has rapid filling properties and is especially suited for use as an internal filling material in a cavity preparation. In addition, it combines the adaptability of mat gold with the surface density of gold foil, making mat foil effective throughout the restoration.

Powdered gold

Manufacture

EZ Gold is a blend of chemically precipitated and atomized pure gold in an organic matrix which is formed into pellets of several sizes and wrapped in pure gold foil (Figs 14-6 and 14-7). Stopfgold is a chemically precipitated gold that is formed into strips in a manner similar to the one used for mat. The common form of powdered gold (EZ Gold, successor to Goldent) consists of small appropriate particles blended with an organic (annealing) indicator, com-

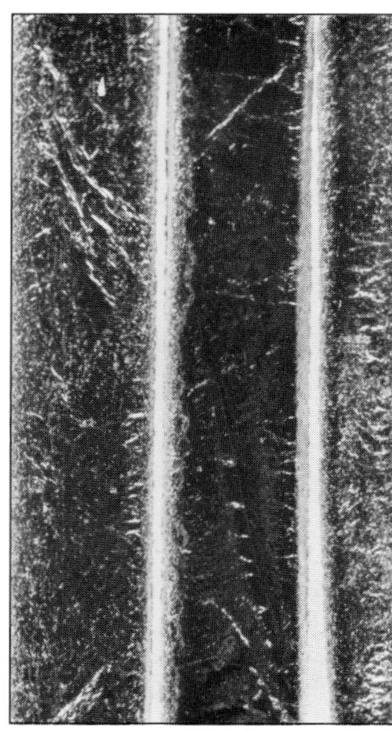

Fig 14-8 Strip of Electraloy RV with an overlay of gold foil.

pressed into small cylinders, cut into various sizes of small spheres, and wrapped in gold foil.

Properties

Powdered gold has greater mass than gold foil. It can be used both internally and on the surface of restorations. However, greater care must be taken to avoid development of surface pits.

Advantages and disadvantages

Because of its density, powdered gold will fill a preparation more rapidly than will other filling materials. Upon condensation, powdered gold spreads laterally from its point of impact. This property is of particular value in the early stages of condensation. Because of powdered gold's rapid filling, it is difficult to prevent "bridging" and surface pits. This advantage may be overcome by taking greater care to systematically step the powdered gold during condensation. This same technique is required with mat gold and mat foil–calcium alloy. It is recommended that powdered gold restorations be overlaid with gold foil.

Alloyed gold

Manufacture

Electraloy RV is a product much like mat foil, but the electrolytic precipitate contains calcium and the strips are thinner than mat foil. The powder manufacture is essentially the same as mat gold with the exception that the anode is an alloy of gold and calcium. As with mat foil, the calcium-containing gold powder is sandwiched between sheets of pure gold foil, sintered, and cut into strips (Fig 14-8).

Properties

Mat foil–calcium alloy has a greater initial density that can be condensed more rapidly than mat gold. Thus, it can be used throughout the restoration, including the final surface condensation.

Advantages and disadvantages

Mat foil–calcium alloy is easy to manipulate. Because its density is greater than that of foil, it will fill a preparation more rapidly. The layer of gold foil on its surface allows this material to be used throughout the complete condensation process. However, mat foil–calcium alloy can cause bridging if improperly stepped and may also create overcontouring during the condensation process.

Clinical processing of direct gold filling materials

Direct gold filling materials require a thoroughly dry field; the use of a rubber dam is imperative. The first step in using direct gold filling materials is referred to as *desorbing*. This term has replaced *annealing* in that it refers to the process of driving off the ammonia from noncohesive foil and other adsorbed gases, such as oxygen or water vapor, from other DFG products. Desorbing may be accomplished by any heating method that raises the temperature above the boiling temperature of water. (EZ Gold needs a different procedure which will be described later.) A natural effect of the heat-treating process used in desorbing is the removal of moisture. Desorbing is accomplished by the alcohol flame method. Powdered gold desorbing still uses the alcohol flame but with a slightly different procedure.

In the past the most popular methods of desorbing (annealing) to direct gold was by the use of a small electric hot plate (Fig 14-9). This method of desorbing was and still is sufficient for pure leaf gold pellets but insufficient for all other types of direct gold. The alcohol flame method is the most reliable for desorbing for all forms of direct gold currently used.

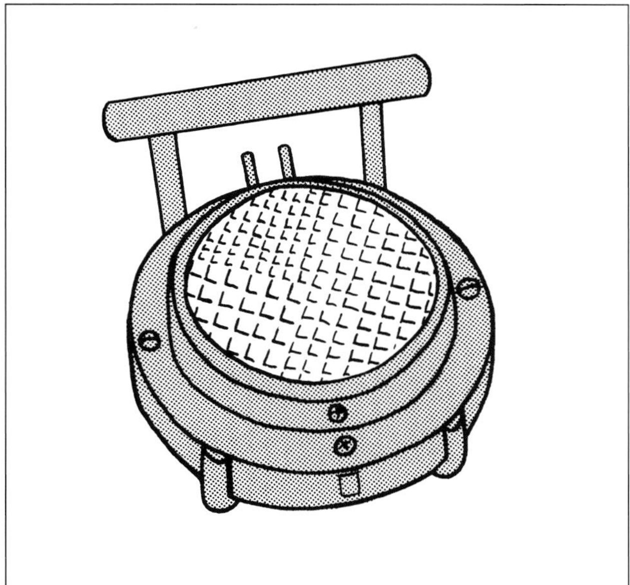

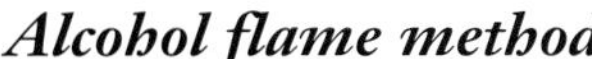

Fig 14-9 Electric hot plate annealer.

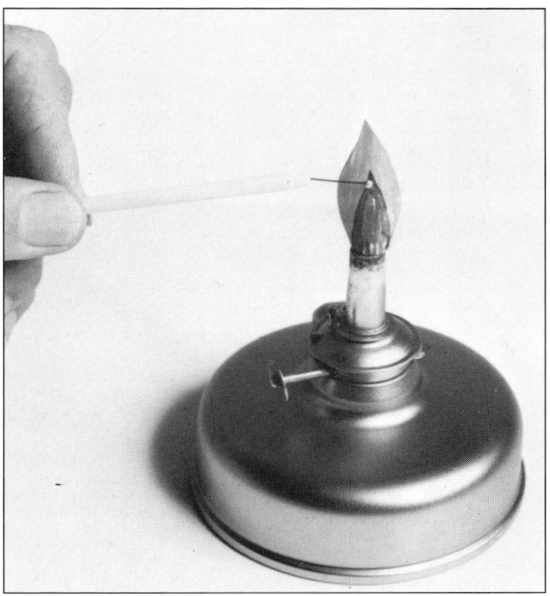

Fig 14-10 Individual gold pellets desorbed over a pure alcohol flame. The gold pellet should be carried through the tip of the inner blue cone.

Alcohol flame method

Individual pellets are heated in a methyl or ethyl alcohol flame. The pellet is held by a pointed nichrome wire or smooth broach and passed through the tip of the inner blue cone of the flame with a slow, continuous motion to allow the gold to acquire a dull red glow (Fig 14-10). Overheating (to a bright red color) makes the gold more difficult to condense. Insufficient heating leaves impurities on the surface of the gold and prevents complete welding. Heating the gold above or below the tip of the inner blue cone may cause some contamination by carbon.

Powdered gold method

Powdered gold requires a slightly different procedure, because the organic (annealing) indicator must be burned off. A pellet is speared with a pointed smooth broach and introduced into the flame of an alcohol lamp. The organic substance contained in each pellet will burst into a yellow flame that will burn for 2 to 3 seconds. After the material has burned out, the pellet will instantly assume a dull red glow, at which time the pellet is removed from the flame, allowed to cool, and carried to the cavity. If left in the flame too long, the pellet develops a hard texture and resists condensation. If not left in the flame long enough, the pellet will break apart and remain powdery.

Condensation

Condensation can be accomplished either manually or mechanically. In manual condensing, a gold foil mallet and condensers are used for hand malleting (Fig 14-11). In mechanical condensing, two types of condensers are available: an automatic electrical high frequency condenser called an *oromatic* and a battery-driven impact mallet (Figs 14-12 and 14-13).

Powdered gold can be adequately condensed by hand pressure as well. Approximately 2.7 to 3.6 kg (6 to 8 lb) of force must be applied through the 0.5-mm^2 instrument to convert the powder into a solid mass. Instruments are available that will transmit the required energy of condensation without penetrating the pellet. Best results are obtained with a convex serrated-faced condenser (Fig 14-14).

There are several controlling factors in the condensation process: (*1*) force of the condensing blow, (*2*) character of the supporting bone's and periodontal membrane's resistance, (*3*) size of the condensing point, and (*4*) proper stepping.

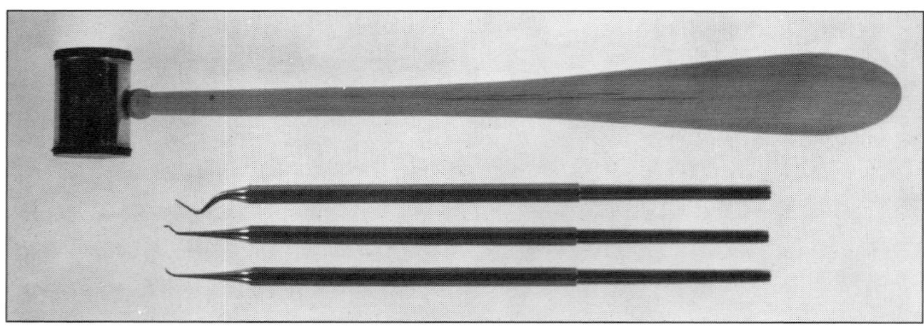

Fig 14-11 Gold foil mallet and selected condensers for hand malleting.

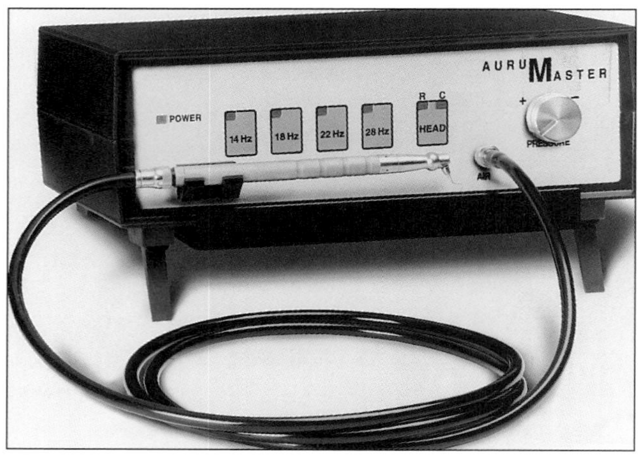

Fig 14-12 *Aurumaster*—a pneumatic condenser designed to condense gold foil. Distributed by Meyer-Haake, Oberursel, Germany.

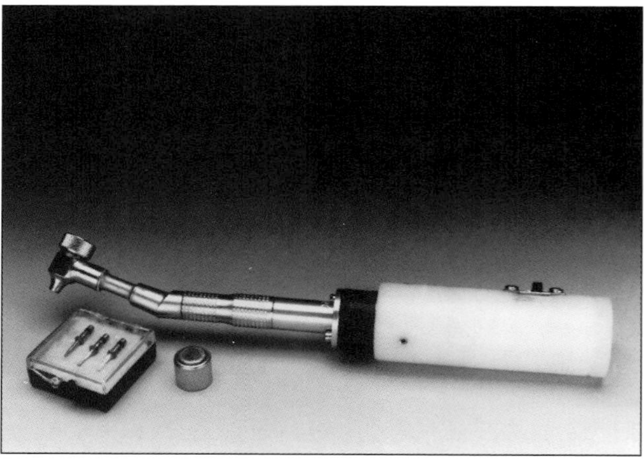

Fig 14-13 Battery-operated gold foil condenser displaying various points. (Courtesy of Dr. Lloyd Baum, LLU School of Dentistry, Loma Linda, CA).

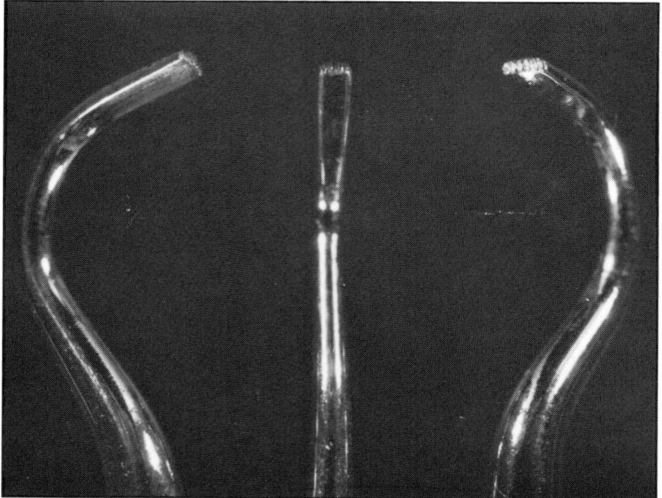

Fig 14-14 Hand condensers showing convex serrated faces.

Finishing

Work hardening of the metal surface is important for the quality of the restoration. The hardness of the metal is increased in direct proportion to the amount of stepping with the condenser and burnishing of the surface after condensation.

Summary of working characteristics

Manipulation

Gold foil Not particularly easy to manipulate, but not difficult either. Miniaturized sheet metal. Can be manipulated through a small cavity orifice.

Platinized gold foil Most difficult of all direct gold filling materials to manipulate. Can be manipulated through a small cavity orifice.

Mat gold Easy to manipulate, not friable, with good spreading qualities.

Mat foil Same manipulation characteristics as mat gold.

Powdered gold Easy to manipulate, comes in a variety of pellet sizes. Tends to be friable, crumbly; needs a larger orifice. Greater mass allows cavity preparation to be filled more rapidly than with gold foil.

Alloyed gold Same manipulation characteristic as mat gold.

Condensation

Gold foil Malleting alone is effective. Will adapt to sharp angles.

Platinized gold foil Malleting alone is most effective. Will adapt to sharp angles. Does not adhere easily during condensation.

Mat gold Hand pressure needed to force large mass into position before actual welding. Malleting effective after positioning. Tendency to bridge.

Mat foil Same condensation characteristics as mat gold.

Powdered gold Hand pressure needed to force large mass of powdered particles into position before actual welding. Malleting alone effective in a small amount, but not in a large mass. Powdered gold needs a wrapping of gold foil such as EZ Gold to keep it confined within the cavity walls. In addition, it has the greatest tendency to bridge of all direct gold filling materials.

Alloyed gold Same condensation characteristics as mat gold; however, it may create overcontouring during condensation.

Finishing

Gold foil Soft; easily workable during finishing.

Platinized gold foil Does not have the surface workability of gold foil. Has BHN greater than gold foil. During surface finishing, the platinum color allows it to blend well with hard casting gold.

Mat gold Produces a more porous surface than gold foil; therefore, it is recommended that the surface of a mat gold restoration be veneered with gold foil.

Mat foil Can be used throughout the restoration, including on the surface, with excellent results.

Powdered gold Difficult to avoid surface pits. Should be overlaid with gold foil. Medium workability. Due to a higher hardness, it is more difficult to obtain contours in the finished restoration.

Alloyed gold Can be used throughout the restoration, including on the surface, with excellent results.

Clinical decision scenarios for direct gold filling materials

This section presents one approach for choosing direct gold filling materials for specific situations. Each of the following scenarios uses the same format as that presented in Chapter 7:

1. The situation is described.
2. Critical factors are listed.
3. Advantages and disadvantages of each material are prioritized using the following codes: * = of minor importance, ** = important, and *** = very important.
4. The situation is analyzed, and the final decision is explained.

Situation Gold foil vs composite restorative material in maxillary anterior tooth (I)

Description For many years, a well-placed gold foil was considered the ultimate dental restoration. Most schools emphasized the foil, and most state boards required performing one of these restorations. Gold foil study clubs were popular, and the ability of a dentist to place a well-done gold foil was considered a mark of superior ability. Esthetic anterior restorations were limited to silicates or unfilled resins, both of which exhibited significant marginal leakage.

With the advent of acid-etched composite restorative materials, esthetic restorations were possible without the leakage problems associated with the silicates or unfilled resins. Many state boards no longer require performance of a foil restoration, and most dental schools have greatly reduced the emphasis on these techniques. Still, the gold foil restoration continues to be considered a respectable restoration.

This clinical situation involves a patient who seeks treatment from the dentist for a small carious lesion on the mesial surface of a mandibular central incisor. He is interested in a restoration that will last a long time, as he does not particularly like to visit the dentist. He has had some three-quarter crowns for several years on his maxillary premolars. Although these restorations show a rim of gold on the incisal edges, he likes the way they have lasted and does not mind the appearance of gold.

Critical factor Durability of the restoration

Advantages

Gold foil

*** 1. Long lasting
** 2. Low marginal leakage

Composite restorative material

* 1. Ease of placement
** 2. Low marginal leakage
** 3. Natural appearance

Disadvantages

Gold foil

* 1. Difficulty of placement
** 2. Unnatural appearance
** 3. Placement may irritate pulp

Composite restorative material

*** 1. Unpredictable durability
** 2. May irritate pulp

Analysis/Decision The dentist chose gold foil in this case. Inasmuch as the patient already displayed gold in the mouth and was more concerned with the durability of the restoration than appearance, the foil was a good choice.

Situation Gold foil vs composite restorative material in maxillary anterior tooth (II)

Description In the same patient, a large mesiofacial carious lesion was present in the maxillary right permanent lateral incisor. It was in such a position that a cast restoration was not practical. Again, the choice was between the foil and the composite restorative material. This time, however, there was the added consideration of support for gold foil condensation. A foil cannot be condensed against unsupported enamel without risk of enamel fracture.

Critical factors Ease of placement, adequate tooth structure to support restoration

Advantages

Gold foil

** 1. Long lasting
** 2. Low marginal leakage

Composite restorative material

*** 1. Ease of placement
** 2. Low marginal leakage
** 3. Natural appearance
*** 4. Adaptable to most cavities

Disadvantages

Gold foil

*** 1. Difficulty of placement
** 2. Unnatural appearance
** 3. Placement may irritate pulp
*** 4. Requires good remaining supporting tooth structure

Composite restorative material

** 1. Unpredictable durability
** 2. May irritate pulp

Analysis/Decision The large carious lesion on the lateral incisor presented a situation in which the remaining tooth structure was so weakened that support for the condensation pressures of a gold foil was questionable. In addition, the size of the restoration made placement very difficult. In light of these two complications, the composite restorative material was chosen even though it did not offer the durability of the foil.

Glossary

annealing The heating of a direct gold filling to remove gaseous impurities from the surface.

bridging The creation of voids and pits in a restoration by improper stepping and condensation.

burnishing Work hardening the surface of the gold restoration.

condensation The compaction of direct gold.

desorbing Removal of adsorbed gases; with direct gold, by means of heating.

electromallet An electrically driven reciprocating hammer.

pneumatic condenser A reciprocating hammer driven by air pressure.

sinter A method of consolidating particles into a more dense agglomerate without melting; takes place during manufacture and during heating to drive off impurities. Shrinkage is proportional to the degree of sintering.

Discussion questions

1. How did the development of dental casting and amalgams lead to a decline in the use of gold foil?
2. What is the metallurgical phenomenon responsible for the densification of direct gold fillings?
3. Why is the direct gold technique so challenging?
4. What are the advantages and disadvantages of direct gold restorations?

Questions and answers

1. **What are the four different types of direct gold?**
   a. foil and platinized
   b. mat foil
   c. mat and Electraloy RV
   d. EZ Gold and Stopfgold
2. **List three areas where direct gold is indicated.** Areas may include small occlusal grooves, buccal and lingual pits, small proximal lesions of the anterior teeth, small proximal lesions in the premolars, gingival erosion, and small carious gingival lesions.
3. **What is used in the manufacture of gold foil to make it temporarily noncohesive?** Ammonia.
4. **What is sintering?** This is a method of consolidating particles into a more dense agglomerate without melting. It takes place during manufacture and during heating to drive off impurities. Shrinkage is proportional to the degree of sintering.
5. **What is the difference between mat gold and mat foil?** Mat foil is mat gold with a sheet of gold foil covering it.
6. **What is the difference between mat foil and Electraloy?** The electrolytically precipitated powder contains a small amount of calcium.
7. **What is the average particle size of powdered gold?** Particles average 80 μm.
8. **(a) How are the particles in powdered gold held together, and (b) what is the heating step that causes some sintering to stick particles together?**
   a. Powdered gold is held together using a Valital organic matrix (pure wax) which is burned off during the desorbing process (annealing).
   b. After burning the organic wax off of the pellet, the pellet is again passed through the alcohol flame and heated to a cherry red color. This takes approximately 2–3 seconds to obtain the proper sintering. This process places the gold into a pure state without impurities.

9. **What is the purpose of combining platinum with gold foil?** Platinum increases the hardness of the finished restoration.
10. **What negative effect does the combining of platinum have upon the working characteristics of the material?** It makes it more difficult to manipulate.
11. **Why is malleability so important in a direct gold restoration?** Malleability enables the restoration to be adapted to a cavity wall.
12. **How can the one-at-a-time desorbing of direct gold pellets be avoided?** A group of pellets may be heated on a nonmetallic tray over a suitable heat source.
13. **What type of alcohol should be used in desorbing individual gold pellets in an open flame?** Methyl alcohol (methanol) or ethyl alcohol (ethanol).
14. **What portion of the flame should be used in heating direct gold?** The tip of the inner blue cone of the flame.
15. **What ill effect occurs when direct gold is underheated? Overheated?** If underheated, the pellet will still have surface impurities. If overheated, the pellet will be hard to condense due to too much sintering.
16. **List three controlling factors of condensation.** Controlling factors include the force of the condensing blow, the character of the resistance of the supporting bone and the periodontal membrane, the size of the condensing point, and the proper amount of stepping.
17. **What does burnishing do to the surface of the restoration?** It smooths off the condenser point irregularities and hardens the surface.
18. **How does gold foil differ from powdered gold in the tooth preparation required?** Foil is used for sharp angles as opposed to rounded angles requiring powdered gold. Foil is also intended for small orifices, whereas powdered gold is used in large openings.
19. **Which type of direct gold is least likely to cause bridging?** Gold foil.

Recommended reading

Gilmore HW, Lund MR. Operative Dentistry. 2nd ed. St Louis: CV Mosby, 1973, 446.

Hollenback GM, Lyons NE, Shell JS. A study of some of the physical properties of cohesive gold. J Calif Dent Assoc 42:9–11, 1966.

Hollenback GM, Collard EW. An evaluation of the physical properties of cohesive gold. J South Calif Dent Assoc 29:280–293, 1961.

Richter WA, Cantwell KR. A study of cohesive gold. J Prosthet Dent 15(4):726, 1965.

Rule RW. Gold foil and platinum centered gold foil; methods of condensation. J Am Dent Assoc 24:1783–1992, 1937.

Schnepper HE. Loma Linda Gold Foil Seminar (brochure). Redlands, CA: Western Printers, 1976.

Schnepper HE. Study of methods of measuring marginal penetration of dental restorations with emphasis on the use of radioactive phosphorus. Master's thesis. Seattle: University of Washington, 1954.

Skinner EW, Phillips RW. The Science of Dental Materials. 8th ed. Philadelphia: WB Saunders, 1982.

Souder WH, Paffenbarger GC. Physical Properties of Dental Materials. National Bureau of Standards circular C433. Washington, DC: US Government Printing Office, 1942; 35.

Thomas JJ. The pulpal effect of gold foil condensation procedure. Master's thesis. Indianapolis: Indiana University, 1966.

Thomas JJ, Stanley HR, Gilmore HW. Effects of gold foil condensation on human pulp. J Am Dent Assoc 78:788, 1969.

Waerhaug J. Histologic considerations which govern where the margins of restorations should be located in relation to gingiva. Dent Clin North Am March 1962; 1619.

Williams RV Jr. As the manufacturer views gold foil. J Am Gold Foil Operators 14:66, 1971.

Chapter 15

Precious Metal Casting Alloys

Since the introduction of investment casting to dentistry by Taggart in 1907, precious metal alloys have traditionally been used for several types of restorations. High-gold-content alloys have been used for inlays and still are because soft alloys that can be burnished are desirable. Full-cast crowns and three-quarter crowns are still cast from gold alloys. However, most crowns and fixed bridgework for the anterior part of the mouth are of the porcelain-fused-to-metal (PFM) type. Alloys for PFM crown-and-bridge work have revolutionized this field and include palladium and nickel alloys, as well as high-gold-content alloys. Another change has been the introduction of lower-gold-content alloys to replace the traditional 18-carat American Dental Association (ADA)–certified alloys developed during the 1930s. The tarnish resistance of these lower-gold-content alloys is sufficient for some oral environments but not others.

Composition and properties

Precious metal casting alloys contain mainly gold, palladium, and platinum (which are classified as noble metals), and silver. They also contain limited amounts of nonprecious alloying elements such as copper, indium, iron, tin, and zinc (Table 15-1). The carat scale expresses the relative amount of gold in an alloy, with 24-carat being pure gold. Twelve- and 18-carat alloys contain 50% and 75% gold, respectively. The fineness of a gold alloy is the percentage gold content multiplied by a factor of 10 (eg, 75% is 750 fine). Fineness is used with dental gold solders, but the carat scale is seldom used in dentistry. Copper, silver, palladium, and platinum generally serve as hardening elements in alloys with high gold content. Iron and tin, at much lower concentrations, are hardening additions in PFM alloys. Indium, iron, and tin also serve to promote bonding of porcelain to PFM alloys by formation of stable, adherent oxides.

High-gold alloys

Traditional dental casting alloys contain 70% by weight or more of gold, palladium, and platinum. American National Standards Institute/American Dental Association Specification no. 5 for Dental Casting Gold Alloy divides these alloys into four types based upon mechanical properties:

Type I—Soft (VHN* 60 to 90)
Type II—Medium (VHN 90 to 120)
Type III—Hard (VHN 120 to 150)
Type IV—Extra hard
(Quenched VHN minimum 150)
(Hardened VHN minimum 220)

See Table 15-2 for currently available alloys and their mechanical properties.

*Vickers hardness number. The Vickers hardness test, or the 136-degree diamond pyramid hardness test, is a micro-indentation method. The indenter produces a square indentation, the diagonals of which are measured. The diamond pyramid hardness is calculated by dividing the applied load by the surface area of the indentation.

Table 15-1 Role of alloying elements in dental gold alloys*

Property	Gold	Platinum	Palladium	Copper	Silver	Zinc	Iridium
Specific gravity	19.32	21.45	12.0	8.96	10.49	7.31	22.4
Melting point °C (°F)	1,063 (1,945)	1,769 (3,224)	1,552 (2,829)	1,083 (1,981)	961 (1,761)	420 (787) BP = 907 (1,663)	2.443 (4.429) BP = 4,200 (7,800)
Atomic diameter (Å)	2.88	2.77	2.74	2.55	2.88	2.66	3.32
Space lattice	Face-centered cubic	Face-centered cubic	Face-centered cubic	Face-centered cubic	Face-centered cubic	Close-packed hexagonal	Face-centered cubic
Chemical activity	Inert	Inert	Mild	Very active	Active	Very active	Active
Color	Yellow	White	White	Red	White	White	White
Approximate content	50%–95%	0%–20%	0%–12%	0%–17%	0%–20%	0%–2%	.005%–.1%
Density (specific gravity)	Increases markedly	Increases markedly	Lowers slightly	Lowers	Lowers	Lowers	Increases slightly
Effect of color on alloy	Lends yellow color	Whitens slowly; 12% required; not pure white	Whitens rapidly; as little as 5%	Lends red color; dark plate high in Cu	Whitens very slowly, counteracts redness of Cu; creates green gold	Percentages too low to have effect	White
Melting	Raises melting point mildly	Raises melting point fairly rapidly	Raises melting point rapidly	Lowers melting point even below its own	Slight effect; may raise or sometimes lower mildly	Lowers melting point rapidly; in most solders	No effect
Tarnish resistance	Essential to good tarnish resistance	Contributes importantly to tarnish resistance	Increases tarnish resistance but less than Au and Pt	Contributes to tarnish in flame or with sulfurous food	Tarnishes in presence of sulfur	Will tarnish, but in low percentage has little effect	Increased
Heat hardening	Contributes importantly with Cu	Increases with Cu	Some increase with Cu	Essential if alloy heat hardens	Increases with Cu	Slight with Cu	No effect
Gas absorption	—	—	Rather high for hydrogen	—	Rather high for oxygen	A good deoxidizer	No effect
Castability	—	—	(Effects not critical)	(Effects not critical)	—	Decreases surface tension and increases fluidity	No effect

*Adapted from Brumfield, 1955.

Table 15-2 Composition and properties of precious metal alloys

Type	Composition (%)				Representative products			Vickers hardness number		Yield strength psi (MPa)		Ductility (% elongation)
	Au	Pt	Pd	Ag	J. F. Jelenko & Co.	J.M. Ney Co.	Williams Dental Co., Inc.	As cast	Hardened	Quenched	Hardened	
I. Soft—one- and two-surface inlays	83.0	—	—	11.5	Special Inlay	ORO A	Harmony Soft	90	—	26,100 (180)		46.0
II. Medium—inlays, MOD, crowns	77.0	—	1.0	13.0	Modulay	ORO A 1	Harmony Medium	120	147	34,000 (234)	43,500 (300)	40.5
III. Hard—inlays, crowns, fixed bridgework	74.0	—	4.0	12.0	Firmilay	ORO B 2	Harmony Hard	130	157	38,000 (262)	48,000 (331)	39.4
	62.0	—	3.0	25.0	Rajah	ORO B 20	XL	142	235	39,400 (272)	79,900 (551)	29.0
IV. Extra-hard—thin crowns, fixed bridgework, partial dentures	68.5	3.0	3.5	10.5	no. 7	ORO 63	Harmony Extra Hard	181	280	56,400 (389)	101,900 (703)	17.0
	63.0	2.0	1.0	16.0	Jel-4	ORO 6	XLS	217	287	64,000 (441)	105,000 (724)	33.0
	40.0	—	4.0	47.0	Forticast	—	Minigold	125	216	47,200 (325)	75,600 (521)	27.5

Type I alloys are weak, soft, and highly ductile. They are useful only in areas not subject to occlusal stress and are not widely used. They do not harden by heat treatment. Type IV alloys are relatively strong, hard, and nonductile. They are intended for high-stress applications such as partial dentures. They also are not widely used at present.

The intermediate Type II and Type III alloys are used for most restorations. Type II alloys are used for inlays in which burnishability of margins is more important than high strength. Type III alloys are used in higher-stress applications for inlays, onlays, and three-quarter crowns, and for bridge retainers and pontics where the restoration design makes burnishability less important than strength.

Typical composition ranges for high-gold alloys are shown in Table 15-2. Iridium in small amounts, around 0.1%, is added as a grain refiner by several manufacturers. Type III and Type IV alloys may contain a high percentage each of palladium and platinum as hardening elements, as shown in the table, while retaining a light gold color. Type III and Type IV alloys are susceptible to heat treatment and may be hardened or softened by appropriate heating cycles (see Table 15-2 for hardness values).

Alloys containing more than 6% palladium are normally white (silver colored). Typical composition ranges of these alloys are given in Table 15-2 also. They are hard, strong, and heat treatable and have mechanical properties characteristic of Type III and Type IV alloys.

Low-gold alloys

Low-gold alloys are composed mainly of gold, silver, and copper, with a small percentage of palladium. Gold content ranges from 45% to 60%. The main incentive for the use of these alloys is financial; when the price of gold increases, the use of low-gold alloys increases relative to that of high-gold alloys.

Few alloys are marketed with gold contents between 55% and 70% because the cost savings are not high enough. Few alloys contain less than 45% gold because of tarnish and corrosion problems with use. There is some tendency for alloys in this group to contain additional palladium to partially make up for low gold content (see Table 15-2).

The mechanical properties of the low-gold alloys generally correspond to the properties of ADA Type III alloys. Thus, the alloys are strong and hard and have only moderate ductility.

Low-gold alloys are rarely used for inlays but can be quite suitable for full-cast crowns.

Palladium-silver alloys

Alloys that have palladium as their main ingredient have several applications. Palladium-silver alloys provide mechanical properties similar to those of Type III gold alloys. An increase in silver content leads to increased ductility and lowered hardness but increases corrosion problems. These alloys are more commonly used for crowns than for inlays. Unless other alloying elements are added, these materials are not heat treatable, because they form only a continuous solid solution at all compositions (Fig 15-1).

High-palladium alloys contain only a small percentage of other precious metals as alloying elements. They have been used as PFM alloys. Such PFM alloys have caused problems with porcelain discoloration owing to the formation of silver oxide and volatilization of the silver.

Porcelain-fused-to-metal alloys

Alloys intended for use as bases for porcelain have special requirements because of the need to develop and maintain strength at the temperature involved in porcelain applications and to provide a firm bond to the applied porcelain. In addition, the designs of many PFM restorations emphasize the need to be able to cast thin sections and the need for high yield strength. Three groups of precious alloys are used for PFM application (see Table 15-2):

1. Type I—Alloys containing over 90% gold, platinum, and palladium with small amounts of iron, indium, and tin as hardening and bonding agents
2. Type II—Alloys containing approximately 80% gold, platinum, and palladium, with trace additions of iron, indium, tin, and silver making up the balance
3. Type III—Palladium-silver alloys

Porcelain-fused-to-metal alloys are the most widely used alloys in commercial laboratories. They constitute approximately 70% of all cast units cur-

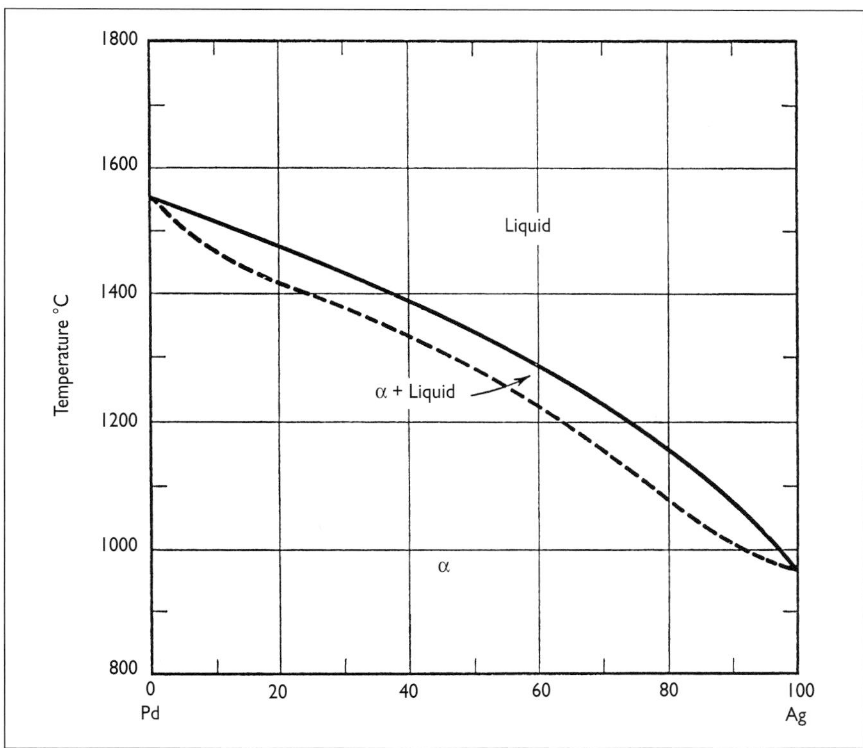

Fig 15-1 Palladium-silver phase diagram about 800°C. In the solid state, a solid solution, α, is formed at all compositions.

rently in use. Precious PFM alloys are now in direct competition with nonprecious PFM alloys.

Properties of importance for PFM alloys include the ability to produce good casting precision in their cross sections, high yield strength, controlled thermal expansion, and suitable surface characteristics for bonding to dental porcelain. Burnishability is a secondary consideration.

Normally, bonding involves the use of a precious metal alloy containing small quantities of iron, indium, and tin. Controlled oxidation of the castings during a "degassing heat treatment" produces an oxide coating on the alloy surface to which the porcelain adheres.

The properties of PFM alloys are improved by heat treatment. A precipitation reaction during the porcelain firing procedure strengthens and hardens the alloys. Iron-platinum and gold-tin phases are common precipitates.

The high-precious-metal alloys are still widely used. Nickel-chromium and other base metal alloys also used for PFM applications are, in general, less desirable because of problems with casting accuracy, fit, finishing, and porcelain bonding.

Heat treatment

Except for Type I and Type II high-gold alloys, precious metal casting alloys respond to heat treatment by changes in properties and microstructure.

Softening (homogenizing) heat treatment consists of heating the alloy to a temperature approximately 75°C below the solidus temperature, holding at that temperature for 10 to 30 minutes, and then quenching to room temperature. Hardening can be produced by one of two methods: slow cooling or a constant-temperature heat treatment. In either case, the important factor is the time spent in a critical temperature range between the softening range and room temperature. This critical temperature varies among alloys; it generally lies about halfway between room temperature and the alloy's softening temperature. Typical cycles for a Type III high-gold alloy are as follows: the softening treatment consists of holding the alloy at 700° to 750°C for 10 minutes, followed by quenching to room temperature. The hardening treatment consists of 10 minutes at 350° to 400°C, followed by quenching or low cooling to room temperature.

High-fusing alloys may require more time as well as higher temperatures for both softening and hardening heat treatments.

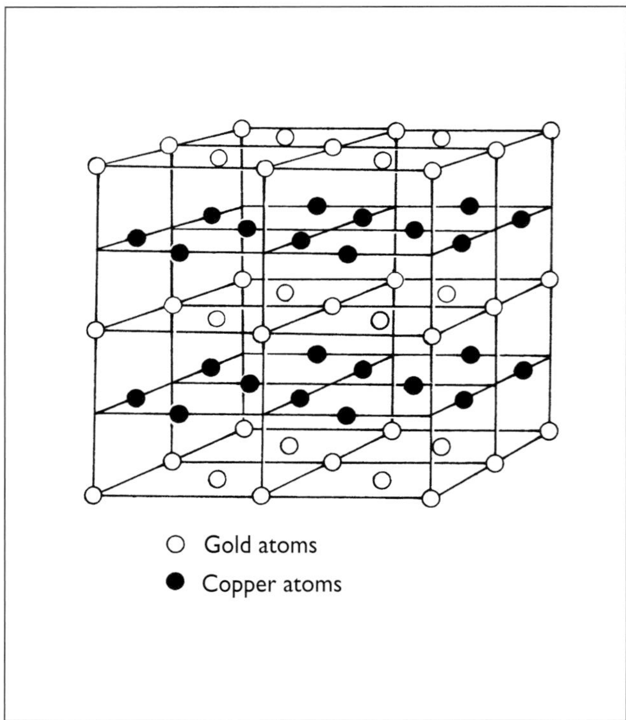

Fig 15-2 The lattice arrangement in an ordered gold-copper alloy with a regular alternation of unlike atoms in layers.

Basic crystal structure

All precious metal casting alloys are based on metallic elements having face-centered cubic crystal structures. With the appropriate homogenizing heat treatment, most of them can be converted to a single phase. Hardening heat treatment results in precipitation of phases with other crystal structures, and hardening alloys may contain several different phases. In many alloys, ordering can occur. This is a rearrangement of atoms within the unit cells of the crystal structure. It can cause a characteristic microstructure to appear. This mechanism is important in the hardening of binary gold-copper alloys but is of only secondary importance in dental alloys (Figs 15-2 and 15-3).

Cast microstructure

Both the cooling and nucleation rates are quite high for most dental castings. Thus, the typical cast structure consists of fine uniform grains. Large-grain structures are found more often with PFM white alloys unless a grain refiner (eg, iridium) is used (Figs 15-4 and 15-5).

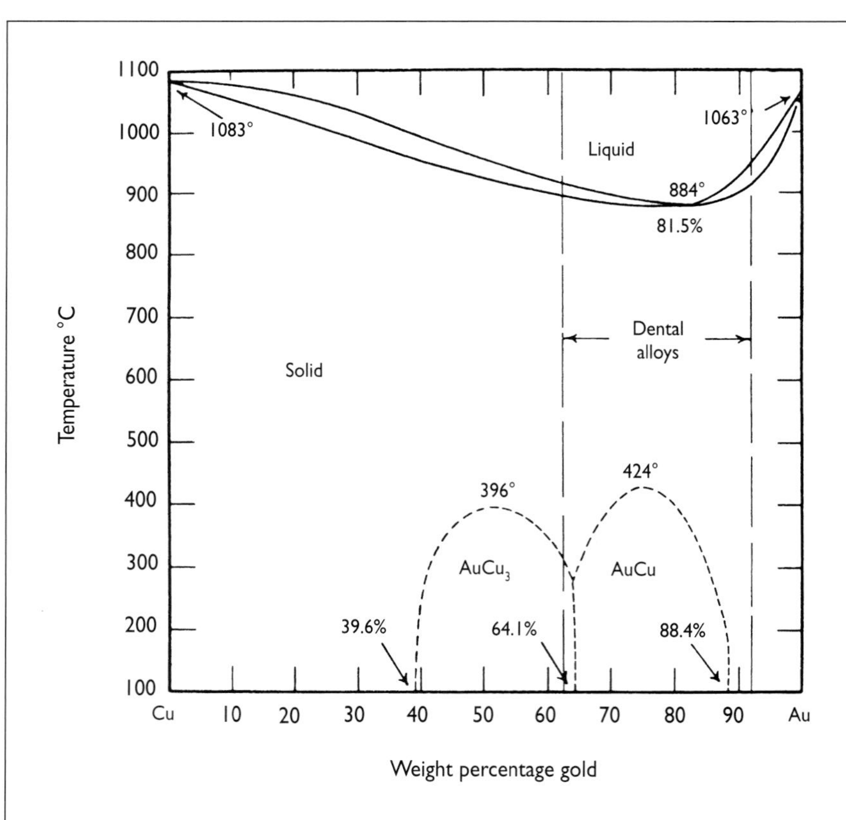

Fig 15-3 The gold-copper phase diagram. The ordered phases $AuCu_3$ and AuCu may be formed by heat treatment. The formation of these phases results in hardening. Quenching from 700°C avoids their formation and hardening.

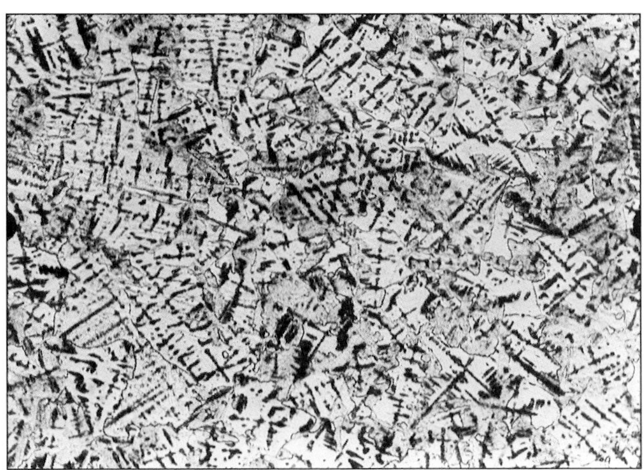

Fig 15-4 Dendritic (skeleton- or needle-shaped) grain structure of precious metal alloy as cast. (Original magnification × 100.)

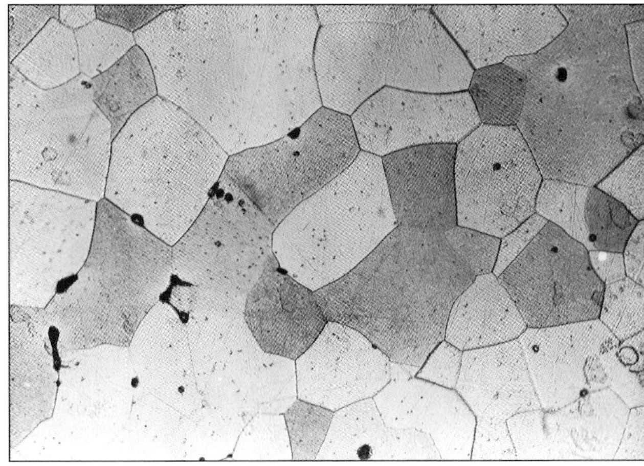

Fig 15-5 Normal grain structure of cast gold alloy after softening heat treatment. (Original magnification × 300.)

Normally, single-phase structures are found in alloys that have received a thorough softening (homogenizing) heat treatment. Hardening produces the appearance of a discontinuous grain boundary precipitate. However, this structure is unrelated to hardening. A submicroscopic continuous precipitate occurring throughout the grains is the primary cause of hardening. This is the result of the separation of silver-rich and copper-rich gold alloy phases. Alloys that undergo ordering during hardening exhibit changes in microstructure.

Glossary

carat A measure of the gold content of an alloy, with 24 carat being 100% gold.

corrosion Attack on a metal surface involving loss of material (eg, rusting of iron).

fineness The percentage of gold content in an alloy multiplied by a factor of 10 (eg, 75% gold is 750 fine).

grain A single crystal of metal as seen in the microstructure.

homogenizing heat treatment A process of heating an alloy to produce a more uniform distribution of elements by diffusion, usually resulting in softening of the alloy.

noble metal A metal that is resistant to oxidation; includes gold, platinum, palladium, and the other platinum group metals.

ordering The regular arrangement of atoms of an element in a lattice structure rather than a random distribution.

precious metal A metal that is relatively high in cost; includes gold, platinum, palladium, and silver.

precipitation The separation of a phase from a solution upon cooling, owing to reduced solubility.

tarnish The formation of objectionable reaction products on the surface of an alloy (eg, black oxides or sulfides on silver).

white gold alloy An alloy containing gold and white metals (eg, silver, palladium) that impart a white appearance to the entire mass.

Discussion questions

1. What is the relationship between carat and platinum metal content and the tarnish of gold restorations?
2. How have the ten-fold increase in the price of gold and the patients' desire for esthetic restorations affected the use of precious metal restorations?
3. What major effect do Ir and Ru have on the microstructure of gold alloys?
4. How would the temperature of quenching a gold casting mold affect its mechanical properties?

Questions and answers

1. **List the elements classified as noble.** Gold and the platinum group metals (platinum, palladium, iridium, rhodium, ruthenium, and osmium).
2. **Which elements contribute to the hardening of dental gold alloys?** Gold, copper, and silver. The platinum metals also contribute some hardening.
3. **Give the main applications of the ADA Type I, II, III, and IV alloys.** Type I alloys are used for one-surface restorations that will be subjected to slight stress; Type II is for two- and three-surface inlays; Type III is for crowns and fixed bridgework; and Type IV is for partial dentures.
4. **Which three elements are added in fractional amounts to harden high-gold-content alloys to be used with porcelain?** Iron, tin, and indium.
5. **What effect does palladium content have on the color of gold alloys?** Palladium has a strong whitening effect on the color of gold alloys.
6. **Describe a softening heat treatment for the ADA Type III and IV alloys.** Heat for 10 minutes at 700°C followed by water quenching for softening.
7. **Describe a hardening heat treatment for the ADA Type III and IV alloys.** Heat for 10 minutes at 350°C followed by water quenching or rapid cooling in air. Cooling a casting in a mold to room temperature (bench cooling) will produce hardening, because the alloy remains in the 350° to 400°C temperature range long enough.
8. **Which element is used as a grain refiner in gold casting alloys? Why is it added?** Iridium. Smaller grains result in a stronger, more ductile and homogeneous casting.
9. **Describe the purpose of the heat treatment given to alloys prior to porcelain application.** The gold alloys containing iron, indium, and tin are heated from about 700°C (1,300°F) to 950°C (1,800°F) in air, and then air cooled. The purpose is to burn off organic contamination and produce an adherent oxide for bonding.
10. **Which five elements are usually present in the white gold alloys used with porcelain (PFM)?** Palladium, silver, gold, tin, and indium.
11. **What is ordering in the gold-copper system?** Ordering is a crystal structure organization in which the atoms of an element (eg, copper) are regularly arranged in a repeating pattern as opposed to a random distribution (ie, disordered).
12. **What process is currently believed to be responsible for the hardening of gold-copper-silver alloys by heat treatment?** The present theory holds that hardening in gold-copper-silver alloys involves a separation of silver-rich and copper-rich gold phases within the grain structure. Ordering of a gold-copper phase also occurs, but is not as important in these ternary alloys. Silver, therefore, is a hardener when used in proper amounts along with copper.

13. **What is the main risk involved in using low-gold-content (less than 45%) crown-and-bridge alloys?** The frequency of tarnish increases as the noble metal content decreases. Laboratory tests indicate that below about 50% palladium or gold, tarnish is very likely.

14. **Which mechanical property is usually considered a measure of the burnishability of a soft inlay alloy?** The ductility or percentage elongation measures the degree to which the alloy can be burnished (spread). Other properties involved are hardness and yield strength, which indicate a resistance to burnishing.

15. **What has been the main problem with high-silver-content alloys for use with porcelain?** Silver produces a green discoloration of the porcelain.

Recommended reading

Brumfield RC. Role of Allowing Elements in Dental Gold Alloys. New York: JF Jelenko & Co, 1955.

Burse AB, et al. Comparison of the in vitro and in vivo tarnish of three gold alloys. J Biomed Mater Res 6:267–277, 1972.

Civjan S, Hugel EF, Marsden JE. Characteristics of two gold alloys used in fabrication of porcelain fused to metal restorations. J Am Dent Assoc 85:1309–1315, 1972.

Civjan S, et al. Further studies on gold alloys used in fabrication of porcelain fused to metal restorations. J Am Dent Assoc 90:659–665, 1975.

Coleman RL. Physical properties of dental materials (gold alloys and accessory materials). US Bur Stand J Res 1(6):867–938, 1928.

Fuys RA, Fairhurst CW, O'Brien WJ. Precipitation hardening in gold-platinum alloys containing small quantities of iron. J Biomed Mater Res 7:471–480, 1973.

Kurnakow NS, Ageew NW. Physicochemical study of the gold-copper solid solutions. Inst Metals J 46:481–501, 1931.

Kurnakow N, Zemezuzny S, Zasadetelev M. The transformation in alloys of gold with copper. Inst Metals J 15:305, 1916.

Leinfelder KF, et al. Hardening of high-fusing gold alloys. J Dent Res 45:393, 1966.

Leinfelder KF, O'Brien WJ, Taylor DF. Hardening of dental gold-copper alloys. J Dent Res 51:900–905, 1972.

Naylor WP. Introduction to Metal Ceramic Technology. Chicago: Quintessence, 1992.

O'Brien WJ, Kring JE, Ryge G. Heat treatment of alloys to be used for the fused porcelain technique. J Prosthet Dent 14:955–960, 1964.

Schoonover IC, Sauder W. Corrosion of dental alloys. J Am Dent Assoc 28:1278, 1941.

Shell JS. Some factors influencing specific gravity determinations of gold cast alloys. J Dent Res 45:337, 1966.

Sims JR, Blumenthal RN, O'Brien WJ. An electrical resistance study of the precipitation reaction in an Au-Pt-Fe alloy. J Biomed Mater Res 7:497–507, 1973.

Smith DL, et al. Iron-platinum hardening in casting golds for use with porcelain. J Dent Res 49:283, 1970.

Swartz ML, Phillips RW, El Tannir MD. Tarnish of certain dental alloys. J Dent Res 37:837, 1958.

Taggart WH. A new and accurate method of making gold inlays. Dent Cosmos 49:1117, 1907.

Valega TM (ed). Alternatives to Gold Alloys in Dentistry. DHEW Pub no. (NIH) 77:1227, Sept 1977.

Wise EM. Cast gold dental alloys. In ASM Metals Handbook. Cleveland: American Society for Metals, 1948; 1120.

Wise EM, Crowell WS, Eash JT. The role of the platinum metals in dental alloys. Tr AIME Inst Metals Div 99:363, 1932.

Wise EM, Eash JT. The role of the platinum metals in dental alloys. III. The influence of platinum and palladium and heat treatment upon the microstructure and constitution of basic alloys. Tr AIME Inst Metals Div 104:276, 1933.

Chapter 16

Alloys for Porcelain-Fused-to-Metal Restorations

In response to the fluctuating prices of gold and other precious metals, many alternative alloys have been introduced into the dental profession. Although the development of these alternative alloy systems was largely motivated by economics, the resultant properties of the alternatives often make them superior choices even when compared with more costly alternatives. Selection of the optimal alloy to use for crowns and fixed partial dentures should be based on a rational appraisal of the properties relevant to the intended use of the alloy. A classification of current alloy systems is given in Fig 16-1, and commercial alloys are listed in Table 16-1.

The proliferation of alloy systems has complicated the dentist's choice of products for specific restorative situations. As a result, many practitioners rely solely on the advice of dental laboratories for their selections. Many laboratories base their choices on cost factors rather than on a material's properties. Additionally, many less significant criteria for alloy selection are used by dentists, for example: alloy color, gold cement, "precious only," high cost, or "looks, feels, or is cast like gold."

Rational selection of a casting alloy for porcelain-fused-to-metal (PFM) restorations should be based on the following:

1. Physical properties
2. Chemical properties
3. Biocompatibility
4. Laboratory workability
5. Porcelain compatibility

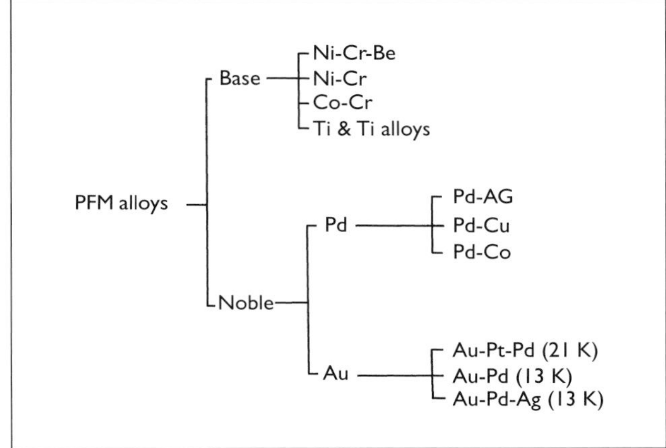

Fig 16-1 A classification of alloys for PFM restorations.

Lastly, in a balanced decision, cost should be considered relative to these criteria. Factors such as single-unit or multiple-unit, presence or absence of metal occlusal surfaces, span length, and porcelain brand often indicate different alloy choices. A practitioner using only one alloy is very unlikely to make an optimal choice in every clinical situation.

Classifications

Before discussing alloy characteristics, it is worth reviewing the terms noble, precious, semiprecious, and nonprecious. *Noble metals* are defined on the basis of their chemical properties; that is, they resist oxida-

Table 16-1 Examples of commercial PFM alloys

Alloys	Representative products	Manufacturer
High gold	Jelenko O	J.F. Jelenko & Co.
	Rx G, Rx Biostar, Rx Y-Ceramic	Jeneric/Pentron Inc.
	Will-Ceram Y	Ivoclar Dental
Gold-palladium (no silver)	Olympia	J.F. Jelenko & Co.
	SFC	Jeneric/Pentron Inc.
	Eclipse	J.M. Ney & Co.
Gold-palladium-silver	Cameo	J.F. Jelenko & Co.
	Rx WCG	Jeneric/Pentron Inc.
	Ceramco-White	Degussa Dental, Inc.
Palladium-copper	Option	J.M. Ney Co.
	Naturelle; Correct-Fit II	Jeneric/Pentron Inc.
	Athenium	Ivoclar Dental
Palladium-silver	Rx 91, Palladent B, Aspen, LTA	Jeneric/Pentron Inc.
	Will-Ceram W1, Protocol	Ivoclar Dental
	Jelstar, Legacy, Legacy XT	J.F. Jelenko & Co.
Nickel-chromium	Neptune	Jeneric/Pentron Inc.
	Lifecast	Ivoclar Dental
	Microbond NP2	Austenal Dental Inc.
Nickel-chromium-beryllium	Rexillium III	Jeneric/Pentron Inc.
	Lifecast B	Ivoclar Dental
	Verabond	Aalba-Dent, Inc.
Cobalt-chromium	Novarex	Jeneric/Pentron Inc.
	Mastercast	Ivoclar Dental
Titanium and Ti-alloys	R1, R4, and R2	Jeneric/Pentron Inc.

tion and are not attacked by acids. Seven metals meet this definition, but only three are widely used in dental alloys: gold, palladium, and platinum. These metals give noble metal alloys their inert properties in the mouth.

The term *precious* refers only to cost, which is controlled by supply and demand. Many elements in the periodic table, including the seven noble metals, are precious by today's standards. In dental advertisements the term *precious* usually refers to silver, a metal that is precious but not noble; silver is usually a major ingredient in most alloys advertised as "precious."

The term *semiprecious* was originally coined for noble metal alloys that contained significant amounts of silver, and it subsequently has been applied to a variety of alloys, some of which are mixtures of precious and nonprecious ingredients. It is advisable to drop the term *semiprecious* from the dental vocabulary, as it is not well defined and leads to much confusion.

Nonprecious alloys are composed of nonprecious ingredients, except for the common inclusion of 1% to 3% beryllium, a precious but ignoble metal. Most nonprecious alloys are based on a combination of nickel and chromium, although cobalt-chromium and iron-based alloys also exist. See Table 16-2 for the compositions of alloys commonly used in PFM restorations.

When an alloy is chosen for a particular clinical situation, a number of characteristics have clinical significance and should be considered. Among the most important of these characteristics are physical and chemical properties, casting accuracy, and porcelain-metal compatibility.

Table 16-2 Composition of alloys for PFM restorations*

Alloys	Percentage							
	Au	Pt	Pd	Ag	Sn	In	Ga	Other metals
High gold	74–88	0–20	0–16	0–15	0–3	0–4	—	Zn <2; Fe <0.5; Ta <1
Gold-palladium (no silver)	45–53	0–1	36–45	—	0–5	2–10	0–3	Zn <4
Gold-palladium-silver	42–55	—	25–32	6–16	0–4	0–3	—	Zn 0–3
Palladium-copper	0–2	0–1	66–81	—	0–8	0–8	3–9	Cu 4–20; Zn 0-4
Palladium-silver	0–6	0–1	50–65	1–40	0–9	0–8	0–6	Zn 0–4; Mn 0-4
Nickel-chromium								Ni 64–68; Cr 10-22
Nickel-chromium-beryllium								Ni 70–80; Cr 12-15; Be 0.6–2
Cobalt-chromium								Co 54–65; Cr 24-32
Titanium								C.P. Grades 2 and 4
Titanium alloys								Ti-6Al–4V; Ti-Nb–Al

*Courtesy of A. Prasad.

Physical and chemical properties

Color is one of the most obvious physical properties of an alloy. Although the color has no biologic significance, it is equated with quality in the minds of many dentists. Sometimes this color factor seems to matter more to the dentist than to the patient.

When the gold content of an alloy is decreased and less costly metals such as silver and palladium are substituted, yellow color is lost. These less yellow dental alloys are not yet widely accepted. In fact, the profession's desire for gold color is so strong that gold-colored semiprecious and nonprecious alloys are commercially available, even though their other physical and chemical properties fall far short of those of even the cheapest white alloys. In some Third World countries, yellow alloys of copper and nickel are currently quite popular.

If an alloy is gold colored, it must contain copper, gold, or both. However, an alloy can contain substantial amounts of gold or copper without appearing yellow. Good examples of this apparent contradiction are jewelers' white gold and some popular gold alloys for PFM restorations (such as Degudent U, Degussa Dental, Inc.; SMG-3, J.M. Ney Co.). The latter products contain more than 80% gold, yet no yellow color is seen because of the strong whitening effects of palladium and platinum.

Color can be a misleading indicator of composition; dentists should consider other physical and chemical properties as more important than color when a casting alloy is selected.

Some important physical and chemical properties to consider when choosing a cast alloy are:

1. *Noble metal content*: the weight (or better, the atomic) percentage of the seven noble metals contained in an alloy
2. *Hardness*: the Vickers hardness number (VHN), a measure of resistance to indentation
3. *Yield strength*: a measure of the stress required to cause permanent deformation under tension
4. *Elongation*: the amount of permanent deformation a metal undergoes when loaded to its fracture point
5. *Fusion temperature*: the approximate temperature at which an alloy separates under its own weight from partial melting

All of these characteristics have clinical significance. The noble metal content determines, to a large extent, the corrosion resistance and inert properties of the alloy. Hardness is important in relation to occlusal wear resistance and finishing and affects polishing properties. Yield strength is necessary in determining load-bearing ability, especially in fixed partial dentures.

Elongation relates to margin-finishing properties, especially important in partial veneer crowns and abutments. It is important to remember that the elongation value for an alloy may be clinically irrelevant if the yield strength is high. To use the potential elongation, stresses exceeding the yield strength must be applied to move the metal. Within each group of alloys, yield strength generally increases with increasing hardness. Fusion temperature is important in relation to solder melting ranges and correlates with sag resistance.

Porcelain-metal compatibility

Thermal expansion, bond strength, and composition are also important properties to consider when choosing among alloys for PFM restorations. These characteristics determine porcelain-metal compatibility.

Thermal expansion is important because a state of zero residual stress is desirable for porcelain in the final restoration. Such a state is achieved when the total expansions and contractions of the porcelain and metal are matched between the porcelain firing temperature and room temperature.

Porcelain-to-metal bond strength ensures retention of porcelain both in the oral environment and during thermal processing, when the induced thermal stresses can be quite high.

Composition is a key factor in porcelain-metal compatibility because some components of an alloy can affect the color of the porcelain, perhaps compromising the esthetics of a restoration. Among the alternative alloys, those containing silver are often associated with porcelain color changes and can cause "greening" of some brands of porcelain. The mechanism for this porcelain discoloration is an exchange between silver from the alloy and sodium from the porcelain. The exchange process requires an oxidizing atmosphere, but a subsequent reducing atmosphere is required to produce the colloidal precipitate responsible for color changes in the porcelain.

Other properties

Because the cross-sectional area of metal used in PFM restorations is usually smaller than that of all-metal restorations, physical properties such as yield strength of the alloy are crucial in design. Stress in turn controls the minimum allowable dimensions of critical areas like connectors. The elastic modulus is equally important because it determines the flexibility of the metal framework. Flexibility is inversely proportional to elastic modulus; an alloy with a high elastic modulus will flex less under load than an alloy of low elastic modulus.

Chemical properties are important because they affect tarnish resistance, corrosion resistance, and thermal stability. Thermal properties are critical in alloys for PFM restorations because the alloy must have a sufficiently elevated melting temperature range to provide dimensional stability during the porcelain firing cycle. Thermal creep results in distortions such as sag in fixed partial denture frameworks and margin opening during the porcelain firing cycles.

Casting accuracy must, of course, be sufficient to provide clinically acceptable castings. In addition to dimensional accuracy (a strong function of technique), the mold-filling ability also contributes to casting accuracy.

Biocompatibility includes a number of factors, among them cytotoxicity and tissue irritation. Potential biologic hazards from the base metal alloys, particularly nickel and beryllium, are controversial. These potential hazards may affect not only the patient but also the dentist or technician who makes the restoration. The lack of data and long-term clinical experience suggests caution in using base metal alloys, particularly for people with known sensitivity to base metals. To date, however, neither experimental data nor clinical experience unequivocally contraindicate the use of alloys containing these potentially toxic elements, even in patients known to be sensitive to them.

The following discussion of each alloy group is intended to be general and not necessarily specific to the proprietary products. The product examples were chosen based on their status as the historical forerunners of each alloy group. Table 16-3 lists properties of alloys used in dentistry and current costs for crowns and copings.

High-gold alloys

Porcelain-fused-to-metal technology was introduced to the dental profession with the introduction of Ceramco No. 1 alloy in 1958. The alloy was a forerunner of the improved high-gold alloys that remain on the market today, such as Jelenko O (J.F. Jelenko & Co.).

The high-gold alloys are composed principally of gold and platinum group metals with minor additions

Table 16-3 Typical properties of alloys for PFM restorations

Group	Vickers hardness number	Elastic modulus psi × 10^6 (GPa)	Yield strength psi (MPa)	Specific gravity
High-gold	182	13 (90)	65,000 (448)	18.3
Gold-palladium (no silver)	220	18 (124)	83,000 (572)	13.5
Gold-palladium-silver	218	16 (110)	63,600 (439)	13.8
Palladium-copper	425	14 (96)	166,000 (1,145)	10.6
Palladium-silver	242	20 (138)	77,000 (531)	11.1
Nickel-chromium	257	29 (207)	58,000 (400)	8.7
Nickel-chromium-beryllium	357	31 (213)	116,000 (800)	7.8

of tin, indium, and iron. Gold content in these alloys varies from 78% to 87% by weight, and total noble metal content is about 97%. Small amounts of tin, indium, and iron are added for strength and to promote a good porcelain bond to metal oxide. Because of their high nobility, these alloys tend to be costly, both in terms of their cost per ounce and their high density, resulting in heavy castings.

High-gold alloys are usually light yellow in color, although some are white. Some are very yellow, apparently in response to the gold mystique previously discussed. The properties of the very yellow alloys are usually inferior to other products in the group, and their low tensile strength in particular makes them a questionable choice for fixed partial dentures.

The hardness of alloys in this group is considered ideal for working characteristics and ease of finishing, and the tensile strength for all but the very yellow products is good. Corrosion resistance is excellent because of high nobility. Porcelain discoloration is not a problem because the alloys contain little or no silver.

Besides cost, the principle disadvantages of the high-gold alloys are low elastic modulus and poor sag resistance during the porcelain firing cycle. These factors are also troublesome for fixed partial dentures and suggest the use of alternative alloys for these situations.

Gold-palladium-silver alloys

Gold-palladium-silver alloys were the first alternative systems, introduced in 1970 as Will-Ceram W (Williams Dental Co., Inc.), and they remain on today's market. The addition of substantial amounts of silver (10% to 15%) and a relatively high palladium content (20% to 30%) reduces the cost of these alloys as compared with the higher-gold-content group. Elastic modulus is higher, and the alloys are less susceptible than the high-gold group to dimensional changes during the porcelain baking cycle. Corrosion resistance and clinical working characteristics are generally good.

The principle disadvantage of these alloys is their tendency to induce color changes in porcelain because of their silver content. Silver transport into the porcelain results in a yellow-green color change, depending on the brand of porcelain.

The gold-palladium-silver group has been largely superseded by silver-free gold-palladium alloys, which eliminate problems with porcelain color change. Although gold-palladium-silver alloys are successfully used by many practitioners and have had excellent commercial success, they are used less since the introduction of the cost-competitive silver-free alloys.

Palladium-silver alloys

The first palladium-silver alloy was introduced to the dental profession in the 1970s, but the one that has remained on the market the longest is Will-Ceram W-1 (Williams Dental Co., Inc.), introduced in 1975, and at one time the largest-selling alloy in the United States.

Palladium-silver alloys usually include 50% to 60% palladium, with most of the balance being silver. The physical and chemical properties are favorable for PFM restorations and are comparable to other noble metal alloys. The 50% to 60% nobility assures a satisfactory degree of tarnish and corrosion resistance and good clinical working characteristics.

The elastic modulus for this group is the most favorable of all the precious metal alloys and results in the least flexible castings. Only nonprecious alloys have superior elastic moduli. Palladium-silver alloys solder well and have the lowest sag tendency of the precious metal alloys. Porcelain bond strength is also excellent.

The principal disadvantage of this group is a porcelain color change to green—which occurs to a greater degree in this group than in alloys with lower silver content, such as the gold-palladium-silver alloys. Color problems vary considerably, depending on the brand of porcelain; with some brands this disadvantage is eliminated. Will-Ceram and Ivoclar (Ivoclar AG) porcelains are more resistant to silver discoloration than others.

Some manufacturers recommend the use of metal surface coupling agents to reduce porcelain color problems. Some of these coupling agents are modified porcelains and others are 24-carat gold. The colloidal gold agents are reasonably effective in reducing surface activity of silver in the alloy, thus preventing diffusion into the porcelain. However, if these gold coupling agents are used in excessive amounts, the gold interferes with surface oxidation necessary for a porcelain-metal bond. Selecting a brand of porcelain that does not change color is a more reliable solution to the problem than using coupling agents.

The palladium-silver group can be a good alternative to the gold-containing group, especially if cost is a major factor in alloy selection. If the porcelain is one that shows minimal (or no) color change in the presence of silver, it is difficult to find fault with these alloys. Mechanical properties are often superior to even the most costly noble metal alloys.

Gold-palladium alloys

The gold-palladium silver-free alloys were developed in the mid-1970s to alleviate the color problems caused by silver. The first silver-free alloy was introduced in 1975 as Olympia (J.F. Jelenko & Co.). These alloys generally contain about 50% gold and 40% palladium. They have had considerable commercial success. Yield strength and hardness are favorable, and elastic modulus is increased significantly compared with high-gold alloys. Cost is comparable to that of the gold-palladium-silver group.

The only recognized disadvantage of the gold-palladium group is thermal expansion incompatibility with some of the higher-expansion porcelains. The silver-free alloys tend to have lower expansion values than the silver-containing group. Some incompatible combinations are well known and are readily acknowledged by the respective manufacturers.

In the absence of thermal expansion incompatibility, there are no disadvantages and several recognizable advantages to using alloys from this group in preference to the high-gold and gold-palladium-silver alloys. Cost per casting (see Table 16-3), is about 40% less than for high-gold alloys. Rigidity is improved for partial dentures, and the porcelain-metal bonds are adequate. Corrosion resistance is excellent because of high nobility. Sag tendencies are about the same as for gold-palladium-silver alloys and, again, much better than for high-gold alloys. Gold-palladium alloys can be an excellent choice when their relatively high cost is not a major consideration.

Recently, small amounts of silver have been added to otherwise silver-free compositions. The resulting alloys are probably superior to the silver-free compositions. Because the silver content is low (usually less than 5%, compared with 10% to 15% in the gold-palladium-silver group previously discussed), no porcelain color problems are evident. However, marketing appeal may be lacking because of the impression created by advertising "silver-free, trouble-free" alloys. Like all new alloys, the best way to test the efficacy of these products is through clinical experience. The new alloys seem promising because thermal expansion is increased and castability is better than with the silver-free alloys. The increase in expansion tends to eliminate the incompatible porcelain-metal combinations previously mentioned.

Palladium-copper alloys

The palladium-copper alloys are a recent development, first introduced to the dental profession in 1982 as Option (J.M. Ney Co.).

Palladium-copper alloys are usually composed of 70% to 80% palladium and contain little or no gold, up to 15% by weight of copper, and around 9% of gallium. Copper was an unusual addition to porcelain-bonding alloys; such large amounts of copper would cause problems with bonding and porcelain color in gold-based alloys, but apparently do not cause these problems in alloys rich in palladium. Because the alloys have no silver, they cause none of the porcelain color problems associated with silver. Some palladium-copper alloys have a rather heavy oxide that is difficult to cover with opaque porcelain. High hardness values in some of the alloys are offset by a relatively low elastic modulus, resulting in better working characteristics than would be expected with a high hardness value. Strength is good, and in some alloys extremely high yield strengths are found.

Palladium-copper alloys generally do not melt or cast as easily as palladium-silver alloys, but they are quite acceptable in this regard. Presoldering has been associated with problems for some, but not all, of these alloys. Additionally, the sag resistance of most of them is not as high as in the palladium-silver alloys, again tending to contraindicate their use in large-span fixed partial dentures.

Clinical use of the relatively new palladium-copper alloys is expected to increase. This clinical experience will determine their overall usefulness in relation to the other groups of alloys. Initial experience is promising.

Palladium-cobalt alloys

Palladium-cobalt alloys, with around 88% palladium and 4% to 5% cobalt by weight, have been in limited use. The main advantages of these alloys is a higher coefficient of thermal expansion that is useful with certain porcelains. However, the main disadvantage is the formation of a dark oxide that may be difficult to mask at thin margins. Also, these alloys may be more susceptible to hot tearing and embrittlement from carbon, if no silver is present. Commercial palladium-cobalt alloys on the market are Jelenko PTM (J.F. Jelenko & Co.) and Jeneric/Pentron APF (Jeneric/Pentron Inc.).

Base metal alloys

Developed in the early 1970s, most of the base metal alloys are based on nickel and chromium, but a few cobalt-chromium and iron-based alloys are also available. Because they are not noble metals, their corrosion resistance depends on other chemical properties. A thin, invisible chromium oxide layer provides a complete and impervious film that passivates the surface of the alloy. The passive layer is so thin, it does not dull the surface finish. A similar passive oxide layer limits surface corrosion in ordinary stainless steel.

In addition to noticeable differences in chemical properties, the nonprecious alloys have different physical properties than the noble metal alloy groups. The most significant of these are high hardness, high yield strength, and high elastic modulus. Elongation is about the same as for gold alloys but is negated by the high yield strength, which makes it difficult or impossible to work the metal.

When used for metal occlusal restorations, the nonprecious alloys have only a few recognizable advantages. They are low in cost, and some have high hardness values, which can be important when wear resistance is needed. Some nickel-chromium alloys in this group, especially those containing beryllium, have mold-filling abilities that are superior to all other groups. This mold-filling ability permits easier casting of thin sections and produces sharp margins on castings.

However, base metal alloys have many disadvantages when used for metal occlusal restorations. Their hardness makes occlusal adjustments, polishing, crown removal, and endodontic opening very difficult. Laboratory labor costs are often higher for crowns made from nonprecious alloys because their hardness increases working time. Increased labor costs offset the slight savings in the cost of material. Although casting accuracy can be excellent, the high casting shrinkage (approximately 2.3%) must be accommodated. This usually requires modification of the casting techniques used for gold alloys, which have a lower casting shrinkage (1.4%). Soldering is unreliable in areas where stresses are involved, although soldering of contacts and minor repairs presents no problem. For the latter, white palladium-based solders work well.

Properties that are considered disadvantages for metal occlusal applications can be used to advantage in porcelain occlusal restorations. Examples include high tensile strength (up to 120,000 psi, or 830 MPa) and high elastic modulus (about 30 million psi, or 200,000 MPa). The high tensile strength permits use of thinner metal sections than would be possible if noble metal alloys were used (with the possible exception of some high-palladium alloys). Nickel-chromium alloys have the highest elastic moduli of all dental alloys, which decreases flexibility to a significant degree. The flexibility of a fixed partial denture framework constructed of nickel-chromium is less than half that of a framework of the same dimensions made from a high-gold alloy. Unlike the relatively thick metal crowns, PFM crowns can be easily removed by penetrating the porcelain with rotary diamond instruments, followed by separating the thin metal with proprietary carbide burs made for this purpose.

The addition of beryllium to some nickel-chromium alloys results in more favorable properties. Beryllium increases fluidity and improves casting performance. Beryllium also controls surface oxidation and results in more reliable, less technique-sensitive porcelain-metal bonds. Generally, these bonds are satisfactory when the alloy contains beryllium but are often questionable when beryllium is lacking. Beryllium-containing alloys require strict control of grinding dust in dental laboratories according to the Occupational Safety and Health Administration (OSHA).

Nickel-chromium alloys show sag resistance that is uniformly superior to all noble metal alloys. This characteristic, along with increased stiffness and high tensile strength, indicates use of these alloys in fixed partial dentures. The problems with presoldering, often necessary for fixed partial dentures, can be easily overcome by using the cast-joining techniques described by Weiss and Munyon (1980).

Some nickel-chromium alloys have been chemically modified to overcome certain objectionable properties of this group as compared with noble metal alloys. Examples include products that are advertised to "feel like gold," "cast like gold," or "process like gold." In general, such modified alloys fall short in mechanical or physical properties, or in casting behavior, when compared with the better nickel-chromium-beryllium alloys in this group. The latter alloys are simply different from gold or other noble metal alloys, and their differences, when taken into account, can be used to advantage.

The allergenic and carcinogenic properties of the base metals, especially nickel, are controversial. Some investigators report no allergic response to nickel, even in known allergic patients, whereas others report a high frequency of allergic reactions in similar patients. A high incidence of respiratory cancer has been well documented in persons who have occupational exposure to nickel. Nickel is also known to induce tumors in rat muscle tissue, whereas other metals, such as manganese, chromium, copper, and aluminum, do not. Until the potential danger from dental alloys is better understood, care should be taken to avoid inhalation of base metal dust, and caution should be exercised when nickel alloy restorations are placed in patients known to be sensitive to nickel.

In summary, base metal alloys are a useful alternative for PFM restorations. Although the properties of alloys in this group are quite different from those of noble metal alloys, these differences can be used to advantage in many PFM situations. Disadvantages associated with metal occlusal restorations are largely overcome when these alloys are used for thin copings under porcelain. Until more long-term data are available, the practitioner should keep in mind the potential biologic hazards associated with base metals and should always follow recommended safety precautions when using these materials. Such precautions include strict control of grinding dust (with suction, masks, etc) and screening patients for allergy to nickel (eg, pierced ear posts and other jewelry).

Titanium alloys

Although titanium is not a noble or precious metal, it is often not classified with the base metals in dentistry due to its high biocompatibility. The main problem with the use of titanium for PFM restorations is difficult processing. Casting of titanium alloys is difficult due to a high casting temperature (2,000°C), rapid oxidation, and reactions with investments. Titanium melting is best done in specially designed furnaces with an argon atmosphere. Investments for use with titanium are described in Chapter 18. A titanium alloy, Ti–6 Al–4V, has been used for PFM restorations with special low expansion porcelains (CE of 9×10^{-6}/°C). Pure titanium is used and is formed by machining and spark erosion with a process developed by Nobelpharma AB for their Procera porcelain. Jeneric/Pentron markets a Ti–Al–V alloy (R/2) with an ultimate tensile strength (UTS) of 1,000 MPa (145,000 psi) and elongation of 9%. Jeneric's pure titanium (R/1) has a UTS of 1,000 MPa (75,000 psi) and elongation of 15%.

Criteria for selecting alloys

Rational selection of a specific alloy should be based on a balanced consideration of cost and the properties relevant to the intended use of the alloy. For single crowns, properties such as strength and sag resistance are less important than they are for fixed partial dentures. Castability, biocompatibility, tarnish and corrosion resistance, porcelain color, and hardness are usually equally important for both alloy uses. For fixed partial dentures, solder and joining behavior, sag resistance, strength, and elastic modulus become increasingly important as the span increases. Porcelain thermal expansion compatibility also increases in importance as the span width increases, because of the complexity of geometry and consequent stress fields due to porcelain and alloy mismatch.

When cost is not a major factor, the clinician has a wide spectrum of alloys from which to choose for PFM restorations. Selection of the best alloy for a particular case depends on a number of factors, including the brand of porcelain selected. Whereas it is difficult to rationalize use of high-gold alloys because of their disadvantages, gold-palladium alloys are considered ideal noble metal alloys by many clinicians and result in a 30% to 40% cost saving over the high-gold alloys. If the clinician were forced to use only one alloy for all PFM restorations, the gold-palladium alloys would probably be the most logical selection. Mechanical and physical properties are good, there are no biologic objections, and cost is moderate. Porcelain compatibility and castability are quite good with minor (less than 5%) silver additions to the gold-palladium alloys.

Gold-palladium-silver alloys are comparable in cost to gold-palladium alloys, but unfortunately they have porcelain color problems due to the substantial silver content (10% to 15%). The silver-free alloys and the very low-silver palladium-gold alloys appear to be better choices in most cases.

When cost is a major factor, the palladium-silver, palladium-copper, and nonprecious nickel-chromium-beryllium alloys are alternative candidates. Considering all factors, including labor, cost is not significantly different among these groups. The nickel-chromium-beryllium alloys are often the alloys of choice where large-span fixed partial dentures are involved, high castability is needed, or esthetic considerations are important. The question of biocompatibility with base metal alloys has yet to be resolved.

Palladium-silver alloys have excellent clinical working characteristics and—provided the porcelain is not one susceptible to discoloration in the presence of silver—have no real disadvantages compared with the more expensive gold alloys. Long-term clinical success is well known with palladium-silver.

The new palladium-copper alloys appear to have many of the advantages of palladium-silver alloys without the porcelain color problems. Limited experience indicates slightly more difficult melting and casting than with palladium-silver but generally good working characteristics and excellent strength. These palladium-copper alloys may replace the palladium-silver alloys as more clinical evidence is accumulated and soldering techniques are developed.

Fixed partial dentures

Rational alloy selections for fixed partial dentures are:

1. Nickel-chromium-beryllium
2. Palladium-silver
3. Gold-palladium, perhaps with minor silver additions

Often irrational selections are:

1. High gold, especially the very yellow ones, due to their high cost, poor sag resistance, and, for the very yellow examples, poor strength
2. Palladium-copper, due to soldering or joining problems
3. Gold-palladium-silver for the combination of cost and porcelain color problems
4. Nickel-chromium without beryllium—because the addition of beryllium greatly enhances its properties without increasing biologic concern to patients

Crowns

Rational selections for single crowns or short-span fixed partial dentures often are:

1. Palladium-copper
2. Palladium-silver
3. Nickel-chromium-beryllium
4. Gold-palladium, perhaps with minor silver addition

Often irrational selections are:

1. Gold-palladium-silver, due to the combination of cost and porcelain color problems
2. High gold, due to cost and lack of desirable properties
3. Nickel-chromium without beryllium, because the addition of beryllium greatly enhances its properties

Some clinicians have found that the very yellow high-gold alloys lead to better porcelain color because their oxides are more readily opaqued with porcelain, allowing thinner opaque porcelain layers and, consequently, better esthetics. In such situations, the lack of strength and poor sag resistance are probably of minor importance and the high-gold yellow alloys should be considered a rational choice for single crowns.

When metal occlusal restorations are present, or when partial veneer abutments are cast in the same alloy, metal hardness and ductility can become important. In these situations, rational alloy choices may be more restricted.

Glossary

alloy A mixture of two or more metals.

base metal A metal that oxidizes readily.

coefficient of thermal expansion A measure of the dimensional change upon heating or cooling, expressed as length change per degree of temperature change.

noble metal A metal that is resistant to oxidation; includes gold, platinum, palladium, and other platinum group metals.

nonprecious metal Relatively inexpensive base metal, such as nickel, chromium, and cobalt.

precious metal An expensive metal; includes gold, platinum group metals, and silver.

Discussion questions

1. Why are the melting temperatures of these alloys so high?
2. What is the role of minor alloying elements in the bonding of these alloys with porcelain?
3. Why does the silver content of these alloys cause a major problem with the color of applied porcelains? What has been done about this?
4. What is the main biological concern with the use of nickel alloys in the mouth?

Questions and answers

1. **What are precious and semiprecious alloys?** The term *precious* refers to higher-cost alloys. The term *semiprecious* has been applied to alloys that are mixtures of precious and nonprecious ingredients.
2. **What are nonprecious alloys?** Nonprecious alloys are composed of nonprecious ingredients, except for small amounts of beryllium. Most are nickel-chromium; some are cobalt-chromium or iron based.
3. **What are the rational considerations for the selection of an alloy?** Rational selection of a specific alloy should be based on a balanced consideration of cost and intended use. For single crowns, strength and sag resistance are less important than they are for fixed partial dentures. Castability, biocompatibility, tarnish and corrosion resistance, porcelain color, and hardness are usually equally important for both alloy uses. For fixed partial dentures, solder and joining behavior, sag resistance, strength, elastic modulus, and the porcelain's thermal expansion compatibility become increasingly important as the span increases.
4. **What is the advantage of palladium-silver alloys?** Excellent clinical working characteristics.
5. **What are the advantages and disadvantages of palladium-copper alloys?** Advantages are good clinical working characteristics, excellent strength, and no porcelain color problems. Disadvantages include slightly more difficult melting and casting than with palladium-silver, and some soldering difficulties.

6. **Which are the base metal alloys to use with porcelain?** Nickel-chromium, cobalt-chromium, and iron-based alloys.
7. **How do nonprecious alloys compare with precious metal alloys?** Nonprecious alloys offer lower cost, higher hardness (more wear resistance), higher tensile strength, and higher elastic modulus. Elongation is about the same as for precious metals, but is negated by the high yield strength, which makes it difficult or impossible to work the metal. Some nickel-chromium alloys, especially those containing beryllium, have mold-filling abilities that are superior to all other alloy groups, permitting easier casting of thin sections and producing sharp margins on castings.
8. **What are gold-palladium alloys, and what are their advantages and disadvantages?** Silver-free alloys containing about 50% gold and 40% palladium. Highly successful commercially, they have favorable yield strength and hardness and higher elastic modulus than high-gold alloys. Cost is comparable to the gold-palladium-silver group. The only disadvantage is thermal expansion incompatibility with some of the higher-expansion porcelains.
9. **What are the necessary precautions for using base metal alloys in place of precious metal alloys?** Strict control of grinding dust (with suction, masks, etc) and screening of patients for possible nickel allergy (eg, pierced ear posts and other jewelry).

Recommended reading

Anusavice KJ. Noble metal alloys for metal-ceramic restorations. Dent Clin North Am 29:789–803, 1985.

Anusavice KJ, et al. Interactive effect of stress and temperature on creep of PFM alloys. J Dent Res 64:1094–1099, 1985.

Baran GR. Selection criteria for base metal alloys for use with porcelain. Dent Clin North Am 29:779–787, 1985.

Bertolotti RL. Calculation of interfacial stress in porcelain-fused-to-metal systems. J Dent Res 59:1972–1977, 1980.

Bertolotti RL, Fukui H. Measurement of softening temperatures in dental bake-on porcelains. J Dent Res 61:180–183, 1982.

Cascone PJ. Effect of thermal properties on porcelain in metal compatibility. J Dent Res 58:263, 1979.

Reese JA, Valega TM (eds). Restorative Dental Materials. London: Quintessence, 1985; 108–133.

Tuccillo JJ, Cascone PJ. The evolution of porcelain-fused-to-metal (PFM) alloy systems. In JW McLean (ed). Dental Ceramics Proc. First Intl Symp. Chicago: Quintessence, 1983; 347–370.

Valega TM Sr (ed). Alternative to Gold Alloys in Dentistry. Conf Proc, 1977. DHEW Publ, no. (NIH) 77–1227; 40–67.

Weiss PA, Munyon RE. Repairs, corrections and additions to nonprecious ceramo-metal frameworks (II). Quintessence Dent Technol 7:45–58, 1980.

Whitlock RP, et al. A practical test to evaluate the castability of dental alloys. J Dent Res 60:404, 1981.

Chapter 17

Casting

The *lost wax casting process*, though one of the oldest existing technologies, is still the preferred and most commonly used method for casting dental restorations. This mode of casting is favored for dental applications because asymmetrical castings incorporating extremely fine detail can be fabricated conveniently and inexpensively compared with other modes of casting.

In brief, a metal casting is made using a refractory mold made from a wax replica or pattern. The procedure includes the following steps:

1. Prepare the tooth or teeth to receive a cast restorative.
2. Make an impression of the prepared tooth.
3. Pour gypsum slurry into the impression to make a positive cast, which is an exact replica of the dental arch from which the individual die(s) representing the prepared tooth or teeth is sectioned.
4. Make a wax pattern that will be representative of the lost tooth structure.
5. Sprue the wax pattern (fix it in space) (Fig 17-1).
6. Invest the wax pattern.
7. Eliminate the wax pattern by burning the wax out of the investment in a furnace, thus making the mold.
8. Force molten metal into the mold using one of a variety of means.
9. Clean the cast.
10. Remove the sprue from casting.
11. Finish and polish the casting on the die.
12. Cement the finished cast restoration on the prepared tooth.

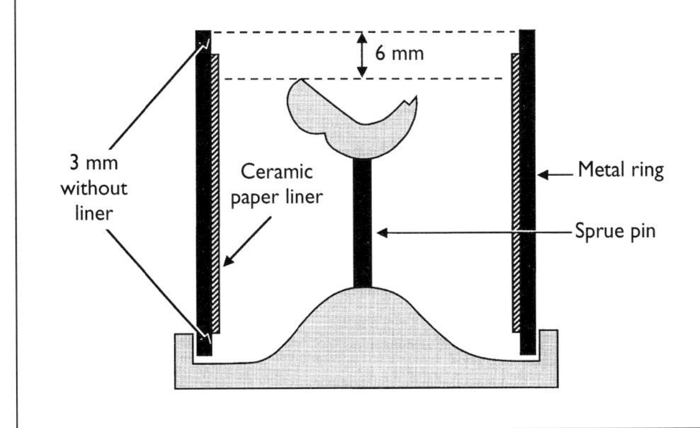

Fig 17-1 Arrangement of a pattern in a ring prior to pouring the investment material. (After Craig and Peyton, 1975.)

When the direct technique—in which the pattern is made on the tooth rather than on the die—is used, steps 2 and 3 are omitted. The desired accuracy of the casting is about 0.1%; therefore, the lost wax procedure requires specially developed materials that compensate for the dimensional changes indicated by the following equation:

wax shrinkage + gold shrinkage = wax expansion + (setting expansion, hygroscopic expansion, and thermal expansion of the investment)

Table 17-1 Expansion requirements of casting

Restoration	Expansion (%)
Thin three-quarter crown	1.80
Classes I and II, small MOD	1.85
Large MOD, three-quarter crown	1.90
Overlay, pin pontic	1.95
Bulky three-quarter crown	2.00
Small Class V, full crown	2.10
Large Class V	2.40

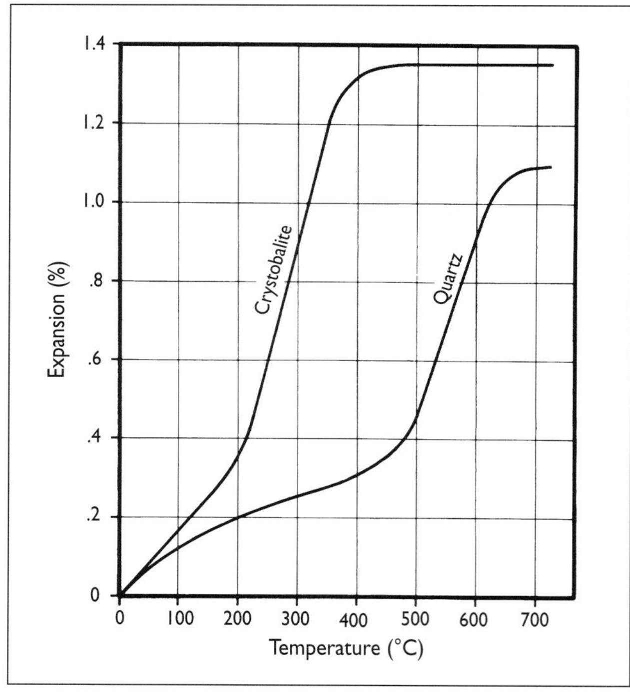

Fig 17-2 Typical thermal expansion curves for cristobalite and quartz.

Thermal shrinkage

Wax

A wax pattern prepared directly in a patient's mouth will shrink about 0.4% when cooled from mouth temperature. In the indirect method of preparing the wax pattern on a die, the wax shrinkage is about 0.2%.

Gold alloy

The casting shrinkage takes place as the solidified metal cools to room temperature. The values for this shrinkage depend upon the geometry of the casting. For example, the gold shrinkage ranges from 1.25% for a thin three-quarter crown to 1.75% for full crowns and 2% for Class V restorations. Table 17-1 summarizes the average amount of mold expansion required for typical types of restorations to compensate for wax and metal shrinkages.

Thermal expansion

High-heat technique

This method employs cristobalite (a high-expansion form of silica) investment materials (Fig 17-2). After the investment has been mixed according to the manufacturer's instructions and allowed to set for at least 45 minutes and no longer than 60 minutes, the mold is placed in a 200°C oven for 20 to 30 minutes to burn out the wax pattern. The temperature of the mold is further elevated by transferring the mold to a second oven and holding at 700°C for no longer than 20 to 30 minutes to obtain the maximum thermal expansion of 1.25% (Table 17-2). Because this type of investment is weak by nature, a metal ring must be used. To increase the setting expansion (SE) of 0.35%, the inside of the ring should be lined with a dampened liner strip that also acts as a cushion against which expansion can take place. This greater expansion caused by the uptake of water from the liner, referred to as hygroscopic expansion (HE), is double the normal SE (see Table 17-2). The HE cited in Table 17-2 includes the SE. Adding the 0.70% HE to the 1.25% thermal expansion (TE) gives the maximum expansion one can expect—about 1.95%. It should be pointed out that most of the compensation is TE that takes place after the wax pattern is eliminated from the mold.

Water-immersion technique (low heat–hygroscopic)

Investments made for water immersion are much stronger than the high-heat types; therefore, a metal ring is not necessary. Instead, a rubber ring is used to

Table 17-2 Mold expansion

Technique	Setting expansion (%)	Hygroscopic expansion (%)	Thermal expansion (%)
High heat (cristobalite)	0.35	0.70†	1.25 (700°C)
Hygroscopic immersion (Beauty Cast*)	0.30	1.50	0.55 (480°C)
Hygroscopic water added (Hygrotrol*)	0.75	2.00	0.55 (480°C)
Phosphate–high heat (Ceramigold*)	0.23–0.50	0.35–1.20	1.33–1.58 (700°C)

*Whip Mix Corp
†Wet liner

contain the mixed investment. Maximum hygroscopic expansion is obtained by immersing the invested pattern and rubber ring, allowing the investment to set under water (hence the name *hygroscopic investment*). In this case, most of the compensatory expansion is HE (1.50%), which again includes the normal SE of 0.3% (see Table 17-2). This expansion takes place with the pattern present in the mold, which may cause distortion in certain pattern configurations (eg, mesio-occlusodistal [MOD]). After the investment has set, the rubber ring is removed from the mold, and the mold is placed directly into a 480°C oven for 30 to 45 minutes to eliminate the wax and acquire the additional necessary TE of 0.55% (see Table 17-2). With a water-immersion investment, one can expect an overall expansion of 2.10% (see Table 17-2).

Phosphate-bonded investment

This type of investment is supplied as a powder containing silica, primary ammonium phosphate ($NH_4H_2PO_4$), and magnesium oxide (MgO). The setting reaction in aqueous solution is:

$$NH_4H_2PO_4 + MgO \rightarrow NH_4MgPO_4 + H_2O$$

A phosphate investment such as Ceramigold (Whip Mix Corp.) may be mixed with a liquid containing a silica sol in water, which increases setting and hygroscopic expansions. The expansion of phosphate investment is adjusted by varying the amount of silica sol liquid used in mixing and by employing hygroscopic and high-heat expansion methods. These investments are employed for high-fusing gold alloys used with porcelain.

Other investment systems

With the advent of alloy systems that do not incorporate any of the noble metals, a very different investment material is required because of the higher fusion or melting temperatures of the alloys. To overcome the decomposition of the gypsum- and phosphate-type investment systems, silicate investments, zircate investments, and various magnesia investments may be used.

Spruing

The purpose of spruing the wax pattern is fourfold:

1. To form a mount for the wax pattern and fix the pattern in space so a mold can be made
2. To create a channel for elimination of wax during burnout
3. To form a channel for the ingress of molten alloy during casting
4. To compensate for alloy shrinkage during solidification

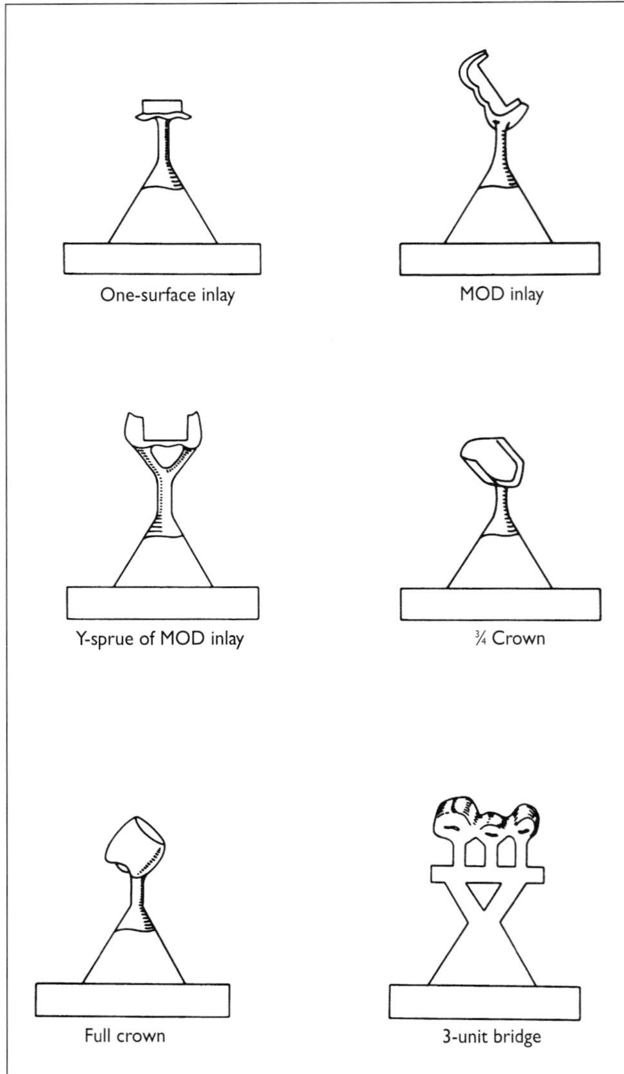

Fig 17-3 Sprue designs for castings (not to scale).

Sprue size and design

The sprue must be large enough so that it remains open until the casting solidifies and short enough to allow rapid filling of the mold cavity. Large and small inlays require sprues that are 14 gauge (4 to 5 mm long) and 16 gauge (3 to 4 mm long), respectively. Large and small crowns require 10-gauge and 12-gauge sprues, respectively, with an average sprue length of 4 to 5 mm.

Point of attachment

Sprue attachment must always be made at the bulkiest portion of the pattern (Fig 17-3). If two bulky portions are separated by a thin cross section (eg, MOD) a Y-shaped sprue (as shown in Fig 17-3) must be used. Turbulence of the molten gold as it enters the mold causes porosity, which is due to entrapped gases and an inappropriate angle of sprue attachment. All attachments, both sprue-pattern and sprue-crucible-former, must therefore be "trumpeted" or "filleted" to eliminate all sharp corners, angles, and instrument marks.

Sprue selection

The wax sprue is the most commonly used. A hollow metal sprue pin is preferable to a solid metal pin because of its stronger attachment. Sticky wax must be used to fill the hollow sprue core before use. Plastic sprues are not recommended because their higher flow temperatures and TE characteristics make it difficult to eliminate the sprue. Since the wax melts at a much lower temperature than the plastic sprue and the TE of the wax is 5 times that of plastic, excessive wax pressure may build up in the mold during burnout before the plastic sprue softens.

Orientation in mold

The wax pattern is mounted on the sprue pin, which in turn is mounted on a clean sprue-crucible-former base, as indicated in Fig 17-1. It is essential that, when the investment ring is placed over the pattern-sprue-crucible-former assembly, the pattern be 6 mm from the end of the ring. If the pattern is less than 6 mm from the end, there is not enough thickness of investment to keep the molten gold from breaking through. If there is more than 6 mm of space, the gold will solidify before the entrapped air can escape, resulting in rounded margins, incomplete casting, or mold fracture.

Liner

A liner is placed inside the ring to allow lateral expansion of the investment. Three millimeters of clearance is allowed at each end of the ring so the mold is sealed and anchored in place. After the liner is placed in the ring, it is dipped in water until saturated, and the excess water is shaken off.

Melting

New metal

Since gold alloys and other alloys change composition during casting, at least one third new gold by weight must be used for each melt.

Contamination

Clean melting crucibles are essential to prevent alloy contamination. Copper-containing gold alloys and noncopper alloys for use with porcelain should not be melted in the same crucible. Previously cast metal must be thoroughly cleaned using appropriate fluxes to remove all gases, oxides, and investment before remelting.

Methods of melting

The various modes available for melting alloys may be grouped into two categories: (*1*) those modes employing a torch, and (*2*) those employing some form of electrical assistance, as shown in Table 17-3. Each mode has its own unique advantages and disadvantages, and in general the modes requiring some form of electrical energy are more costly than those requiring a torch.

Torch melting

The natural gas/air method is the most common for melting gold alloys intended for inlays and crown-and-bridge purposes. Such alloys require the maximum heat production that a gas/air torch is capable of generating (Fig 17-4). For gold alloys with higher fusion temperatures, such as those intended for porcelain-fused-to-metal (PFM) applications, palladium alloys and some base metal alloys can be melted by the higher temperatures provided by the natural gas/oxygen torch.

Air/acetylene and oxygen/acetylene generate much higher temperatures, with the latter providing the hottest flame. Although air/acetylene and oxygen/acetylene modes have the advantage of melting the alloys faster than gas/air or gas/oxygen modes, the disadvantages outweigh their advantages for the following reasons:

Table 17-3 Methods of alloy melting

Torch	Electrical
Gas/air	Resistance
Gas/oxygen	Induction
Air/acetylene	Electric arc
Oxygen/acetylene	

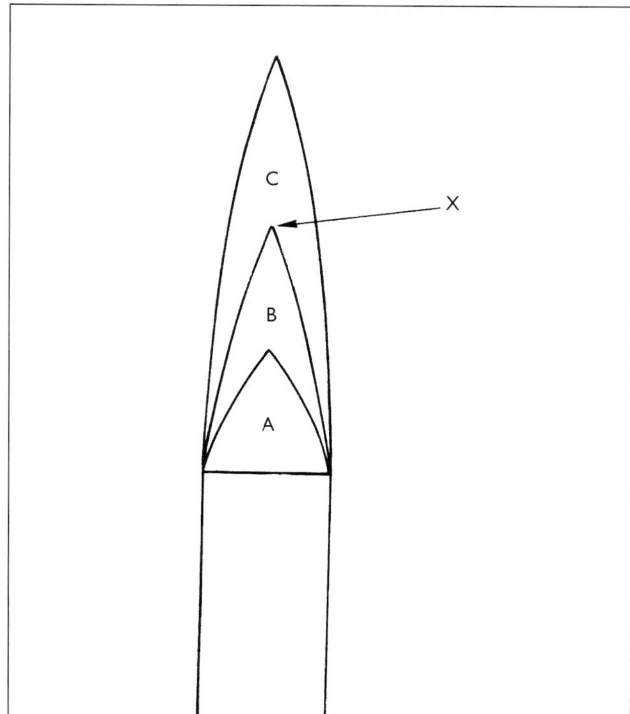

Fig 17-4 Zones of torch flame. The innermost cone (A) consists of unburnt gases and is not hot enough to melt gold. The second cone (B) is blue with burning gases and forms a reducing atmosphere. Point X is best for melting or soldering, because it is the hottest zone of the flame. The outer cone (C), which contains burnt gases, forms an oxidizing atmosphere and should be avoided.

1. Excessive heat may distill lower melting components, thus changing the composition of the alloys.
2. Overheating some alloys allows environmental gases to be dissolved in the melt, resulting in porous castings.

3. Some alloys, particularly base metal, may be excessively hardened and made too brittle due to the uptake of carbon from the acetylene flame.
4. Since the environment cannot be controlled, the extremely high temperature may cause excessive oxidation of the alloy. In fact, the newer titanium alloys cannot be melted by torch. The best practice is to leave the use of the air/acetylene and oxygen/acetylene modes to a highly skilled technician.

Electrical melting

The electric mode of melting includes electric resistance melting, which is suitable for all gold alloys, as well as induction melting and electric arc melting, which are capable of melting cobalt-chromium and titanium alloys. Gold and palladium alloys require a reducing atmosphere as supplied by the use of the middle blue cone of the torch (see Fig 17-4), with flux being added to the melt. A greater convenience is afforded by the electrical resistance furnace, which uses a carbon (rather than ceramic) crucible, thus providing a reducing environment throughout the melting regime.

The electrical resistance furnace also provides the best means of temperature control. The torch adjustment is always variable with no means of monitoring the temperature, and the induction and electric arc modes are less controllable than the resistance mode because melting is achieved so rapidly. Attempts to control the melt temperature when using induction or electric arc require a pyrometer to be focused on the melt. However, since each alloy has its own unique emissivity, the pyrometer is only reliable when calibrated to a given alloy; when a different alloy is used, the pyrometer must be recalibrated.

Casting machines

Casting machines provide the means for transferring the molten alloy from the melting crucible to the mold. They vary greatly, from the most elementary to the complex, with corresponding variations in cost. The casting machines can be divided into two broad categories: (*1*) those employing pneumatic forces, and (*2*) those that provide primarily centrifugal forces to transfer the molten alloy to the heated mold.

Pneumatic forces

A very old method still used to a limited extent throughout the world today uses steam pressure to drive the melt into the mold. The alloy is melted in the sprue-crucible-former part of the mold. A simple handheld device fitted with a wet asbestos plug is quickly placed over the melt, making a seal with the mold ring. When the device is pressed down firmly the wet asbestos makes contact with the molten alloy, generating sufficient steam pressure to complete the casting.

The pressure/vacuum casting machine produces pressure over the molten alloy. A vacuum is applied to the bottom of the mold; thus, the molten alloy is "pushed and sucked" simultaneously into the mold. In variance, the vacuum/pressure types of casting machines first evacuate the melting chamber to reduce oxidation and then apply air pressure uniformly about the casting ring, forcing the alloy into the mold. An innovative variation of the pneumatic mode is the jet casting machine, which depends on combustion gas to provide the casting force.

Casting results from these three machines are comparable. One factor must be taken into consideration when using the pneumatic-type casting machines: They all provide good castings when a porous gypsum investment is used, but when more dense investment—such as a phosphate investment or an investment that tends to sinter on heating—is used, castings may be incomplete. Since the melting procedure is usually done directly in the sprue-crucible-former part of the investment mold, which may be subject to thermal decomposition, thin sprues must be used to prevent premature entrance of the alloy into the sprue opening of the mold during melting.

Centrifugal forces

Two considerations are fundamental to any casting procedure: (*1*) the casting force, be it pneumatic pressure or centrifugal (speed of the rotating arm), and (*2*) the rate of time required to fill the mold. In most cases the two are inversely related—the greater the casting force used the less time required to fill the mold.

The *castability* of an alloy—its ability to completely fill the mold—is determined by a number of variables: its melting range, the mold temperature, and the initial acceleration of the casting machine or applied force, among them. Although the rotation speed of the spring-driven casting machines can be increased by increasing the number of windings of the casting arm, and the vertical rotating casting machines reach their maximum revolutions per minute before the horizontal rotating casting machines, the time required to fill the mold is significantly greater than when pneumatic modes are employed. Even more time is required to fill the mold with the motor-driven casting machine because of the longer time needed to achieve maximum rotation. A large posterior full crown, whose occlusal surface cross section is thick with large adjoining cusps and whose margins are feathered, can hinder the maximizing of the casting force. As the molten metal under a given centrifugal force enters the thickest cavernous area of the mold, a pressure drop is realized before the molten alloy is forced into the feathered margin area. The greatest difficulty in the overall casting regime is in the initial acceleration of the casting machine's arm. To improve the castability of an alloy, one must increase the initial acceleration of the rotation so the mold is filled quickly and the ultimate rotation speed of the casting machine becomes relatively unimportant compared with the initial acceleration.

The traditional centrifugal casting machine has been modified (Airspin Pneumatic Caster, Airspin Manufacturing Co.) to enhance or improve the initial acceleration. It is a vertical-motion centrifugal casting machine that is rapidly accelerated by activating a pneumatic cylinder and piston. Compressed gas is applied to the piston to move it within the cylinder, and a connected drive chain engages a drive wheel coupled to the casting arm. Movement of the piston through the drive stroke is thereby coupled to rotate the casting arm and provide such rapid acceleration that the mold is filled with molten metal before any significant cooling can take place.

With the advantage of increased acceleration, casting of finer detail and thinner cross sections can be made. This has clinical significance because the ability to cast thin sections is critical for maximum marginal integrity and is especially important with alloys intended for porcelain bonding. When casting alloys with a high modulus of elasticity are used, a coping thickness of only 0.1 mm will provide sufficient strength to support the porcelain and allow increased thickness of body porcelain to cover the opaque porcelain, thus greatly improving the esthetics.

Cleaning and finishing the casting

After the casting has been made, the mold is removed from the cradle of the casting machine as soon as the arm stops rotating. It is immersed in cold water when the button (the excess gold left in the crucible above the sprue) turns a dark red. This softens the gold casting, which can then be hardened in a controlled manner by heat treatment. As the mold is plunged into the water, the water in contact with the mold boils, breaking most of the investment away from the casting. The rest can be removed easily by the careful use of any suitable hand instrument or brush.

The cleaned casting may have a dark or tarnished appearance owing to oxide or sulfide deposits on the surface. The deposits are removed by immersing the casting in a pickling solution. Such a solution is usually an acid or a combination of acids with a HCl base. It is highly recommended that the pickling solution be acquired from the alloy supplier, because their formulations are usually nonfuming and emanate no corrosive vapors.

The casting is placed in a small porcelain casserole and just enough solution is added to cover the casting. The solution may be heated carefully until the characteristic gold luster develops. The pickling solution is flushed from the casserole with copious quantities of tap water. Plastic or quartz tongs are not required for this method, eliminating the chance of dropping the casting; also, since only a small quantity of solution is needed (10 mL), new pickling solution can be used each time.

Never use pickling solution if the color has changed even slightly, and never use metal tongs. Never heat the gold casting directly or indirectly in a flame prior to immersing it in pickling solution, because the casting may be dropped or become distorted, or the margins may become rounded from overheating. Furthermore, grain growth is possible, making the casting weak and difficult or impossible to polish. Ultrasonic cleaners and abrasive spray devices (sandblasting) can also play a useful role in the overall cleaning procedure.

Polishing is the final step after precision of fit and marginal integrity have been established on the die. Rubber, rag, or felt wheels impregnated with abrasives are used in the initial stages of finishing. Final polishing is accomplished with various oxides of tin and aluminum used in conjunction with a small rag or chamois buffing wheel, followed with an iron oxide rouge. Since these oxides are often supplied in stick form for convenience of handling and confining the abrasive to the wheel, residual traces of the rosin or waxlike matrix must be removed with a suitable solvent or "polishing compound remover" followed by a hot, soapy water rinse.

Other casting alloys

The metals used for partial denture frameworks are usually alloys of cobalt, with chromium being the primary additive. Lesser amounts of nickel, molybdenum, and carbon are also added in varying amounts. Gold alloys have been used for this purpose; however, since they possess a relatively low modulus of elasticity and proportional limit, are relatively soft, and have a density about twice that of the cobalt alloy, the gold alloys are not preferred for partial denture fabrication. Both alloys, however, possess excellent corrosion resistance properties.

The casting technique for cobalt alloys is very similar in most respects to that described for gold alloys. Although the demands for accuracy may not be as stringent, the principles set forth for gold casting are still valid. Only the primary differences between the gold and cobalt alloy techniques will be presented here. Because the general practitioner is not likely to have the appropriate casting facilities, further details of the actual casting technique should be obtained by reading technical manuals supplied by the manufacturers.

The investment used must be of the phosphate- or silica-bonded type. Cobalt allows melt in the temperature range of 1,250° to 1,450°C (2,280° to 2,640°F), well above the decomposition temperature of calcium sulfate; gypsum investment therefore cannot be used.

Induction is the preferred method for melting cobalt alloys. An oxygen/acetylene torch may be used, but the control of the flame is critical. If the flame is acetylene-rich, carbon is picked up by the alloy, embrittling it; if the flame is oxygen-rich, the metal is oxidized. The melting range of these alloys is well above the upper limits of an air/gas or an oxygen/gas flame, and therefore these mixtures cannot be used. Because of the relatively great hardness of the cobalt alloys, sandblasting and electrolytic polishing techniques are used. Rouges can often be used for final polishing.

Nickel alloys used for crown-and-bridge restorations are melted with gas/oxygen or acetylene/oxygen torches or by electrical induction. Phosphate-bonded investments are required, since these alloys are cast at about 1,260°C (2,300°F). They are handled similarly to the cobalt-chromium alloys. Titanium-based alloys must be melted in a highly controlled inert environment (ie, argon or nitrogen) using either the induction or electric arc mode. Because titanium alloys have such extremely high fusion temperatures, only zircate or magnesia investments can be used.

Titanium and titanium casting are discussed in Chapter 19.

Gold casting troubleshooting

1. Problems with accuracy
   a. *Water/powder ratio* Higher values reduce setting, thermal, and hygrocopic expansions, giving smaller casting.
   b. *Spatulation* Increased spatulation increases setting expansion, giving larger castings.
   c. *Burnout temperatures* Lower temperatures result in less thermal expansion and smaller castings.
   d. *Immersion time* Delay results in decreased hygroscopic expansion and smaller castings.
   e. *Water-added technique* Decreased amounts of water added to investment result in decreased hydroscopic expansion and smaller castings.
   f. *Water bath* Temperatures below 37°C (100°F) reduce hygroscopic expansion and result in smaller castings.
2. Problems with distortion
   a. *Wax too hot* Excessive shrinkage results upon cooling.
   b. *Wax too cool* The pattern undergoes stress release with a change in shape.
   c. *Insufficient pressure during waxing* The pattern distorts because of thermal shrinkage.
   d. *Delayed investment* The sooner the investment is complete, the less distortion there will be.
   e. *Heating pattern during spruing* This may create distortion.
   f. *Overheating casting during soldering procedure* This warps or melts the margins.
3. Problems with bubbles
   a. *Inadequate vacuum or ineffective painting procedure* The vacuum must have at least 26 in. of mercury for vacuum investing.
   b. *Water/powder ratio* If the investment is too thick it will not cover the pattern completely.
   c. *Excessive vibration of the ring* This produces small nodules.

4. Problems with surface roughness
   a. *Water/powder ratio* A high ratio increases the roughness of the mold.
   b. *Excess wetting agent or salivary contamination* This may form a film on the pattern surface and be reproduced on the casting surface. Generally the roughness is localized on the exterior and is masslike in appearance.
   c. *Prolonged heating or overheating of the mold* Prolonged heating may cause investment disintegration, whereas overheating may cause a reaction between the alloy and casting investment. Roughness appears general and feels sharp.
   d. *Premature heating of casting investment* Wait a minimum of 45 minutes for burnout.
5. Problems with fins on the surface or margins
   a. *Prolonged heating* This may produce cracks in the investment that radiate out from the surface of the pattern.
   b. *Heating rate is too rapid* Cracks may appear in the investment, caused by nonuniform heating of investment.
   c. *Water/powder ratio* A high ratio produces a weak investment that may crack.
   d. *Excessive casting pressure* Metal impact may cause investment fracture.
   e. *Cooling of the investment prior to casting* This may produce cracks in the investment.
6. Problems with short, rounded margins
   a. *Investment or alloy is too cold* In this case, solidification is completed prior to completion of the mold.
   b. *Casting pressure* The casting pressure is inadequate to fill the mold because of trapped air. The situation depends on the pattern position and the porosity of the investment.
   c. *Incomplete burnout* This may result in residual carbon at peripheral portions of the pattern.
7. Problems with miscasting
   a. *Casting is nearly or entirely missing* The pattern detached from the sprue pin, owing to excessive vibration.
   b. *Pattern fractured during investing*
   c. *Gold alloy was too cold during casting*
   d. *Incomplete burnout*
   e. *Sprue pin was too small* If the sprue freezes before the alloy fills the mold completely, incomplete casting results.
8. Problems with pits
   a. *Inclusions of investment, asbestos, or other debris are carried to the margin by molten alloy* Pits generally exhibit angular edges. They may be rounded if they are the result of flux inclusion.

Internal porosity

9. Problems with localized shrinkage porosity
   a. *Sprue pin diameter is too small* The sprue channel solidifies simultaneously with or before the casting. Additional molten alloy is prevented from entering the mold to compensate for solidification shrinkage.
   b. *Alloy or mold temperature is too low* Rapid solidification of the alloy results here.
10. Problems with subsurface porosity
    a. *Short, thick sprue pin* Rapid entry of the alloy causes skin formation; the bulk of alloy pulls away, forming subsurface porosity.
    b. *Alloy or mold temperature is too high* The first portion of gold to contact the investment will solidify and form a thin skin. The alloy behind it shrinks during solidification and pulls away, forming small porosities.
11. Problems with microporosity
    a. *Alloy or mold temperatures are too low* If solidification occurs more rapidly than normal, shrinkage may develop throughout the casting.

External porosity

12. Problems with back pressure porosity
    a. *Insufficient alloy mass* Air is entrapped in the solidifying alloy.
    b. *Insufficient turns on the casting machine* The denser the investment, the greater the force needed to eliminate the gas within the mold chamber.
    c. *Pattern is too far away from the end of the ring* The situation is aggravated by dense investments and lower burnout temperatures.

Glossary

die A replica of a tooth or prepared tooth onto which a wax pattern is formed. The die is usually made of a gypsum material.

gypsum The hydrated product formed when plaster is mixed with water: $CaSO_4 \cdot 2H_2O$.

investment A molding material that surrounds the pattern and subsequently hardens and forms the mold after the wax pattern is eliminated.

refractory Any material that has an extremely high melting point. In gold casting, some form of silica (usually cristobalite) would be the refractory.

Discussion questions

1. For an inlay casting, how close is the tolerance at the margins?
2. If an inlay or crown casting is too small, what factors in the process may be responsible?
3. How can porosity, which is a problem in polishing, be reduced?
4. Compare the advantages and disadvantages of the high heat and hygroscopic mold expansion techniques.
5. Why are the properties of the wax pattern so important in the accuracy of the lost wax process?

Questions and answers

1. **Describe the lost wax technique of casting.** A wax pattern is used to form a refractory mold for the casting of a molten metal.
2. **What equation must be satisfied in order to make a casting that will fit?** Wax shrinkage + gold shrinkage = setting expansion + hygroscopic expansion + thermal expansion of the investment + wax expansion.
3. **What are the two primary techniques used in fabricating a wax pattern?**
   a. The direct technique, in which the wax pattern is formed directly on the prepared tooth
   b. The indirect technique, in which the wax pattern is fabricated on a gypsum replica of the prepared tooth
4. **What primary factor determines the amount of gold shrinkage?** Geometry of the casting, or more specifically the surface/volume ratio, is the primary factor.
5. **What is cristobalite?** A high expansion form of silica.
6. **Why is it necessary to use an asbestos liner when making a cristobalite investment?** To increase the setting, hygroscopic, and thermal expansions.
7. **Name four commonly used investing techniques.** High heat, water immersion (low heat hygroscopic), controlled water added, and phosphate bonded.
8. **Which investment is designed for the higher-fusing casting golds, as used in porcelain-fused-to-gold techniques?** Phosphate bonded.
9. **How can the expansion of phosphate investment best be controlled?** By varying the amount of the silica sol component of the liquid mixed with the phosphate-bonded investment powder.
10. **What are the four primary functions of the sprue?**
    a. As a mount for wax pattern
    b. As a channel for wax escape during burnout
    c. As a channel for filling the mold with molten gold
    d. As a compensation for shrinkage during solidification.

11. **Why must gold alloys be cleaned by melting on a charcoal block before being used for the second time?** To remove oxides, sulfides, and particles of investment that were formed or added during the first melt.

12. **Name three types of casting machines commonly used in gold casting.** Centrifugal, pressure, and pressure/vacuum.

13. **What is the nature of pickling solutions used for cleaning gold alloys?** These solutions comprise acids or a combination of acid with a HCl base.

14. **What are the primary components of the base metals used for partial denture frameworks?** Cobalt, chromium, nickel, molybdenum, and carbon.

15. **Why is gold not the metal of choice for fabricating a partial denture framework?** Gold alloys possess a relatively low modulus of elasticity and proportional limit. They are relatively soft, and their density is about twice that of the cobalt-chromium alloys.

16. **Name two types of investment used for casting cobalt-chromium alloys.** Phosphate-bonded investments and silica-bonded investments.

Recommended reading

Asgar K, Arfaei AH. Castability of crown and bridge alloys. J Prosthet Dent 54:60, 1985.

Asgar K, et al. Further investigations into the nature of hygroscopic expansion of dental casting investments. J Prosthet Dent 8:673, 1958.

Craig RG, et al. Strength properties of waxes at various temperatures and their practical applications. J Dent Res 46:300, 1967.

Craig RG, Peyton FA. Restorative Dental Materials. 5th ed. St Louis: CV Mosby Co, 1975.

Delgado VP, Peyton FA. The hygroscopic setting expansion of a dental casting investment. J Prosthet Dent 3:423, 1953.

Docking AR. The hygroscopic setting expansion of dental casting investments. Parts I–IV. Aust Dent J Jan 1948, 6; May 1948, 160; Sept 1948, 320; Sept 1949, 261.

Donovan TE, White LE. Evaluation of an improved centrifugal casting machine. J Prosthet Dent 53:609, 1985.

Dootz ER, et al. Influence of investments and duplicating procedures on the accuracy of partial denture castings. J Prosthet Dent 15:679, 1965.

Eames WB, MacNamara JF. Evaluation of casting machines for ability to cast sharp margins. Oper Dent 3:137, 1978.

Earnshaw R. Investments for casting cobalt-chromium alloys. Br Dent J 108:1, 1960.

Ida K, Tsutsumi S, Togaya T. Titanium or titanium alloys for dental casting. Microfilmed Paper no. 397. Delivered at the Annual Meeting of the International Association for Dental Research, Dental Materials Group, Osaka, Japan, June 5–7, 1980.

Ida K, et al. Casting force in several casting methods. Part I. Casting pressure produced by gaseous pressure casting apparatus and speed of revolution of centrifugal casting machine. J Osaka Univ Dent Sch 10:35, 1970.

Ida K, Kuroda T, Yamaga R. Casting force in several casting methods. Part II. Comparison of casting time in several casting methods. J Osaka Univ Dent Sch 10:47, 1970.

Jones DW, Wilson HJ. Variables affecting the thermal expansion of refractory investments. Br Dent J 125:249, 1968.

Jørgensen KD. Study of the setting expansion of gypsum. Acta Odontol Scand 21:227, 1963.

Mahler DB, Ady AB. An explanation for the hygroscopic setting expansion of dental gypsum products. J Dent Res 39:576, 1960.

Mahler DB, Ady AB. The effect of the water bath in hygroscopic casting techniques. J Prosthet Dent 15:1115, 1965.

Mahler DB, Ady AB. The influence of various factors on the effective setting expansion of casting investments. J Prosthet Dent 13:365, 1963.

Mahler DB, Asgarzadeh K. The volumetric contraction of dental gypsum materials on setting. J Dent Res 32:354, 1953.

Peyton FA, et al. Controlled water-addition technic for hygroscopic expansion of dental casting investment. J Am Dent Assoc 52:155, 1956.

Ryge G, Fairhurst CW. Hygroscopic expansion. J Dent Res 35:499, 1956.

Chapter 18

High-Temperature Investments

The main use of these investments is for casting dental alloys that need to be heated to casting temperatures in excess of about 1,200° to 1,300°C (2,192° to 2,372°F).* Alloys that fit this description include many high-gold and palladium-based alloys used for the fabrication of porcelain-veneered fixed partial dentures and those dental alloys based on nickel, cobalt, or titanium. These investments are also used for creating fixtures that hold sections of prostheses in proper apposition while joining them together during soldering, brazing, or welding operations. Another application is for making dies that are employed for the fabrication of porcelain facial tooth veneers.

These investments are not gypsum based, as are those used for the casting of alloys that have casting temperatures less than approximately 1,200°C (2,192°F), but instead have a variety of basic formulations that are better suited to withstand exposure to high temperatures. The predominate compositions, used for the casting of high-temperature alloys and for creating veneering dies, are based on the use of a phosphate binder. Silicate-bound systems are also used (Kondic, 1960), but because of their difficult handling, their use tends to be restricted to the casting of cobalt-chromium alloys at temperatures above 1,425°C (2,600°F).

Either entirely new systems or modifications of the aforementioned ones have been needed for the casting of titanium-based alloys. These alloys require special investments because they are cast from higher temperatures than the others and are also highly reactive. They can easily degrade the more conventional molds at elevated temperatures and, as a result, produce poor surface finishes. Further, they can be contaminated by degradation of the investment components, such as silica and carbon, and by oxygen and nitrogen present in the atmosphere. These contaminations serve to harden and embrittle the surface of titanium castings. Because of the more recent developments of investments for the casting of titanium alloys for dental applications, a separate section is devoted to this subject.

*Casting temperature is approximately 65° to 150°C (150° to 300°F) above the top of the melting range for most dental alloys.

Phosphate-bonded investments

Applications

Phosphate-bonded investments have been used for many years in dentistry to make molds into which high-melting-temperature dental alloys were cast. There are two types of casting investments. Type I traditionally has been employed for the casting of inlays, crowns, and other restorations (especially for alloys based on gold, platinum, and palladium to which porcelain is fused in the construction of aesthetic fixed partial dentures). Type II is used for the casting of removable partial dentures. These uses continue to the present day, but the alloy applications have grown. The Type I phosphate-bonded investments are now also used for the casting of cobalt-chromium and nickel-chromium alloys, primarily used for porcelain-veneered fixed par-

Table 18-1 Properties of phosphate-bonded investments used for high-temperature operations with dental materials (except titanium alloys)

Casting investments	
Compressive strength	2.5 MPa/min, Type I (for inlays, crowns, etc)* 10 MPa/min, Type II (for removable appliances)*
Setting expansion (linear)	Within 15% of manufacturer's stated value* With use of full-strength liquid about 0.4% can be attained with some; when a hygroscopic technique is used, about another 0.6% to 0.8% can be realized†
Thermal expansion	Within 15% of manufacturer's stated value* About 0.8% can be attained with a 50:50 mixture of liquid and water; about 1% to 1.2% can be attained with the use of undiluted liquid†
Modulus of rupture	0.1 to 0.5 MPa (14.4 to 72.5 psi); green, about 0.8 MPa (116 psi), as fired†
Refractory die stones	
Compressive strength	13 MPa/min
Setting expansion (linear)	Within 30% of manufacturer's stated value*
Thermal expansion	Within 15% of manufacturer's stated value* Manufacturers state that their materials are designed to be compatible with their porcelain at temperatures in the vicinity of the glass-transition temperature. Values of about 12 to 13 × 10^{-6}/°C^{-1} would be expected.

*According to current status of working draft for ISO #9694 (November 17, 1993).
†Approximate values attainable with some of the commercial brands.

tial dentures. Some variations are used for cast titanium alloys, discussed later in this chapter.

Another traditional use of phosphate-bonded investments is to make "soldering" fixtures that hold prosthetic components in alignment while they are being joined with solders, brazing alloys, or welding alloys. More recently (since around 1980) modifications have been used to make refractory dies for the fabrication of custom veneer facings from dental porcelains.

Composition

These investments are available as two component systems that react to form a solid when mixed together (Takahashi et al, 1990). One component consists of a powder, and the other is an aqueous solution stabilized with colloidal silica. The powder has a variety of ingredients. There are particles of refractory materials such as silica glass, quartz, and cristobalite to control thermal expansion and, along with other metal oxides, provide bulk and help control the surface finish of a casting. There is also powdered ammonium dihydrogen phosphate, $NH_4H_2PO_4$, (provided in excess) which, in reaction with water in the presence of calcined magnesium oxide (MgO) powder (another ingredient), provides for the binding of the particles at ambient temperatures. The liquid provides the water needed for the room-temperature setting reaction. The setting reaction of the $NH_4H_2PO_4$ with calcined magnesium oxide in the presence of water is:

$$n\,NH_4H_2PO_4 + MgO + 5H_2O \rightarrow NH_4MgPO_4{\cdot}6H_2O + (n-1)\,NH_4H_2PO_4$$

After a mixed slurry sets to form a mold, it is fired to burn out consumable patterns (mostly waxes, but some polymers are used also).

Properties

Important properties of phosphate-bonded investments are given in Table 18-1. High-temperature mold strength is achieved by the formation of complex silicophosphates from the reaction of some of the silica with the excess dihydrogen phosphate. Thermal expansion is raised by the remainder of the silica. Liquid that is supplied with the investment may be used either full strength or diluted with water to provide some degree of control over the setting and thermal expansions.

Although the basic binding reaction is the same for all of the phosphate-bonded investments, there are some important differences in properties due to composition. Those used for the casting of high-temperature alloys and for making dies used in the fabrication of porcelain veneers contain quartz and cristobalite to achieve expansion, which compensates for the shrinkage (contraction) of either the cast alloy or the porcelain veneer during cooling from elevated temperatures. The die materials also contain finer particles to provide smoother surfaces where contact with the porcelain is made. Soldering investments, however, do not require especially fine powders and are designed without high-expansion fillers. The latter is to keep parts that are to be joined from shifting while they and the surrounding investment are heated to the joining temperature. Graphite is found in some investments to render them more permeable after burnout and/or to provide a reducing atmosphere.

Advantages and disadvantages

There are several advantages associated with phosphate-bonded investments. They have both high green and as-fired strengths. This makes them easy to handle without breaking before they are placed in a furnace for the wax burnout process and strong enough afterward to withstand the impact and pressure of centrifugally cast molten alloy. They can also provide setting and thermal expansions high enough to compensate for the thermal contraction of cast-metal prostheses or porcelain veneers during cooling. Finally, they have the ability to withstand the burnout process (~1 to 1.5 hours) with temperatures that reach 900°C (1,650°F), and they can withstand temperatures up to 1,000°C for short periods of time (useful for fabricating porcelain veneers or performing metal-joining operations).

These investments are at a disadvantage when used with higher-melting alloys, those with casting temperatures greater than about 1,375°C (2,500°F). These temperatures coupled with high mold temperatures result in mold breakdown and rougher surfaces on castings. The high strength of these investments, although an advantage during casting, can make divesting (removal of the casting from the investment) a difficult and tedious task without the use of a simple tool, such as a press to force the investment out of the metal casting ring (when a casting ring is used). Further, when higher expansion is required, more of the silica liquid is used with the result that a more dense and less porous mold is produced. This can result in incomplete castings if a release for trapped gases is not provided.

A disadvantage when the powder is supplied in bulk form—rather than in sealed, premeasured packages—is a reaction over time with moisture in the air and a loss of the ability to either set to a strong mass or expand during setting.

Ethyl silicate–bonded investments

Applications

Ethyl silicate–bonded investments comprise the second type of investment used in dentistry. These investments have been used since the early 1930s to make molds for the casting of removable partial dentures of cobalt-chromium alloys. This continues to be their primary use, although they are occasionally used for the casting of nickel-based alloys.

Composition

Ethyl silicate–bonded investments (ESBIs) rely on binding by the formation of a gel from silicic acid which is derived from the hydrolysis of tetraethyl orthosilicate, $Si(OC_2H_5)_4$. It is from this derivation that these investments got their name. As with the phosphate-bonded investments, ESBIs are supplied as a powder that requires mixing with a liquid to bind the mixed mass via a setting reaction at room temperature. The powder consists of refractory particles of silicas and glasses in various forms along with calcined magnesium oxide and some other refractory oxides in minor amounts.

The liquid that is used for the setting reaction may be supplied as a stabilized alcohol solution of silica gel, or it may be formed from two liquids that are supplied. When the system uses two liquids, one is ethyl silicate and the other may be an acidified solution of dena-

Table 18-2 Properties of ethyl silicate–bonded investments used for high-temperature operations with dental materials

Casting investments	
Compressive strength	1.5 MPa/min*
Setting expansion (linear)	There is no requirement for setting expansion Setting contractions of 0 to 0.4% has been reported This value will depend on the method of measurement One manufacturer reports virtually no (0 to 0.05%) contraction†
Thermal expansion	Within 15% of manufacturer's stated value* About 1.5% to 1.8% can be attained between room temperature and 1,000° to 1,177°C (1,800° to 2,150°F)†

*According to current status of working draft for ISO #11246 (November 17, 1993).
†Approximate values attainable with some of the commercial brands.

tured ethyl alcohol. Three component systems also exist and may consist of stabilized colloidal silica, ethyl silicate, and denatured ethyl alcohol. Regardless of the number of liquids provided, the active species is the hydrated silica that is formed by the reaction of ethyl silicate with water in the presence of the acid (or a base) according to the reaction:

$$Si(OC_2H_5)_4 + 4H_2O \text{ acid/base} \rightarrow SiOH + 4C_2H_5OH$$

Binding is by the reaction of the hydrated silica in the presence of MgO to form a gel according to

$$nSi(OH)_4 + MgO \rightarrow MgO[Si(OH)_4]_n$$

A wetting agent is added to at least one of the liquid components to reduce the formation of gaseous bubbles on the surface of a pattern.

Properties

The most important property of the ESBIs is their ability to withstand higher temperatures than the phosphate-bonded investments and to achieve sufficient expansion to compensate for the cooling shrinkage from the higher solidification temperatures of the higher-casting-temperature alloys with which they are used (ie, cobalt-chromium alloys). During the vibration of the investment slurry into a casting ring around a pattern, a separation occurs between the finer and coarser particles. The finer particles of the investment rise to the top of the mold where the slurry acquires more liquid. As a result, the top of the mold (near the bottom of the pattern, opposite the sprue end) is prone to cracking due to great drying shrinkage from the evaporation of the ethyl alcohol that results from the formation of the silica gel. These cracks must be removed prior to the firing process. Otherwise, when the mold is heated to burn out a pattern and achieve thermally induced expansion, the cracks will grow and result in faulty castings. To overcome this problem, a sufficient header of investment is provided to allow for removal of the cracked portion by grinding. The remaining investment itself undergoes virtually no solidification shrinkage and is free of critical cracks. The expansion of the investment is all due to thermal expansion. Thus, distortion of patterns (such as those that can occur with setting expansion) is minimized, and these investments are well suited for producing large, precise castings.

Because of the low dimensional changes during setting (Table 18-2), models made from these investments may be articulated directly against gypsum models of opposing dentition. However, the green strength of these investments is low, and refractory models are best handled by reinforcing them with a resin dip. A fine-grained surface coat is sometimes applied to the reinforced model and to the pattern on the model in order to achieve a superior surface finish on the cast appliance.

Advantages and disadvantages

These investments offer the ability to cast high-temperature cobalt-chromium and nickel-chromium alloys, and attain good surface finishes, low distortion, and high thermal expansion (good fit). They are less

Table 18-3 Titanium investments available in Japan and Germany

Mold-casting temperature (°C)	Binder	Refractory	Burnout temperature (°C)	Country
RT*	MgO, phosphate	Al_2O_3, ZrO_2	900	Japan
RT*		Al_2O_3, ZrO_2	1,100	Japan
800		Al_2O_3, ZrO_2	1,150–1,200	Japan
RT*		Al_2O_3, SiO_2	900–1,000	Japan
200		Al_2O_3, SiO_2	1,100	Both
500		Al_2O_3, SiO_2	950	Both
100		$ZrSiO_4$, SiO_2	1,100	Japan
RT*		Al_2O_3, $LiAlSi_2O_6$	1,050	Japan
600–700	Ethyl silicate	MgO, Al_2O_3	900	Japan
600–700		MgO, SiO_2, Al_2O_3	900	Japan
100		MgO, Zr†	850	Japan
100	Aluminous cement	MgO, Zr†	850	Japan
600–700		MgO, Al_2O_3	900	Japan

*RT= room temperature.
†Addition for oxidizing expansion.

dense (more permeable) than the phosphate-bonded investments, and thin sections with fine detail can be reproduced. Their low fired strength makes divesture easier than with phosphate bonded investments.

Their disadvantages lie primarily in the added processing attention (resin-model reinforced dies, pattern coats) and the extra precaution needed in handling the low-strength fired molds. The low strength and high thermal expansion require a more precise burnout process and firing schedule to avoid cracking and, hence, destruction of a mold.

Other systems

Applications

These investments are aimed at the casting of titanium and titanium-based alloys, although the possibility of applications for the casting of other alloys or for refractory pattern coats becomes apparent from some of the properties shown in the following section.

Recently, efforts to cast dental appliances in Japan, Europe, and the United States from titanium or titanium-based alloys have shown that the conventional phosphate-bonded investments and ethyl silicate-based investments are deficient for that purpose. This is because molten titanium is highly reactive with oxygen and is capable of reducing some of the oxides commonly found in those investments. Titanium can also dissolve residual oxygen, nitrogen, and carbon from the investment; these elements can harden and embrittle titanium in the solid state. As a result, either modifications of existing refractory formulations and binders or new refractory formulations and binder systems are required.

Composition

A variety of investment formulations for the casting of titanium have been developed over the past several years (Table 18-3) (Togaya, 1993; Miyazaki and Tamaki, 1993). These investments might be classified as phosphate-bonded, ethyl silicate–bonded, and "cemented" according to the source of the binder. Many kinds of refractories such as silica (SiO_2), alumina (Al_2O_3), magnesia (MgO), and zirconia (ZrO_2) have been used.

Properties

Standards do not exist, nor are they in development for investments for the casting of titanium and titanium alloys for dental purposes. It is reasonable to expect that those mechanical properties being contemplated for the conventional phosphate and ethyl silicate-based binders would apply here as well.

New refractory compositions and binders have been investigated for the casting of titanium prostheses. The objectives have been to reduce breakdown of the investment and the contamination of titanium. One approach to reducing the reaction with investment is to employ molds that have been expanded by the burnout process and then cooled back to near ambient temperatures prior to the casting process. This reduces the time that the alloy is in contact with the mold at elevated temperatures, and the overall reactivity is reduced. However, lowering of the mold temperature requires that either nonreversible expanders, such as metals that expand by oxidation at the elevated temperatures, be used or that the temperature of the mold be kept just above the temperature where a reversal of expansion due to crystalline phase changes takes place.

In order to avoid contamination of titanium by oxygen through the reduction of refractory oxides of the investment, refractory materials that are less easily reduced by titanium should be used. The Gibbs free energy of formation (FEF) (Chase et al, 1985) of titanium oxide (TiO) at 1,727°C is –716 KJ/mol of oxygen, and that for titanium dioxide (TiO_2) at 1,727°C is –580 KJ/mol of oxygen. The corresponding FEFs of SiO_2 in the forms of cristobalite and quartz are –550 and –549 KJ, respectively. From this, it is clear that titanium may be expected to be oxidized by SiO_2, which is reduced.

Some modifications of phosphate-bonded investments have been explored for the purpose of rendering them more compatible with molten titanium metals. One investment consisting of a phosphate binder, magnesia, and quartz was developed under the hypothesis that quartz would not be as reactive as silica (Takahashi, 1993). On the basis of FEFs, there is little advantage in the use of one form of SiO_2 over another, and any advantages of one form over another would have to lie elsewhere (perhaps their decomposition kinetics are sufficiently different). This investment was recommended for use as a room-temperature mold, ostensibly to reduce reaction with titanium. However, contamination of castings by reaction with the investment was still encountered, as would be expected from the previous discussion on FEFs.

To make use of the setting expansion of a phosphate binder, alumina (FEF = –687 KJ/mol of O_2 at 1,727°C) and magnesia (FEF = –640 KJ/mol of O_2 at 1,727°C), both of which have good heat resistance, can be used as refractories; however, the thermal expansions of these oxides is low. If either of their powders are mixed with colloidal silica to raise the expansion, some contamination from the silica again becomes a problem.

In order to achieve expansion without the use of reactive powders, a phosphate investment that contains *both* magnesia and alumina as refractories was developed. This investment can attain large expansion by the spinel reaction of alumina and magnesia ($MgO + Al_2O_3 \rightarrow MgO - Al_2O_3$) when it is burned out at 1,150° to 1,200°C. The spinel is, of course, also highly refractory. The spinel-forming temperature can also be reduced by mixing with magnesia acetate. Another approach to obtaining the needed expansion is through the use of spodumen ($Li_2O - Al_2O_3 - SiO_2$) (Okuda, et al, 1991). Spodumen expands irreversibly upon heating through the temperature range of 900° to 1100°C.

Reaction of ethyl silicate–bonded investments with liquid titanium has been reported to be somewhat less than that of phosphate-bonded investments; this is most likely due to the use of highly refractory oxides in the powder (Table 18-3). Regardless, these investments require a more complex procedure for their use.

A more recent development is an investment using magnesia bonded by an aluminous cement ($CaO - Al_2O_3$) and containing 5% zirconium powder by weight (Togaya, 1985). The aluminous cement serves as a binder for the magnesia refractory, and it sets by mixing with water. Oxidation of the zirconium powder to zirconia during the burnout process provides irreversible expansion to compensate for shrinkage of the casting during cooling from the solidification temperature. The zirconia formed is highly stable, it has an FEF of –728 KJ/mol of oxygen, and it should not contaminate the titanium. Titanium castings from this investment were reported to have smooth surfaces free of contamination from mold reaction.

Glossary

articulation Joining or meeting of the maxillary and mandibular dentition or of a replica of it.

calcined Rendered a powdery, friable, dry substance by the application of heat.

colloidal The state of finely divided particles that are in suspension in a liquid. The particles acquire special properties (electrical, gelatinous, etc.) as a result of their fine size and interaction with each other and the liquid. Colloidal silica consists of fine particles of hydrated silicas that can form a gel and bind larger particles of noncolloidal nature.

exothermic Heat-releasing.

fired strength The strength of an investment following a burnout process. This strength is often measured by resistance to breaking under three point loading or bending.

fixture A device that is firmly fastened in place in a mechanical sense, often used to secure other devices.

green strength The prefired strength of an investment, acquired through some chemical reaction at or near room temperature. (See fired strength.)

hydrolysis Decomposition of a compound by water, or the interaction of positive and negative ions of a salt with hydroxyl and hydrogen ions to form an acid and a base.

hygroscopic Pertaining to the absorbing of water.

investment A refractory used to form a mold around a wax pattern.

mold A cavity into which molten metal is cast.

refractory A heat resistant material.

ring A thin-walled structure used to contain an investment slurry before it sets: also provides support for set or fired investments that have poor strength.

setting expansion The volumetric or linear increase in physical dimensions of an investment, caused by the chemical reactions that occur during hardening to a rigid structure.

shelf life The period of time during which an investment (or other compound) retains its useful characteristics.

slurry A thin mixture of liquid and powder.

soak period The time during which an investment mold is allowed to remain at any given temperature during the burnout process.

surface coat The first coating that is applied to a wax pattern or the surface of the mold that comes into direct contact with a cast metal.

thermal expansion The increase in dimension of a set investment due to temperature increase during burnout.

Discussion questions

1. Which developments in clinical dentistry have led to a switch from the use of gypsum to more refractory materials?
2. What are the matrix compositions of the two major high heat investments?
3. How can additional expansion be obtained with magnesia and ethyl silicate investments?
4. Which of the two high heat investments gives more accurate models?

Questions and answers

1. **Given a multicomponent system that includes ethyl silicate as a reacting component, how can the reaction time for hydrolysis be altered?** (a) Changing the temperature of the reacting components (higher temperature results in faster reactions); (b) changing the acidic concentration or the amount of water available (lower concentrations of these ingredients result in slower reaction rates).
2. **By cooling hydrated ethyl silicate to 4.4°C (40°F), its shelf life is extended.**
   a. **Would the shelf life be extended by refrigeration to lower temperatures?** Yes.
   b. **To what extent may the liquid be cooled without encountering adverse effects?** The temperature may be lowered until the liquid begins to freeze, at which point precipitation of gelled silica hydrate renders the liquid incapable of properly binding investment particles via a gelation process. The temperature of 4.4°C has practical significance, as this is a temperature achieved in the main storage compartment of a refrigerator.
3. **Why is denatured ethyl alcohol used rather than 95% ethyl alcohol as a component of an ethyl silicate system?** To avoid higher costs because of the federal tax on spirits, and to eliminate the chance it will be imbibed.
4. **List advantages and disadvantages of phosphate-bonded investments.**

   Advantages:

   1. Rapid setting rate.
   2. Useful for lower burnout temperatures because much of the expansion is achieved as a result of the setting reaction rather than temperature increase.
   3. High green strength.
   4. High as-fired strength, which results in less mold cracking and fewer fins on castings.
   5. Liquid formed by mixing colloidal silica with water may be used immediately.

   Disadvantages:

   1. The investment powder will react with moisture, imposing limitations on the shelf life of opened containers.
   2. High setting expansion is an impediment to using the investment for producing refractory models that will be used for articulation against "stone" models (the high expansion results in a model that will not properly match the opposing model of stone).
   3. High tendency for reaction with nonprecious alloys, producing oxides that are difficult to remove from castings.
   4. Lower permeability, which yields a tendency to produce short castings in a gas entrapment.
   5. The colloidal silica liquid cannot be shipped under conditions that would result in freezing of the liquid and agglomeration of colloidal silica.
   6. Higher-temperature castings (investment temperature greater than 980°C [1,800°F]) have poorer surfaces owing to refractory loss.
5. **List advantages and disadvantages of ethyl silicate-bonded investments.**

   Advantages:

   1. High permeability yields sharply defined dental castings.
   2. Low setting expansion (contraction) renders refractory partial denture models that may be articulated against stone models.
   3. A nearly flat expansion vs temperature curve at high temperature (approx. 1,150° [2,100°F]) and a low expansion vs time effect at that temperature make possible precise control of total expansion.
   4. The investment is more refractory, which results in smoother castings.
   5. Lower burnout strength results in easier removal of castings and cleaning of oxides from the casting.

   Disadvantages:

   1. Limited shelf life of liquid.
   2. Must wait substantial period of time prior to using freshly mixed liquid.
   3. Potential of cracking during burnout owing to high thermal expansion.

6. **For the casting of nonprecious crown-and-bridge alloys, which technique would be recommended with a phosphate-bonded investment?** The hygroscopic technique to generate the maximum expansion of the investment, thereby helping to compensate for the greater shrinkage of nonprecious alloys as opposed to gold.

7. **What is the investment of choice for casting the following alloys?**
   a. **Ceramic gold alloy?** Phosphate
   b. **Cobalt-chromium partial denture alloy?** Ethyl silicate or mixed ethyl silicate, colloidal silica, phosphate-bonded
   c. **Nickel-based crown-and-bridge alloy?** Phosphate

8. **List at least three approaches to altering the fit of a casting.**
   a. Increased colloidal silica for phosphate-bonded systems, increased ethyl silicate for ethyl silicate system—both increase expansion
   b. Hygroscopic technique (phosphate)
   c. Higher burnout temperatures
   d. Increased soak time
   e. Modification of the grain size of the investment
   f. Alteration of the basic mineral composition of the investment, ie, more cristobalite or increased glass content

9. **What might be an advantage of a mixed colloidal silica–ethyl silicate system?**
   a. Lower setting shrinkage (possible expansion) than a straight ethyl silicate system.
   b. Smoother casting surfaces without the need for pattern precoats, because the fine colloidal silica yields a loss of refractory capability, causing sintering of particles on the mold cavity surface.

10. **A carbon-filled and a noncarbon-filled phosphate investment are available to you for casting ceramic alloys. Which would you use (and why) for casting: a gold alloy or a nonprecious alloy?** Use a properly burned out carbon-filled investment for each alloy. However, if the investment is made by a laboratory, this control is difficult. A carbon mold for the gold alloy reduces oxides on the casting.

    For the nonprecious alloy, a noncarbon investment would be advised if control of burnout is difficult, since carbon can interact rapidly with the nonprecious alloys. This may reduce the strength of the PFM bond and could also increase hardness of a nickel alloy.

Recommended reading

Chase MW, et al (eds). JANAF Thermochemical Tables. Vol 14, Suppl #1. National Bureau of Standards, American Chemical Society, and American Institute of Physics, 1985.

Kondic V. Metallurgical Principles of Foundry. Amsterdam: Elsevier, 1960;193.

Miyazaki T, Tamaki Y. Current situation of investment materials for casting of titanium, QDT (extra issue): 25–30, 1993 (in Japanese).

Okuda R, Satou H, Satou M, Matsui A. Assessment of an experimental investment specified for titanium casting by the observation of the castings. Dent Jpn 28:71–83, 1991.

Takahashi J. Can we use phosphate-bonded silica investment for casting pure titanium? QDT (extra issue):24, 1993 (in Japanese).

Takahashi J, Kimura H, Lautenschlager EP, Lin JHC, Moser JB, Greener EH. Casting pure titanium into commercial phosphate-bonded SiO_2 investment molds. J Dent Res 69(112):1800–1805, 1990.

Togaya T. Selection of investments for improving fits of titanium castings. Shika Gikou 21(9):909–917, 1993 (in Japanese).

Togaya T, Suzuki M, Ida K, Nakamura M, Uemura T. Studies on magnesia investment for casting of titanium—improvement of fitness on castings by utilizing an expansion due to oxidation of additive Zr powder in the investment. J Dent Mater 4(4):344–349, 1985.

Chapter 19

Base Metal Casting Alloys

Chromium-containing base metal casting alloys have been used in dentistry for almost 70 years. The attractiveness of these materials stems from their corrosion resistance, high strength and modulus of elasticity (stiffness), low density, and low cost.

Chromium-type alloys are the principal materials used in the fabrication of removable partial denture frameworks, and they enjoy wide use in fixed prosthodontic procedures. Alloys of similar composition to those used in removable and fixed dental restorations are available for use in dental, maxillofacial, dental, and orthopedic implants. Figure 19-1 indicates which chromium-containing alloys are recommended for these procedures.

Partial denture alloys

Alloys based on cobalt or nickel and containing a substantial amount of chromium are suitable for the construction of removable partial denture frameworks, full denture bases, and temporary toothborne surgical and periodontal splints. Table 19-1 shows the base metal partial denture alloys that are currently available commercially.

Cobalt-chromium

The major constituents of most available materials are about 60% cobalt and 25% to 30% chromium, which

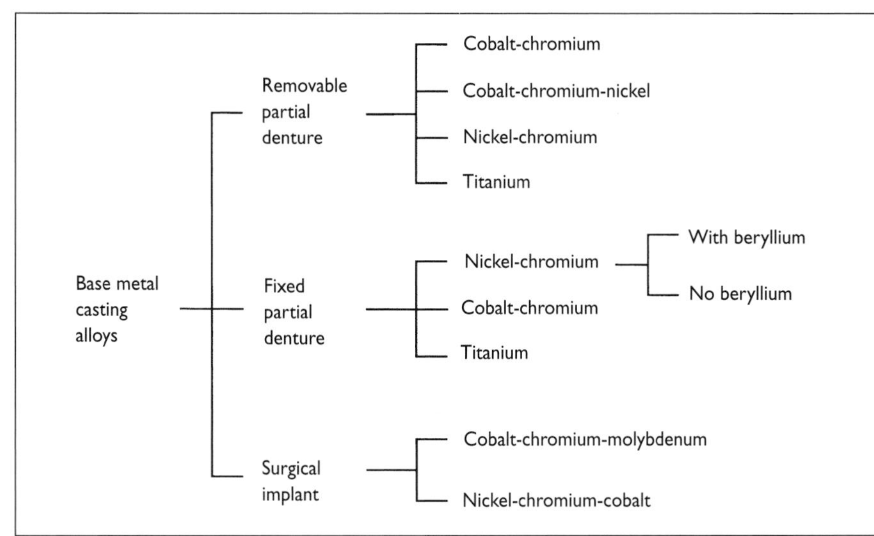

Fig 19-1 A classification of base metal casting alloys.

Table 19-1 Chromium-type partial denture alloys

Alloy	Manufacturer
Vitallium	Austenal Dental, Inc.
Vitallium 2	Austenal Dental, Inc.
Dentorium	Dentorium Products Co., Inc.
Regalloy	Dentsply International, Inc.
JD Alloy: LG Alloy	J.F. Jelenko & Co.
Neoloy "N" Partial Alloy-Regular	Neoloy Products, Inc.
Nobilium Alloy	Nobilium/American Gold
Ticonium Premium 100*	Ticonium Co.
Premium Hard	Ticonium Co.
Master Tech	Williams Dental Co., Inc.

*Nickel-chromium based alloy.

impart corrosion resistance. They may also contain minor quantities of molybdenum, aluminum, tungsten, iron, gallium, copper, silicon, carbon, and platinum. Manganese and silicon enhance fluidity of the molten alloys, and molybdenum, tungsten, and carbon are the principal hardening and strengthening elements.

Cobalt-chromium-nickel

The base of one variant of the cobalt-chromium system consists of about 50% cobalt, 25% chromium, 19% nickel, and minor components that are found in other cobalt-based products. However, the variant's molybdenum level of about 3.7% and carbon level of about 0.2% are significantly lower than those of the more conventional cobalt-chromium alloys.

Nickel-chromium

One representative proprietary nickel-chromium alloy contains about 70% nickel and 16% chromium. Important minor components are about 2% aluminum and 0.5% beryllium. Aluminum and nickel form an intermetallic compound (Ni_3Al) that contributes to strength and hardness, and beryllium lowers the melting range, enhances fluidity, and improves grain structure. Other minor elements include molybdenum, tungsten, manganese, cobalt, silicon, and carbon.

Physical properties

Melting temperatures of the base metal partial denture alloys are significantly higher than those of dental golds; a fusion temperature range of 1,399° to 1,454°C (2,550° to 2,650°F) is common. Polished cobalt-chromium and nickel-chromium prostheses are lustrous and silvery white. Chromium-type casting alloys are lighter than their gold alloy counterparts. Densities of the cobalt-chromium and nickel-chromium materials lie between 8 and 9 g/cm^3. Lightweight materials are especially useful for the construction of large and bulky maxillary removable appliances. Linear casting shrinkage is relatively high, 2.05% to 2.33%.

Mechanical properties

Chromium-containing partial denture alloys are about 30% harder than Type IV golds. Usually, indentation hardness is measured on the Rockwell superficial hardness scale (R-30N), and a Vickers (diamond pyramid) number of 370 is typical. Appliances cast from alloys exhibiting such hardness values must be finished and polished with special laboratory equipment.

Ultimate tensile strength values range from 90,000 to 120,000 psi (621 to 828 MPa). Values for yield strength fall between 60,000 to 90,000 psi (414 and 621 MPa) and are comparable to the yield strengths of Type IV golds. When comparing yield strengths of base metals with those of golds, the amount of offset (0.1% or 0.2%) used in analysis of stress-strain diagrams must be the same for both types of materials. Use of a 0.2% offset in the evaluation of base metals is common; resulting values may be as much as 10% higher than those obtained with a 0.1% offset.

The modulus of elasticity (stiffness) of cast base metal alloys is approximately twice that of cast dental gold alloys. Thus, under a given load within the elastic limit, a structure cast from a chromium type alloy will be deflected only half as much as a structure of comparable thickness cast from a gold alloy. Modulus of elasticity values of the cobalt-chromium and nickel-chromium partial denture alloys approach 30 million psi (207 GPa).

Chromium-type alloys are quite brittle. Elongation values are dependent upon casting temperature and mold conditions. Available cobalt-chromium alloys exhibit elongation values of 1% to 2%, whereas cobalt-chromium-nickel alloy, which contains lesser amounts of molybdenum and carbon than the other cobalt-based materials, shows an elongation of 10%.

The mechanical properties of cobalt-chromium-based partial denture alloys can be neither improved nor controlled by heat treatment. On the other hand, the strength and ductility of some nickel-chromium alloys can be altered markedly by high-temperature heat treatment. A softening treatment (15 minutes at 982°C [1,800°F] followed by water quenching) may be used to improve workability, and subsequent rehardening (15 minutes at 704°C [1,300°F] followed by water quenching) will increase the toughness of dental castings.

Chemical properties

Clinical experience has shown that partial denture alloys containing a total of no less than 85% by weight chromium, cobalt, and nickel exhibit a reasonable degree of intraoral corrosion resistance. The surfaces of these alloys are made passive in air by the spontaneous development of a thin, transparent, and contiguous chromium oxide film. The presence of the protective film reduces the corrosion rate to a relatively low level. Chromium-containing alloys are attacked vigorously by chlorine; household bleaches should not be used for cleaning appliances made from chromium-type alloys.

Manipulation

Alloys melting above 1,300°C (2,372°F) should not be cast in gypsum investments. High-fusing alloys require the use of ethyl silicate– or phosphate-bonded investment materials. These investments preclude the possibility of harmful sulfonation of the cast alloy, which could occur upon breakdown of a conventional gypsum (calcium sulfate dihydrate) investment. The thermal expansion of ethyl silicate– and phosphate-bonded investments compensates, in part, for the relatively high linear casting shrinkage of cobalt-chromium alloys. The manufacturer of one high-fusing nickel-chromium partial denture alloy suggests that this product be cast into molds made from a special oxalate-protected gypsum-bonded investment.

Entrapped gases can produce voids in large castings. Care must be exercised to ensure adequate spruing and mold venting, complete wax elimination, and proper melting and casting practices to facilitate the escape of mold gases.

High-temperature equipment (oxygen/acetylene, oxygen/natural gas, or electric induction) is required. An induction melting unit equipped with an optical pyrometer provides the most reliable means for attaining proper melting and casting temperatures. Oxidation of the metal and the formation of embrittling nitrides must be avoided.

Casting temperatures affect the microstructure and mechanical properties of chromium-type alloys. Excessive temperatures and overheating can lead to the production of casting porosity and interaction between the alloy and constituents of the investment.

Simple "broken-arm" machines are not recommended for the centrifugal casting of lightweight, base metal removable partial denture frameworks. The most satisfactory results are obtained with more complex equipment that allows for adjustment and control of acceleration, centrifugal force, and speed.

Cast molds should be set aside and bench cooled to room temperature before further handling. Investment molds can be cleaved with a small pneumatic mallet for retrieval of the castings. Oxide coatings and remnants of investment should be removed by liquid honing or abrasive blasting, rather than by "pickling" in mineral acids.

High hardness and strength make necessary the use of high-speed laboratory equipment for sprue removal and grinding and finishing operations. Special stones and abrasive wheels are available.

Disadvantages

Allergic responses to the constituents of base metal alloys, especially nickel, are observed occasionally. Most adverse tissue reactions attributed to the wearing of a base metal removable prosthesis, however, are manifestations of improper design or poor fit.

Although certain physical and mechanical features of the chromium-type alloys are superior to those of partial denture golds, clinical application of the chromium-containing materials may be burdened by the following occurrences:

1. Clasps cast from relatively nonductile base metal alloys can break in service; some break within a short period of time.
2. Minor but necessary adjustments required upon delivery of a base metal partial denture can be made difficult by the alloy's high hardness and

Table 19-2 Chromium-type crown-and-bridge alloys

Alloy	Manufacturer	Major elements	Contains beryllium
Vera Bond	Aalba-Dent, Inc.	Ni-Cr	Yes
Vera Soft	Aalba-Dent, Inc.	Ni-Cr	Yes
Beta	Amp-Sterngold	Ni-Cr-Mo	Yes
Microbond NP2*	Austenal Dental, Inc.	Ni-Cr-Ga	No
Vi-Comp	Austenal Dental, Inc.	Co-Cr-Mo	No
Calloy	California Dental Products, Inc.	Co-Cr	No
Calloy 1210	California Dental Products, Inc.	Ni-Cr	No
Biobond II	Dentsply International, Inc.	Ni-Cr-V	Yes
Neptune	Jeneric Industries, Inc.	Ni-Cr-Mo	No
Novarex	Jeneric Industries, Inc.	Co-Cr-W	No
Rex V	Jeneric Industries, Inc.	Ni-Cr-Mo	Yes
Rexalloy	Jeneric Industries, Inc.	Ni-Cr-Mo	No
Rexillium III	Jeneric Industries, Inc.	Ni-Cr-Mo	Yes
Crown Cast*	Jeneric Industries, Inc.	Co-Cr-Si	No
Albond	Jensen Industries, Inc.	Ni-Cr-Mo	No
Unitbond	Jensen Industries, Inc.	Ni-Cr-Mo	Yes
Neobond II	Neoloy Products, Inc.	Co-Cr-W	No
Neobond II Special	Neoloy Products, Inc.	Co-Cr-W	No
NPX III*	Nobilium/American Gold	Ni-Cr	Yes
NuPent	Pentron Corp.	Co-Cr-W	No
Pent V	Pentron Corp.	Ni-Cr-Mo	Yes
Pentillium	Pentron Corp.	Ni-Cr-Mo	Yes
PNP	Pentron Corp.	Ni-Cr-Mo	No
Safety Bond	Pentron Corp.	Ni-Cr-Mo	No
Wonder White*	Pentron Corp.	Co-Cr-Si	No
T-3*	Ticonium Co.	Ni-Cr	Yes
Ticon*	Ticonium Co.	Ni-Cr	Yes
Servalloy	United Dental Service	Ni-Cr-Mo	Yes
Ultra NP	Unitek Corp.	Ni-Cr	No
Ultra 100	Unitek Corp.	Co-Cr	No
Will-Ceram Litecast B	Williams Dental Gold Co., Inc.	Ni-Cr-Mo	Yes
Will-Ceram Litecast	Williams Dental Gold Co., Inc.	Ni-Cr-Mo	No

*Not used with fused porcelain.

strength, and accompanying low elongation. Such adjustments consume inordinate amounts of the dentist's valuable chair time.

3. High hardness of the alloy can cause excessive wear of restorations or natural teeth that contact the cast framework.

Crown-and-bridge alloys

Castings of chromium-containing alloys are used as substructures for porcelain-veneered fixed restorations and, to a lesser extent, as all-metal restorations. Numerous varieties of chromium-type alloys are available for crown-and-bridge applications. They are listed in Table 19-2.

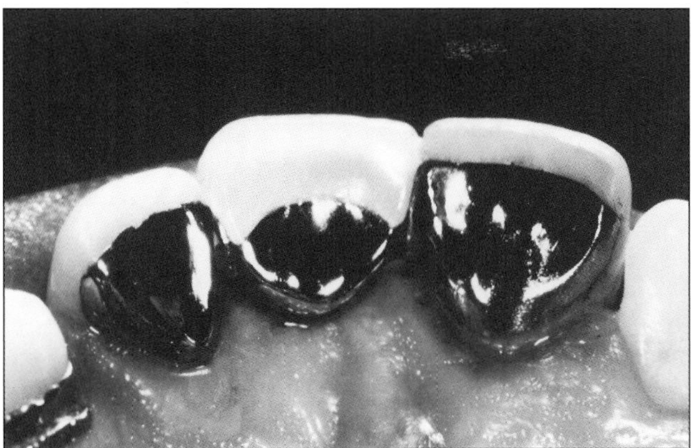

Fig 19-2 A Maryland bridge with abutments bonded to enamel. (Courtesy of Dr. Van P. Thompson.)

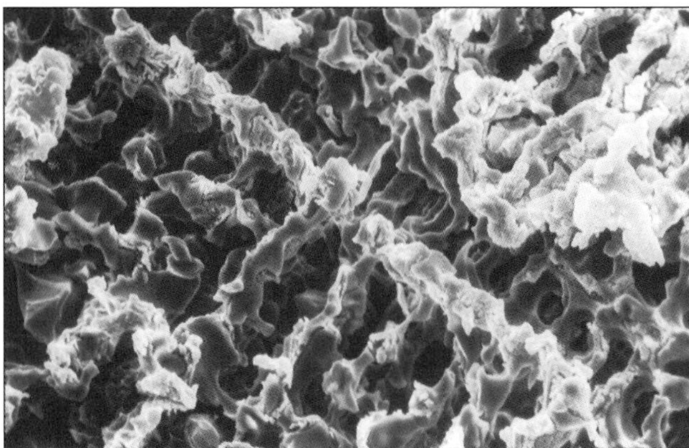

Fig 19-3 The microstructure of an etched Ni-Cr-Mo-Al-Be alloy showing dendritic structure. (Courtesy of Dr. Van P. Thompson.)

Minor compositional differences can produce significant variations in the microstructures and properties of chromium-type crown-and-bridge alloys. So previous experience with one commercial product cannot be used to predict the handling characteristics and clinical behavior of another.

Nickel-chromium alloys

Available nickel-chromium products contain 62% to 82% nickel and 11% to 22% chromium. Common minor constituents are molybdenum, aluminum, manganese, silicon, cobalt, gallium, iron, niobium, titanium, and zirconium. Beryllium, in amounts ranging from 0.5% to 2% by weight, is a constituent of several commercial alloys.

The ease with which certain nickel-chromium alloys can be etched electrochemically has led to the wide clinical use of resin-bonded fixed prostheses known as "Maryland bridges." A Maryland bridge is shown in Fig 19-2.

Electrochemical etching creates a large bonding area for a composite resin and thereby precludes the concentration of occlusal stresses in narrow tags of luting medium that protrude from perforated frameworks. Also, etching minimizes exposure of the resin luting medium to untoward events that may lead to abrasion or microleakage between the resin and the metal framework. The etched surface of a chromium-type crown-and bridge-alloy is shown in Fig 19-3.

Cobalt-chromium alloys

Typically, these products contain about 53% to 65% cobalt and about 27% to 32% chromium. Some members of the cobalt-chromium alloy family contain 2% to 6% molybdenum. Other minor components include tungsten, iron, copper, silicon, tin, manganese, and ruthenium, a platinum group metal.

Properties

Melting ranges of the nickel-chromium and cobalt-chromium alloys are between 1,232° and 1,454°C (2,250° and 2,650°F). When polished, the surfaces of nickel-chromium and cobalt-chromium castings are lustrous and silvery white. These alloys are light, with densities slightly greater than 8 g/cm^3.

Available chromium-type alloys for casting single- and multiple-unit fixed restorations offer broad ranges of hardness and strength. Most, however, are harder and stronger than their noble metal crown-and-bridge counterparts. Typical Rockwell and Vickers hardness values are in the vicinity of 50 and 300, respectively. Ultimate tensile strength ranges from 80,000 to 150,000 psi (552 to 1,034 MPa), and yield strength is between 32,000 and 110,000 psi (221 and 779 MPa).

Modulus of elasticity values are close to 30 million psi (207 GPa). High stiffness coupled with relatively high yield strength suggests the usefulness of chromium-type alloys for the fabrication of long-span fixed prostheses. The elongation of most chromium-containing crown-and-bridge alloys is low (2% to 3%).

Measured bond strengths of many base metal–porcelain combinations are comparable to those of noble alloy–porcelain couples. Nonetheless, bonding of porcelain to some chromium-type products is inhibited by thick oxides that accrue on the underlying cast framework.

Some nickel-chromium and cobalt-chromium alloys have higher in vitro corrosion rates than dental golds. The clinical significance of this finding, however, is not known.

Manipulation

The alloys' high melting and casting temperatures mandate the use of phosphate-bonded investments. Burnout temperatures of 732° to 927°C (1,350° to 1,700°F) are employed, with 815°C (1,500°F) being the most popular temperature.

The thermal expansion of some available "high-heat" investments does not compensate adequately for the casting shrinkage of chromium-type crown-and-bridge alloys. Often, copings and crowns tend to be undersized. Many of the problems encountered in the adjustment and seating of undersized, tight-fitting copings and crowns, however, can be obviated by the judicious use of a so-called die spacer.

High-temperature equipment (acetylene/oxygen, natural gas/oxygen, or electric induction) is required for melting. Oxides that form during heating of the alloy prevent coalescing of the molten ingots. After casting, the lightweight oxides formed upon melting the alloy will remain in the crucible as slag.

High hardness and strength necessitate the use of high-speed laboratory engines and special abrasive disks and stones for sprue removal and finishing. The use of inappropriate equipment and metal removing instruments is time-consuming and ineffective.

The refractory oxides that form on chromium-type alloys, especially those containing beryllium, make soldering a difficult task. Solder joints exposed to high masticatory forces are unreliable. Thus, care should be exercised in the design of fixed prostheses to make possible the use of one-piece castings whenever possible.

Surface preparation of substrate castings is critical. The porcelain-bearing surface of the cast framework must be ground and finished with successively finer ceramic-bonded aluminum oxide stones. The use of resin-bonded disks and other resin-bonded metal removal devices may deposit a resin-rich layer of debris on the metal's bonding surface, which may preclude the future development of the proper surface oxide.

The ground surfaces of the framework should be pressure blasted with clean, unrecycled fine-grit aluminum oxide until all scratches made by grinding are obliterated. Then the framework must be cleaned ultrasonically in an industrial detergent. The use of household detergents for the cleaning of cast frameworks should be avoided because they tend to bleach unwanted surface debris rather than facilitate its removal.

After cleaning, the frameworks should be transferred with a hemostat to a beaker containing deionized water and rinsed ultrasonically. All subsequent handling of the cleaned and rinsed framework must be accomplished with a clean metallic instrument to prevent contamination of the bonding surface by organic materials.

Manufacturers' instructions regarding thermal conditioning ("desorbing" or "degassing"), choice of porcelain, and fusion procedure should be followed explicitly.

Biologic effects

The biocompatibility of chromium-type alloys, especially those that contain nickel, is controversial. Whereas some researchers report no allergic responses to nickel-containing crown-and-bridge alloys, even in known nickel-sensitive patients, others report a high incidence of adverse response in similar patients.

The high incidence of malignant neoplastic disease of the lung and nasal sinuses found among workers engaged in the production of nickel alloys is well documented. Similarly, nickel is known to produce sarcoma when implanted subdermally in Wistar rats.

To date, however, neither substantial data nor clinical experience unequivocally contraindicates the use of nickel-based crown-and-bridge alloys. Conversely, the lack of sufficient, appropriate, and reliable long-term biologic data has precluded definite demonstration of the safety of these materials. Until the potential risks associated with nickel-containing alloys are better understood, care should be taken to avoid inhalation of nickel-containing dust, and caution should be exercised in using nickel alloys in restorations for nickel-sensitive patients.

Dusts from grinding beryllium-containing alloys should be avoided. Work areas should be equipped

Table 19-3 Mechanical properties of surgical alloys*

Property	Cobalt-chromium	Nickel-chromium-cobalt
Tensile strength (psi)	130,000	68,000
Yield strength† (psi)	100,000	48,000
Proportional limit (psi)	69,000	38,000
Modulus of elasticity ($\times 10^6$ psi)	36	29
Elongation (%)	2	20
Hardness (R-30N)	54	19

*After Civjan et al (1972).
†0.2% offset.

with adequate air-exchange systems and kept free from dust. Additionally, laboratory personnel should be equipped with individual respirators.

Advantages and disadvantages

The nickel-chromium alternatives to noble crown-and-bridge alloys offer high strength, stiffness, and hardness at a seemingly low cost. Nonetheless, some significant disadvantages accompany their selection and clinical application. High hardness complicates occlusal adjustment, polishing, restoration removal, and endodontic opening. Usually, laboratory labor is more costly for base metal fixed restorations than for noble alloy restorations because the former's properties and technique sensitivities increase working time. Often, material cost savings are negated by increased labor costs.

Surgical alloys

Presently, most permanent dental implants are being machined from highly biocompatible, commercially pure titanium. Nonetheless, chromium-type casting alloys exhibiting a sufficient degree of electropassivity are available for use in bone surgery as plates, screws, intermedullary bars and trays, and posts for anchorage of fixed and removable dental prostheses.

Two alloy systems are available. One is based on about 60% cobalt and 32% chromium (Vitallium, Austenal Dental, Inc.); the other contains about 54% nickel, 25% chromium, and 15% cobalt (Surgical Ticonium, Ticonium Co.).

Chromium-type surgical alloy systems employ about 4% molybdenum, 0.5% silicon, and 0.6% iron. Both contain manganese and carbon. For the cobalt-chromium–based alloy, however, the content of manganese (about 0.7%) and carbon (about 0.4%) are 24 and 30 times greater, respectively, than in the nickel-chromium-cobalt alloy.

Properties

Liquidus temperatures of chromium-type surgical alloys are in the vicinity of 1,554°C (2,650°F). When highly polished, the surfaces of cast surgical devices are lustrous and silvery white. Most implant devices, however, are left with a dull matte finish. The surgical alloys are light; their densities (about 8 g/cm^3) are comparable to those of chromium-type partial denture alloys.

Commercially available chromium-type surgical alloys offer a wide choice of mechanical properties as outlined in Table 19-3.

Chemically, these alloys are not inert. However, in vivo and in vitro testing has shown that these materials are more resistant to corrosion than many stainless steels used as implants. Insertion of cast-screws and pins requires the use of instruments made from the same alloy to prevent corrosion by the interaction of dissimilar metals.

Manipulation

The same factors that are important to the proper handling of chromium-containing partial denture alloys need to be considered with respect to the selection of investment materials, melting and casting techniques, and finishing procedures for chromium-type surgical grade alloys.

Biologic effects

Implanted metallic bodies can stimulate both generic and specific local responses. A generic response is evidenced by fibrous encapsulation of the implant. This reaction may be a manifestation of rejection or merely a reparative response to surgical trauma. Specific responses are induced by identifiable chemical, physical, and mechanical factors.

Chemical responses are traceable to corrosion of the implant. Regardless of alleged corrosion resistance, any metal or alloy placed in contact with tissue will exhibit some degree of ionization or solubility. The severity of a chemical response is related directly to the concentration of metal ions released into the tissue. Ions present in local tissues can be transported to various distant organs, particularly the lungs, liver, and spleen, regardless of the implant site.

Mass, size, and configuration of the implant device can influence biologic tolerance. The availability of casting alloys suitable for implantation has encouraged the use of massive forms with greater surface areas. Large surface areas create potential spaces at implant-tissue interfaces, which can be transformed into adventitious bursae. Large metallic implants are more likely to elicit signs of clinical failure than are smaller ones.

Sharp edges and protuberances can injure intervening soft tissue. Movement of the implant resulting from improper stabilization may produce painful bursae and decubitus ulcers.

The formation of an adventitious bursa is an early sign of implant rejection. Continued irritation by corrosion or movement can cause pain, swelling, and necrosis, thereby necessitating removal of the implant. Complete rejection is manifested by the formation of fistulae or by frank extrusion.

Advantages and disadvantages

The availability of surgical casting alloys makes possible the on-site preoperative construction of customized replacements for various parts of the mandible and the facial bones. Cobalt-chromium-molybdenum, the most commonly used chromium-type surgical alloy, is especially suited for the management of situations with high strength requirements. On the other hand, the nickel-chromium-cobalt–based material offers good ductility and lower hardness and yield strength. These features may facilitate adjustment or shaping often required during the insertion of cast implant devices.

Over the years, problems associated with surgical alloy-tissue interaction have catalyzed the search for alloplasts exhibiting a greater degree of inertness. Today, the need for this desirable feature in a dental endosteal implant is being met by the remarkable metal, titanium.

Commercially pure titanium

The following features make commercially pure (c.p.) titanium an attractive alternative to chromium-type partial denture and crown-and-bridge alloys: low cost, low density, nonstrategic geopolitical status, mechanical properties that resemble those of hard and extra hard casting golds, high corrosion resistance, and remarkable biocompatibility.

"Commercially pure" disclaims 100% purity and acknowledges that small amounts of oxygen (0.18% to 0.40% by weight) and iron (0.20% to 0.50% by weight) are combined with titanium. On the basis of varying oxygen and iron contents, c.p. titanium is obtainable in four different grades.

Titanium crowns, multiple-unit fixed restorations, and removable partial denture frameworks are being cast in research laboratories and in a few commercial dental laboratories. Irrefutable is the proposition that recent improvements in melting and casting technologies and mold fabrication procedures make feasible the production of titanium dental devices.

Nonetheless, missing from the titanium puzzle is a keystone cadre of titanium users with the hands-on experience needed to develop definitive, cost-effective solutions to problems encountered in casting a low density (4.5 g/cm^3) metal that melts at temperatures in the vicinity of 1,700°C (3,092°F); possesses a strong affinity for oxygen, hydrogen, and nitrogen; and reacts with the components of most investment materials. These factors reduce casting efficiency by adversely affecting the filling of molds with molten metal and the soundness of castings.

Intolerable macro- and microporosity are frequently observed features of dental restorations cast from titanium. Often, an inordinate amount of difficulty is experienced in producing a relatively thin casting. To make a suitable titanium coping for a porcelain-metal restoration, the pattern is usually waxed to a thickness of about 0.6 mm. This practice makes necessary the machining of the resultant casting to the desired thickness. When heated in air at temperatures in the vicinity of 750°C (1,382°F), titanium becomes embrittled through the absorption of oxygen, hydrogen, and nitrogen. Such embrittlement may cause thin margins of restorations to fracture during burnishing.

When heated at temperatures below 800°C (1,472°F) for short periods, titanium of high purity or commercial purity forms a compact, adherent oxide scale. At higher temperatures and extended periods of heat treatment, however, titanium forms a porous and poorly adherent scale.

During a few successive firings of a low fusing (750°C), low expansion (= 7.1 x 10^{-6}/°C on cooling) porcelain to titanium, the smooth adherent oxide produced on degassing at 750°C thickens and becomes flaky. An oxide of this type precludes attainment of a reliable porcelain-to-metal bond.

Properties

At room temperature, the lattice configuration of virgin, c.p. titanium is hexagonal close-packed. This atomic arrangement known as alpha phase (α) persists until the metal is exposed to high temperatures. Upon reaching its transus temperature of 833°C (1,531°F), titanium's entire habit becomes cubic body-centered. This crystal lattice is known as beta (β) phase. Fabricated titanium structures consisting mainly of beta phase are stronger but less ductile than comparable structures with a dominant alpha (α) phase. So, to obtain consistently reproducible mechanical properties, the solidified metal's cooling rate and the time and temperature of subsequent heat treatments must be controlled.

The tensile strength and elongation of pure titanium are about 36,250 psi (250 MPa) and 50%, respectively. It is known, however, that seemingly slight variations in oxygen and iron content exert substantial and lasting effects on titanium's properties. Generally, as oxygen or iron content increases, strength increases and ductility decreases.

Furthermore, the consequences of titanium-oxygen interactions seem to vary according to melting and casting practices. When melted and cast with the use of an argon arc–centrifugal casting machine, yield strength (0.2% offset), ultimate tensile strength, and elongation for grade 1 c.p. titanium are about 84,000 psi (579 MPa), 101,600 psi (701 MPa), and 18%, respectively. Comparatively, castings made in an argon-tungsten arc vacuum pressure machine exhibit greater ductility (elongation = 31%), but yield strength and tensile strength fall to 11,300 psi (285 MPa) and 53,000 psi (365 MPa), respectively.

Titanium's elastic modulus of about 17 million psi (117 GPa) is higher than those of Type III and Type IV casting golds (~100 GPa), but lower than those of most chromium-type alloys (171 to 218 GPa). The Vickers hardness of cast c.p. titanium is 210.

Titanium alloys

Presently, titanium alloys are not being used in the United States for the commercial production of fixed or removable dental prostheses. Nevertheless, a high level of interest in such alloys exists within the dental research community. Titanium alloys of interest include Ti-30Pd, Ti-20 Cu, Ti-15V, and Ti-6Al-4V.

Alloying other metals with titanium enables attainment of the benefits of lower melting and casting temperatures. Also, it provides a means to stabilize, or expand, either the alpha phase field or the beta phase field. In Ti-13Nb-13Zr, niobium and zirconium expand the beta phase field by decreasing the (alpha + beta) transus temperature. Conversely, in Ti-6Al-4V, aluminum is an alpha stabilizer because it increases the (alpha + beta) to beta transformation temperature and thereby expands the alpha phase field.

Accordingly, Ti-13Nb-13Zr is a near-beta alloy with a substantially lower beta transus (735°C) than Ti-6 Al-4 V (1,000°C) which has an (alpha + beta) structure.

The effects of interactions with atmospheric gases during melting, casting, and other high-temperature laboratory procedures are as devastating to titanium alloys as they are to unalloyed titanium. Thus, the problems encountered in producing cast dental restorations from titanium alloys are not unlike those experienced with titanium of high or commercial purity.

Properties

The ultimate tensile strength, 0.2% offset yield strength, and modulus of elasticity of various titanium alloys range from 101,500 to 142,800 psi (700 to 985

MPa); 81,200 to 124,700 psi (560 to 860 MPa); and 16 million to 17 million psi (110 to 117 GPa), respectively. Except for modulus of elasticity, the tensile properties of titanium alloys are quite similar to those of chromium-type alloys.

Biologic effects

The corrosion resistance and biocompatibility of titanium at room, oral, and body temperatures are attributed to the formation of a stable oxide film with a thickness of less than 1 nm (10^{-9} meter). If the film is scratched or abraded, the involved area repassivates within a few nanoseconds (10^{-9} seconds). At high temperatures, the oxide film is not protective because it thickens and becomes nonadherent.

Numerous reports document the superior biocompatibility of titanium. The reaction of tissue that contacts titanium or its alloys, Ti-6Al-4V and Ti-13Nb-13Zr, is extremely mild, and direct bone ingrowth or osseointegration does occur. See Chapter 23 for further information on osseointegration with titanium.

Titanium's remarkable biocompatibility perpetuates the insatiable desire to develop simple, reliable, and reasonably priced technology that would make possible in any dental laboratory the routine production of titanium dental restorations. Perhaps this desire will be fulfilled not by further modification of melting and casting-art practices, but by exploitation of computer-aided design (CAD) and computer-aided manufacturing (CAM). These technologies are being used routinely to produce customized titanium-valvular and titanium-hip prostheses.

Glossary

adventitious bursa Fluid-filled cyst formed between two parts as a result of friction.

base metal alloy An alloy composed of metals that are neither precious nor noble.

decubitus ulcer Superficial loss of tissue on the surface of skin or mucosa, usually with inflammation, caused by pressure.

embrittlement To render susceptible to breakage under slight bending.

ethyl silicate investment A silica refractory bonded by hydrolysis of ethyl silicate in the presence of hydrochloric acid.

generic tissue response A reaction that cannot be attributed to a specific characteristic of a foreign body or substance.

implant Material inserted into intact tissues of a host.

intermedullary Between bone marrow spaces.

intermetallic compound A definite combination by weight between metals. These compounds have specific, reproducible physical characteristics.

low-fusing alloys Alloys molten below 1,315 °C (2,400 °F) and that may be cast in a special gypsum investment.

optical pyrometer A device to measure temperature by matching the color of an electrically heated wire to the color of the surface being tested. The current required is calibrated against temperature.

phosphate-bonded investment Used in casting high-melting alloys. Contains a mixture of silica with a metallic oxide and a phosphate that combine to bind the silica together. On heating, forms complex silicophosphates that increase the strength.

Rockwell superficial hardness scale (R-30N) An indication of resistance to penetration of balls or metal cones of differing diameters under different loads.

specific tissue response A reaction caused by a definite characteristic of a foreign body or substance.

Discussion questions

1. What are the biocompatibility problems associated with high nickel alloys?
2. What are the advantages and disadvantages of Ni-Cr alloys for porcelain-fused-to-metal restorations?
3. Compare the relative clinical advantages and disadvantages of gold and Co-Cr alloys for partial dentures.
4. What are the advantages and disadvantages of titanium as porcelain-fused-to-metal crown and bridge alloys?

Questions and answers

1. **What are the three major types of chromium-containing dental casting alloys?** The chromium-type dental casting alloys include cobalt-chromium, nickel-chromium, and cobalt-chromium-nickel.
2. **How do the mechanical properties of chromium-type crown-and-bridge alloys differ from those of dental gold alloys?** Most chromium-type alloys are harder and stronger than conventional gold crown-and-bridge alloys. Strength and hardness of some materials are comparable to those of chromium-type partial denture alloys.
3. **Which properties of the chromium-type alloys make these materials suitable for the fabrication of long-span bridges?** High modulus of elasticity (stiffness) and yield strength (resistance to permanent deformation) suggest the usefulness of chromium-type alloys for the fabrication of long-span fixed appliances.
4. **What effect do excessive surface oxides have on the bonding of porcelain to chromium-type alloys?** Excessive oxidation of substrate castings inhibits porcelain-to-metal bonding.
5. **How do the tensile properties of cast titanium alloys compare with those of chromium-type alloys?** The ultimate tensile strength, 0.2% offset yield strength, and modulus of elasticity of various titanium alloys range from 101,500 to 142,800 psi (700 to 985 MPa), 81,200 to 124,700 psi (560 to 860 MPa), and 16 million to 17 million psi (110 to 117 GPa), respectively. Except for modulus of elasticity, which is relatively low, the tensile properties of titanium alloys are quite similar to those of chromium-type alloys.

Partial denture alloys: true/false statements

1. **Certain minor components strengthen cobalt-chromium-based alloys.** True: Principal strengthening elements are molybdenum, tungsten, and carbon.
2. **The performance potential of cobalt-chromium castings is enhanced by nitride inclusions and excessive metallic carbides.** False: Nitride inclusions and excessive metallic carbides can cause alloy embrittlement.
3. **Low density is a useful characteristic of chromium-type partial denture alloys.** True: Low density makes chromium-type alloys especially useful for the fabrication of large maxillary appliances. Lighter devices are more resistant to displacement by gravitational forces and are, therefore, less likely to subject abutment teeth to unnecessary stresses.
4. **The hardness and strength of chromium-type partial denture alloys are essentially the same as those of type IV gold alloys.** False: Chromium-type partial denture alloys are about 30% harder than Type IV golds. Strengths of the chromium-type alloys and Type IV gold alloys, however, are comparable.

5. **In function, a chromium-type removable partial denture framework is more likely to flex than one cast from a Type IV gold.** False: The modulus of elasticity (stiffness) of chromium-type partial denture alloys is about twice that of the Type IV golds. Thus, sufficient stiffness can be obtained with the use of relatively thin chromium-type castings.
6. **Chromium-containing removable prostheses should be cleaned regularly in household bleaches.** False: Strong oxidizing agents should not be used for cleaning appliances fabricated from chromium-containing alloys.
7. **Gypsum investments are not recommended for the casting of cobalt-chromium alloys.** True: Ethyl silicate– or phosphate-bonded investments are required for the casting of alloys with fusion temperatures higher than 1,315°C (2,400°F).
8. **Casting temperatures for cobalt-chromium alloys must be controlled carefully.** True: Casting temperature affects microstructure and mechanical properties.
9. **Conventional laboratory equipment and techniques can be used to finish cobalt-chromium and nickel-chromium castings.** False: The alloys are very hard. Conventional equipment and procedures consume excessive amounts of time and are relatively ineffective.
10. **Sensitivity to one or more alloy components accounts for a significant incidence of adverse tissue response among wearers of chromium-type partial dentures.** False: Improper design and fit of chromium-type appliances are the major causes of adverse tissue reactions.

Crown-and-bridge alloys: true/false statements

1. **Chromium-containing crown-and-bridge alloys are based entirely upon the nickel-chromium system.** False: Chromium-type crown-and-bridge alloys employ the cobalt-chromium as well as the nickel-chromium system.
2. **The mechanical properties of the chromium-type crown-and-bridge alloys are slightly inferior to the properties of dental gold alloys.** False: Chromium-type alloys are harder and stronger than conventional gold crown-and-bridge alloys. Strength and hardness of some materials are comparable to those of chromium-type partial denture alloys.
3. **Certain properties of chromium-type alloys make them suitable for fabrication of long-span fixed restorations.** True: High modulus of elasticity (stiffness) and relatively high yield strength (resistance to permanent deformation) suggest the usefulness of chromium-type alloys for the fabrication of long-span fixed appliances.
4. **Except for modulus of elasticity, the tensile properties of some titanium alloys are comparable to those of chromium-type alloys.** True: The tensile strength and yield strength of some titanium alloys are similar to those of chromium-type crown-and-bridge alloys. When compared to chromium-type alloys, modulus of elasticity values for titanium alloys are relatively low.
5. **The ability of chromium-type alloys to form surface oxides when exposed to temperatures employed in the porcelain firing cycle ensures the development of a strong and reliable porcelain-to-metal bond.** False: Excessive oxidation of a substrate casting can inhibit porcelain-metal bonding.
6. **The biocompatibility of c.p. titanium, certain titanium alloys, and chromium-type crown-and-bridge alloys is well documented.** False: The biocompatibility of titanium and some titanium alloys is well documented, but the long-term biocompatibility of chromium-type crown-and-bridge alloys remains to be determined.

Surgical casting alloys: true/false statements

1. **The tensile properties and hardness of nickel-chromium-cobalt and cobalt-chromium surgical alloys are comparable.** False: The nickel-chromium-cobalt base alloy (Surgical Ticonium) is much softer and much more ductile. The cobalt-chromium–based material (Vitallium) is exceptionally strong and hard.
2. **Chemical factors alone influence tissue response to alloy implants.** False: Physical and mechanical factors also influence biologic tolerance to alloy implants.

3. **Metallic ions liberated from an alloy implant can be transported to distant organs.** True: The lungs, liver, and spleen are principal target organs for metallic ions.
4. **The surface area of a metallic implant plays a prominent role in biologic acceptance.** True: Large implants are more prone to failure than smaller ones. Large surface areas create spaces between the implant and the tissue that may be transformed into undesirable bursae.
5. **Certain clinical signs signal complete rejection of an implant device.** True: Complete rejection is characterized by development of fistulae or frank exposure of the implant.

Recommended reading

Chromium-type partial denture alloys

Asgar K, Techow BO, Jacobson JM. A new alloy for partial dentures. J Prosthet Dent 23:36, 1970.

Bates JF. Studies related to the fracture of partial dentures: flexural fatigue of a cobalt-chromium alloy. Br Dent J 118:532, 1965.

Carter JJ, Kidd JN. The precision casting of cobalt-chromium alloys. Part I. The influence of casting variables on dimensions and finish. Br Dent J 118:383, 1965.

Civjan S, et al. Effects of heat treatment on mechanical properties of two nickel-chromium based casting alloys. J Dent Res 51:1537, 1972.

Earnshaw R. Further measurements of the casting shrinkage of dental cobalt-chromium alloys. J Dent Res 39:1101, 1960.

Evitmore E, Aliksiera K. Some physical properties of the chrome-cobalt-molybdenum and nickel-chromium alloys. Stomatologija (Sofia) 48:18, 1966.

Osborne J. Improvement in cobalt-chromium alloys. Rev Belge Med Dent 21:303, 1966.

Paffenbarger GC, Caul HJ, Dickson G. Base metal alloys for oral restorations. J Am Dent Assoc 30:825, 1943.

Taylor DF, Leibfritz WA, Alder AG. Physical properties of cobalt-chromium alloys. J Am Dent Assoc 56:343, 1958.

Taylor TD, Morton TH Jr. Ulcerative lesions of the palate associated with removable partial denture castings. J Prosthet Dent 66:213, 1991.

Chromium-type crown-and-bridge alloys

American Dental Association; Council on Dental Materials, Instruments, and Equipment. Report on base metal alloys for crown and bridge applications: benefits and risks. J Am Dent Assoc 111:479, 1985.

Anusavice KJ, Shafagh I. Inert gas presoldering of nickel-chromium alloys. J Prosthet Dent 55:317, 1986.

Bertolotti RL. Alternative casting alloys for today's crown-and-bridge restorations. Part I. All metal restorations. J Calif Dent Assoc 11:37, 1983.

Huget EF, Dvivedi N, Cosner HE Jr. Properties of two nickel-chromium crown-and-bridge alloys for porcelain veneering. J Am Dent Assoc 94:87, 1977.

Huget EF, Vilca JM, Wall RM. Characterization of two ceramic-base metal alloys. J Prosthet Dent 40:637, 1978.

Livaditis GJ, Thompson VP. Etched castings: An improved retentive mechanism for resin-bonded retainers. J Prosthet Dent 47:52, 1982.

Moffa JP, et al. An evaluation of nonprecious alloys for use with porcelain veneers. Part II. Industrial safety and biocompatibility. J Prosthet Dent 30:432, 1973.

Moffa JP, Jenkins WA. Status report on base-metal crown and bridge alloys. J Am Dent Assoc 89:652, 1974.

Moffa JP. Physical and mechanical properties of gold and base metal alloys. Alternatives to Gold Alloys in Dentistry. US Department of Health, Education, and Welfare, Public Health Service, National Institutes of Health. DHEW publication no. (NIH) 77-1227, 1977; 81–87.

Morris HF, et al. Veterans Administration Cooperative Studies Project No. 14 7/242. Part VII: The mechanical properties of metal ceramic alloys as cast and after simulated porcelain firing. J Prosthet Dent 61:160, 1989.

Morris HF, et al. Casting alloys: The materials and the clinical effects. Advances in dental research (Effects and side effects of dental restorative materials). National Institutes of Health Technology Assessment Conference, National Institute of Dental Research, International Association for Dental Research. Vol 6. Washington DC: NIDR, 1991; 28–31.

Sandrick JL, et al. Biocompatibility of nickel-base dental alloys. Biomater Med Devices Artif Organs 2:31, 1974.

Sarkar NK, Greener EH. In vitro corrosion resistance of new dental alloys. Biomater Med Devices Artif Organs 1:121, 1973.

Sced IR, McLean JW. The strength of metal-ceramic bonds with base metals containing chromium. A preliminary report. Br Dent J 132:232, 1972.

Vermilyea SG, et al. Observations on nickel-free, beryllium-free alloys for fixed prostheses. J Am Dent Assoc 106:36, 1983.

Winkler S, Morris HF, Monterio JM. Changes in mechanical properties and microstructure following heat treatment of a nickel-chromium base alloy. J Prosthet Dent 52:821, 1984.

Chromium-type surgical alloys

Civjan S, et al. Properties of surgical casting alloys. J Prosthet Dent 28:77, 1972.

Cohen J. Corrosion of orthopaedic implants. J Bone Joint Surg 44:307, 1962.

Ferguson AB, et al. Characterization of trace ions released from embedded metal implants in the rabbit. J Bone Joint Surg 44:323, 1962.

Ferguson AB, et al. Metal ion concentration in the liver, spleen and lung of normal rabbits. J Bone Joint Surg 48:567, 1966.

Hicks JH, Carter WH. Minor reactions due to modern metal. J Bone Joint Surg 44:122, 1962.

Huget EF, Vermilyea SG. Base metal dental and surgical alloys. In DC Smith, DF Williams (eds). Biocompatibility of Dental Materials. Vol IV. Boca Raton, FL: CRC Press, Inc, 1982; 37–49.

Jergensen F. Metallic surgical implants—principles and mechanical factors. J Bone Joint Surg 46:401, 1964.

Mears DC. Electron-probe microanalysis of tissue and cells from implant areas. J Bone Joint Surg 48:567, 1966.

Pappas AM, Cohen J. Toxicity of metal particles in tissue culture. Part I. A new assay method using cell counts in the phase of replication. J Bone Joint Surg 50:535, 1968.

Titanium and titanium alloys

Adachi M, et al. Oxide adherence and porcelain bonding to titanium and Ti-6Al-4V alloy. J Dent Res 69:1230, 1990.

Albrektsson T, et al. Osseointegrated titanium implants. Acta Orthop Scand 52:155, 1981.

Davidson JA, Mishra AK, Kovacs PT. A new low-modulus, high-strength, biocompatible Ti-13Nb-13Zr Alloy for orthopaedic implants. Trans Soc Biomat, Vol. XVI, 145 (1993).

Donachie MJ (ed). Titanium. A Technical Guide. Metals Park, OH: ASM International, 1988; 11, 105.

Goodman SB, et al. The local and systemic response to cylinders of a low modulus titanium alloy (Ti-13Nb-13Zr) and a wear resistant zirconium alloy (Zr-25Nb) implanted in the rabbit tibia. Transactions of Society for biomaterials, Vol. XVI, 76 (1993).

Hamanaka H, et al. Dental casting of titanium and Ni-Ti alloys by a new casting machine. J Dent Res 68:1529, 1989.

Hero H, Syverud M, Waarli M. Mold filling and porosity in castings of titanium. Dent Mater 9:15, 1993.

Lintner F, Zweymuller K, Brand G. Tissue reactions to titanium endoprostheses. Autopsy studies in four cases. J Arthroplasty 1:183, 1986.

Lyman WS. Titanium, properties of pure metals. In Baker H, Benjamin D (eds). Metals Handbook. 9th ed. Vol 2. Metals Park, OH: ASM, 1979; 815.

Menis DL, Moser JB, Greener EH. Experimental porcelain compositions for application to cast titanium. J Dent Res 65(Abstr no. 1565):343, 1986.

Sunnerkrantz P, Syverud M, Hero H. Effects of casting atmosphere on the quality of Ti-crowns. Scand J Dent Res 98:268, 1990.

Chapter 20

Orthodontic Wires

In recent years, the orthodontic manufacturers have introduced new body-temperature shape-memory nickel-titanium wires, ion-implanted beta-titanium and nickel-titanium wires, and ceramic/plastic wires. The objective of this chapter is to provide information about the wide variety of orthodontic wires commercially available, in order to assist the clinician in making rational selections for patient treatment. A general classification of the alloy systems used for the metallic orthodontic wires is provided in Fig 20-1.

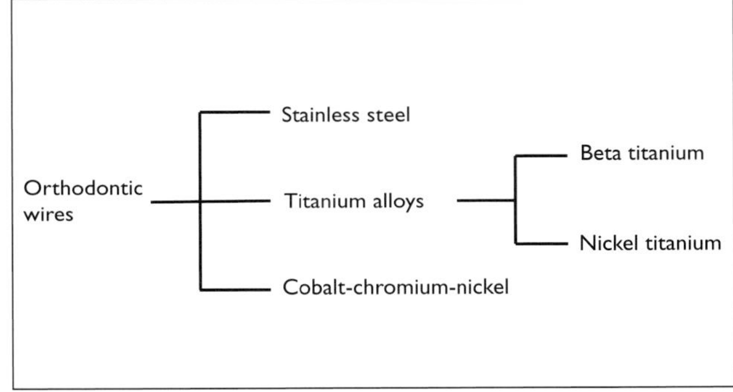

Fig 20-1 Classification of the alloy systems used for metallic orthodontic wires.

Mechanical properties

Manufacturing of orthodontic wires

Metallic orthodontic wires are manufactured by a series of proprietary steps, typically involving more than one company. Initially, the wire alloy is cast in the form of an ingot, which must be subjected to successive deformation stages, until the cross section becomes sufficiently small for wire drawing. Several deformation stages and intermediate heat treatments are required because considerable work hardening of the alloy occurs during wire manufacturing. Important proprietary details include the rate of drawing, the amount of cross-section reduction per pass, the nature of intermediate heat treatments, the die material and lubricant in contact with the wires, and the ambient atmosphere, which would be important for the reactive titanium-containing wire alloys. In general, the casting of the starting ingot and the initial mechanical deformation stages are not performed by the orthodontic materials companies that market the wires.

Whereas round orthodontic wires are manufactured by drawing through dies, rectangular cross-section wires are fabricated from round wires by a rolling process using a Turk's head, which contains pairs of rolls. The resulting rectangular or square cross-section wires will necessarily have some degree of rounding at the corners, which varies with the specific wire type and the manufacturer. This edge bevel can be of clinical significance for the actual torque delivered by the arch wire–bracket combination. Moreover, the surface roughness of the wire, which has a clinically significant effect on the arch wire–bracket sliding friction, varies considerably among the various products and is generally greater for the beta-titanium and nickel-titanium wires.

As a result of the wire-drawing sequence, orthodontic wires have a characteristic wrought microstructure. The original equiaxed grain structure of the starting cast ingot is completely eliminated, and when a polished and etched wire specimen is viewed through the optical or scanning electron microscope, the wrought grain structure appears as a series of closely spaced lines parallel to the original direction of drawing. It is well known that this microstructure is essential for an orthodontic wire to maintain the desired temper (springiness) or optimal mechanical properties for clinical use. For example, heat treatment of stainless steel wires at temperatures of 700°C (1,300°F) and higher causes rapid softening and loss of the wire structure due to recrystallization. Optimum heat treatments would involve only the recovery stage of annealing. In practice, clinicians perform heat treatments using electrical resistance (spot) welding apparatus, and the stainless steel, cobalt-chromium-nickel, and nickel-titanium wires may be advantageously heat treated.

The properties of a metallic orthodontic wire are thus derived from two principal origins. First, there are four general wire alloys in significant current use: austenitic stainless steel, cobalt-chromium-nickel, beta-titanium, and nickel-titanium. The basic alloy composition will determine the broad range of inherent general properties for each metal type. Second, the particular nature of the drawing, rolling, and other special processes, including heat treatments by the manufacturer and clinician, will have further significant effects on the specific wire properties and arch wire–bracket torque delivery characteristics.

In general, an orthodontist should consider the following aspects in the selection of wires: force delivery characteristics, elastic working range, ease of joining individual segments to fabricate more complex appliances, corrosion resistance and biocompatibility in the oral environment, and cost. In a practical sense, wire costs represent a significant concern for the clinician, and there is a considerable difference between stainless steel arch wires and beta-titanium and nickel-titanium arch wires. However, these more expensive alloys offer unique properties that should be carefully considered when selecting orthodontic wires.

Bending tests and mechanics principles

In order to understand the mechanical properties of primary importance when comparing different wire types and sizes, it is first necessary to review the underlying principles and terminology. Typically, the mechanical properties of orthodontic wires are determined from some type of bending test, because this mode of deformation is considered more representative of clinical conditions than the tension test conventionally used for metals. The cantilever bending test in American National Standards Institute/American Dental Association (ANSI/ADA) Specification no. 32 for orthodontic wires not containing precious metals has been strongly criticized, and the ANSI/ADA Specification Subcommittee is currently developing a new bending test that better simulates clinical interbracket distances and is more suitable for the very low elastic modulus nickel-titanium wires than the present test which uses the Olsen stiffness tester.

All bending tests involve the measurement of angular or linear deflection of an arch wire segment resulting from a bending moment or an applied force. The bending moment or force and the deflection are represented on the vertical and horizontal axes, respectively, of a graphic plot that is generally a straight line at the force levels for elastic deformation of clinical interest. The exception is when very short test spans are used. Although orthodontists typically activate wires somewhat into the permanent deformation range, the bending property concepts are based upon elastic deformation. Although clinical interest is obviously in the unloading characteristics of activated arch wires, investigators have generally determined mechanical properties during the initial loading stage. The elastic loading and unloading plots differ for the nickel-titanium orthodontic wires, although they do not differ for the other alloy types.

There are several basic mechanical properties of orthodontic wires that are determined from the bending test plot:

1. The *rate of force delivery* is the slope of the initial straight line and is the amount of force or bending moment required for unit activation. This property is termed the *stiffness* of the wire and is the inverse of the property of flexibility.
2. The *moment at yielding* is the bending moment that corresponds to a designated small amount of permanent deformation; for example, 2.9 degrees in the bending test for the ANSI/ADA specification. This property is analogous to the yield strength (*YS*) for the tension test, and the analogous value of stress in bending is termed the *flexural yield strength*.

3. The *maximum bending moment* considers the permanent deformation range (curved portion) of the bending plot. This property is less relevant for the clinician than the moment at yielding, because only elastic deformation is desired for tooth movement.
4. The maximum amount of elastic activation before the onset of permanent deformation is the value of linear or angular deflection corresponding to the maximum elastic force or moment. This property is known as the *elastic range* or *working range* of the wire.

Wire stiffness or elastic force delivery is dependent on two fundamental factors: (*1*) the composition and structure of the wire alloy, reflecting both the basic metallurgy and the manufacturing sequence, and (*2*) the wire segment geometry, that is, the cross-section shape and size and the segment length. The basic metallurgy contribution of the wire alloy is given by the modulus of elasticity (E), or Young's modulus, which relates tensile and compressive elastic stress and strain independent of the specimen cross-section area and length. The elastic modulus values determined from bending and tension tests should be the same, provided that the bending deformation is properly analyzed.

The resistance of a cross-section shape to elastic bending is given by the *moment of inertia* (I). For a round wire of diameter (d), the moment of inertia is given by

$$I = \frac{\pi d^4}{64}$$

whereas for a rectangular wire of width (w) and thickness (t) in the plane of bending,

$$I = \frac{wt^3}{12}$$

The stiffness of an arch wire is also proportional to the segment length (l), so that if the length is doubled the wire flexibility or elastic deflection will be doubled for the same applied force or bending moment. Summarizing these contributions, the elastic stiffness or force delivery characteristics are given by the following expressions:

$$\text{Round wire: } \frac{Ed^4}{l}$$

$$\text{Rectangular wire: } \frac{Ewt^3}{l}$$

There are two additional very useful mechanical properties for orthodontic wires, which are obtained by combining the basic mechanical properties previously discussed (Table 20-1):

1. The *modulus of resilience* or *resilience* is the area under the elastic force-activation plot and represents the total biomechanical energy per unit volume available for tooth movement when the wire is loaded to the maximum elastic stress or bending moment or, equivalently, unloaded from this level. The modulus of resilience for an orthodontic wire is usually written as $(YS)^2/2E$, as the yield strength is generally used to represent the onset of permanent deformation because of the difficulty in precisely locating the proportional limit (PL) on a bending test plot. The formal expression in materials science for the modulus of resilience is $(PL)^2/2E$. It follows that the resilience is much more strongly affected by changes in yield strength or proportional limit than elastic modulus, which is important for the heat treatment response of cobalt-chromium-nickel and stainless steel wires.
2. The *springback* for an arch wire after unloading is given by the expression YS/E, which is approximately equal to the maximum elastic strain or working range of the wire. (The formal expression from materials science for springback would be PL/E.) Since the unloading curve from the permanent deformation range for well-behaved orthodontic wire alloys (ie, other than nickel-titanium wires) is parallel to the elastic loading curve, the value of YS/E represents the approximate amount of elastic strain released by the arch wire on unloading.

Numerous articles listed in the references discuss the mechanics of bending tests for orthodontic wires.

Orthodontic wire alloys

Stainless steel

Stainless steel continues to be the most popular wire alloy for clinical orthodontics because of an outstanding combination of mechanical properties, corrosion resistance in the oral environment, and cost. The wires used

Table 20-1 Summary of conventional terminology for important mechanical properties of orthodontic wires*

Basic property	Location on bending plot	Equivalent terms
Rate of force delivery (stiffness)	Slope of elastic loading curve or unloading curve	$\frac{EI}{l}$
Moment at yielding or flexural yield strength	Bending moment for designated small amount of permanent deformation (vertical axis of graph)	$YS^{\dagger}$
Working range	Maximum value of purely elastic deformation (horizontal axis)	—
Modulus of resilience (resilience)	Area under elastic loading curve or unloading curve	$\frac{(YS)^{2\dagger}}{2E}$
Springback	Elastic strain recovered on unloading from permanent deformation range	$\frac{YS^{\dagger}}{E}$

*The expressions are applicable for tension tests and for bending tests with well-behaved wire alloys and sufficiently long specimens. In these cases, the elastic loading curve of clinical interest is essentially the same as the initial linear plot for elastic loading. For short loading spans and the nonsuperelastic nickel-titanium alloys, the unloading curves are nonlinear and it is difficult to define a modulus of elasticity. (Terms from Thurow, 1982; Popov, 1968.)

†For the idealized definitions, the yield strength (*YS*) should be replaced everywhere by the proportional limit (*PL*). Other symbols have their usual meanings: *E* - modulus of elasticity, *I* - moment of inertia (proportional to d^4 for round wire and wt^3 for rectangular wire), *l* - segment length, *d* - diameter, *w* - width, *t* - thickness in plane of bending.

Table 20-2 General compositions for four major classes of orthodontic wire alloys not containing precious metals

Wire alloy	Weight percentage of elements
Austenitic stainless steel*	17%-20% Cr, 8%-12% Ni, 0.15% C maximum, balance principally Fe (approx. 70%)
Cobalt-chromium-nickel† (Elgiloy)	40% Co, 20% Cr, 15% Ni, 15.8% Fe, 7% Mo, 2% Mn, 0.15% C, 0.04% Be
Beta-titanium (TMA)‡	77.8% Ti, 11.3% Mo, 6.6% Zr, 4.3% Sn
Nickel-titanium§ (Nitinol)	55% Ni, 45% Ti (approx. and may contain small amounts of Cu or other elements)

*Data from ASM (1961).
†Data from Phillips (1991).
‡Data from Burstone and Goldberg (1980).
§Data from Civjan et al (1975), Khier (1988), and Quo et al (1994).

in orthodontics are generally American Iron and Steel Institute (AISI) types 302 and 304 austenitic stainless steels, with similar nominal compositions, although the use of 17-7 precipitation-hardening stainless steel has been explored. Type 302 is composed of 17% to 19% chromium, 8% to 10% nickel, and 0.15% maximum carbon. Type 304 contains 18% to 20% chromium, 8% to 12% nickel, and 0.08% maximum carbon. The balance of the alloy composition (Table 20-2) is essentially iron (approximately 70%). These are the well-known "18-8" stainless steels, so designated because of the percentages of chromium and nickel in the alloys.

Research has shown that the modulus of elasticity in tension for stainless steel orthodontic wires, where values are more reliable than bending tests, ranges from about 160 to 180 GPa. These values depend on the manufacturer and temper, and are indicative of differences in alloy compositions, wire drawing procedures, and heat treatment conditions. It was not appreciated until recently that the elastic modulus for stainless steel orthodontic wires can be significantly decreased below the 190 to 210 GPa range given in standard physical metallurgy textbooks for annealed stainless steel, although this reduction in elastic modulus was well known over four decades ago for heavily cold-worked industrial austenitic stainless steel alloys.

Table 20-3 Range of mechanical properties in tension of principal clinical importance for four major orthodontic alloys and as-received wires*

Wire alloy	Modulus of elasticity (GPa)	Yield strength (MPa)
Stainless steel (resilient temper)	160–180	1,100–1,500
Cobalt-chromium-nickel (Elgiloy-soft temper)	160–190	830–1,000
Beta-titanium (TMA)	62–69	690–970
Nickel-titanium (nitinol)	34	210–410

*The data for modulus of elasticity and yield strength are for round wires with diameters from 0.016 to 0.020 inch and for rectangular wires with cross-section dimensions from 0.017 inch × 0.025 inch to 0.019 inch × 0.025 inch. (Data from Asgharnia and Brantley, 1986, and Drake et al, 1982.)

Note that 1 MPa = 145 psi and 1 GPa = 145,000 psi.

X-ray diffraction has shown that austenitic stainless steel arch wires do not necessarily have the single-phase austenitic structure in the as-received condition from the manufacturers. The microstructural phases in these stainless steel wires depend upon the manufacturer, temper, and cross-section size; the fundamental factors are the AISI type (particularly carbon content) and thermomechanical processing during manufacturing.

The yield strength for the stainless steel arch wires shows a much wider variation than the elastic modulus and has been found to range from approximately 1,100 to 1,500 MPa for a resilient temper from a single manufacturer and several cross-section sizes. The yield strength was increased to about 1,700 MPa for several wire sizes after heat treatment. The range in values of mechanical properties in tension for as-received stainless steel wires of clinically important sizes is summarized in Table 20-3. Heat treatment of these wires also causes significant decreases in residual stress and modest increases (~10%) in resilience. Springback (*YS/E*) was found to range from 0.0060 to 0.0094 for eight different sizes of as-received stainless steel wires and from 0.0065 to 0.0099 after heat treatment.

The use of heat treatment to eliminate residual stresses that might cause fracture during manipulation of stainless steel appliances can be important under clinical conditions. However, austenitic stainless steel alloys can be rendered susceptible to intergranular corrosion when heated to temperatures between 400° and 900°C, due to the formation of chromium carbides at the grain boundaries. These precipitates deplete the amount of chromium near the grain boundaries in the bulk stainless steel below the level needed for corrosion resistance. Since the stainless steel alloys must be heated within this temperature range for soldering, clinicians are cautioned to minimize the time required for this process.

Cobalt-chromium-nickel

Cobalt-chromium-nickel orthodontic wires are very similar in appearance, mechanical properties (Table 20-3), and joining characteristics to stainless steel wires, but have a much different composition and considerably greater heat treatment response. Table 20-2 shows that the most commonly used alloy, Elgiloy (Rocky Mountain Orthodontics) has a complex composition of 40% cobalt, 20% chromium, 15% nickel, 15.8% iron, 7% molybdenum, 2% manganese, 0.15% carbon, and 0.04% beryllium, which is somewhat similar to that for some base metal casting alloys for removable partial dentures.

Cobalt-chromium-nickel wires are available in four tempers: soft, ductile, semiresilient, and resilient. The differences in mechanical properties arise from proprietary variations in the wire manufacturing process. The soft-temper wires are popular with clinicians because they are easily deformed and shaped into appliances, then heat treated to provide substantially increased values of yield strength and resilience. Increases of 20% to 30% in the yield strength of Elgiloy-soft wires after heat treatment have been reported, and similar heat treatment responses appear to occur for the soft, ductile, and semiresilient tempers. The large increases in modulus of resilience principally arise from the dependence on $(YS)^2$ (see Table 20-1). The effect of heat treatment on mechanical properties has been attributed to complex precipitation processes. Springback for the Elgiloy-soft alloy was found to range from 0.0045 to 0.0065 for five different sizes of as-received wires and from 0.0054 to 0.0074 after heat treatment.

The other tempers are less popular than the soft temper because wires made from them have lower formability and are somewhat higher in cost than stainless steel. For Elgiloy-soft, the elastic modulus in tension ranges from about 160 to 190 GPa for as-received wires (Table 20-3), and from about 180 to 210 GPa after heat treatment. The corresponding ranges in yield strength are approximately 830 to 1,000 MPa in the as-received condition, and 1,100 to 1,400 MPa after heat treatment. It is important to emphasize that the elastic force delivery is very nearly the same for stainless steel and Elgiloy-soft arch wire segments of the same size and length, as indicated in Table 20-3. A common misconception is that the elastic force delivery is much less for soft-temper cobalt-chromium-nickel arch wires because of the "feel" of these wires. In reality, the yield strength and elastic range are the properties that are diminished relative to the more resilient stainless steel alloys.

Beta-titanium

A beta-titanium orthodontic alloy, TMA (Ormco/Sybron), was introduced to the orthodontic profession about 15 years ago. The nominal composition of TMA (*t*itanium-*m*olybdenum *a*lloy) is 77.8% titanium, 11.3% molybdenum, 6.6% zirconium, and 4.3% tin (Table 20-2). The presence of molybdenum causes the elevated temperature body-centered cubic beta polymorphic phase of titanium to be metastable at room temperature, rather than the hexagonal close-packed alpha phase. This results in excellent formability or capability for permanent deformation. The beta-titanium alloy has somewhat less than half the elastic force delivery (E ranging from about 62 to 69 GPa) of stainless steel wires, with the yield strength ranging from approximately 690 to 970 MPa (Table 20-3). Springback for four different sizes of as-received beta-titanium wires was found to range from 0.0094 to 0.011.

Another noteworthy characteristic is that beta-titanium is the only orthodontic wire alloy that possesses true weldability. (Welded joints that are fabricated from stainless steel and cobalt-chromium-nickel alloys must be built up with the use of solders to maintain adequate strength.) Optimum conditions for welding TMA with commercial apparatus have been published. Heat treatment by the clinician is not recommended for TMA, although this beta-titanium alloy does respond to a precipitation hardening procedure. Solution heat treatment (SHT) between approximately 700° and 730°C, followed by water quenching, then aging at approximately 480°C results in a peak value for the YS/E ratio.

The physical metallurgy of the beta-titanium alloys is complex, and systems other than the titanium-molybdenum-zirconium-tin alloy may also be suitable for orthodontic applications.

Nickel-titanium

The fourth wire alloy, nickel-titanium, has remained a strong focus of materials research, as well as considerable marketing activity by manufacturers. The name *nitinol* is derived from the *ni*ckel and *ti*tanium composition, along with the *N*aval *O*rdnance *L*aboratory where these alloys were originally developed.

Nickel-titanium orthodontic alloys are based upon the intermetallic compound NiTi, which has weight percentages of 55% nickel and 45% titanium (Table 20-2). Chemical analyses of two nickel-titanium alloys revealed similar nickel-rich compositions (59 to 60 weight percent nickel), with other trace elements in amounts less than 0.01 weight percent. In contrast, recently reported X-ray energy-dispersive analyses of two nickel-titanium alloys indicated titanium-rich compositions (51 to 52 atomic percent titanium) containing 1.6 to 1.8 atomic percent copper.

Although the shape-memory effect (SME) associated with these nickel-titanium alloys was not available in the original nitinol wire (Unitek/3M), there are two features of considerable importance for clinical orthodontics:

1. The very low elastic modulus (E about 34 GPa in tension) for nitinol corresponds to about one fifth of the force delivery for stainless steel arch wires and half the force delivery for beta-titanium wires having the same cross-section dimensions and length.
2. Because of the extremely wide elastic working range, 12.5-mm segments in the clinically important size ranges retain a permanent set of not more than 5 degrees, after bending 90 degrees by the ANSI/ADA

specification test procedure and release of the applied moment. The yield strength for the nitinol wires generally ranges from about 210 to 410 MPa. Springback for six different sizes of as-received wires was found to range from 0.0058 to 0.016.

New Chinese nickel-titanium orthodontic wire (now marketed as Ni-Ti by Ormco/Sybron), was compared with nitinol and stainless steel wires, using a cantilever bending test and 5-mm span lengths appropriate to clinical interbracket distances. The nonlinear activation characteristics of clinical interest are quite evident. However, whereas the average unloading stiffness (ratio of bending moment to amount of deactivation in degrees) is the same for all activations of nitinol, the unloading curves for Chinese nickel-titanium wires are dependent on the level of activation (amount of bending deflection). These latter unloading curves have relatively high values of unloading stiffness for the initial and final stages (under 10 degrees) of deactivation; through the middle range of deactivation, the unloading stiffness is much smaller and approaches constant force delivery. The average stiffness of Chinese nickel-titanium wire from these unloading curves was found to increase considerably on going from the largest to smallest activations; with the 5-mm test spans, the springback of Chinese nickel-titanium wire was over 4 times that for stainless steel and more than 50% greater than that for nitinol wire.

A new Japanese nickel-titanium wire (now marketed as Sentalloy by GAC International) was subsequently introduced. The stress-strain curves in tension and the load-deflection curves for three-point bending of 14-mm test spans were compared for 0.016-inch diameter wires of this alloy, nitinol, stainless steel, and Elgiloy. The tension and bending tests confirmed the existence of superelastic behavior in the Japanese nickel-titanium wires. After a certain level of tensile strain or bending deflection, further deformation (up to about 10% tensile strain or 2 mm deflection for a 0.016-inch diameter wire) takes place at nearly constant tensile stress or bending force. The unloading characteristics exhibit initial and final regions of relatively steep slope, along with an extensive intermediate region where there is little change in stress or force.

When the Japanese nickel-titanium wire was heat treated at 500°C from 5 minutes to 2 hours, the bending force remaining during the superelastic region of the deactivation curve could be varied over a wide range. This behavior has been exploited (GAC International) to develop commercial nickel-titanium wires that can deliver low, medium, or high levels of force. A highly convenient electric resistance method has been developed for the heat treatment of Japanese nickel-titanium wires, and a commercial apparatus (GAC International) is available that enables the clinician to heat treat superelastic nickel-titanium arch wires as desired for the treatment of individual patients.

The bending properties of several nickel-titanium wire products with both round and rectangular cross-sections have been compared, using cantilever specimens with 6-mm test spans. The bending test plots indicated that the Chinese nickel-titanium wire and nitinol SE (Unitek/3M) possessed superelastic behavior (Fig 20-2) very similar to that for the Japanese nickel-titanium wire and that the original nitinol wire (Fig 20-3) should be classified as nonsuperelastic. The three superelastic wire products evaluated exhibited responses to vacuum heat treatment for 10 minutes and 2 hours at 500° and 600°C (Fig 20-4) which were similar to those reported for Japanese nickel-titanium wire. The constant bending moment in the superelastic deactivation range was decreased after heat treatment at 500°C, and loss of superelastic behavior occurred after heat treatment at 600°C. In contrast, the bending properties of the three nonsuperelastic wire products evaluated were essentially unaffected by heat treatment.

Shape-memory characteristics of the nickel-titanium alloys are associated with a reversible transformation between the austenitic and martensitic NiTi phases, which occurs by a twinning process. The martensitic phase forms from the austenitic phase over a certain transformation temperature range (TTR) or when the stress is increased above some appropriate level. The austenitic phase forms from the martensitic phase over the TTR, or when the stress is decreased below the appropriate level. The shape-memory characteristics of several commercial nickel-titanium wires have been evaluated by measuring the final length of segments that had been permanently deformed approximately 7% in tension below the TTR reported by the manufacturers for the transformation to austenite and then heated above the TTR to 150°C. The deformed alloys evaluated exhibited excellent shape (length) recovery ranging from 89% to 94%.

Nickel-titanium alloys with shape-memory behavior activated at body temperature have been recently introduced by manufacturers.

Decreases in the mechanical properties of nickel-titanium wires after long-term deflection have been reported, and time-dependent relaxation of bending

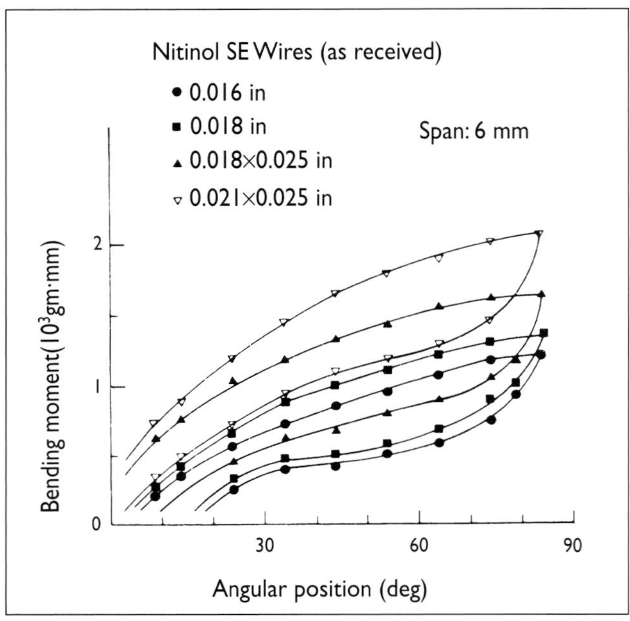

Fig 20-2 Cantilever bending plots for 6-mm test spans of four different sizes of as-received nitinol SE (Unitek/3M), a superelastic wire. (Reprinted from Khier et al, 1991, with permission from American Journal of Orthodontics and Dentofacial Orthopedics.)

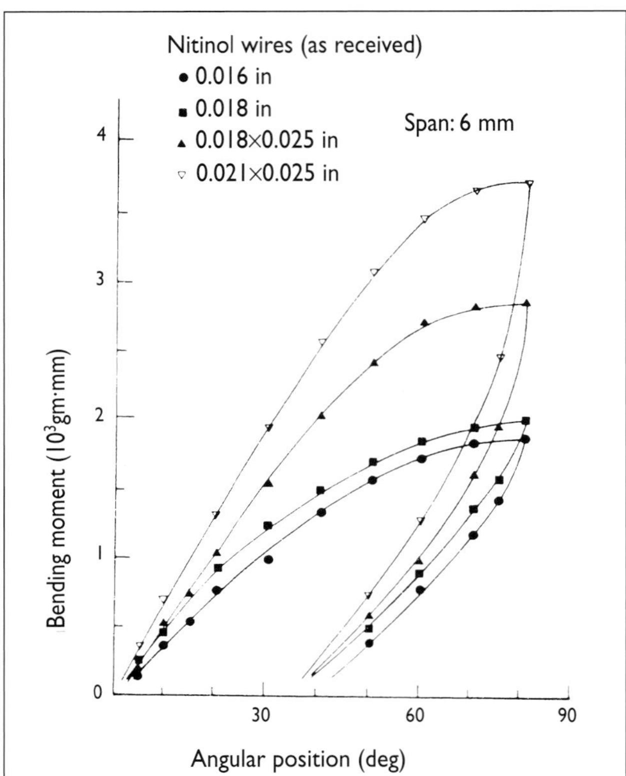

Fig 20-3 Cantilever bending plots for 6-mm test spans of four different sizes of as-received nitinol (Unitek/3M), a nonsuperelastic wire. (Reprinted from Khier et al, 1991, with permission from American Journal of Orthodontics and Dentofacial Orthopedics.)

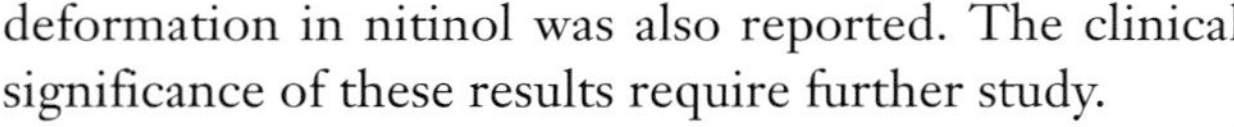

deformation in nitinol was also reported. The clinical significance of these results require further study.

Nickel-titanium arch wires with ion-implanted surfaces to obtain reduced bracket friction have been recently introduced (GAC International).

Considerations for selection

Although the stainless steel arch wires are still the most widely used in orthodontics and cobalt-chromium-nickel wires are selected by many clinicians, the nickel-titanium and beta-titanium wires have become very popular. The gold alloy wires, while still available commercially, are relatively expensive and have minimal clinical use. Each of the four major non-precious orthodontic wire alloys has distinct advantages for selection by the clinician, along with some areas or potential areas of concern, as summarized in Table 20-4.

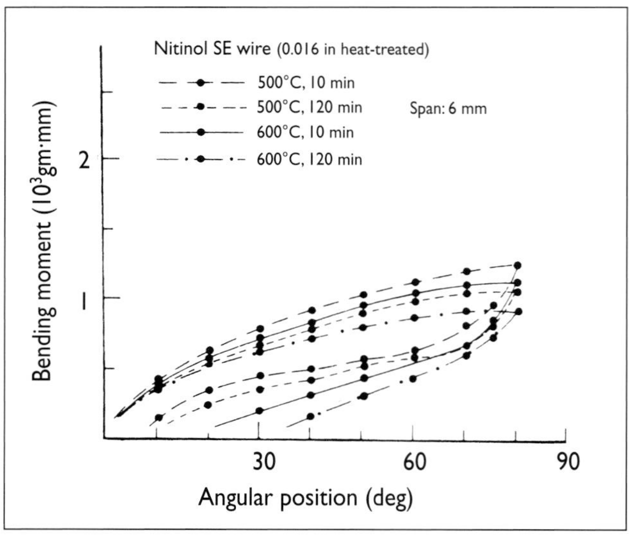

Fig 20-4 Cantilever bending plots for 6-mm test spans of 0.016-inch diameter nitinol SE wires subjected to heat treatments of 10 minutes and 2 hours at 500° and 600°C. (Reprinted from Khier et al, 1991, with permission from American Journal of Orthodontics and Dentofacial Orthopedics.)

Table 20-4 Advantages and disadvantages of each of the four major orthodontic wire alloys

Stainless steel

Advantages

Lowest cost of the wire alloys
Proven biocompatibility from extensive clinical use
Excellent formability for fabrication into orthodontic appliances
Can be soldered and welded, although welded joints may require solder reinforcement

Disadvantages

High force delivery
Relatively low springback in bending compared to beta-titanium and nickel-titanium alloys
Can be susceptible to intergranular corrosion after heating to temperatures required for joining

Elgiloy (soft temper)

Advantages

Relatively low cost, although greater than stainless steel
Proven biocompatibility from extensive clinical use
Outstanding formability in as-received condition (heat treated to increase YS and resilience)
Can be soldered and welded, with joining characteristics similar to stainless steel
Excellent in vivo corrosion resistance

Disadvantages

High elastic force delivery, similar to that for stainless steel
Lower springback than stainless steel (using YS/E values from tension test)

Beta-titanium

Advantages

Intermediate force delivery between stainless steel or Elgiloy and nickel-titanium
Excellent formability and only orthodontic wire alloy with true weldability
Excellent springback characteristics (using YS/E values from tension test)
Excellent biocompatibility from high titanium content demonstrated by clinical use

Disadvantages

Expensive
High arch wire–bracket friction with original TMA (decreased for new ion-implanted product)

Nickel-titanium

Advantages

Lowest force delivery of the four orthodontic wire alloys
Excellent springback in bending, particularly for superelastic and shape-memory alloys
Superelastic alloys can be heat treated by clinician to vary force delivery characteristics

Disadvantages

Expensive, particularly for newest products
Second highest arch wire–bracket friction after TMA (decreased for new ion-implanted product)
Difficult to place permanent bends and cannot bend wire over sharp edge or into complete loop
Wires cannot be soldered and must be joined by mechanical crimping process
Lowest in vitro corrosion resistance of wire alloys (may be concern about in vivo nickel release)

The stainless steel and cobalt-chromium-nickel wires offer the advantages of relatively low cost, known biocompatibility from extensive clinical usage, and excellent formability for the fabrication of orthodontic appliances. However, these wires have much higher force delivery (elastic modulus) than the beta-titanium and nickel-titanium wires, and the force delivery is increased after heat treatment by the clinician to increase resilience (particularly in Elgiloy-soft) and relieve residual stresses.

The relatively high cost of the beta-titanium orthodontic wires is offset by the intermediate force delivery, excellent formability, and true weldability of this alloy. The clinician may select beta-titanium arch wires because they more nearly fill the bracket slots, compared with the wire sizes that would be selected for a stainless steel alloy. The formability or ductility of beta-titanium provides the orthodontist with the capability of fabricating arches or segments with complicated loop configurations not possible with the nickel-titanium alloys. Clinical examples include the alignment of teeth in an arch during finishing, the rotation and changing of the axial orientation of teeth, the use of specialized springs or auxiliaries such as an intrusive arch or a canine root spring, and the fabrication of closing loops that may contain helices. The direct welding of auxiliaries to arch wires enable hooks, tie backs, and finger springs to be easily prepared with commercial welding apparatus. The recently introduced ion-implanted beta-titanium alloys with reduced arch wire–bracket friction should become popular, as the relatively high bracket friction was a disadvantage of the original TMA alloy.

It is well known from histologic studies on tooth movement that light, continuous, nearly constant forces represent optimum biomechanical conditions. The Chinese and Japanese nickel-titanium wires with excellent springback (range of elastic action), low stiffness, and nearly constant force delivery during deactivation, provide these desirable mechanical properties better than stainless steel, cobalt-chromium-nickel, beta-titanium, and original nitinol wire alloys.

Another interesting feature is the increase in force delivery that occurs when an appliance is removed and then retied (ligated) with Chinese nickel-titanium wire. These results would be anticipated with the other superelastic alloys. Superelastic nickel-titanium alloy coilsprings have also been developed for orthodontic applications.

Corrosion resistance of the orthodontic wires is provided by a chromium oxide film for the stainless steel and cobalt-chromium-nickel alloys, and a titanium oxide film for the beta-titanium and nickel-titanium alloys. Clinical experience is that corrosion of orthodontic wires is of minimal concern, and immersion of wires in a 1% sodium chloride solution for periods up to 11 months caused no significant changes in the bending mechanical properties of nitinol wire segments. When the cyclic potentiodynamic polarization behavior (–500 mV to 300 mV) of stainless steel, cobalt-chromium-nickel, beta-titanium, and nitinol wires in a 1% sodium chloride solution was compared, breakdown of the surface oxide and pitting were observed only for nitinol and appeared to be accompanied by the selective dissolution of nickel. Research has shown that nickel dissolution does occur at sites of surface damage in nickel-titanium wires. Nickel hypersensitivity reactions to nickel-titanium wires have been observed in orthodontic patients who are nickel-sensitive, although such cases are rare. Recent in vitro studies using human epithelial (He La) cells have shown noncytotoxic responses from nickel-titanium alloys. Moreover, a survey of orthodontic practices did not yield any significant relationship between the usage of nickel-containing wires (stainless steel, cobalt-chromium-nickel, and nickel-titanium) and the development of skin lesions. The greater cost of the nickel-titanium arch wires and the considerable recent interest in infection control procedures have stimulated several studies on orthodontic wires. These studies suggest that sterilization and clinical recycling only have small effects on the mechanical properties of the nickel-titanium wires.

A transparent nonmetallic orthodontic arch wire (Optiflex, Ormco/Sybron) with a silica core, a silicone resin middle layer, and a stain-resistant outer layer has recently been developed and successfully used in patient treatment. Although sharp bends cannot be placed because of the brittle core, this ceramic/polymer wire is highly resilient and undergoes minimal permanent deformation under clinical conditions. Future developments of nonmetallic wires are anticipated.

Clinical scenario

This section presents an approach for choosing materials and a system for a specific situation. It uses the same format as that presented in Chapter 7:

1. The situation is described.
2. Critical factors are listed.
3. Advantages and disadvantages of each material/system are prioritized using the following codes: * = of minor importance, ** = important, and *** = very important.
4. The situation is analyzed, and the final decision given.

Situation Superelastic NiTi wire vs stainless steel wires†

Critical factors Good esthetics, speed of completion

	Superelastic nickel-titanium wires NiTi	Stainless steel wires
Advantages	*** 1. Produces lower moments and forces	*** 1. Less expensive
	*** 2. Constant force over wide range of deflection	2. Good formability
	3. Low stiffness	3. High resilience
	** 4. High spring back	* 4. Can be soldered or welded
	** 5. High stored energy	** 5. Good in final detailing
	* 6. More effective in initial tooth alignment	** 6. Great for arch coordination
	7. Shape memory	*** 7. Good torque control
	*** 8. Less patient discomfort	8. Relatively predictable biomechanical properties
Disadvantages	* 1. Cannot be soldered or welded	** 1. More chair time
	** 2. Cannot be easily formed or bent	2. Resilience depends on diameter
	*** 3. Tendency for dentoalveolar expansion	3. No shape memory or superelasticity
	*** 4. Costly	** 4. Poor deflection range
	5. Poor torque control	
	*** 6. Patient discomfort with larger activation	

†Prepared by Dr. David E. Wacker, 1995.

Glossary

activation Bending a wire that will produce an elastic force for tooth movement.

austenite phase The face-centered cubic solid solution structure of iron, chromium, nickel, and carbon for stainless steels, or the body-centered cubic structure of NiTi for the nickel-titanium alloys.

force delivery The force produced by an orthodontic wire against a tooth.

martensitic phase A body-centered cubic phase in austenitic stainless steels or a phase (reported as monoclinic, triclinic, or hexagonal) in nickel-titanium alloys that forms as a result of quenching or cold working the austenite phase.

shape memory A property of certain wires that will permit shaping at a higher temperature, followed by deformation at a lower temperature, and a return to the original shape by reheating.

temper The spring character of an orthodontic wire, which is related to the mechanical properties of yield strength and resilience.

weldability Having the capability of being joined by the passage of a strong electric current.

working range The maximum deflection of a wire within the elastic range.

Discussion questions

1. What phenomenon is responsible for the force delivery to teeth by deformed wires?
2. How is it possible to obtain different mechanical properties from the same wire?
3. Which type of orthodontic wire is most susceptible to welding?
4. What is shape memory, and which wires have it?

Questions and answers

1. **What are the types of orthodontic wires in current use?** Stainless steel, cobalt-chromium-nickel, beta-titanium, and nickel-titanium.
2. **What are the main criteria for the selection of an orthodontic wire?** Force delivery characteristics, elastic working range, ease of manipulation by permanent deformation to desired shapes, capability of joining individual segments to fabricate more complex appliances, corrosion resistance and biocompatibility in the oral environment, and cost. The relatively new beta-titanium and nickel-titanium arch wires are more than ten times as costly as the traditional stainless steel alloys; but they offer unique properties that should be carefully considered when selecting wires.
3. **What determines wire stiffness or elastic force delivery?** (a) The composition and structure of the wire alloy, and (b) the wire segment geometry—cross-section shape and size and the length.
4. **What are the advantages of stainless steel wires?** Bioinertness and corrosion resistance in the oral environment, and low cost.
5. **What is Elgiloy?** A cobalt-chromium-nickel alloy very similar in appearance, physical properties, and joining characteristics to the stainless steel wires, but with a much different composition and considerably greater heat treatment response. Available in four tempers: soft, ductile, semiresilient, and resilient.
6. **What is the composition of the beta-titanium wire?** Titanium, 77.8% molybdenum, 11.3%; zirconium, 6.6%; and tin, 4.3%. The addition of alloying elements to pure titanium causes the body-centered cubic beta polymorphic phase to be metastable at room temperature, rather than the hexagonal close-packed alpha phase, which results in excellent formability or the capability for permanent deformation.
7. **What are the disadvantages of nickel-titanium alloy wires?** The values of yield strength are much less than those for tensile strength. Special techniques are required for permanent bending, and the wires cannot be bent over a sharp edge or into a complete loop. The wires cannot be soldered or welded but must be joined by a mechanical crimping procedure. Heat treatment is not recommended.
8. **What are the advantages of beta-titanium orthodontic wire?** An intermediate force delivery between stainless steel or cobalt-chromium-nickel and nickel-titanium wires, excellent formability, and true weldability. Beta-titanium arch wires can more nearly fill the bracket slots. The ductility allows arches or segments with complicated loop configurations, which are not possible with nickel-titanium alloys.

Recommended reading

Altuna G, Lewis DW, Chao I, Rourke MA. A statistical assessment of orthodontic practices, product usage, and the development of skin lesions. Am J Orthod Dentofac Orthop 100:242–250, 1991.

American Dental Association specification no. 32 for orthodontic wires not containing precious metals. J Am Dent Assoc 95:1169–1171, 1977.

Andreasen GF, Brady PR. A use hypothesis for 55 nitinol wire for orthodontics. Angle Orthod 42:172–177, 1972.

Andreasen GF, Hilleman TB. An evaluation of 55 cobalt substituted nitinol wire for use in orthodontics. J Am Dent Assoc 82:1373–1375, 1971.

Andreasen GF, Morrow RE. Laboratory and clinical analyses of nitinol wire. Am J Orthod 73:142–151, 1978.

Angolkar PV, Kapila S, Duncanson MG Jr, Nanda RS. Evaluation of friction between ceramic brackets and orthodontic wires of four alloys. Am J Orthod Dentofac Orthop 98:499–506, 1990.

Asgharnia MK, Brantley WA. Comparison of bending and tension tests for orthodontic wires. Am J Orthod 89:228–236, 1986.

ASM Committee on Wrought Stainless Steels. Wrought stainless steels. In Metals Handbook. 8th ed. Vol 1. Metals Park, OH: American Society for Metals, 1961.

Backofen WA, Gales GF. Heat treating stainless steel wire for orthodontics. Am J Orthod 38:755–765, 1952.

Bass JK, Fine H, Cisneros GJ. Nickel hypersensitivity in the orthodontic patient. Am J Orthod Dentofac Orthop 103:280–285, 1993.

Bradley TG, Brantley WA, Culbertson BM. Differential scanning calorimetry (DSC) analyses of superelastic and nonsuperelastic nickel-titanium orthodontic wires. Am J Orthod Dentofac Orthop 109:589–597, 1996.

Bradley TG, Mitchell JC, Brantley WA. Surface composition and microtopography of nickel-titanium orthodontic wires. J Dent Res 75 (IADR Abstracts):61, 1996.

Brantley WA. Comments on stiffness measurements for orthodontic wires. J Dent Res 55:705, 1976.

Brantley WA, Augat WS, Myers CL, Winders RV. Bending deformation studies of orthodontic wires. J Dent Res 57:609–615, 1978.

Brenner J, Brantley W, Conover J. Effects of heat treatment on mechanical properties of orthodontic wires. J Dent Res 60 (IADR Abstracts):439, 1981.

Brick RM, Pense AW, Gordon RB. Structure and Properties of Engineering Materials. 4th ed. New York: McGraw-Hill, 1977; Chap 10 and 14.

Buckthal JE, Kusy RP. Effects of cold disinfectants on the mechanical properties and the surface topography of nickel-titanium arch wires. Am J Orthod Dentofac Orthop 94:117–122, 1988.

Buehler WJ, Gilfrich JV, Riley RC. Effect of low-temperature phase changes on the mechanical properties of alloys near the composition of TiNi. J Appl Phys 34:1475–1477, 1963.

Buehler WJ, Wang FE. A summary of recent research on the nitinol alloys and their potential application in ocean engineering. Ocean Eng 1:105–120, 1968.

Burstone CJ. Variable-modulus orthodontics. Am J Orthod 80:1–16, 1981.

Burstone CJ, Goldberg AJ. Beta-titanium: a new orthodontic alloy. Am J Orthod 77:121–132, 1980.

Burstone CJ, Goldberg AJ. Maximum forces and deflections from orthodontic appliances. Am J Orthod 84:95–103, 1983.

Burstone CJ, Qin B, Morton JY. Chinese NiTi wire—a new orthodontic alloy. Am J Orthod 87:445–452, 1985.

Chen R, Zhi YF, Arvystas MG. Advanced Chinese NiTi alloy wire and clinical observations. Angle Orthod 62:59–66, 1992.

Chen RS, Vijayaraghavan TV, Schulman A. Electric spot welding of nickel-titanium (Titanal) wires. J Dent Res 69(IADR Abstracts):312, 1990.

Civjan S, Huget EF, DeSimon LB. Potential applications of certain nickel-titanium (Nitinol) alloys. J Dent Res 54:89–96, 1975.

Craig RG (ed). Restorative Dental Materials. 9th ed. St Louis: Mosby, 1993; 400–402, 435–445.

Craig RG, Slesnick HJ, Peyton FA. Application of 17-7 precipitation-hardenable stainless steel in dentistry. J Dent Res 44:587–595, 1965.

Dieter GE. Mechanical Metallurgy. 3rd ed. New York: McGraw-Hill, 1986; Chap 8 and 19.

Di Giovanni J, Staley RN, Jakobsen JR. Effect of electric heat treatment on martensitic-active nickel titanium. J Dent Res 73(IADR Abstracts):413, 1994.

Donovan MT, Lin JJ, Brantley WA, Conover JP. Weldability of beta-titanium arch wires. Am J Orthod 85:207–216, 1984.

Drake SR, Wayne DM, Powers JM, Asgar K. Mechanical properties of orthodontic wires in tension, bending and torsion. Am J Orthod 82:206–210, 1982.

Edie JW, Andreasen GF, Zaytoun MP. Surface corrosion of nitinol and stainless steel under clinical conditions. Angle Orthod 51:319–324, 1981.

Fariabi S, Thoma PE, Abujudom DN. The effect of cold work and heat treatment on the phase transformations of near equiatomic NiTi shape memory alloy. Proc ICOMAT-1989.

Fillmore GM, Tomlinson JL. Heat treatment of cobalt-chromium alloys of various tempers. Angle Orthod 49:126–130, 1979.

Fletcher ML, Miyake S, Brantley WA, Culbertson BM. DSC and bending studies of a new shape-memory orthodontic wire. J Dent Res 71(IADR Abstracts):169, 1992.

Fukuyo S, Nakazato H, Masukawa T, Sachdeva R, Fukuyo S. Cytotoxicity studies on TiNi alloy using tissue culture agar overlay test (AOT). J Dent Res 70(IADR Abstracts):398, 1991.

Funk AC. The heat-treatment of stainless steel. Angle Orthod 21:129–138, 1951.

Goldberg J, Burstone CJ. An evaluation of beta-titanium alloys for use in orthodontic appliances. J Dent Res 58:593–599, 1979.

Goldberg AJ, Vanderby R Jr, Burstone CJ. Reduction in the modulus of elasticity in orthodontic wires. J Dent Res 56:1227–1231, 1977.

Goldstein D, Kabacoff L, Tydings J. Stress effects on nitinol phase transformations. J Metals 39:19–26, 1987.

Greppi L, Smith DC, Woodside DG, Varrela T, Lugowski S. Nickel hypersensitivity reactions in orthodontic patients. J Dent Res 70(IADR Abstracts):361, 1991.

Harris EF, Newman SM, Nicholson JA. Nitinol arch wire in a simulated oral environment: changes in mechanical properties. Am J Orthod Dentofac Orthop 93:508–513, 1988.

Howe GL, Greener EH, Crimmins DS. Mechanical properties and stress relief of stainless steel orthodontic wire. Angle Orthod 38:244–249, 1968.

Hudgins JJ, Bagby MD, Erickson LC. The effect of long-term deflection on permanent deformation of nickel-titanium archwires. Angle Orthod 60:283–288, 1990.

Hurst CL, Duncanson MG Jr, Nanda RS, Angolkar PV. An evaluation of the shape-memory phenomenon of nickel-titanium orthodontic wires. Am J Orthod Dentofac Orthop 98:72–76, 1990.

Kapila S, Angolkar PV, Duncanson MG Jr, Nanda RS. Evaluation of friction between edgewise stainless steel brackets and orthodontic wires of four alloys. Am J Orthod Dentofac Orthop 98:117–126, 1990.

Kapila S, Haugen JW, Watanabe LG. Load-deflection characteristics of nickel-titanium alloy wires after clinical recycling and dry heat sterilization. Am J Orthod Dentofac Orthop 102:120–126, 1992.

Kapila S, Reichhold GW, Anderson RS, Watanabe LG. Effects of clinical recycling on mechanical properties of nickel-titanium alloy wires. Am J Orthod Dentofac Orthop 100:428–435, 1991.

Kapila S, Sachdeva R. Mechanical properties and clinical applications of orthodontic wires. Am J Orthod Dentofac Orthop 96:100–109, 1989.

Khier SE. Structural Characterization, Biomechanical Properties, and Potentiodynamic Polarization Behavior of Nickel-Titanium Orthodontic Wire Alloys. PhD dissertation. Milwaukee, WI: Marquette University, 1988.

Khier SE, Brantley WA, Fournelle RA. Structure and mechanical properties of as-received and heat-treated stainless steel orthodontic wires. Am J Orthod Dentofac Orthop 93:206–212, 1988.

Khier SE, Brantley WA, Fournelle RA. Bending properties of superelastic and nonsuperelastic nickel-titanium orthodontic wires. Am J Orthod Dentofac Orthop 99:310–318, 1991.

Khier SE, Brantley WA, Fournelle RA, Ehlert T. XRD and DSC studies of NiTi orthodontic wire alloys. J Dent Res 68(AADR Abstracts):386, 1989.

Kohl RW. Metallurgy in orthodontics. Angle Orthod 34:37–52, 1964.

Kusy RP. On the use of nomograms to determine the elastic property ratios of orthodontic arch wires. Am J Orthod 83:374–381, 1983.

Kusy RP. Nitinol alloys: so, who's on first? (Letter to the editor) Am J Orthod Dentofac Orthop 100:25A–26A, Sept 1991.

Kusy RP, Dilley GJ. Elastic modulus of a triple-stranded stainless steel arch wire via three- and four-point bending. J Dent Res 63:1232–1240, 1984.

Kusy RP, Greenberg AR. Effects of composition and cross section on the elastic properties of orthodontic wires. Angle Orthod 51:325–341, 1981.

Kusy RP, Greenberg AR. Comparison of the elastic properties of nickel-titanium and beta-titanium arch wires. Am J Orthod 82:199–205, 1982.

Kusy RP, Stevens LE. Triple-stranded stainless steel wires—evaluation of mechanical properties and comparison with titanium alloy alternatives. Angle Orthod 57:18–32, 1987.

Kusy RP, Tobin EJ, Whitley JQ, Sioshansi P. Frictional coefficients of ion-implanted alumina against ion-implanted beta-titanium in the low load, low velocity, single pass regime. Dent Mater 8:167–172, 1992.

Kusy RP, Whitley JQ. Coefficients of friction for arch wires in stainless steel and polycrystalline alumina bracket slots. I. The dry state. Am J Orthod Dentofac Orthop 98:300–312, 1990.

Kusy RP, Whitley JQ, Mayhew MJ, Buckthal JE. Surface roughness of orthodontic archwires via laser spectroscopy. Angle Orthod 58:33–45, 1988.

Kusy RP, Whitley JQ, Prewitt MJ. Comparison of the frictional coefficients for selected archwire-bracket combinations in the dry and wet states. Angle Orthod 61:293–302, 1991.

Lee JH, Park JB, Andreasen GF, Lakes RS. Thermomechanical study of Ni-Ti alloys. J Biomed Mater Res 22:573–588, 1988.

Leu L, Fournelle R, Brantley W, Ehlert T. Evidence of R structure in superelastic NiTi orthodontic wires. J Dent Res 69 (IADR Abstracts):313, 1990.

Lopez I, Goldberg J, Burstone CJ. Bending characteristics of nitinol wire. Am J Orthod 75:569–575, 1979.

Mayhew MJ, Kusy RP. Effects of sterilization on the mechanical properties and the surface topography of nickel-titanium arch wires. Am J Orthod Dentofac Orthop 93:232–236, 1988.

Melton KN. Ni-Ti based shape memory alloys. In Duerig TW, Melton KN, Stöckel D, Wayman CM (eds). Engineering Aspects of Shape Memory Alloys. London: Butterworth-Heinemann, 1990; 21–35.

Mitchell JC, Bradley TG, Brantley WA. Elemental analyses of six commercial nickel-titanium orthodontic wires. J Dent Res 75(IADR Abstracts):168, 1996.

Miura F, Mogi M, Ohura Y, Hamanaka H. The super-elastic property of the Japanese NiTi alloy wire for use in orthodontics. Am J Orthod Dentofac Orthop 90:1–10, 1986.

Miura F, Mogi M, Ohura Y. Japanese NiTi alloy wire: use of the direct electric resistance heat treatment method. Eur J Orthod 10:187–191, 1988.

Miura F, Mogi M, Ohura Y, Karibe M. The super-elastic Japanese NiTi alloy wire for use in orthodontics. Part III. Studies on the Japanese NiTi alloy coil springs. Am J Orthod Dentofac Orthop 94:89–96, 1988.

Nakazato H, Fukuyo S, Masukawa T, Sachdeva R, Fukuyo S. Cytotoxicity studies on shape memory TiNi alloy. J Dent Res 70(IADR Abstracts):397, 1991.

Nelson KR, Burstone CJ, Goldberg AJ. Optimal welding of beta-titanium orthodontic wires. Am J Orthod Dentofac Orthop 92:213–219, 1987.

Nikolai RJ. Bioengineering Analysis of Orthodontic Mechanics. Philadelphia: Lea and Febiger, 1985.

Nikolai RJ, Anderson WT, Messersmith ML. Structural responses of orthodontic wires in flexure from a proposed alternative to the existing specification test. Am J Orthod Dentofac Orthop 93:496–504, 1988.

Novak C. Structure and constitution of wrought austenitic stainless steels. In Peckner D, Bernstein IM (eds). Handbook of Stainless Steels. New York: McGraw-Hill, 1977; Chap 4.

Oshida Y, Miyazaki S, Sachdeva R. Microanalytical studies of orthodontic NiTi archwire. J Dent Res 69(IADR Abstracts):313, 1990.

Otsuka K. Introduction to the R-phase transition. In Duerig TW, Melton KN, Stöckel D, Wayman CM (eds). Engineering Aspects of Shape Memory Alloys. London: Butterworth-Heinemann, 1990; 36–45.

Phillips RW. Skinner's Science of Dental Materials. 9th ed. Philadelphia: Saunders, 1991; Chap 28.

Popov EP. Introduction to Mechanics of Solids. Englewood Cliffs, NJ: Prentice-Hall, 1968; Chap 6.

Prososki RR, Bagby MD, Erickson LC. Static frictional force and surface roughness of nickel-titanium arch wires. Am J Orthod Dentofac Orthop 100:341–348, 1991.

Quo SD, Marshall SJ, Marshall GW. Chemical and phase contents analysis of Ni-Ti wires. J Dent Res 73(IADR Abstracts):413, 1994.

Sachdeva RCL, Miyazaki S. Superelastic Ni-Ti alloys in orthodontics. In Duerig TW, Melton KN, Stöckel D, Wayman CM (eds). Engineering Aspects of Shape Memory Alloys. London: Butterworth-Heinemann, 1990; 452–469.

Sarkar NK, Redmond W, Schwaninger B, Goldberg AJ. The chloride corrosion behaviour of four orthodontic wires. J Oral Rehab 10:121–128, 1983.

Schwaninger B, Sarkar NK, Foster BE. Effect of long-term immersion corrosion on the flexural properties of nitinol. Am J Orthod 82:45–49, 1982.

Sebanc J, Brantley WA, Pincsak JJ, Conover JP. Variability of effective root torque as a function of edge bevel on orthodontic arch wires. Am J Orthod 86:43–51, 1984.

Smith GA, von Fraunhofer JA, Casey GR. The effect of clinical use and sterilization on selected orthodontic arch wires. Am J Orthod Dentofac Orthop 102:153–159, 1992.

Talass MF. Optiflex archwire treatment of a skeletal Class III open bite. J Clin Orthod 26:245–252, 1992.

Thayer TA, Bagby MD, Moore RN, De Angelis R. X-ray diffraction of nitinol orthodontic arch wires. Am J Orthod Dentofac Orthop 107:604–612, 1993.

Thurow RC. Edgewise Orthodontics. 4th ed. St Louis: Mosby, 1982; Chap 3–5, 17.

Todoroki T, Tamura H. Effect of heat treatment after cold working on the phase transformation in TiNi alloy. Trans Japan Inst Metals 28:83–94, 1987.

Wang FE, Buehler WJ, Pickart SJ. Crystal structure and a unique martensitic transition of TiNi. J Appl Phys 36:3232–3239, 1965.

Wang FE, Pickart SJ, Alperin HA. Mechanism of the TiNi martensitic transformation and the crystal structures of TiNi-II and TiNi-III phases. J Appl Phys 43:97–112, 1972.

Wayman CM, Duerig TW. An introduction to martensite and shape memory. In Duerig TW, Melton KN, Stöckel D, Wayman CM (eds). Engineering Aspects of Shape Memory Alloys. London: Butterworth-Heinemann, 1990; 3–20.

Williams BR, Caputo AA, Chaconas SJ. Orthodontic effects of loop design and heat treatment. Angle Orthod 48:235–239, 1978.

Wilson DF, Goldberg AJ. Alternative beta-titanium alloys for orthodontic wires. Dent Mater 3:337–341, 1987.

Yoneyama T, Doi H, Hamanaka H, Okamoto Y, Mogi M, Miura F. Super-elasticity and thermal behavior of Ni-Ti alloy orthodontic arch wires. Dent Mat J 11:1–10, 1992.

Yoshikawa DK, Burstone CJ, Goldberg AJ, Morton J. Flexure modulus of orthodontic stainless steel wires. J Dent Res 60:139–145, 1981.

Zapffe CA. Stainless Steels. Cleveland: American Society for Metals, 1949; Chap 6.

Chapter 21

Dental Porcelain

Porcelain has been used for denture teeth since 1790. Today the major use is for porcelain individual jacket crowns and for veneering metal crowns and bridgework. Porcelain has also been used to fabricate inlays, but this has fallen into disuse.

The main advantages of porcelain, responsible for its wide acceptance, are its excellent appearance properties, durability, and biocompatibility. Most attention today is centered on comparisons of the porcelains used to fabricate porcelain-fused-to-metal (PFM) crown-and-bridge work and the new, stronger ceramics used for all-ceramic jacket crowns. There is also growing interest in use of porcelain for veneers bonded to teeth to cover unsightly areas.

Porcelain is defined as a white, translucent ceramic that is fired to a glazed state. Dental porcelains are classified according to fusion temperature as follows:

High fusing	1,288° to 1,371°C (2,350° to 2,500°F)
Medium fusing	1,093° to 1,260°C (2,000° to 2,300°F)
Low fusing	871° to 1,066°C (1,600° to 1,950°F)

Denture teeth

The raw materials for porcelain denture teeth are mainly feldspar, with about 15% quartz and 4% kaolin clay to improve moldability. A plastic mass made from this mixture and additional pigments is formed into metal molds and fired under vacuum to reduce porosity. During firing the porcelain teeth are glazed by the glass produced from the feldspar. Metal pins or holes are placed in the teeth during manufacture for mechanical attachment to the denture base. Acrylic denture teeth have been steadily improved, and their use has grown as an alternative to porcelain.

Advantages

Advantages of porcelain teeth include:

1. Excellent biocompatibility
2. Natural appearance
3. High resistance to wear and distortion

Disadvantages

There are also several disadvantages to porcelain dentures:

1. Brittle
2. No bond to acrylic denture bases; requires mechanical attachments
3. Produces clicking sound on contact
4. Cannot be polished easily after grinding
5. Higher density increases weight of teeth
6. Mismatch in coefficient of thermal expansion produces stresses in acrylic denture base

Porcelain enamels used with metals

Composition

Dental porcelains are used to bond with metals for an outer layer of natural-appearing porcelain, as shown in Fig 21-1. These porcelains were developed during the 1950s by raising the coefficient of thermal expansion of feldspar porcelain to match the values of gold alloys, which are 13 to 14 × 10^{-6}°C. This was accomplished by heating orthoclase feldspar with alkali metal carbonates (eg, K_2CO_3, Li_2Co_3) to approximately 1,093°C (2,000°F) to form a glass and a high-expansion ceramic phase identified as leucite ($K_2O \cdot Al_2O_3 \cdot 4SiO_2$) (O'Brien and Ryge, 1964). An analysis of several of these high-expansion porcelain enamels is given in Table 21-1.

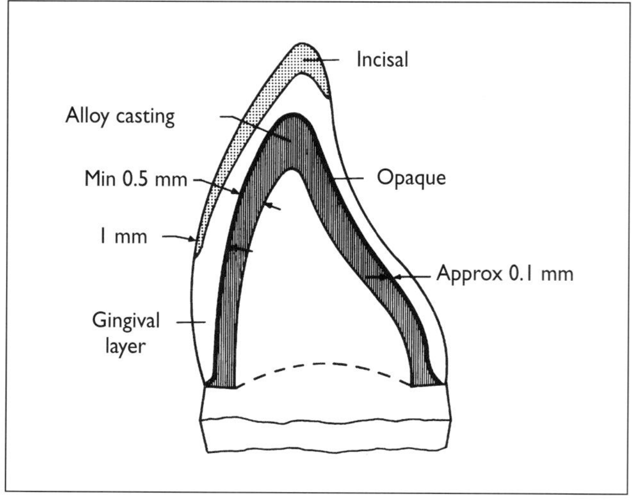

Fig 21-1 Cross section of a ceramic metal crown with full coverage.

During manufacture, the fused glass containing the leucite is quenched or "fritted" in water, freezing it in an amorphous state. The frit is then ground up by ball milling and pigmented with colored ceramic compound such as iron oxide to shade the porcelain. Each kit of porcelain supplied to dental technicians contains about a dozen shades of porcelain in at least three translucency levels for forming layers in building up the crown. The opaque porcelain contains approximately 15% tin oxide, zirconium oxide, or titanium dioxide. These opaque porcelains screen out the underlying metal oxide surface color, even in very thin layers. The main layer above the opaque layer is known as the *body* or *dentin* layer. Finally, a highly translucent porcelain called *incisal* or *enamel* gives the crowns a natural translucent appearance at the incisal edge.

Condensation and sintering

The anatomy of a porcelain crown is built up by hand by applying a paste of porcelain powder (applied to a metal casting or a platinum foil matrix with a small

Table 21-1 Chemical analysis of dental porcelains*

Compound	Biodent opaque	Ceramco opaque	VMK opaque	Biodent dentin	Ceramco dentin	VMK dentin
SiO_2	52.0 %	55.0 %	52.4 %	56.9 %	62.2 %	56.8 %
Al_2O_3	13.55	11.65	15.15	11.80	13.40	16.30
CaO	—	—	—	0.61	0.98	2.01
K_2O	11.05	9.6	9.9	10.0	11.3	10.25
Na_2O	5.28	4.75	6.58	5.42	5.37	8.63
TiO_2	3.01	—	2.59	0.61	—	0.27
ZrO_2	3.22	0.16	5.16	1.46	0.34	1.22
SnO_2	6.4	15.0	4.9	—	0.5	—
Rb_2O	0.09	0.04	0.08	0.10	0.06	0.10
BaO	1.09	—	—	3.52	—	—
ZnO	—	0.26	—	—	—	—
UO_3	—	—	—	—	—	0.67
B_2O_3, CO_2 and H_2O	4.31	3.54	3.24	9.58	5.85	3.75

*Data from Nally and Meyer, 1970.

brush). Generally, distilled water or special liquids are used to form the paste with the porcelain powder on a glass slab. As each layer of paste is added, most of the water is removed by vibrator and contact with an absorbent tissue paper. This gives the wet crown more strength and increases the density of the compact.

As each layer of the crown is built up, it is fired in a porcelain furnace. The wet crown is first dried in front of the furnace to remove the residual water and then fired under vacuum. As the porcelain is heated, adjacent particles bond together in a process called *sintering*. Although there is no meeting of the porcelain powder particles, they join together by flow on contact as a result of surface energy, as illustrated by Fig 21-2.

Firing in a vacuum furnace greatly reduces the porosity of the final product, as shown in Figs 21-3a and 21-3b. The first firing of porcelain is called the *bisque* or *biscuit bake*. After the incisal layer is added, the porcelain is brought to the final stage, called the *glaze bake*. Upon reaching the glazing temperature of the porcelain, a layer of glass is formed on the surface. After glazing, the crown is removed from the furnace and cooled under an inverted glass or beaker. An alternative approach is to add a thin layer of a low-fusing glass or glaze to the surface and fire to the flow temperature of the glaze.

Properties

Porcelain enamels have a vitreous structure consisting of an irregular network of silica produced by the presence of large alkali metal ions, such as sodium, potassium, and lithium (Fig 21-4a). This amorphous structure produces physical properties typical of a glass, including brittleness and lack of a definite melting

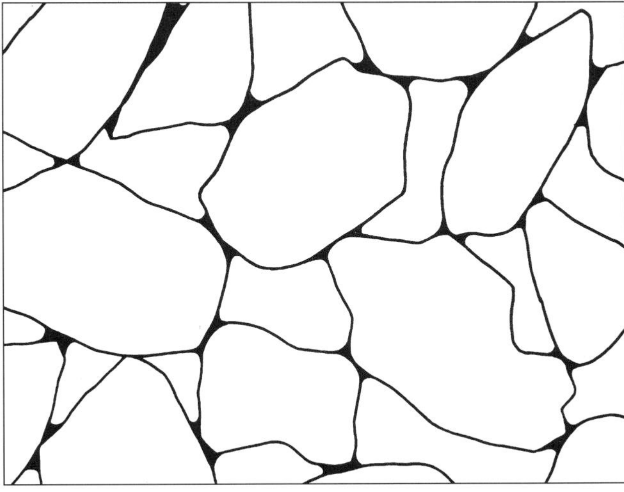

Fig 21-2 Biscuit stage of vitreous sintering, involving flow of glass to form bridges between particles. (From Van Vlack, 1959.)

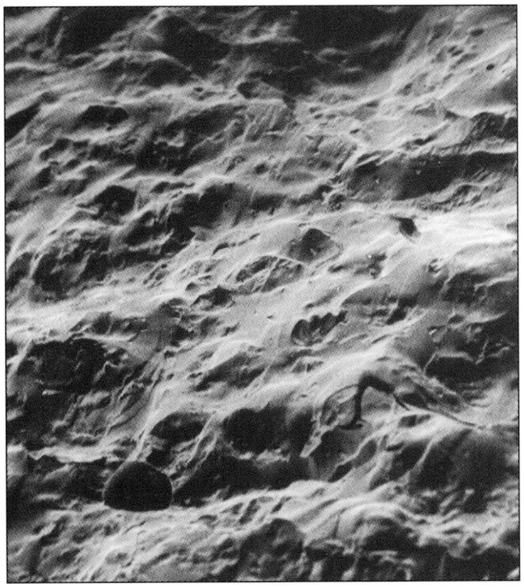

Fig 21-3a Fracture surface of gingival porcelain fired under vacuum. (Scanning electron micrograph, original magnification × 300; from Meyer et al, 1976.)

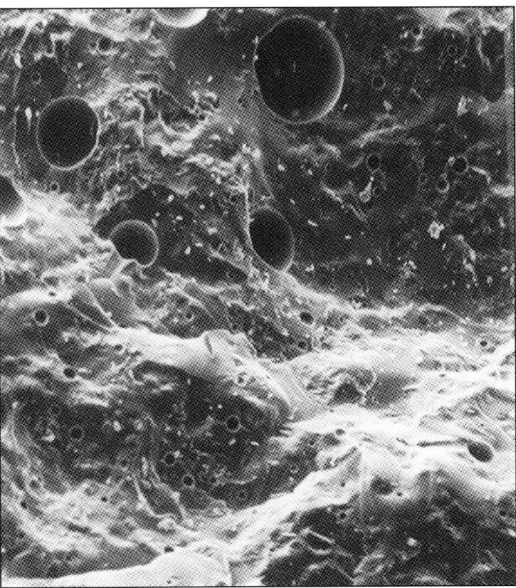

Fig 21-3b Fracture surface of gingival porcelain fired under normal atmospheric pressure. (Scanning electron micrograph, original magnification × 300; from Meyer et al, 1976.)

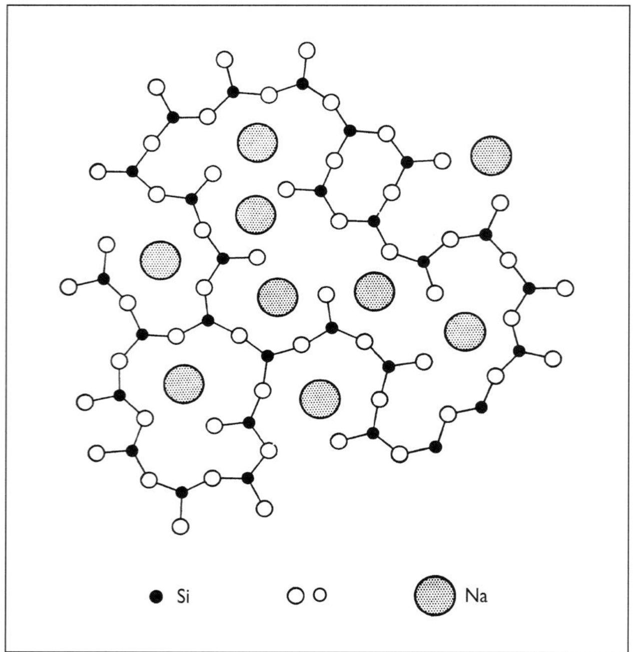

Fig 21-4a Irregularity of glass structure due to the presence of large alkali cations. (After Warren, 1941.)

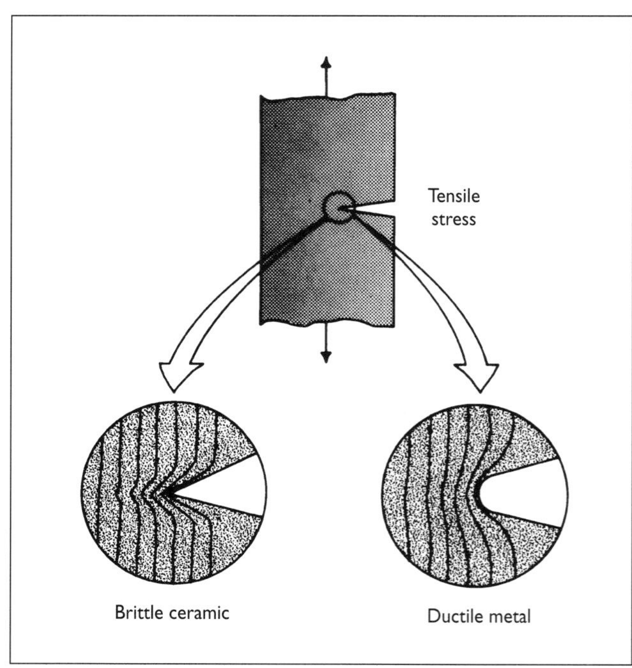

Fig 21-4b Effects of tensile and compressive forces on crack propagation in ceramics, resulting in high compressive strength and low tensile strength.

temperature. Glasses are brittle due to the irregular structure and the absence of slip planes present in a true crystalline material. The strength of glasses and brittle materials is actually governed by the presence of small flaws or cracks. When stressed in tension, according to the crack propagation theory, small flaws tend to open up and propagate, resulting in a low tensile strength. This is less of a factor with ductile metals because stress concentration around the tip of flaws is reduced by elongation of the metal, as illustrated in Fig 21-4b. However, glasses are much stronger in compression, because compressive stresses tend to close up flaws. Therefore, the tensile strengths of vitreous dental porcelains are around 5,000 psi (35 MPa) as compared with compressive strengths of 75,000 psi (517 MPa).

The strength of dental porcelains is traditionally tested in flexure as a beam and reported as *modulus of rupture*. The modulus of rupture of a vitreous body or enamel porcelain is about 13,000 psi (90 MPa). The strengths of vacuum-fired porcelains are higher due to fewer flaws.

Vitreous dental porcelains do not have a definite melting temperature but undergo a gradual decrease in viscosity when heated. A sharp decrease in viscosity occurs around the glass-transition temperature, T_g, as shown in Fig 21-5. Below T_g, the glass has the properties of a solid. Above T_g, glass flows more readily, and vitreous sintering takes place.

A typical thermal expansion (TE) curve of a porcelain bar is shown in Fig 21-6. The TE is linear up to around T_g. Above T_g there is a rapid increase in the rate of expansion when the glass has a more liquid structure. If heating is continued, the bar will reach the softening temperature and collapse. The TE of dental porcelains for bonding to metals is especially important in relation to the TE of the metal involved. Generally, the metal and porcelain should be matched in coefficients of TE values. If the TE curves of the metal and porcelain are too far apart, undesirable thermal stresses will result in fracture of the porcelain, which is the weaker material. The porcelain and metal are therefore said to be incompatible.

Adhesion to metals

Several factors have been identified as promoting good adhesion or bonding of a porcelain enamel to a metal, including wetting, adherent oxide, and mechanical retention.

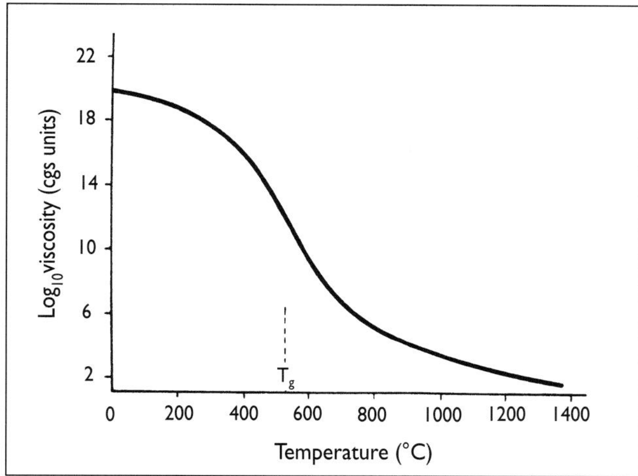

Fig 21-5 Viscosity (rigidity) increasing rapidly below glass-transition temperature. (From Jones GO. Glass. London: Methuen, 1956.)

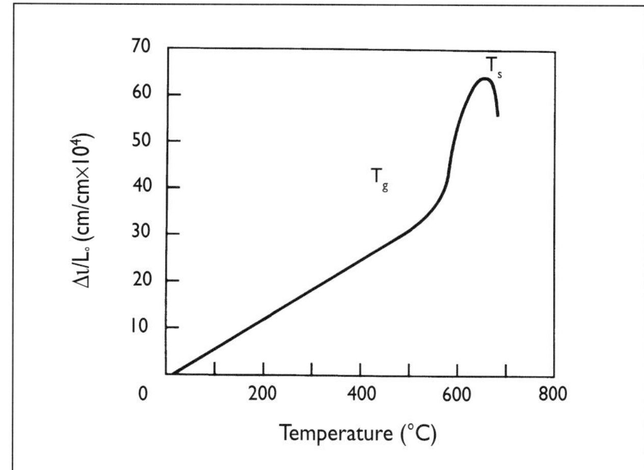

Fig 21-6 Thermal expansion curve for glass with a glass-transition temperature (Tg) and softening temperature (Ts).

Wetting

Good wetting of the porcelain on the metal is indicated by a low contact angle of a drop of the porcelain when fired on the solid, as shown in Fig 21-7. Good wetting promotes penetration of the glass into surface irregularities and, therefore, a greater area of contact. Good wetting also indicates chemical compatibility between the porcelain and the metal.

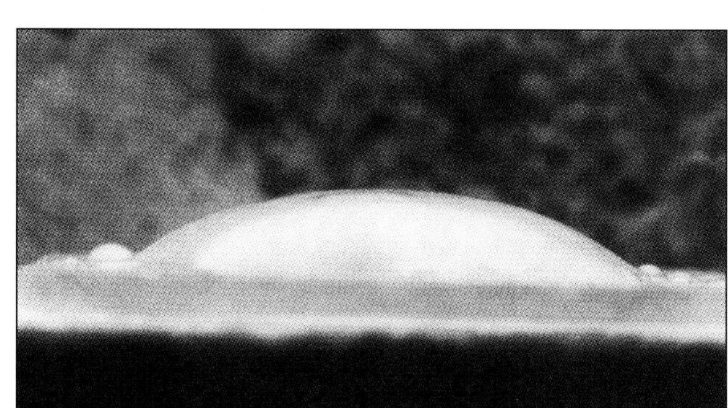

Fig 21-7 Good wetting of molten porcelain on alloy.

Adherent oxide

The presence of an adherent oxide on the metal surface that is wet by the porcelain provides a beneficial transition layer. Diffusion of atoms from the metal and porcelain into this oxide usually can be detected and is cited as evidence of a chemical bond. A nonadherent oxide can lead to a weak boundary failure.

Mechanical retention

The presence of surface roughness on the metal oxide surface can result in mechanical retention on a microscopic level, especially if undercuts are present.

Bond failure classification

The several types of failure possible are shown in Fig 21-8. A Type I failure, shown in Fig 21-9, was the result of using a thick, pure gold coating agent on the alloy surface. Such a coating blocks formation of the trace metal oxide layer necessary for strong bonding.

Figure 21-10 shows a clinical failure found in a nickel-chromium alloy, which is classified as Type V. If the oxide layer on nickel alloys becomes too thick, a weak boundary layer is formed. Figure 21-11 shows a nickel alloy surface with microscopic cohesive attachment sites where the bond was stronger than the porcelain. The relation between the density of these sites to bond strength is shown in Fig 21-12.

When density is low, mixed types of bond failure are observed. However, when the cohesive plateau is reached, the bond strength is equal to the strength of the porcelain, S_p, and cohesive failure is observed. Because the bond strength in tension has been found to be about 5,000 psi (35 MPa) with properly oxidized gold alloys, and the tensile strength of the porcelain has been measured to be about the same, higher bond strengths lack practical significance. Shear bond

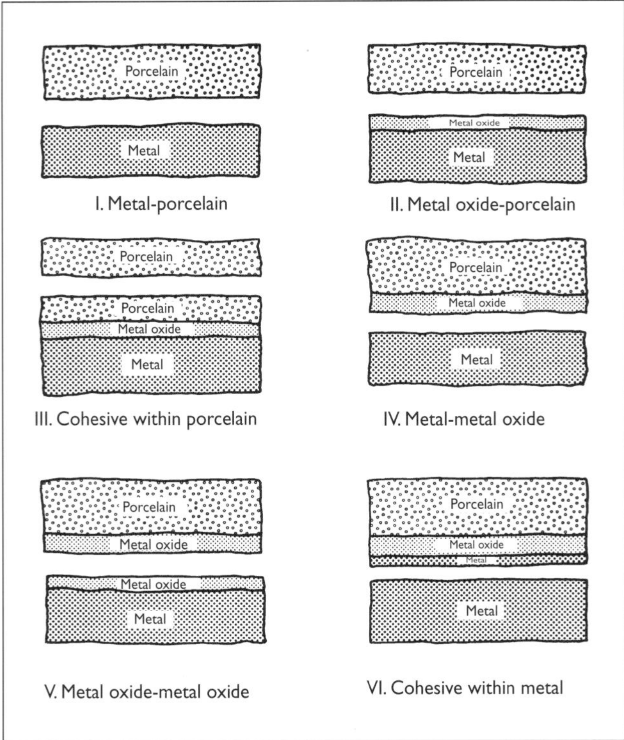

Fig 21-8 Classification of porcelain enamel failures according to interfaces formed. Type III represents cohesive failure indicative of a proper bond. (From O'Brien, 1977.)

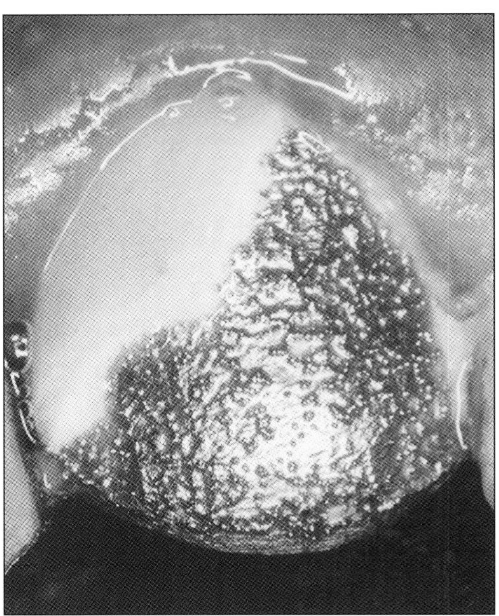

Fig 21-9 Type I failure in gold casting coated with pure gold.

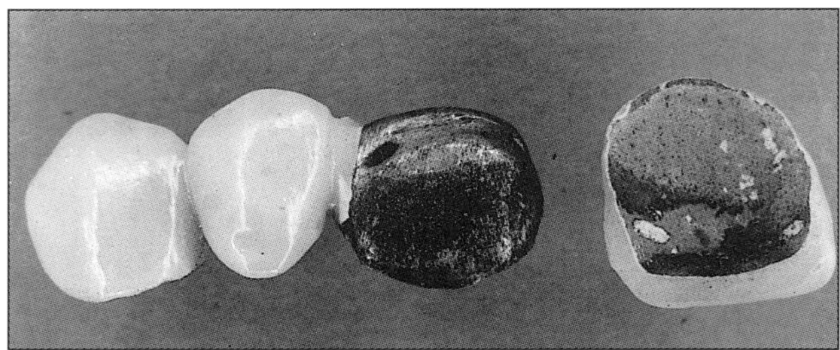

Fig 21-10 Example of Type V failure with fracture through oxide layer of nickel-chromium alloy.

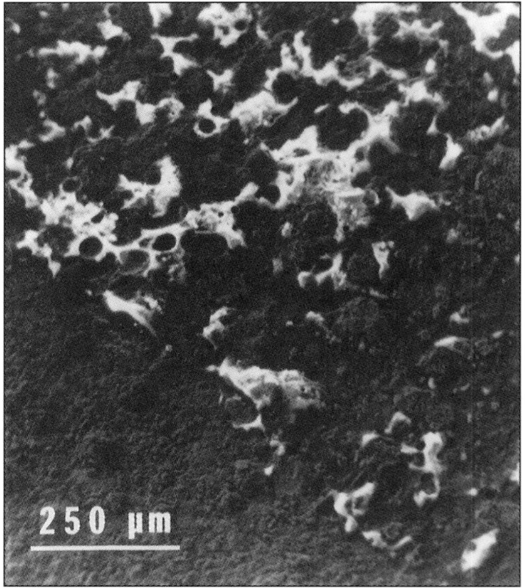

Fig 21-11 Microscopic cohesive attachment sites on fracture interface between nickel alloy and porcelain; a mixed failure.

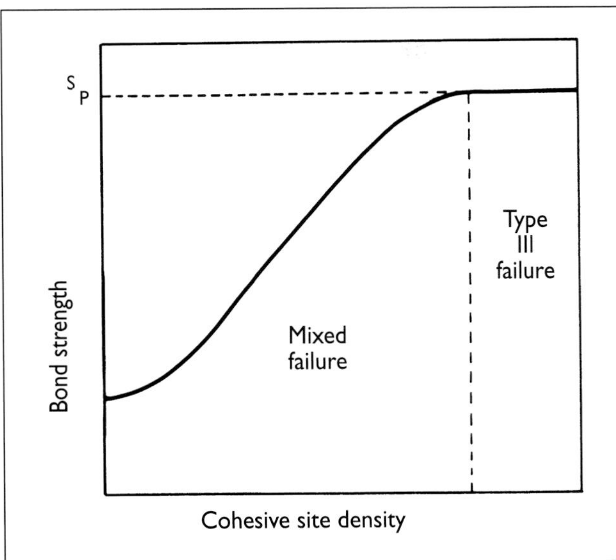

Fig 21-12 Relation between density of cohesive attachment sites and observed bond strengths.

strength tests indicate values of 16,000 psi (111 MPa) to 21,000 psi (147 MPa), as these represent the shear strengths of the porcelains.

Advantages

The advantages to bonding porcelain enamels to metal include:

1. High strength
2. Makes bridgework possible
3. Excellent fit

Disadvantages

Some of the disadvantages of these restorations are:

1. Appearance of metal margins
2. Discoloration by metal
3. Difficulty producing an appearance of translucency
4. Bond failure with metals
5. Possible disadvantages of alloy used

All-ceramic crowns

A classification of porcelain crowns according to composition is shown in Fig 21-13. The *jacket crown* is the traditional and still-valid term for all-ceramic crowns used for restoring the entire clinical crown portion of a tooth.

The most significant developments in dental ceramics within the past few years have been in new materials and processes for fabricating ceramic jacket crowns. Porcelain jacket crowns have been used widely in dentistry since Land developed the platinum foil technique in 1903. They were fabricated with high-fusing feldspathic porcelains and were known for natural esthetics resulting mainly from high translucency and the specialized laboratory skills used. However, they have not been used extensively for the past 15 years. Failures of these porcelain crowns include breakage or fracture. It has been suggested that failures are caused by the low strength of the porcelain or possibly poor adaptation to the tooth, resulting in high-stress areas; however, this has not been documented.

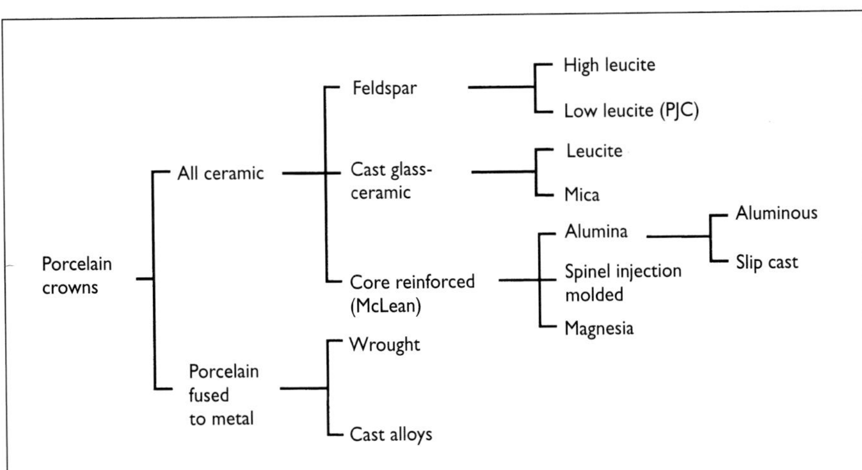

Fig 21-13 A classification of porcelain crowns according to composition.

In 1965, alumina-reinforced porcelain crowns were introduced. These crowns are constructed of a coping or core of a ceramic material containing 40% to 50% alumina with an outer layer of translucent porcelain. The alumina ceramic core material has a flexure strength of approximately 131 MPa (19,000 psi), which is twice that of feldspathic porcelain. The clinical failure rate for anterior crowns made with alumina ceramic cores has recently been established to be below 2%, which is considered an acceptable risk. However, the failure rate for molar crowns was 15.2%, which is unacceptable. Therefore, core materials for anterior crowns should have flexure strengths not significantly below 131 MPa (19,000 psi), and the strength required for posterior crowns is still to be determined.

Interest in all-ceramic crowns in the United States has developed recently for many reasons. First, the all-ceramic crown has greater potential for more esthetic anterior restorations. In the PFM crown, the alloy structure produces an opaque appearance and the metal margins are often visible. Also, the selection of alloys for PFM has become a confusing issue for many dentists. The high-gold-content alloys are relatively expensive, and the alternatives may have disadvantages such as risk of metal allergy, bond failure, or porcelain discoloration. In addition, the number of available alloys is extensive, and noble metal content alone is not indicative of clinical performance. Currently, alloys that are classified as acceptable or provisionally acceptable by the American National Standards Institute/American Dental Association (ANSI/ADA) range from high-noble alloys to nickel alloys.

Spinel injection-molded core material

The injection molding process is used for the coping of an all-ceramic crown. The rest of the crown is built up by hand and fired in the same way as alumina-reinforced porcelain jacket crowns. Its advantages are the elimination of the platinum foil step in forming the crown and improved marginal adaptation. The molding material is a low-shrinkage alumina magnesia spinel ceramic. The low shrinkage from the unfired (green) state to the fired state is obtained by controlling the time and temperature of the firing cycle in a special furnace.

Injection molding of core material was recommended for single anterior or posterior crowns. Tooth preparation for the margin is either a full 90-degree shoulder with rounded gingivo-axial line angle, or a 135-degree chamfer. Tooth reduction is 1.2 to 1.5 mm for facial, lingual, and interproximal surfaces; 1.5 to 2 mm for incisal edges; and 2 mm for occlusal surfaces. In some applications, such as for mandibular incisors, 1-mm shoulders may be prepared. All sharp angles should be rounded to avoid stress concentration.

An impression is taken using a nonaqueous elastomeric impression material such as polysulfide, polyether, silicone, or selected polysiloxane. A polysiloxane impression material that releases gases during polymerization should not be used. An epoxy model is poured and cured, and a die is prepared. The epoxy die is used for waxing a coping to a uniform thickness (0.5 mm for anterior crowns, 0.8 mm for posterior crowns). A die stone mold of the coping incorporating the master epoxy die is prepared. The volume intended for forming the coping is obtained by the lost wax process. A plastic composition containing alumina, magnesia, wax, glass, and a silicone resin is heated to 180°C (356°F) and injection molded into the mold under air pressure to form the new coping.

After the sprue is removed, the core material is fired in a special furnace for several hours (usually overnight) to a peak temperature of 1,300°C (2,372°F). During the firing procedure, complex reactions in the ceramic compensate for the normal firing shrinkage, resulting in greater accuracy. Special veneer porcelains are then fired on the core coping for a good esthetic appearance and to complete the anatomy of the crown. The flexure strength of the original core material is 118 MPa (17,110 psi), which is not significantly different from that of the alumina-reinforced core material. A second-generation material has a higher strength.

The advantage of the process is greater potential accuracy of the fit of the coping on the master die. Of course, the accuracy of the fit to the prepared tooth will depend on the accuracies of the impression, the die, and the manipulation. There is a greater potential for better esthetics because the metal coping is absent. However, the final appearance depends on the usual factors of shade matching by the dentist and technical skill in building up the outer layers of the crown.

Other possible advantages include radiolucency and good biocompatibility. The main disadvantage is

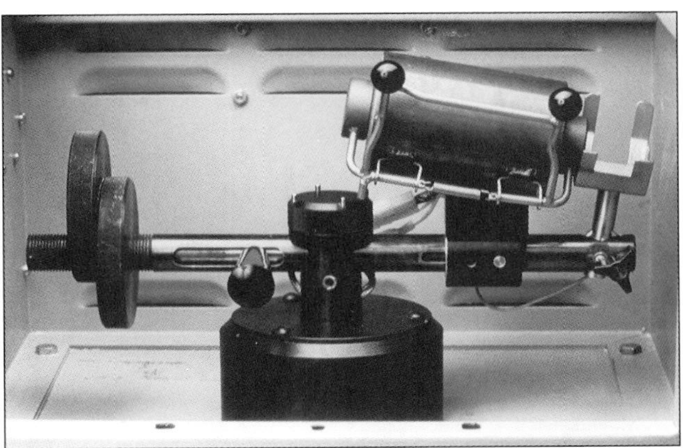

Fig 21-14 Centrifugal casting machine for castable ceramic crowns (Dicor system).

the complexity and cost of the process, making the final crown as expensive as a PFM crown. High cost, complexity, and lack of demand apparently led to this type of crown being withdrawn from the market. However, it could possibly reappear at a later time and is therefore included here.

Castable ceramic

Castable ceramic systems are used to cast crowns by the lost wax process. Indication for use is in single anterior and posterior crowns. Tooth preparation is either a 90-degree shoulder with a rounded internal line angle or a 120-degree chamfer with adequate tooth reduction—from 1 mm minimum on the gingivo-axial surfaces to 1.5 to 2 mm incisally and occlusally.

Impressions, models, and dies are made in the usual manner. The restoration is waxed on the die, and the wax pattern of the crown is invested in a phosphate-bonded investment following the same procedure used for some metal crowns. An ingot of the ceramic material is placed in a special crucible and melted and cast with a motor-driven centrifugal casting machine at 1,380°C (2,500°F) (Fig 21-14). The cast crown is a clear glass that must be heat treated to form a crystalline ceramic, which is essentially a fluorine mica silicate. The crystallization procedure takes several hours in a heat-treating or "ceramming" furnace, with a final temperature of 1,075°C (1,967°F).

The fired ceramic crown has a "universal" white shade with a translucency of around 50%. It has a flexure strength of 152 MPa (22,000 psi) and a coefficient of TE of 7.2×10^{-6}/°C. Final shading is achieved using a series of light coats of colored surface porcelains. Shaded zinc phosphate cements are suggested by the manufacturer. As the entire crown is translucent, these colored cements may also be used to achieve the final shade. Before seating the crown, tight contacts may be adjusted with an abrasive stone or wheel and then polished with rubber wheels.

A second cast ceramic (Cerapearl, Kyocera America, Inc.) based on a calcium-phosphate glass has been introduced. This system also involves casting by the lost wax process and heat treatment to convert the cast glass into a ceramic. Transverse strength values between 17,000 and 43,500 psi (116 to 300 MPa) are reported. However, experience and documentation of the properties of this new system are limited at this time compared with the fluorine-mica system.

Magnesia core material

Magnesia core material is compatible with the high-expansion porcelains normally bonded to metals. This is a major advantage because technicians are already familiar with handling these porcelains. Also, shade matching with adjacent PFM bridges is simpler.

Magnesia rather than alumina is used as the basis of the high-expansion core material because it has a coefficient of TE of 13.5×10^{-6}/°C for magnesia. This higher TE is explained on the basis that magnesia has a face-centered cubic structure, whereas alumina has a hexagonal, close-packed structure. Strengthening is achieved by dispersion of the magnesia crystals in a vitreous matrix, and also by crystallization within the matrix. These mechanisms are both necessary to achieve the required strength. The microstructure is shown in Fig 21-15 and crown design in Fig 21-16.

The magnesia core material has a modulus of rupture strength of 19,000 psi (131 MPa) after firing and a coefficient of TE value of 14.5×10^{-6}/°C. Its strength can be doubled by applying a glaze to a value of 39,000 psi (269 MPa). The glaze strengthens by two mechanisms: (*1*) It penetrates into surface pores to fill in these points of high stress; and (*2*) it places the surface layer in compression. The strength of the core material in relation to other dental ceramics is given in Fig 21-17.

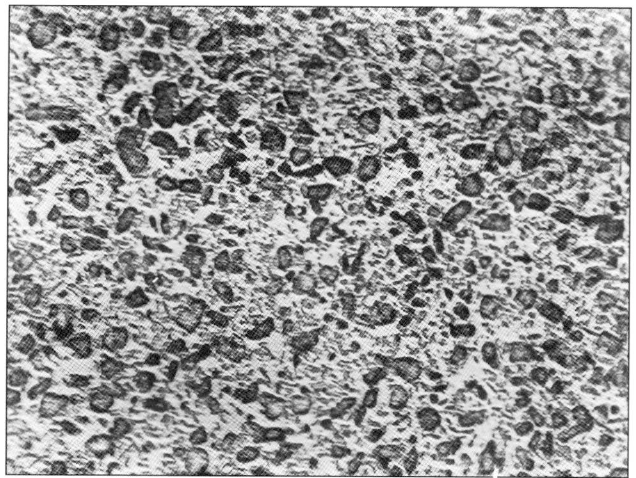

Fig 21-15 The microstructure of the high-expansion magnesia core material.

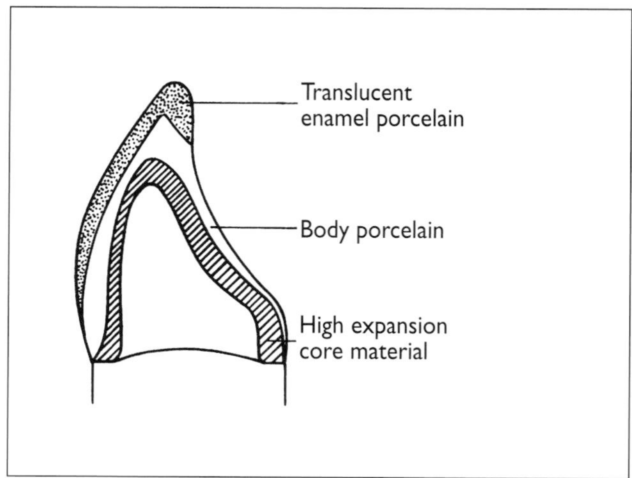

Fig 21-16 Magnesia-core crown.

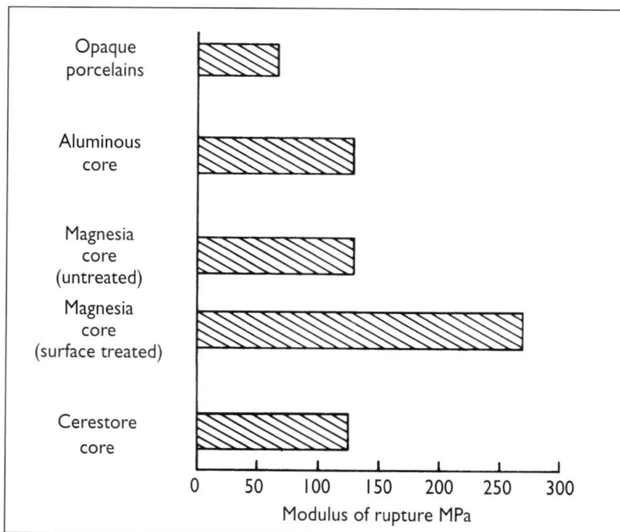

Fig 21-17 Comparison of strengths of porcelains for jacket crowns.

Advantages

Reasons to use this material include:

1. Adequate strength for most anterior crowns
2. Esthetics superior to PFM for a given shade and technician (eg, no metal margins, discoloration, etc)
3. No risk in choosing alloy

Disadvantages

These disadvantages are worthy of consideration as well:

1. Not used for bridges
2. Requires learning to do good shoulder preparation (new instruments available)

Injection-molded high-leucite porcelain

In this process (Empress, Ivoclar) high-leucite porcelain ingot cylinders are heated to 115°C to produce a plastic state. Then, the ingots are pressure-injected into investment molds formed by the lost wax process for crowns, inlays, onlays, and veneers (Fig 21-18). Due to the relatively high leucite content and pressure forming process, the flexural strength of porcelain formed by this process is around 200 MPa. The advantages of the process are good fit and higher strength for the resulting restorations.

Alumina slip casting

This is a process for forming alumina cores that gives very high strength values (around 500 MPa).

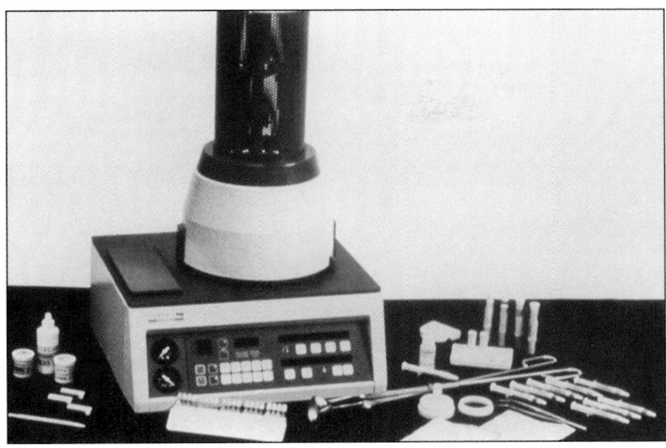

Fig 21-18 Injection-molding oven for high-leucite Empress porcelain.

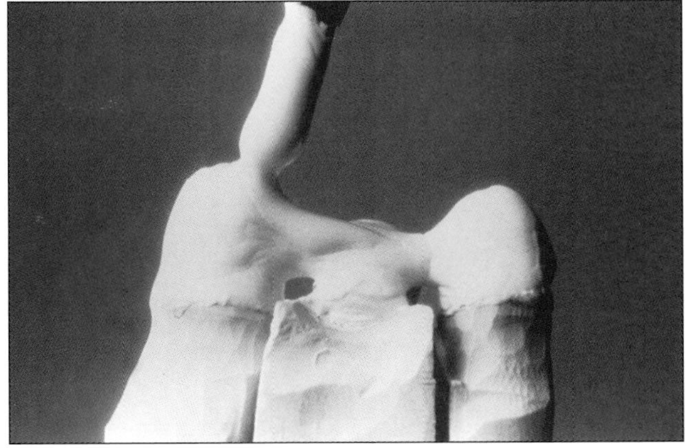

Fig 21-19 Application of alumina-liquids slip to plaster cast that absorbs water by capillary action. (Courtesy of Vident, Inc.)

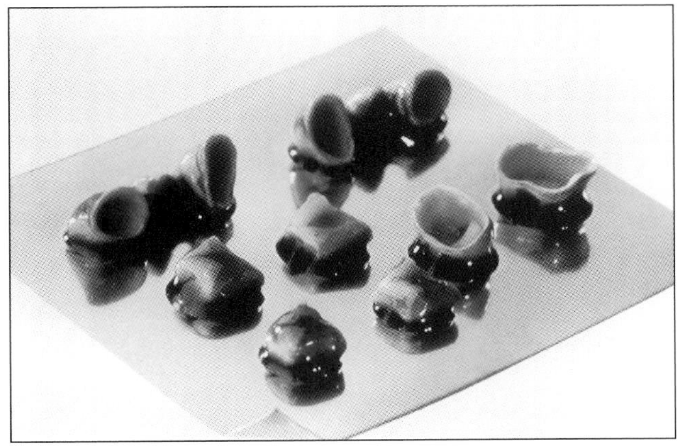

Fig 21-20 Glass infiltration of alumina copings fired on platinum foil.

To form the alumina cores, a slurry of fine alumina particles is painted on plaster dies, which absorb the water to form a green state core. The alumina is then sintered at 1,120°C to form a dense mass. Glass is then applied and fused at 1,100°C for 4 hours to allow glass infiltration (Figs 21-19 and 21-20). The rest of the crown is then formed by firing a body porcelain over the cores by traditional firing. The advantages of this process are high strength and good fit. The disadvantages are the high initial cost, long processing time, and lack of bonding to the tooth structure. Although the strength of the glass-infiltrated alumina cores is high, the alumina cannot be etched and silane treated for resin bonding.

Milled ceramic restorations

A number of systems for machining ceramics to produce inlays, onlays, and veneers have been introduced. One system uses *computer-assisted designs and computer-assisted manufacturer* (CAD/CAM) technology and comes from the manufacturing industry. In making an inlay with the Cerec CAD/CAM chairside system, the following sequence is carried out. First, a powder is applied to the patient's prepared tooth to provide contrast for the optical scanner. Next, the prepared tooth is scanned with an optical probe, and the image is stored in a computer (see Fig 21-21). The inlay is designed on a monitor screen with computer assistance. The proximal surfaces are generated by the computer. After the restoration is designed, a bloc of a machinable glass-ceramic is selected by shade. With information from the computer, the inlay is milled in a few minutes in a compartment of the chairside unit. The inlay is then acid-etched, and a silane agent is applied in preparation for bonding to the tooth preparation. After cementing with a resin cement, the occlusal and then the main surfaces are contoured with a diamond contour instrument and polished. The main advantage of the Cerec CAD/CAM system is the elimination of sending work to an outside laboratory for processing. This allows ceramic restorations to be made and cemented in a single visit. The major disadvantages are high initial equipment costs and a lack of marginal accuracy. The average marginal fit with the Cerec system varies from 50 µm to 260 µm, which is much higher than the accepted 30 to 40 µm requirement for a proper fit. However, since a resin cement and enamel ceramic bonding are used, the

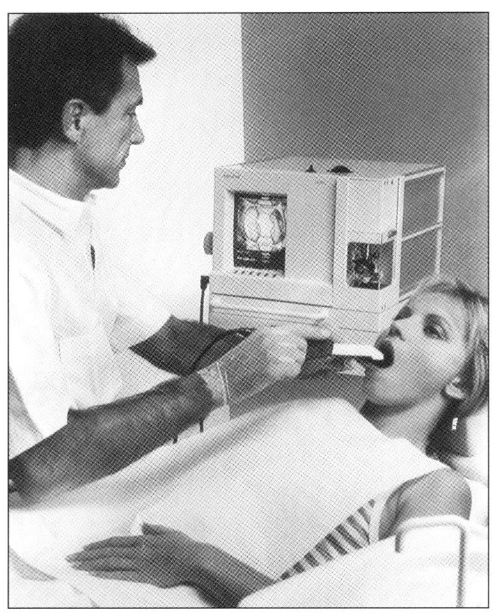

Fig 21-21 The Cerec CAD/CAM system for chairside inlay fabrication. (Courtesy of Siemens, Inc.)

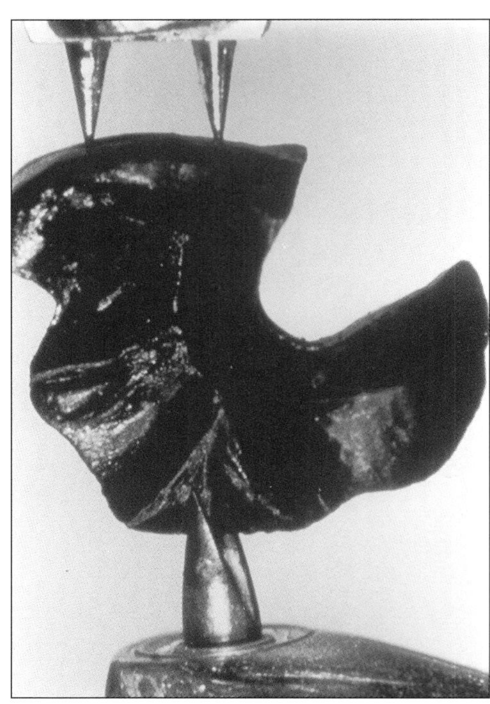

Fig 21-22 Composite materials pattern for copy milling. (Courtesy of Vident, Inc.)

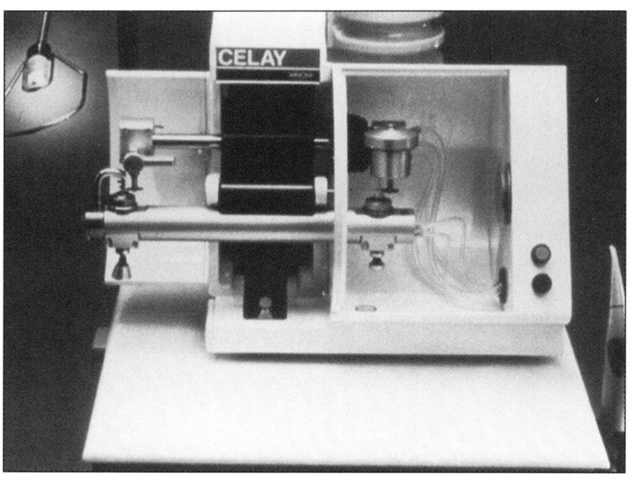

Fig 21-23 The Celay copy-milling machine. (Courtesy of Vident, Inc.)

older standard of marginal fit may be too stringent. Although the resin cement is worn down considerably during the first year, it appears to stop thereafter. A third disadvantage of this system is that around 50% of the time required for a restoration is spent in creating the occlusion and polishing by hand. Less time is usually required for this step when an inlay is made from an elastomeric impression using the traditional technique.

Another system for machining ceramic blocks into inlays, onlays, and veneers is copy milling, known as the Celay system (Vident, Baldwin Park, CA). In this system, a pattern is made with a waxlike modeling material on a traditional die (Fig 21-22). The modeling material is then hardened by light curing. This pattern is then used in a copy-milling machine (see Fig 21-23). As the outline of the pattern is traced on one side, a block of ceramic is milled to duplicate it simultaneously in a process analogous to key duplication. This equipment is less expensive than the CAD/CAM system, and the occlusal surface is produced by the milling based on the handmade pattern. The disadvantages vis-á-vis CAD/CAM are that an impression and extra visit are required because copy milling is not a chairside, one-visit procedure.

Copy milling has been shown to produce marginal accuracy values in the range of 80 to 100 μm, which is close to values for conventional laboratory sintering techniques. However, the Cerec inlays have reported values of 200 to 260 μm for marginal gaps, as shown in Figures 21-24a and 21-24b. There is more variability in marginal openings reported in studies.

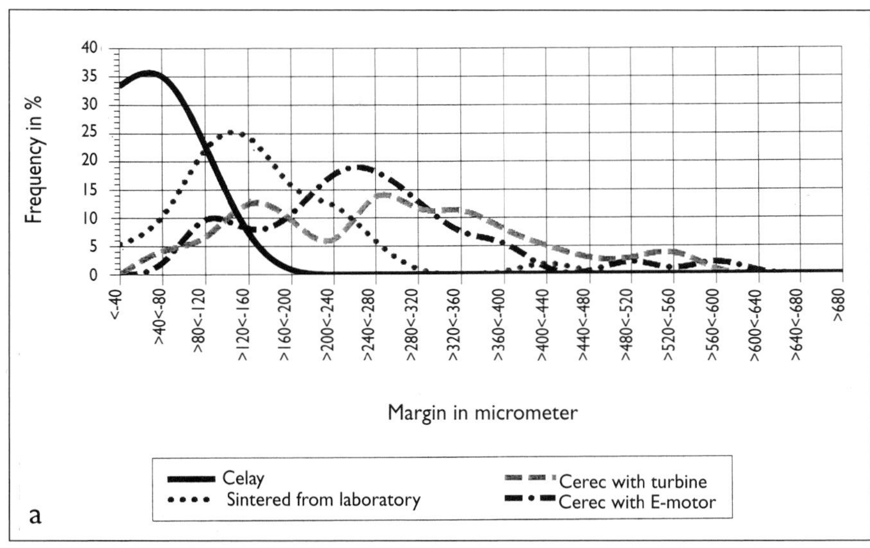

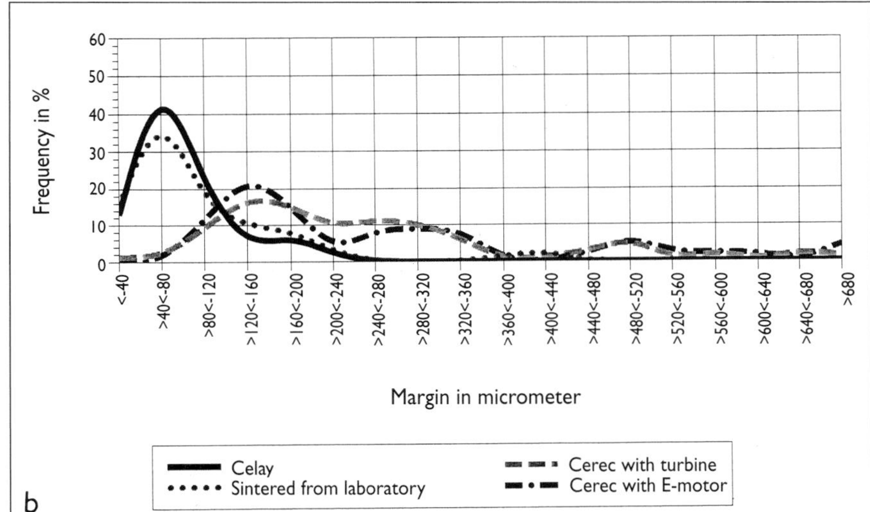

Fig 21-24 The marginal gap distribution found for mesio-occlusodistal porcelain inlays procedures: (a) approximal, (b) occlusal. (From Siervo et al, 1994.)

Clinical scenario for dental porcelain manufacture

This section presents an approach for choosing materials and a system for a specific situation. It uses the same format as that presented in Chapter 7:

1. The situation is described.
2. Critical factors are listed.
3. Advantages and disadvantages of each material/system are prioritized using the following codes: * = of minor importance, ** = important, and *** = very important.
4. The situation is analyzed, and the final decision given.

Situation: CAD/CAM or Vita InCeram inlays versus Empress inlays to improve esthetics in fewer appointments

A patient has had a number of routine restorations placed over the years. They consist basically of Class I and II amalgam restorations and some anterior composites. The patient has been very satisfied with the results of these restorations, but is now seeking more esthetic, but still long-lasting, alternatives to replace her amalgams. She also indicates that she is leaving on vacation in two weeks, and that she would like to have all the dental work done before that.

Situation CAD/CAM inlays vs Empress inlays†

Critical factors Good esthetics, speed of completion

Advantages

CAD/CAM inlays

*** 1. Good esthetics
*** 2. Can be completed in one appointment
*** 3. No impressions required
*** 4. No temporization required
*** 5. Not dependent on lab availability
* 6. No lab fee

Empress inlays

*** 1. Excellent esthetics
** 2. Good marginal adaptation

Disadvantages

CAD/CAM inlays

* 1. Expensive equipment
** 2. Variability in marginal adaptation

Empress inlays

*** 1. At least two appointments required for completion
*** 2. Impressions required
*** 3. Temporization required
*** 4. Dependent on lab availability
* 5. Lab fee

†Courtesy of Gisele de Faria Neiva.

Situation IPS Empress vs Vita InCeram†

Critical factors Etch ability, cost, and flexural strength

Advantages

IPS Empress

*** 1. Ability to be etched
** 2. Marginal fidelity of <50 μm
*** 3. Flexural tensile strength of 95 to 195 MPa
** 4. Versatility (anterior crowns, veneers, inlays, and onlays)
*** 5. Twenty-five shades in the Chromascop system, including Vita hues
** 6. Three-dimensional color, translucency, and opalescence from leucite porcelain substructure, if layered
** 7. Relatively simple technique using lost wax technique modified for this system
*** 8. Wears almost like tooth enamel
** 9. Biocompatible

Vita InCeram

*** 1. Flexural tensile strength of 450 to 600 MPa
** 2. Marginal fidelity of 20 to 25 μm
*** 3. Versatility (single crown; three anterior fixed partial dentures; and inlays, onlays, and veneers with Spinel InCeram)
*** 4. Vita Lumin Vacuum shade guide
** 5. Three-dimensional color, translucency, and opalescence from its aluminous porcelain substructure and Vitadur Alpha superstructure
** 6. No thermal sensitivity
** 7. Biocompatible
** 8. Flexibility of provisional cementation

Disadvantages

IPS Empress

*** 1. Expensive system (EP 500)—laboratory's initial set-up cost is $17,200 with training and support services—slightly more than PFM
** 2. Learning period required for technicians
* 3. Dependent on dentist's knowledge of dentin bonding and resin cement use
*** 4. Longevity (market life span has increased since 1992)

Vita InCeram

*** 1. Expensive system—laboratory's initial set-up cost is $15,906 with training and support services
*** 2. Learning period required for technicians, because of the complexity of slip-cast fabrication, a relatively new concept
*** 3. Nonetchable
*** 4. Time and labor-intensive
*** 5. Longevity (market life span needs more clinical service)
*** 6. Questionable wear

†Courtesy of Waletha Wasson, DDS, MS.

Analysis/Decision

Because of the patient's request for long-lasting restorations and also because of the urgency for treatment completion, posterior composites were ruled out. Therefore the decision was between CAD/CAM, or Vita InCeram or laboratory-processed Empress inlays.

Because time was so important, the CAD/CAM system was chosen.

Glossary

bisque (biscuit bake) The first firing of a porcelain.

cohesive plateau strength The apparent bond strength between porcelain and alloy equal to the strength of the porcelain, attained when the bond is stronger than the porcelain.

crack propagation theory The theory that glasses and other brittle materials fail by the propagation of minute flaws or cracks when under stress.

feldspar A crystalline mineral of the general formula $X_2O \cdot Al_2O_3 \cdot 6SiO_2$, where X may be sodium or potassium.

frit A powdered glass.

glass-transition temperature The temperature below which a glass behaves like a solid.

glaze The shiny layer of surface glass produced on a porcelain by firing. The glass may either come from within the porcelain or be added to the surface before the final firing.

jacket crown An all-porcelain crown.

modulus of rupture The flexure strength of a material determined by loading a beam-shaped specimen.

opacifiers White oxides added to decrease the transparency of the porcelain. Usually tin oxide or titanium dioxide.

porcelain A white, ceramic-containing glass with a glazed surface.

porcelain, aluminous A porcelain-containing alumina (Al_2O_3) as an opacifier and strengthener.

residual stresses Stresses frozen in a material that are independent of an applied force.

sintering The densification of a powdered material, usually by heating.

vitreous Glasslike in properties.

Discussion questions

1. What is the biocompatibility of porcelain to soft and hard tissues that it contacts?
2. Compare the advantages of porcelain-fused-to-metal and all-ceramic crowns.
3. What is the nature of the bond between porcelain and metal?

Questions and answers

1. **What is the difference between vitreous and crystalline ceramics?** Crystalline ceramics have an orderly, repetitive arrangement of atoms. Vitreous ceramics have an amorphous structure without the orderly pattern of a crystal.
2. **Which ions form glasses by their incorporation into silicate systems?** Alkali ions (ie, Na^+, K^+, Li^+) disrupt the silicate structure to form glasses.
3. **What is the nature of the coloring agents used in dental porcelains?** Metallic oxides are added for color in dental porcelains.
4. **How is a frit made?** A frit is powdered glass made by fusing the constituents together in a furnace and then quenching and grinding.
5. **How does sintering differ from complete fusion?** Sintering involves increasing the density of a powdered mass by bonding at points of contact rather than by melting particles.

6. **What is the role of surface tension in sintering?** The driving force for sintering is the reduction of surface area by the force of surface tension. Therefore, a fine particle size and high glass surface tension promote rapid sintering.
7. **Why are porcelains fired under vacuum?** To reduce porosity created by entrapped air.
8. **Why is glazing not produced during the biscuit bake?** The porcelain is not heated enough to produce glazing until the final bake in order to limit firing shrinkage. Excessive glazing also produces a rounding of edges.
9. **How much shrinkage occurs during the firing of porcelain?** About 30%–40%.
10. **Define glass-transition temperature.** The temperature below which glass becomes very rigid or behaves like a solid.
11. **Why are glasses considerably weaker under tensile stresses than under compressive stresses?** Glasses and other brittle solids fail by crack propagation. Tensile stresses cause cracks to spread, whereas compressive stresses do not.
12. **Why can residual stresses in ceramics be either beneficial or harmful?** Residual compressive stresses at the surface of a ceramic inhibit surface-crack propagation and increase strength. Tensile stresses at the surface lower strength. Therefore, the location and direction of residual stresses determine their effect on properties.
13. **How does the bond strength of porcelains to alloys compare with the strength of the feldspar glass alone?** According to the cohesive plateau theory, the maximum measurable bond strength is equal to the cohesive strength of the porcelain (ie, 5,000 psi [35 MPa] in tension).
14. **What effect does the addition of oxide-forming elements to gold have on the wetting and bonding of porcelain enamels?** The nature and thickness of the oxide layer formed on alloys are critical to the bond strength. Bonding to pure gold produces only a relatively weak bond. Tin, indium, and iron oxides adhere strongly to a gold-alloy surface, reduce the contact angle, and produce cohesive porcelain fractures.

Recommended reading

Denry IL. Recent advances in ceramics for dentistry. Crit Rev Oral Biol Med 7:134–143, 1996.

Felcher FR. Dental porcelains. J Am Dent Assoc 19:1021, 1932.

Hodson JT. Some physical properties of three dental porcelains. J Prosthet Dent 9:235, 1959.

Kelly M, Asgar K, O'Brien WJ. Tensile strength determination of the interface between porcelain fused to gold. J Biomed Mater Res 3:403–408, 1969.

Lewis AF, Natarajan RT. Adhesion Science and Technology. New York: Plenum Press, 1975.

McLean JW. A higher strength of porcelain for crown and bridge work. Br Dent J 119:268, 1965.

McLean JW. The Science and Art of Dental Ceramics. Vol I. The Nature of Dental Ceramics and Their Clinical Use. Chicago: Quintessence Publishing Co, 1979.

Meyer JM, O'Brien WJ, Yu R. The sintering of dental porcelain. J Dent Res 52:580, 1976.

Mumford G. The porcelain fused to metal restorations. Dent Clin North Am 9:241, March 1965.

Nally JN, Meyer JM. Recherche expérimentale sur la nature de la laison céramo-métallique. Schweiz Monatsschr Zahnheilkd 80:250, 1970.

O'Brien WJ (ed). Ceramics. Dent Clin North Am Vol 29. Philadelphia: WB Saunders Co, 1985.

O'Brien WJ. Dental porcelains. In RG Craig (ed). Dental Materials Review. Ann Arbor: University of Michigan Press, 1977; 123–135.

O'Brien WJ, Ryge G. Contact angles of drops of enamels on metals. J Prosthet Dent 15:1094, 1965.

O'Brien WJ, Ryge G (eds). Dental Ceramics. Engineering and Science Proc. Columbus, OH: American Ceramic Society, Jan-Feb 1985.

O'Brien WJ, Ryge G. Relation between molecular-force calculations and observed strengths of enamel-metal interfaces. J Am Ceramic Soc 47:5–8, 1964.

Preston JD (ed). Perspectives in Dental Ceramics. Proceedings of the Fourth International Symposium on Ceramics. Chicago: Quintessence, p. 53, 1988.

Rekow ED. A review of the developments in dental CAD-CAM systems. Curr Opin Dent 2:25, 1992.

Ryge G. Current American research on porcelain-fused-to-metal restorations. Int Dent J 15:385, 1965.

Shell JS, Nielsen JP. A study of the bond between gold alloys and porcelain. J Dent Res 41:1424–1437, 1962.

Sherrill CA, O'Brien WJ. The transverse strength of aluminous and feldspathic porcelains. J Dent Res 53:683, 1974.

Shoher I, Whiteman A. Captek—a new capillary casting technology for ceramometal restorations. Quintessence Dent Technol 18:9, 1995.

Siervo S, Pampalone A, Siervo P, Siervo R. Where is the gap? Machinable ceramic systems and conventional laboratory restorations at a glance. Quintessence Int 25:773–776, 1994.

Van Vlack LH. Elements of Materials Science. Reading, MA: Addison-Wesley, 1959.

Vergano PJ, Hill DC, Uhlmann DR. Thermal expansion of feldspar glasses. J Am Ceram Soc 50:59, 1967.

Vines RF, Semmelman JO. Densification of dental porcelains. J Dent Res 36:950, 1957.

Warren BE. J Am Ceram Soc 24: 256, 1941.

Weinstein M, Katz S, Weinstein AB. Fused porcelain-to-metal teeth. US Patent No. 3,052,982, September 11, 1962; and Weinstein M, Weinstein AB. Porcelain-covered metal-reinforced teeth. US Patent No. 3,052,983, September 11, 1962.

Chapter 22

Soldering, Welding, and Electroplating

Soldering

Soldering is often used in the construction of dental appliances. Larger fixed partial dentures are frequently cast in parts that are soldered together after careful fitting to the master cast. This procedure improves dimensional accuracy. Wrought-wire clasp arms can be soldered in place for partial dentures using investment soldering techniques. Orthodontic wires and bands are often soldered together. Soldering can be used to build up certain regions of crowns and inlays where the dimensions should be increased, such as for missing contact points. Some casting defects can be corrected with soldering.

Clean oxide-free metal surfaces brought into intimate contact will bond together as a consequence of metallic bonding forces. However, this does not occur in most practical situations due to surface contamination and/or oxidation. Additionally, metallic bonding forces are of a very short range compared with the surface roughness of even polished flat surfaces. Only small areas will be sufficiently close for bonding to occur, even when clean and oxide free.

The basic technique of soldering is first to obtain metal surfaces that are free of contamination. This is accomplished by cleaning and by using fluxes, which also prevent oxidation during the soldering process. Second, a metal or alloy with a lower melting point than the parts to be joined must be chosen. Third, the parts and solder should be brought to the solder's melting temperature. If the molten metal wets the solid metal, it will spread between the flux and the metal part, providing intimate contact. Upon solidification, the solder will still be in contact and metallic bonding will be established. Solder penetrates joints by capillary action.

Solder compositions

Usually the fineness of a solder is less than that of the alloy being soldered. The proportion of pure gold in gold solders is specified by its fineness. Some manufacturers give a carat designation indicative of the gold alloy for which the solder is to be used (eg, an 18-carat solder is intended for soldering an 18-carat alloy); the proportion of gold in the solder may be less than 18 carat. The compositions of several solder alloys are given in Table 22-1.

Copper is added to a solder to lower the fusion temperature, improve its strength, and make it amenable to age hardening. Silver in a larger proportion than copper improves the wetting (spreading and penetration) of gold solders. Also, silver whitens the alloy. Tin and zinc are present in relatively fixed amounts (2% to 4%) to lower the fusion temperature. Nickel may be added instead of copper if a white alloy is desired.

Preceramic solders for soldering of PFM appliances must withstand the high sintering temperatures of porcelain and so contain more noble metals and less tin and zinc. Copper is not used because it colors the porcelain green, as does silver.

Table 22-1 Composition and melting ranges of dental gold solders*

Solder no.	Composition (wt %)					Melting range	
	Gold	Silver	Copper	Zinc	Tin	°C	°F
A	65.0	16.3	13.4	3.9	1.7	765–800	1,410–1,470
B	65.4	15.4	12.4	3.9	3.1	745–785	1,375–1,445
C	66.1	12.4	16.4	3.4	2.0	750–805	1,385–1,480
D	72.9	12.1	10.0	3.0	2.0	755–835	1,390–1,595
F	80.9	8.1	6.8	2.1	2.0	745–870	1,375–1,595

*From Coleman (1928).

Silver solders contain 10% to 80% silver, 15% to 50% copper, 4% to 35% zinc, and small amounts of cadmium, tin, and phosphorus to lower the fusion temperature.

Flux and antiflux compositions

Borax flux for soldering gold can be made from dehydrated borax ($Na_2B_4O_7$), boric acid (H_3BO_3), and silica (SiO_2). The fused borax flux produces oxide-free surfaces over which the solder will flow easily. The flux can be applied as a powder, a liquid (flux mixed with alcohol), or a paste. A paste gives the most control in application and is formed by mixing the powdered flux with petrolatum or a similar inert base.

Fluoride fluxes are used for soldering alloys containing chromium because fluorides dissolve the chromium oxide. A flux consisting of potassium fluoride, boric acid, borax glass, and sodium carbonate or silica is typical. The ingredients are fused and ground to fine powder, which is used either directly or as a liquid in alcohol or a paste in petrolatum.

An antiflux prevents flow of solder and is used to confine the solder to the work area. Graphite from a lead pencil is a convenient antiflux; however, it is removed by oxidation at higher temperatures. An effective antiflux for prolonged heating or higher temperatures can be made from a suspension of rouge (ferric oxide) or chalk (calcium carbonate) in alcohol.

Investment materials

Soldering investments should not expand as much as for casting investments because soldering requires lower temperatures than casting. Consequently, quartz-based, rather than cristobalite-based, gypsum investments are used for soldering with typical low-fusing gold solders. Phosphate-bonded soldering investments are used for preceramic soldering.

Manipulation of solder

Selection is made on the basis of the solder's corrosion resistance, strength, fusion temperature, and color (to give an inconspicuous joint). The fusion range of the solder must be at least 100°C (212°F) below that of the parts to be soldered. Additionally, selection of solder is based upon how permanent the appliance will be and if the appliance can be removed for cleaning. A solder of 580 fineness has been suggested as the lowest fineness to be used in permanent restorations; higher-fineness solders are generally recommended. Removable appliances can be removed for cleaning and polishing so a lower-fineness solder may be used.

In soldering appliances, such as orthodontic wires and bands, recrystallization or softening of the wires must be avoided. Lower-melting-point solders such as silver solders or low-fineness gold solders, which also improve the mechanical properties of the joint, are preferable. Silver solders are used for stainless steel and other base metal wires. Gold solders used with nickel-chromium and cobalt-chromium-nickel wires are generally about 450-fine and seldom above 650-fine. Higher-fineness solders have inferior mechanical properties.

Cleaning

Surface films of inorganic gases, organic material, and metallic oxides separate the two surfaces and prevent the solder from wetting the metal's surfaces. These must be removed by cleaning and using fluxes, which also prevent oxidation during the soldering process.

Parts must be thoroughly clean in order to obtain a good joint. Casting oxides are removed by pickling in acids. If the parts are polished prior to soldering, they must be thoroughly washed with soap and water then pickled to remove residual polishing materials. Rubber-bonded finishing wheels and points are useful for removing oxides and contamination from the region to be soldered.

Investment soldering

Investment soldering is recommended for precise arrangement of parts for bridgework or partial dentures with wrought-wire clasp arms. The general procedure is as follows:

1. To prevent warping or porosity; the parts are placed on the master cast so that the "gap distance" between them is at least 0.1 mm. Excessive gap distance can lead to distortion and pitting. A typical business card, which ranges in thickness from 0.20 to 0.34 mm, can be used as a gauge for maximum gap distance. Sheets of paper should not be used as a gauge because they are often too thin, ranging from 0.05 to 0.1 mm in thickness.
2. The parts are securely fastened together with sticky wax before removal from the master cast and subsequent placement in the soldering investment.
3. Investment should cover metal parts not to be soldered, but no investment should be at the joint.
4. Antiflux may be applied to confine the flow of solder.
5. In order to obtain dimensional accuracy, the investment is preheated to eliminate moisture and to provide enough thermal expansion to compensate for the thermal expansion of the crowns. Overheating may cause sulfur contamination.
6. Flux can be applied to the joint area before or after preheating.
7. Soldering is accomplished with a reducing flame when the parts are at 750° to 870°C (1,382° to 1,598°F), giving them a yellowish red color. The solder should immediately flow smoothly into the joint area if the surfaces are clean.
8. The investment and appliance are allowed to cool for about five minutes before quenching. This allows some age hardening to occur and prevents warping that could result if the investment were quenched immediately. Total bench cooling would make the solder too brittle through age hardening.
9. The flux cools to a glass that can be removed through pickling. Generally, finishing instruments should not be used to remove the flux because the glass is harder than the metal, and surrounding metal will be removed along with the flux. Small amounts of flux can, however, be chipped or crushed off with a hard instrument (#7 spatula or knife).

Free-hand soldering

Soldering of orthodontic appliances is generally accomplished without the use of an investment. Orthodontic torches can be placed on the bench so that both hands are free to hold the parts in position. Solder is generally melted onto one of the parts; then they are held together and the joint is heated.

Thin wire parts must be held in contact to avoid narrowing of the joint caused by the surface tension of the solder. This decrease in diameter concentrates stress and is much more significant than for larger appliances.

The wires can easily be overheated, with deterioration of mechanical properties resulting. Orthodontic torches, which develop small needlelike flames, are used to limit the heating to a small area around the joint. Quenching prevents embrittlement of the solder by age hardening. Overheating of stainless steel wires can lead to carbide precipitation, which may soften the wire.

Defective soldering

Overheating of wrought wires during soldering can lead to diffusion between solder and wire, and to recrystallization and grain growth. Microstructural changes, surface pitting, and internal porosity all result in a weak joint. Microstructural changes result from prolonged heating or overheating.

When the solder does not flow properly, resulting in an incomplete joint, it is usually due to one or more of the following:

1. The parts were too cool when the solder was applied.
2. If the parts were not at similar temperatures, the solder would flow over the hotter part leaving an incomplete joint.
3. Flux was insufficient to cover the joint.
4. Contamination was present owing to improper cleaning, poor placement of flux, sulfur released from overheated investment, oxidation from an improperly adjusted torch, or oxidation caused by removing the reducing portion of the flame from the joint before the solder flows.

Table 22-2 Tensile properties of gold solders*

Solder no.†	Heat treatment	Proportional limit		Tensile strength		Elongation
		kg/cm^2	psi	MPa	psi	(%)
A	Soft	2,100	30,000	302	44,000	9
	Hard	5,400	77,000	632	92,000	<1
B	Soft	1,890	27,000	283	42,500	14
	Hard	3,850	55,000	431	63,000	1
C	Soft	2,060	29,500	306	44,500	12
	Hard	5,420	77,500	573	83,500	<1
D	Soft	1,680	24,000	247	36,000	7
	Hard	4,300	61,500	480	70,000	<1
E‡	Soft	1,440	20,500	257	37,500	18

*From Coleman (1928).
†Composition given in Table 22-1.
‡No appreciable age hardening.

5. The gap distance was too small (<0.1 mm) for the solder to penetrate between the parts. The joint may appear complete but there will be a void at the center of the soldered joint which could result in premature failure.
6. If the gap distance was too large, the solder may not bridge the gap or, if it does, the diameter of the joint will be too small for adequate strength. Parts should be shaped to fit together with a proper sized gap separating them.

Properties of solder

Fusion temperature

The melting ranges of several gold solders are given in Table 22-1. The difference in melting range between high- and low-fineness solders is not great. Silver solders begin to melt between 600° and 700°C (1,112° and 1,292°F) with a range of about 10° to 40°C.

Mechanical properties

Gold solders have different properties in their soft and hard conditions (Table 22-2). The proportional limit can be doubled for these solders at the expense of elongation and, therefore, toughness. Age-hardened solder joints are very brittle.

Silver solders have mechanical properties comparable to gold solders in the soft condition.

Corrosion resistance

Since there is a composition difference between the solder and the parts, the joint is susceptible to galvanic corrosion.

Interfacial properties

The relationship of the interfacial energies between the metal parts, solder, and flux determines how well the solder will flow. The fluxes used in dentistry will remove surface oxides and protect the parts from further oxidation. Solders penetrate the flux and wet the metal surfaces beneath.

Soldering of metal ceramic bridges

Metal ceramic bridges can be soldered together prior to placement and firing of the ceramic (preceramic soldering) or after firing of the ceramic (postceramic soldering). The two methods require different procedures and materials.

In preceramic soldering, a high-fusing precious metal solder must be used to avoid melting or distortion during firing of the porcelain. Usually a single-orifice gas/oxygen torch is used for soldering. Except for using a phosphate-bonded soldering investment, the procedure is similar to the previously described investment soldering.

A lower-fusing gold solder is used for postceramic soldering so as to avoid thermal damage to the porcelain or its shape. To avoid overheating the porcelain, the parts are oven soldered. Except for the oven heating, the procedure is the same as for investment soldering. Following oven drying and fluxing, the correct amount of solder is placed on the joint and the dried invested pieces are placed in a furnace heated to the upper fusion range of the solder.

Preceramic and postceramic soldering have been successfully used with base metal ceramic bridges. The main difference between soldering of gold and base metal alloys is that special fluoride fluxes must be used for the latter to dissolve the chromium oxides. However, not all fluoride fluxes work equally well. It is important to use the manufacturer's recommended fluxes for these alloys.

Infrared soldering

Dental appliances can also be soldered using an infrared light source. The process is similar to investment soldering except that a focused light beam is used in place of the torch. The invested appliance is preheated in an oven before rapid placement in the infrared soldering apparatus. At the push of a button, a reflector collects and focuses the light from a high-intensity light bulb at the spot where the solder and joint are placed. The light supplies the sufficient heat to bring the parts to the soldering temperature and melt the solder. Infrared soldering devices for soldering dental appliances are no longer readily available.

Commercial soldering materials

A number of companies supply gold ranging from 450 to 800 in fineness (eg, Degussa Corp; Ivoclar Williams, a branch of Ivoclar North America, Inc.; J.F. Jelenko & Co.; J.M. Ney Co.). In addition, most companies carry white gold solders for soldering white gold. Some companies also have special gold solders (eg, Balance Line Solder, J.M. Ney Co.) made to match the colors of certain of their gold alloys with the same names (eg, Balanced Line Gold).

High-Fusing Ceramic Gold Solder (Ivoclar Williams); SMG 1, 2, 3, or YW (J.M. Ney Co.), Jelenko O and Olympia Presolder (J.F. Jelenko & Co.), and Degussa WPG Solder (Degussa Corp.) are examples of preceramic solders. While manufacturers of preceramic solders also make postceramic solders, the lower-fusing gold solders of the previous paragraph can be used for postceramic soldering.

Soldering Flux (J.F. Jelenko & Co.), which comes in a paste or powder, and Solder Flux (J.M. Ney Co.) are examples of fluxes for soldering of gold alloys. A liquid flux, "T" Flux (Degussa Corp.), is recommended for both postceramic and conventional soldering of precious metal alloys.

Speed-E Soldering Investment (Whip Mix Corp.) is recommended for soldering of low-fusing gold alloys. Some examples of high temperature investments for preceramic soldering are Biovest Soldering Investment (Dentsply/York Division) and Hi-Heat Soldering Investment (Whip Mix Corp.). High Heat Solder Investment #2400 (3M) and Place-It #2 (American Dental Supply Inc.), which comes in a tube, are two investments recommended for both preceramic and postceramic soldering.

Orthodontic supply companies have silver solders and fluxes for soldering chromium alloys. Some examples are RMO Silver Solder Wire and Tru-Chrome Flux (Rocky Mountain Orthodontics Inc.) and Formula No. 6 Silver Solder and Unitek Flux (Unitek Corp.).

Welding

Bonding will occur between two metallic surfaces placed in contact if they are free of surface films (including oxides and films of adsorbed gases) and surface roughness. The three methods of welding used in dentistry achieve metal-to-metal contact differently.

Spot welding

The two clean metal surfaces to be welded are placed together under pressure (Fig 22-1). Metal-to-metal contact is obtained by passing a current through the joint to cause interfacial melting. If a pulse of sufficient voltage and duration is applied by means of copper electrodes, melting will begin at the interface between the parts and spread outward to form a weld. The equation

$$\text{Heat} = I^2R$$

gives the amount of heat in watts generated per second by a current of I amperes passing through a structure

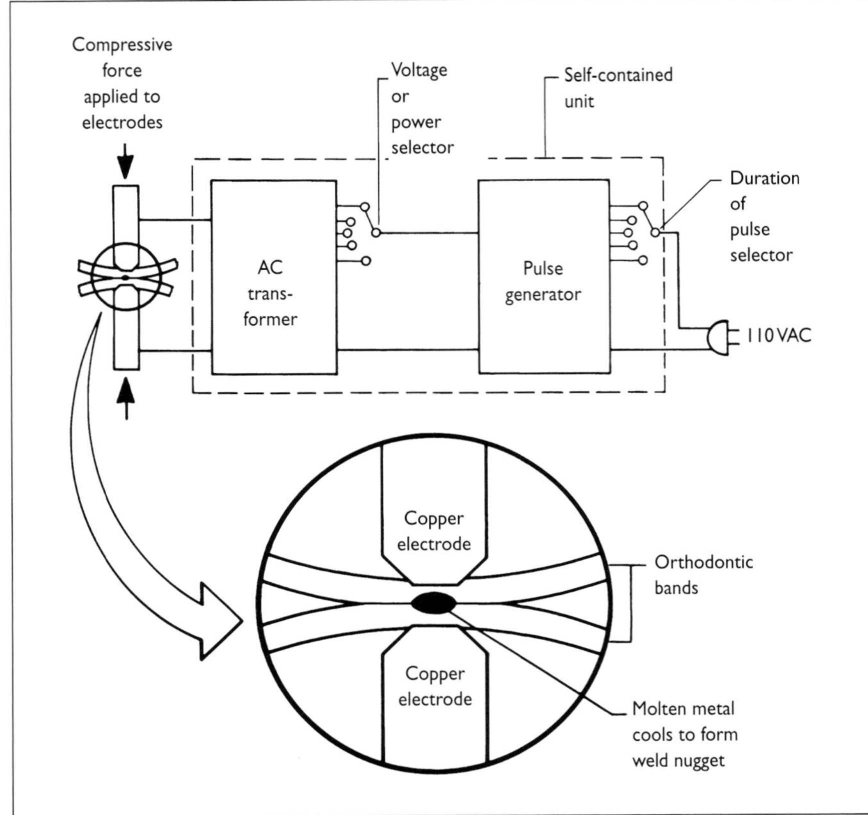

Fig 22-1 Diagrammatic representation of a dental spot welder. Adjustable parameters are the magnitude and duration of the pulse, electrode size and shape, and pressure applied at the electrodes. Typical pulse parameters are 2 to 6 V for 1/25 to 1/50 of a second, which generally results in an applied current of 250 to 750 amperes, depending on the metal, size, and shape of the work, electrodes, and pressure.

having a resistance of *R* ohms. The resistance of the joint is much higher than that of the rest of the parts because of the small contact area at the joint and the surface films present. Because the current is constant, more heat will be generated at the contact areas than in the interior parts. Therefore, the metal will melt first at the contact points.

Liquid contact is established because of the applied pressure and the expansion upon melting. Molten areas spread because the resistance of the metal in its liquid state is greater than in its solid state. Similar conditions exist at the electrode interface, but a higher-energy pulse would be required to cause melting because of the low resistance and high thermal conductivity of copper.

Small welds are generally considered better, because bonding is achieved with a minimum of change in the original grain structure.

Pressure welding

If two metal parts are placed together and a sufficiently large force is applied perpendicular to the surface, pressure welding occurs. Pure gold is extremely malleable and, in the form of thin foils, can be pressure welded by hand. Pure gold has no surface oxides but adsorbed gases prevent metal-to metal contact. The applied force must be sufficiently large to produce permanent distortions parallel to the surface so as to expose film-free metal. The force must be applied rapidly so the exposed surfaces can be compressed together before surface gases adsorb. In pressure welding, the problems of surface roughness are overcome by compressive forces.

Laser welding

A laser generates a coherent, high-intensity pulse of light that can be focused. By selecting the duration and intensity of the pulse, metals can be melted in a small region without extensive microstructural damage to surrounding areas. In laser welding, the beam is focused at the joint to melt the opposing surfaces. Owing to expansion from the locally high temperature and the change of state, the two liquid surfaces contact and form a weld on solidification.

Welding manipulation

Spot welding

Spot (resistance) welding is used to join flat structures, such as orthodontic bands and brackets, and to join orthodontic wires. The work is pressed together between two copper electrodes and an electrical pulse is applied. The magnitude of the pulse depends on the metals and their size and shape at the welding point, and on the size of the electrodes. Typical values for the pulse are 2 to 6 V for $\frac{1}{25}$ to $\frac{1}{50}$ seconds at 250 to 750 A.

Pressure welding

Gold foil (foil, mat, or powdered pure gold) restorations are pressure welded by hand or mechanical condensers, as described in Chapter 14.

Laser welding

Light from a laser can be focused on small regions and can apply high energy to these regions in a very short amount of time. The intensity and duration of the laser pulse is such that sufficient energy can be added to a joint to melt the adjoining metals and achieve a weld before much heat is conducted away. This means that there is very little heating of the total appliance, except at the point of application. Consequently, the procedures can be performed on the master cast.

Properties of welds

Strength

In engineering applications, spot and pressure welds have strengths comparable to other forms of joining metals, such as soldering or arc welding. Laser welds are comparable to soldered joints between cast structures. Spot welding of work-hardened structures, such as bands and wires, destroys the grain structure and softens the metal at and around the weld.

Corrosion resistance

In general, welds are more susceptible to corrosion than are the metals surrounding them. Spot welding in dentistry has been confined to temporary appliances, where the results have been satisfactory. Pressure-welded gold foil restorations are not subject to corrosion in the oral environment.

Commercial welders

The 660 Multi-Purpose Welder (Rocky Mountain Orthodontics Inc.) and Orthodontic Welder Model 1071 (Unitek Corp) are examples of commercial orthodontic welders.

Electroplating

Dies formed by electroplating are used in the construction of ceramic and PFM restorations particularly for full mouth reconstruction. The chances for abrasion of the die surface are higher for construction of appliances involving ceramics than for all-metal ones. Consequently, a more durable die is desired when ceramic restorations are involved. Metal-plated dies are more abrasion resistant than stone dies and are, therefore, often used for making PFM restorations. Metal-plated dies are also utilized in the construction of platinum-bonded alumina crowns.

There is a relationship between electroplating and galvanic corrosion. In galvanic corrosion, the anode is corroded by oxidation and ionic dissolution. Under proper conditions—dependent upon electrolyte, composition, potential difference between electrodes, and the metals involved—the dissolved ions from the anode can plate onto the cathode.

Plating solutions vary in their ability to plate concave surfaces, such as tooth surfaces of impressions. This plating ability is referred to as *throwing power*. Considering the size, depth, and shape of impressions of teeth, solutions with considerable throwing power are required for dental applications.

Plating manipulation

The basic procedure for construction of *electroformed* dies, dies formed by electroplating, is to plate an impression with an appropriate metal, which is then poured in stone or acrylic. The impression is removed, leaving the metal firmly attached to the die material. Impressions from compound or elastomeric materials can be electroplated. Generally, compound impressions are plated with copper whereas silver is used for elastomeric impressions. Nickel is also used as plating metal for impressions.

A copper wire is threaded through nonvital regions of the impression in order to establish electrical contact with a direct current power supply and the inner surface of the impression. The impression is made electrically conductive by a process called *metallizing*, whereby a camel's-hair brush is used to burnish a fine powder of metal onto the impression. Wax is applied over areas that need not be plated.

The proper plating solution containing the same metal ion as the plating electrode is chosen. The impression is made cathodic to the plating anode by connection to a direct current power supply. At the proper voltage—dependent upon the size of the impression and the materials involved—the process requires about 10 to 15 hours. Approximately 1 mm of metal is deposited on the impression. The impression is rinsed thoroughly in running water and other appropriate solutions to neutralize the plating electrolytes. The impression is poured in stone or acrylic, then removed as usual, leaving the metal attached to the stone or acrylic.

There are potential inaccuracies associated with electroformed dies that do not occur for properly made stone dies. The plating process is of sufficient duration that the impression can distort. The plated metal layer can also slightly distort the impression's surface. Potential inaccuracies may occur if self-curing acrylic is used instead of stone. Curing shrinkage of the acrylic may distort the metal.

Platinum-bonded alumina crown

Jacket crowns are generally made by firing porcelain to a thin platinum coping that has been adapted to a die. This coping is not bonded to the porcelain and must be removed before cementation, which results in a thick cement layer between crown and tooth. Electroplating the platinum coping with tin has been found to produce a surface conducive to bonding. The electroplated coping is oxidized in a furnace, producing a tin oxide layer to which the alumina core will adhere. This process allows the platinum coping to be left in place during cementation and likely improves the strength of the crown.

Electroformed gold copings

Nearly pure gold copings for PFM restorations can be made by an electroplating process similar to that used to make electroplated dies. In this case, however, an accurate die is metallized and plated with gold to a thickness of 0.2 to 0.3 mm. The die material is then removed from the gold by grinding and dissolving the remainder in an acid solution. The gold is trimmed and fitted to the master die to give an accurate coping. Gold particles and organic binders are then applied to the outer surface of the coping before it is electroplated with tin so as to obtain a good bond with dental porcelains that have fusion temperatures below 927°C. Thin, accurate-fitting gold copings can be made by this process. These copings are too weak to support porcelain bridges.

Commercial products

Standard or Imperial Electroforming Units (Teledyne Water Pik) are examples of commercial copper electroplating units made for dental use. Teledyne Water Pik is a source of copperplating solutions. Silverplating solutions are difficult to obtain. They contain silver cyanide and, therefore, should only be used under a hood. Most large cities have precious metal electroplating businesses where plating solutions and advice can be obtained. These businesses will also do plating for dentists. However, one must remember that impressions distort with time, and arrangements should be made for immediate plating of the impressions.

Apparatus and materials for making electroformed gold copings are available from Gramm GmbH, Germany (Electroformed Gold) and Leach & Dillon, United States (Captek).

Glossary

antiflux Material placed on the work before the flux to confine the flow of solder.

fluoride flux Fluoride-containing flux for chromium alloys.

flux A substance that promotes the flow of solder over the metal parts by cleaning the surfaces and removing oxides.

free-flowing solder Solder that flows readily over clean metal surfaces and penetrates small openings and joints by capillary action.

gap distance Space between parts to be soldered, which will be filled with solder.

laser welding A form of welding in which the heat for melting the metal is supplied by a focused beam of light generated by a laser.

metallizing Coating an impression material with a powdered metal to make it electrically conductive.

pressure welding A form of welding in which the weld is made by pressure.

solder Metal or alloy melted to unite adjacent, less fusible metal parts.

soldering investments Similar in composition to quartz casting investments, which may be used for soldering.

spot welding A form of welding in which the heat for melting the metal is generated by the flow of electricity through the parts to be welded.

sticky wax Brittle wax-containing resin used to hold metal parts in investment soldering. It fractures rather than deforms under stress.

throwing power A measure of the uniformity in plating thickness of irregular surfaces.

welding The joining of metal surfaces directly by the application of heat or high compressive forces.

Discussion questions

1. Why do dental bridges often fail clinically at solder junctions?
2. How do the processes of soldering and welding differ on a basic level?
3. What precautions need to be taken when soldering or welding wrought metals?
4. What problems might be expected in the clinical use of pure electroplated gold porcelain-fused-to-metal crowns and bridges?
5. What are the consequences of using too much solder or making too large a spot weld when joining orthodontic wire?

Questions and answers

1. **What are the two main components of gold solder, besides gold, and why are they added?** Copper will lower the fusion temperature, increase the strength, and make it susceptible to age hardening. Silver is added primarily to improve the free-flowing qualities of the solder.
2. **What would be expected to happen if a porcelain-gold appliance was presoldered with an ordinary gold solder?** The appliance would probably come apart at the joint during firing of the porcelain because of the high temperatures. In addition, the porcelain near the joint would have a greenish tinge because of the copper.
3. **Why is a special fluoride flux required to solder alloys containing chromium?** The fluoride flux is required to remove the chromium oxide coating, which gives the alloy its corrosion resistance. Regular borax flux will not remove chromium oxide.
4. **What is an antiflux?** Solder will not wet a surface covered with antiflux. Antiflux can be used to confine the solder to a given region.
5. **Give two examples of an antiflux.** Graphite from a lead pencil; iron rouge suspended in alcohol.
6. **To avoid melting the gold parts, what fineness does the solder usually have relative to the parts?** The fineness of the solder should be less than the fineness of the parts.

7. **What is the suggested minimum fineness recommended for soldering permanent restorations?** 580-fine.

8. **Why is silver solder recommended for soldering stainless steel wires?** Silver solder has a sufficiently low fusion temperature so that carbide precipitation can be minimized or avoided with proper soldering procedures.

9. **Why is cleaning the parts important to successful soldering?** Solder will not wet a surface covered with thick casting oxides and organic films. These films must be removed prior to soldering, since the action of the flux is not sufficient to remove them.

10. **When is investment soldering recommended?** Investment soldering is used whenever exact positioning of parts is required.

11. **What would happen with investment soldering if the sticky wax fractured but the soldering operations were continued?** Fracture of the sticky wax indicates that the parts have been moved in relationship to each other, and that the finished appliance probably will not fit.

12. **What is the purpose of preheating the investment, and what will happen if it is overheated?** Preheating eliminates moisture and provides thermal expansion to compensate for the expansion of the metal. Underheating the investment will lead to poor fit of the appliance. Overheating the investment could fracture it, leading to a poorly fitting appliance, and it could release sulfur, which would contaminate the surface and prevent the flow of solder over the parts.

13. **How does one determine if all parts are at the proper temperature for soldering?** All regions of the appliance adjacent to the joint will be yellowish red.

14. **Why is it important to have uniform heating at the joint?** If one part is significantly hotter than the other, the solder will flow to and wet the hot surface and not the other surface.

15. **What are some of the major differences between investment soldering of relatively large parts and free-hand soldering of wires?** Because of the small size of wires, greater care must be exercised to avoid overheating. Wires should be in contact, compared with the 0.1-mm gap distance recommended for larger parts.

16. **What microstructural changes are expected if wrought wires are overheated?** Diffusion between solder and wire, recrystallization, and grain growth are all possible if a wire is overheated. Overheated stainless steel wires can lead to excessive carbide precipitation.

17. **What difficulties might occur if soldering were performed in a dark room?** If allowance is not made for the fact that an object at a given temperature will appear much brighter in a dark room than in subdued light, the parts are likely to be too cool for the solder to flow. The lack of flow could, mistakenly, be attributed to contamination. If the torch is concentrated on the solder, it could become overheated before the parts come to the proper temperature.

18. **A soldered joint of an appliance that failed in service had the following defects: (a) surface porosity, (b) flux incorporated into the solder, and (c) a large pore at the center of the joint. What were the likely causes?** Surface porosity was probably due to overheating. Excessive use of flux probably resulted in the incorporation of the flux into the solder. The large pore at the center of the joint probably indicates that the parts were in contact in this area.

19. **If a joint becomes oxidized during soldering, what will happen?** The solder will not wet the oxidized surfaces, so that if soldering operations are continued, overheating of the work is likely.

20. **What are causes of oxidation?** Oxidation is due to one or more of the following:
    a. Insufficient flux
    b. Improperly adjusted torch
    c. Using the oxidizing portion of the flame
    d. Removing the flame before soldering operations are completed

21. **What errors in soldering procedure could lead to a poorly fitting appliance?** A poorly fitting appliance could be caused by one or more of the following: fracturing of the sticky wax, fracturing of the investment by improper heating, failure to preheat the investment, and using a high water/powder ratio for the investment.

22. **Why is flux important to successful soldering?** A flux is required to remove surface oxides and helps to protect the parts and solder from oxidation at soldering temperatures.

23. **Referring to Table 22-2, what property of solders is seriously reduced by age hardening, and how is this avoided in the investment soldering procedure?** The large reduction of elongation upon age-hardening indicates that the solder has become considerably more brittle. The work is quenched after 5 minutes to prevent it from staying at the age-hardening temperature too long. Waiting 5 minutes allows some hardening, but the increased proportional limit is more important than the slight increase in brittleness.

24. **Why would it be impractical to spot weld flat copper structures together using orthodontic spot welders?** Because the copper parts to be welded and the copper electrodes have similar resistances, the electrodes are likely to be welded to the work.

25. **Why is it unlikely that thin foils of copper could be pressure welded by gold foil condensers?** A greater amount of distortion would be required for copper because of its surface oxides. In addition, the stress and energy required for this distortion would be much higher because copper has a higher proportional limit and lower malleability than pure gold.

26. **Why can laser welding be accomplished on the master cast?** With a laser, the region of heat input can be localized to a very small area, and the time of application can be reduced so the total heat required for melting the metal at the junction is insufficient, when dissipated throughout the parts, to produce a temperature high enough to cause distortion or destruction of the cast.

27. **Can pressure welding be applied to nongold alloys?** From the discussion of the theory of pressure welding, it is, in principle, possible to weld other metals or alloys besides pure gold. In practice, the stresses are considerably higher than those required for pure gold, and in many cases heat is also required to obtain good welds.

28. **Why might an organic film prevent welding during spot welding of orthodontic appliances?** It would increase the resistance of the contact areas and reduce the current, which varies inversely with the resistance. Since the heat generated is proportional to the square of the current and only directly proportional to the resistance, a large reduction in current could make the available heat insufficient to melt the metal.

29. **What is the main application of electroplating in dentistry?** Electroplated dies for crown-and-bridge restorations.

30. **What are the advantages and disadvantages of electroplated dies?** Electroplated dies are more abrasion resistant. However, electroplating takes 10 or more hours for completion, requires special equipment and solutions, and may introduce distortions of the impression's surface. Some plating solutions are very toxic and should only be used under a hood.

31. **Why is the throwing power of a plating solution important?** A solution with a high throwing power will produce more uniform plating of an impression and therefore preserve accuracy.

Recommended reading

Bailey JH, Donovan TE, Preston JD. The dimensional accuracy of improved dental stone, silverplated, and epoxy resin die materials. J Prosthet Dent 59:307, 1988.

Coleman RI. National Bureau of Standards Research Paper no. 32. J Res Nat Bur Stand 1:894, 1928.

Coleman RI. Some effects of soldering and other heat treatment on orthodontic alloys. Int J Orthod 19:1238, 1933.

Crowell WS. Dental gold solders. In T Lyman (ed). Metals Handbook. 5th ed. Cleveland: ASM, 1948; 1104.

Gordon TE, Smith DL. Laser welding of prostheses—an initial report. Quintessence Int 3:63, 1972.

Mc Lean JW. The Science and Art of Dental Ceramics. Vol II. Bridge Design and Laboratory Procedures in Dental Ceramics. Chicago: Quintessence Publishing Co, 1980.

Meyer FS. The elimination of distortion during soldering. J Prosthet Dent 9:441, 1959.

Milner DR, Apps RI. Introduction in Welding and Brazing. New York: Pergamon Press, 1968.

O'Brien WJ, Hirthe WM, Ryge G. Wetting characteristics of dental gold solders. J Dent Res 42:675, 1963.

Peyton FA, Craig RG. Restorative Dental Materials. 4th ed. St Louis: CV Mosby Co, 1971.

Phillips RW. Skinner's Science of Dental Materials. 8th ed. Philadelphia: WB Saunders Co, 1982.

Rogers OW. The dental application of electroformed pure gold. I. Porcelain jacket crown technique. Aust Dent J 24:163, 1979.

Ryge G. Dental soldering procedures. Dent Clin North Am, Nov 1958; 747–757.

Sloan RM, Reisbick MH, Preston JD. Post-ceramic soldering of various alloys. J Prosthet Dent 48:686, 1982.

Smith DL, Burnett AP, Gordon TE Jr. Laser welding of gold alloys. J Dent Res 51:161, 1972.

Stade EH, Reisbick MH, Preston JD. Preceramic and postceramic solder joints. J Prosthet Dent 34:527, 1975.

Vrijhoef MMA, Spanauf HJ, Renggli HH, Wismann H, Somers GA. Electroforming as an alternative to casting: A preliminary report. Restor Dent 1:143, 1985.

Willis LM, Nicholls JI. Distortion in dental soldering as affected by gap distance. J Prosthet Dent 43:272, 1980.

Zietsman ST, Fidos H. Electrical resistance welding or orthodontic wires. J Dent Assoc S Afr 37:880, 1982.

Chapter 23

Dental Implant Materials

Overview of the problem of the edentulous patient

A critical problem in dentistry is treating the edentulous patient. A recent survey by the National Institute for Dental Research (NIDR) has shown that 42% of the population over the age of 65 is totally edentulous, and that a substantial number of other patients are partially edentulous, having an average of 10 missing teeth. Although removable dentures and fixed bridges offer effective treatments for many edentulous patients, those who have lost substantial tooth-bearing portions of bone and cannot manage prostheses or cannot masticate properly can improve their oral function through the use of dental implants. The use of implants as a means of treating these patients has accelerated in the last decade, and there are now over 300,000 dental implants in use in the United States. A 1988 conference on dental implants led to the conclusions that they can be effective in providing long-term total and partial support for restorations. Despite the expanded use of implants, however, they can only be evaluated on a largely qualitative level. To better understand and quantify the clinical effectiveness of dental implants, a greater understanding of the parameters governing the long-term success of this complex material/tissue aggregate is needed.

In this chapter, the parameters important to implantology are presented. Following an overview of general implantology concepts and indications for implant use, osseointegration is defined and discussed. Next, methods of achieving osseointegration are presented and parameters important to achieving implant success are reviewed, with a primary focus on biomaterials and biomechanical factors.

Indications for dental implant use

The general requirement for use of dental implants is available bone to support the implant. Available bone means there is adequate bone to support the implant with the physiological parameters of width, height, length, contour, and density. Note that the importance of these parameters varies, depending on the specific implant type (Table 23-1). Despite the "glamour" of

Contraindications for dental implant use*

- Unattainable prosthodontic reconstruction
- Patient sensitivity to implant component(s)
- Debilitating or uncontrolled disease
- Pregnancy
- Inadequate practitioner training
- Conditions, diseases, or treatments that may compromise healing (ie, radiation therapy)
- Poor patient motivation/hygiene
- Perceived poor patient compliance
- Unrealistic patient expectations

*Adapted from NIH Consensus Development Conference, J Dent Res 52:824, 1988.

Table 23-1 Summary of dental implant types and indications for each*

Implant type	Indications
Endosseous	
Root form	Adequate bone to support implant—width and height of primary concern Maxillary and mandibular arch locations Completely or partially edentulous patients
Blade (plate) form	Adequate bone to support implant—width and length of primary concern Maxillary and mandibular arch locations Completely or partially edentulous patients
Ramus frame	Adequate anterior bone to support implant—width and height of primary concern Mandibular arch location Completely edentulous patients
Subperiosteal	
Complete	Atrophy of bone, but adequate and stable bone to support implant
Unilateral	Maxillary and mandibular arch locations
Circumferential	Completely and partially edentulous patients
Transosteal	
Staple	Adequate anterior bone to support implant—width and height of primary concern
Single pin	Anterior mandibular arch location
Multiple pin	Completely and partially edentulous patients

*Adapted From NIH Consensus Development Conference, J Dent Res 52:824, 1988.

implant dentistry, a conservative treatment protocol must be stressed. Unsatisfactory treatment with removable dentures or fixed bridges remains an important indication for implant use. In other words, dental implants are not a first-treatment option. A number of other contraindications for implant use also exist.

Types of implants

In general, dental implants are classified as (*1*) endosseous, (*2*) subperiosteal, or (*3*) transosteal (Fig 23-1), and are subdivided according to Table 23-1. *Endosseous implants* are embedded in mandibular or maxillary bone and project through the oral mucosa covering the edentulous ridge. Subperiosteal implants rest on the surface of the bone beneath the periosteum. *Transosteal implants* penetrate the inferior mandibular border and also project through the oral mucosa covering the edentulous ridge. *Root-form endosseous screw-threaded implants* are the most commonly used implants in clinical practice today. This class of implants is the only one for which good long-term (eg, 10- to 15-years) clinical tracking of large patient populations is available. Results indicate success rates for mandibular implants of approximately 96%, 94%, and 86% at 5, 10, and 15 years, respectively. For maxillary implants, success rates are 88%, 82%, and 78% at these same times. Breaking down the data based on oral location indicates the following 5-year success rates: anterior mandible, 99%; posterior mandible, 94%; anterior maxilla, 92%; posterior maxilla, 75%. The clinician's expertise and surgical technique are more important than the specific implant and are the primary factors dictating clinical outcome.

Osseointegration

Unlike many biomaterials, which strive to replace as much of a tissue's natural structure and function as possible, dental implants do not restore function by mimicking the natural function of the periodontal ligament (Fig 23-2). Instead, *osseointegration*, as originally

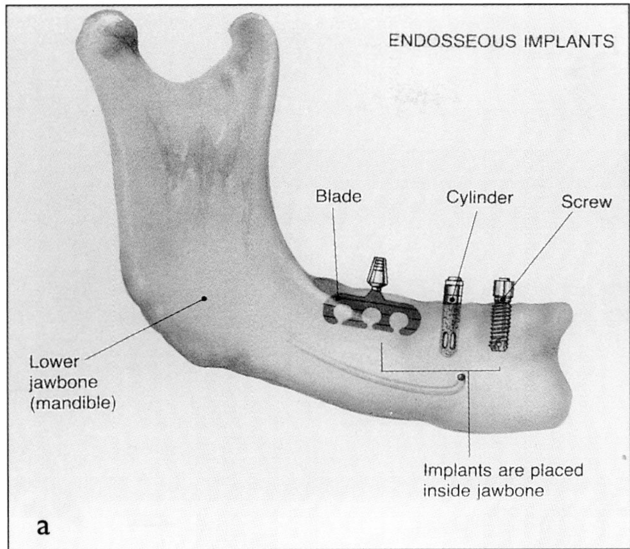

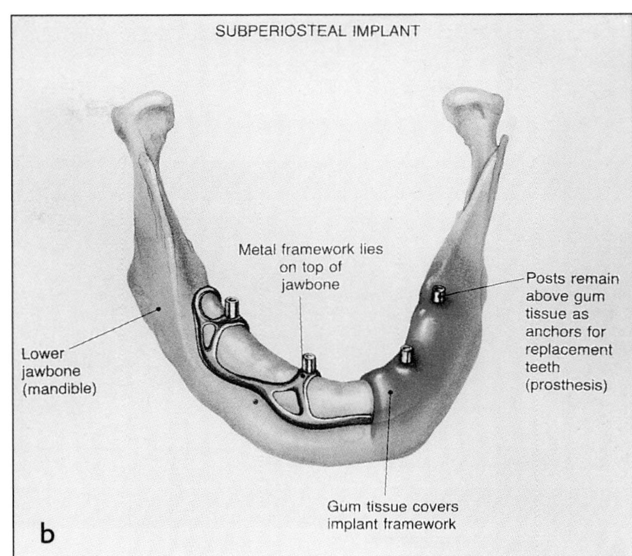

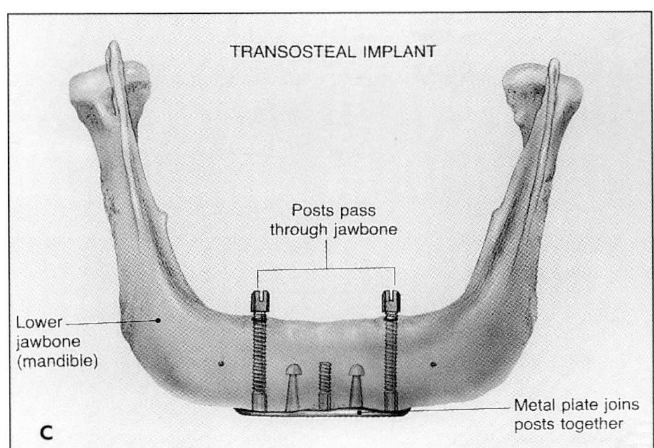

Fig 23-1 Three main classes of dental implants: (a) endosseous, (b) subperisoteal, (c) transosteal. (From Taylor, 1990.)

defined, was intended to provide a direct structural and functional connection between ordered, living bone and the surface of a load-carrying implant. This definition was originally based on retrospective radiographic and light microscopic observations, and has since been modified based on scanning and transmission electron microscopic observations. However, the general working definition of osseointegration is fundamentally the same—the host bone responds, in a safe, predictable, and versatile manner, to surgery and placement of an implant in a sterile wound, with a healing cascade leading to interfacial osteogenesis and immobility of the implant (Fig 23-3). In a well-functioning implant, interfacial osteogenesis and clinical immobility are achieved (Fig 23-4a). In comparison, poorly differentiated connective tissue adjacent to an implant leads to clinical mobility and implant failure (Fig 23-4b).

There are a multitude of interrelated clinical, biological, and engineering factors that control the oral cavity's response and dictate the success of osseointegration. These factors are discussed in the remainder of this chapter.

Mechanisms for achieving and enhancing implant/tissue attachment

An implant must be capable of carrying occlusal stresses. Additionally, stresses must be transferred to the adjacent bone. Not only must stresses be transferred, but they must be of a "correct" orientation and magnitude so that tissue viability is maintained in as near a physiological state as possible. The ability to transmit stress is largely dependent on attaining interfacial fixation. Thus, two further requirements are that

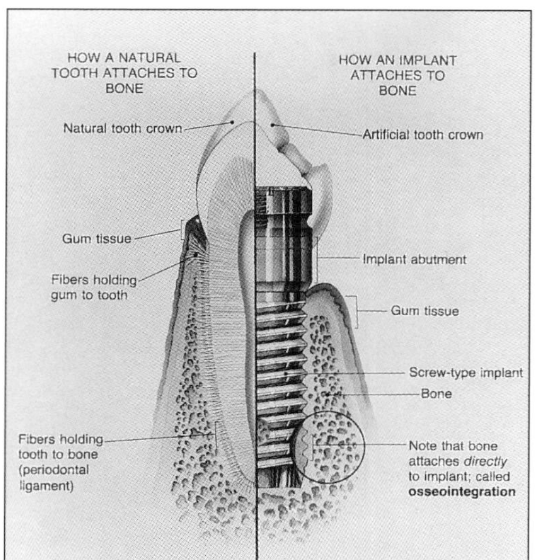

Fig 23-2 Schematic of natural tooth vs implant attachment to bone. (From Taylor, 1990.)

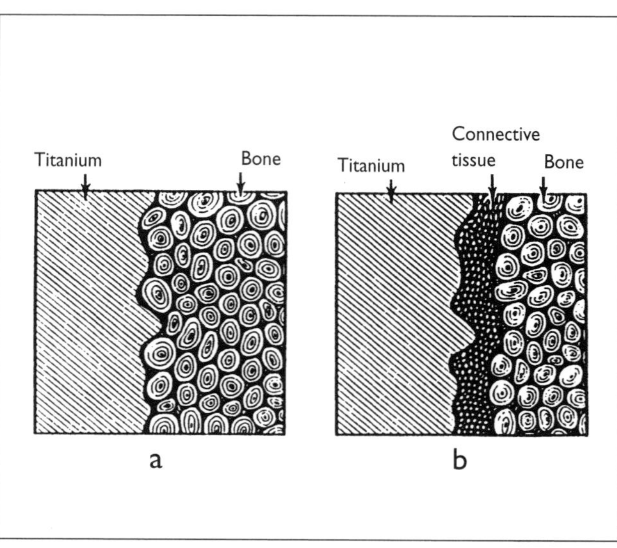

Fig 23-3 Schematic of localized sections of interfacial zone, showing (a) osseointegrated and (b) fibrous-integrated tissue adjacent to implant surface. Conditions (a) and (b) might occur with minimized (a) and excess (b) tissue/implant relative motion. (From Brånemark et al, 1987.)

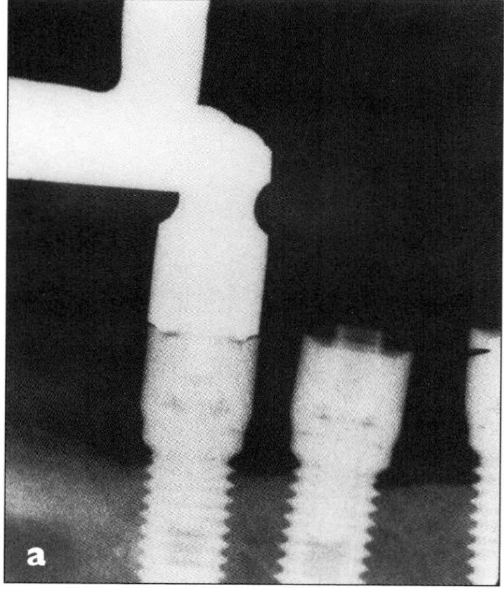

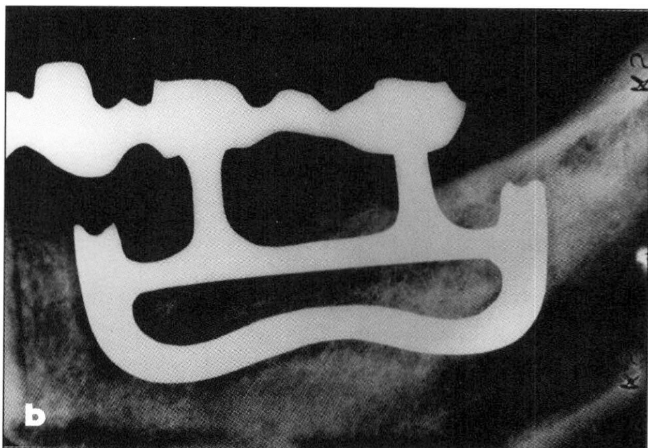

Fig 23-4 Radiographic example of (a) well-functioning and (b) failing dental implants. In (a), a well-osseointegrated interfacial zone led to clinical immobility, whereas in (b), poorly differentiated interfacial connective tissue led to mobility and failure.

the interface stabilize in as short a time postoperatively as possible and that, once stable, the interface remain stable for as long a time as possible.

In an ideal situation, such as the situation that can be achieved with commercially pure titanium (c.p. Ti), calcified tissue can be observed within several hundred Angstroms of the implant surface. A layer of proteoglycans, 200 to 400 Å thick, lies adjacent to the metal oxide, and collagen filaments can be observed about 200 Å from the surface (Fig 23-5). Less than optimal surgical techniques, implant surface chemistry, and relative motion can lead to a thicker zone of proteoglycans, soft connective tissue, and disordered bone.

Developing an "optimal" implant that meets all of these objectives requires the integration of material, physical, chemical, mechanical, biological, and

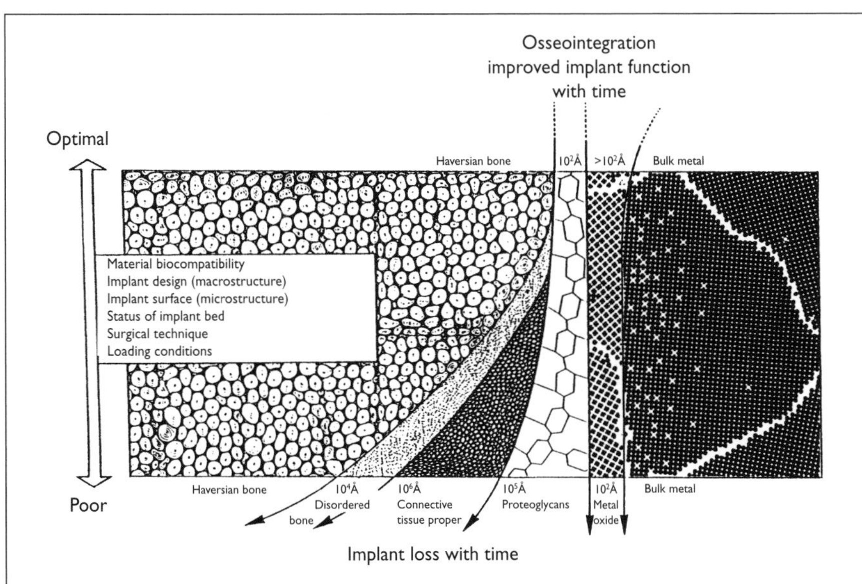

Fig 23-5 Schematic of interfacial zone, showing constituents: bulk metal, metal oxide, proteoglycans, connective tissue, disordered and ordered bone, and relative proportions of each for good and poor osseointegration. (From Brånemark et al, 1987, with permission.)

economic factors. It should be pointed out that while all of these properties are important, they cannot all be optimized in a given design. In fact, optimization of one property often detracts from another. Thus, in implant design, a ranking of requirements and objectives is necessary.

The approach taken to meet a specific property objective should be based on a materials science approach, in that the synergistic relationships between processing, composition, structure, and properties are characterized. Altering any one of these four entities may alter the other three. For example, it is too simplistic to regard all hydroxyapatite (HA)-coated dental implants as similar.

Because of the need to develop a stable interface prior to loading, it is desirable to accelerate tissue apposition to dental implant surfaces. Materials developments that have been implemented in clinical practice include the use of surface-roughened implants and ceramic coatings. Other, more experimental techniques include electrical stimulation, bone grafting, and growth factors and bone proteins.

A variety of surface configurations have been proposed as means of improving the cohesiveness of the implant/tissue interface, maximizing load transfer, minimizing relative motion between implant and tissue, minimizing fibrous integration, and ultimately minimizing loosening and lengthening the service life of the construct. For metal implants, these surface configurations include those that are smooth, textured, screw threaded, plasma sprayed, or porous coated. By far, the most common surface configuration is the screw-threaded dental implant. Osseointegration around screw-threaded implants occurs through tissue ongrowth, or direct apposition between tissue and the implant surface. Alternative methods of implant fixation, based on tissue ingrowth into roughened or three-dimensional surface layers, yield higher bone/ metal shear strength than other types of fixation. Increased interfacial shear strength results in a better stress transfer from the implant to the surrounding bone, a more uniform stress distribution between the implant and bone, and lower stresses in the implant. In principle, the result of a stronger interfacial bond is decreased implant loosening.

Bioceramics can have four different surface types and tissue attachment mechanisms:

1. Fully dense, inert ceramics that attach to bone by either a press fit or bone ongrowth onto a roughened surface
2. Porous inert ceramics, into which bone ingrowth occurs, creating a mechanical attachment
3. Fully dense surface-active ceramics, that attach to bone via a chemical bond
4. Resorbable ceramics that integrate with and are eventually replaced by bone

A progression of surfaces from the lowest implant/ tissue shear strength to the highest is as follows: smooth, textured, screw threaded, plasma sprayed, and

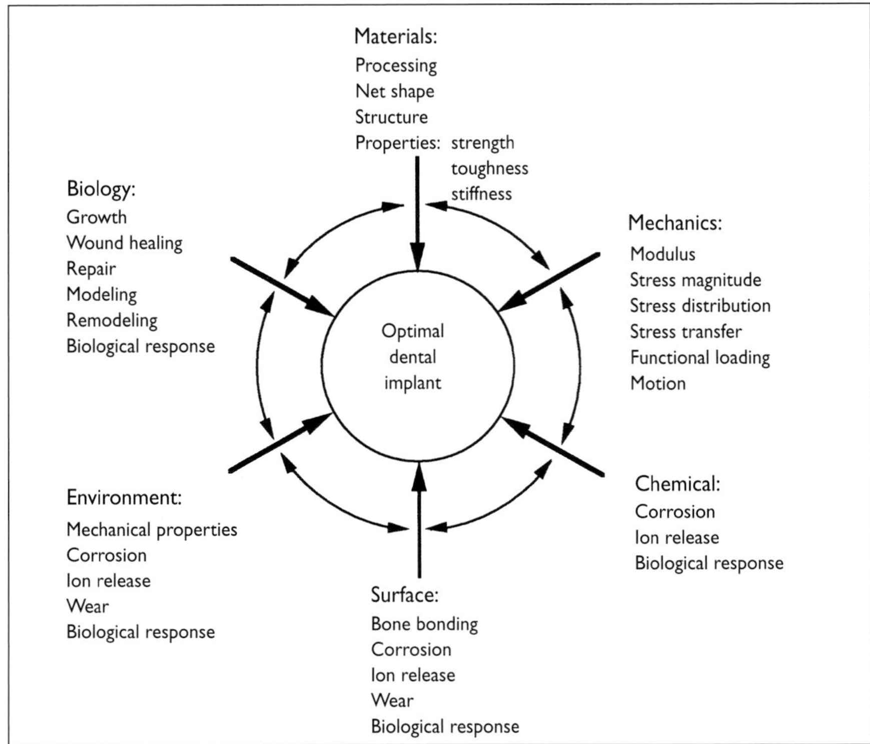

Fig 23-6 Schematic of interdependent engineering factors affecting the success of dental implants. (From Kohn, 1992, with permission.)

porous surfaced. Two factors must be stressed. First, different surface structures necessitate different osseointegration times. Second, surface roughening, particularly of titanium-based materials, results in reduced fatigue strength. Thus, improvements in implant/tissue attachment strength are often countered by a loss of structural strength and must be met with design compromises to avoid metallurgic failure.

Criteria for successful dental implants

Three aspects of an implant/tissue system are important in determining success: (*1*) the implant material(s) and adjacent tissue(s), (*2*) the interfacial zone between the implant and tissue, and (*3*) the effect of the implant and its breakdown products on the local and systemic tissues. Although the interfacial zone is composed of a relatively thin heterogeneous metallic oxide, proteinacious layer, and connective tissue, it has an effect on the maintenance of interfacial integrity. Furthermore, interfacial integrity is dependent on material, mechanical, chemical, surface, biological, and local environmental factors, all of which change as functions of time in vivo. In addition, implant "success" is dependent on the patient's overall medical and dental status, the surgical techniques employed, and the extent and time course of tissue healing. The focus of this chapter is on the biomaterial and biomechanical factors, which are summarized in Fig 23-6.

Surgical parameters

Adequate preparation of bone is critical for bone-cell survival, well-ordered connective tissue apposition close to an implant surface, the establishment of a reliable bone anchor, and long-term implant and tissue viability. Poor surgical technique or premature functional loading may result in an inability to achieve osseointegration, fibrous adaptation, and early implant failure. The standard clinical protocol therefore calls for a two-stage surgical procedure. The first stage involves the careful preparation of the implant bed in a manner that minimizes trauma and optimizes healing and interfacial osteogenesis. Certain thermal limits should not be exceeded during surgery. If these temperatures are exceeded, thermal necrosis can occur, resulting in a thicker layer of soft tissue directly apposing the implant surface and jeopardizing osseointegration. Following the initial surgery, the implants are sealed in situ and remain unloaded for 3 to 6 months. During this period, ordered, living bone, with the potential for ultimately carrying occlusal loads, develops within the interfacial zone.

Surface chemistry and biological response

Implant materials may corrode and/or wear, leading to the generation of micron- or sub–micron-sized debris that may elicit both local and systemic biological responses. Metals are more susceptible to electrochemical degradation than ceramics. Therefore, a fundamental criterion for choosing a metallic implant material is that the biological response it elicits is minimal. Titanium-based materials are well tolerated by the body because of their passive oxide layers. The main elemental constituents, as well as the minor alloying constituents can be tolerated by the body in trace amounts. However, larger amounts of metals usually cannot be tolerated. Therefore, minimizing mechanical and chemical breakdown of implant materials is a primary objective.

Linked to biological response are nine questions that must be considered:

1. Is material released?
2. What material is released?
3. What is the form of the material released?
4. How much material is released?
5. What is the rate of release?
6. In what subsequent reactions are the release products involved?
7. What percentage of release products are excreted/retained?
8. Of the percentage that is retained, where do they accumulate?
9. What biological response(s) result from the retained fraction?

Local accumulation of material around an implant may include membrane-bound ions, particles released due to wear or fatigue processes or insoluble reaction products. Excessive metal ion accumulation can lead to metallosis or tissue discoloration and also to reduced phagocytosis and cytoxicity.

Understanding implant surface chemistry is important to ensure a twofold requirement. First, implant materials must not adversely affect local tissues, organ systems, and organ functions. Second, the in vivo environment must not degrade the implant and compromise its long-term function. The interface zone between an implant and the surrounding tissue is therefore the most important entity in defining the biological response to the implant and the response of the implant to the body.

The success of any implant is dependent on its bulk and surface properties, the site of implantation, tissue trauma during surgery, and motion at the implant/tissue interface. The surface of a material is almost always different in chemical composition and morphology than the bulk material. These differences arise from the molecular arrangement, surface reactions and contamination. In this regard, the interface chemistry is determined primarily by the properties of the metal oxide and not as much by the metal itself. There is little or no similarity between the properties of the metal and the properties of the oxide, but adsorption and desorption phenomena can still be influenced by the properties of the underlying metal. Therefore, characterization of surface composition, binding state, and morphology are important in the analysis of implant surfaces and implant/tissue interfaces. Surface analysis aids in material characterization, determining structural and composition changes due to processing, and in identifying biologically induced surface reactions.

Metallic oxides dictate the type of cellular and protein binding at the implant surface. Surface oxides are continually altered by the indiffusion of oxygen, hydroxide formation, and the outdiffusion of metallic ions. Thus, a single oxide stoichiometry does not exist. The surface potential may play an important role in osseointegration, and it has been postulated that oxides with high dielectric constants inhibit the movement of cells to an implant surface. It has also been demonstrated that the type and orientation of cells attaching to metal surfaces is influenced by the microscopic geometry of the substrate surface.

Mechanical Parameters

Mechanical properties important in designing implant materials include stiffness, yield and ultimate strengths, fracture toughness, and fatigue strength. Stiffness, or modulus of elasticity, dictates, to a large extent, the ability of the implant to transmit stresses to the adjacent tissue and maintain tissue viability over time. Static and fatigue strengths obviously are impor-

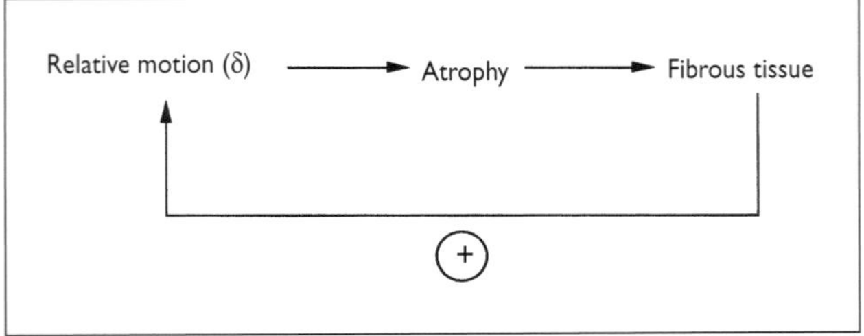

Fig 23-7 Schematic of positive feedback mechanisms leading to implant loosening. (From Kohn, 1992, with permission.)

tant in minimizing material failures. Fracture toughness is a gauge of the energy needed to cause failure in the presence of existing damage.

Three points about mechanical properties must be emphasized. First, for many materials, including titanium, optimum strength (tensile and fatigue) and optimum ductility (elongation and toughness) require different microstructural morphologies and therefore different thermal processing. Second, depending on the surface configuration, properties differ in their ranked importance. For example, fatigue of smooth-surfaced implants is governed by the initiation stage, whereas fatigue of surface-roughened implants is governed by propagation. Therefore, different microstructures and thermal-processing techniques are desirable for different surface conditions. Third, if any surface coatings are used, the mechanics become more difficult, as there are now effectively three materials of interest—the substrate material, the substrate/coating composite, and the substrate/coating interface.

Implants are subjected to axial, shear, bending, and torsional loads, so, in addition to the magnitude of the loading, directionality must also be considered. With the above-mentioned considerations and only a qualitative knowledge of "stability"—the maximum allowable displacement at an implant/tissue interface that will still result in osseointegration and bone maintenance—it must be stressed that the postimplantation time at which an implant can begin to undergo loading is most likely implant- and location-specific and generally unknown.

Although rare, material failure of implants, generally by fatigue, does occur. Failure of implant structures or abutments should be not disregarded or viewed as isolated instances. Fatigue of implant materials is clinically important for several reasons. First, fatigue properties of implant materials should be accurately quantified so implants may be designed intelligently. Second, the stress distribution between an implant and surrounding bone tissue is dependent on the section size of the implant as well as the elastic moduli of both the implant and tissue. Third, coated implants may undergo local fracture processes that do not necessarily compromise the integrity of the implant, but do compromise its functionality and ability to transmit stress to tissue.

Implant design

The design of dental implants is based on many interrelated factors, including the geometry of the implant, how this geometry affects mechanical properties, and the initial and long-term stability of the implant/tissue interface. There is no one design criterion. Implants can be designed to maximize strength, interfacial stability, or load transfer, with each of these criteria requiring different material and interface properties. Two goals of any implant design are to maximize initial stability (ie, through implant design and surgical precision, create as tight a fit as possible at the time of surgery and accomplish osseointegration in as short a time as possible following implantation) and minimize loosening (ie, maintain osseointegration for as long a time as possible following achievement of stability).

To ensure osseointegration and achieve the potential benefits of biological fixation, the interface must be stable (ie, relative motion must be minimized) prior to loading and throughout the service life of the device. It should be reiterated, however, that the quantification of stability is unknown. In general, if excessive relative motion at the implant/tissue interface occurs, a positive feedback system is created in which relative motion leads to bone atrophy, the formation of a fibrous tissue layer, and further increased displacements (Fig 23-7).

Quantifying stresses and strains in implants, tissues, and implant/tissue interfaces is important for understanding mechanically mediated response mechanisms and for implant design. Implant and tissue geometry, elastic properties, loading, boundary conditions, interface conditions, and local stresses and strains are all important.

Since most dental implant clinical failures initiate in the interfacial zone, it is the local properties of this region that are the most important. It has been hypothesized that the local material and tissue (including bone and fibrous tissue) microstructure within the

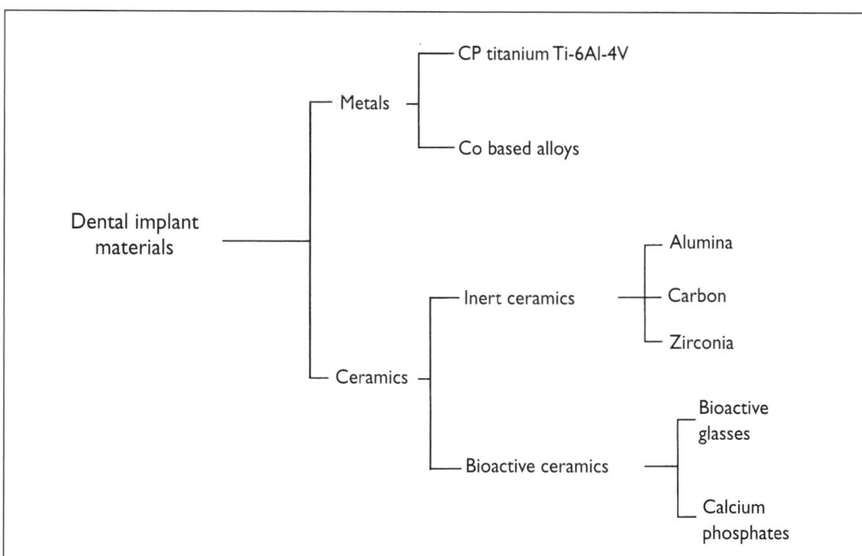

Fig 23-8 Classification of dental implant materials.

implant/tissue interfacial zone is the major factor determining the local stresses and therefore regulates tissue integration and adaptation and the success of implants. Rationale for this hypothesis is provided by the fact that osseointegration is not uniform.

Biological parameters and properties of tissues

As discussed earlier, osseointegration is a direct structural and functional contact between loaded, viable bone and an implant surface. Perhaps more important is the corollary that the creation and maintenance of osseointegration depends on the understanding of the tissue's healing, repair, and remodeling capacities. Dental implant design and function, therefore, are not only based on material considerations, but also on the properties of the surrounding tissue.

The microstructure of the mandible is complex, consisting of secondary Haversian bone, regular and irregular primary lamellar bone, and plexiform lamellae of varying orientations. In general, the mandible is composed of basilar and alveolar bone, with no well-defined boundary between the two. The basilar bone forms the body of the mandible. Alveolar bone, formed in conjunction with tooth eruption, is a thin lamella that surrounds the tooth roots, attaches to the periodontal ligament fibers, and is surrounded by another layer of bone that supports the tooth sockets. In both humans and animals, the type and orientation of tissue microstructure are regionally dependent, as are density and mechanical properties. For example, compressive strength changes with tissue organization, morphology, and density and progressively increases with increasing numbers of osteons, numbers of lamellar plates, plate density, plate orientation with respect to the stress axis, amount of ground substance, and mineral content. Thus, even within the mandible of one species, held constant with respect to age, sex, and metabolic state, there are substantive differences in architecture and physical/mechanical properties. Location-dependent properties might imply a structure-function relationship in the mandible.

In general, the material and mechanical properties of mandibular bone are nonuniform and vary as functions of anatomic location, age, sex, and metabolic state. Variations in these properties are functions of variations in composition and microstructure at a local level. The processing-composition-structure-property synergy and mechanistic understanding of synthetic materials at an atom level, discussed previously, holds true for tissue also. In biological materials, it is necessary to understand mechanisms at the cellular and molecular levels. An understanding of regional properties will provide a better understanding of localized bone regeneration, repair, modeling, remodeling, and disease states and possibly facilitate the design of site-specific dental implants and bone augmentation materials.

Materials used in dental implantology

In general, two basic classes of materials—metals and ceramics—are used in dental implantology, either alone or in hybrid fashion (Fig 23-8). Metallic implant materials are largely titanium based—either commercially pure Ti or Ti-6Al-4V alloy. However, as already stated, it is essential to recognize that the synergistic relationship between processing, composition, structure, and properties of both the bulk metals and their surface oxides effectively leaves more than two metals. Casting, forging, and machining of metal implants, densification of ceramics, deposition of ceramic and metal coatings onto metal implants, as well as cleaning and sterilization procedures, can all alter the microstructure, surface chemistry, and properties. Thus, the many material-processing sequences necessary to yield a dental implant strongly influence implant properties and functionality, primarily through temperature and pressure effects.

Metals

Although cobalt-based alloys have been used experimentally in dentistry, metallic dental implants are almost exclusively titanium based. A good deal of the knowledge about titanium stems from the extensive aerospace and metallurgy literature. Many requirements of an aerospace component, primarily high strength and corrosion resistance, are characteristic properties needed in a dental implant. Thus, titanium has been called the "material of choice" in dentistry because of its strength and the minimal biological response it elicits. The strength of titanium is due to its hexagonal close-packed crystal lattice and crystallographic orientation, whereas its biocompatibility (corrosion resistance) is attributed to its stable, passive oxide layer.

Titanium-based implants are in their passive state (ie, their oxide is stable) under typical physiological conditions and breakdown of passivity should not occur. Both c.p. Ti and Ti-6Al-4V possess excellent corrosion resistance for a full range of oxide states and pH levels. It is the extremely coherent oxide layer and the fact that titanium repassivates almost instantaneously through surface-controlled oxidation kinetics that renders titanium so corrosion resistant. However, even in its passive condition, titanium is not inert. Titanium ion release that does occur results from chemical dissolution of titanium oxide. However, the low dissolution rate and near chemical inertness of titanium dissolution products allow bone to thrive and therefore osseointegrate with titanium. Surface potential may also play an important role in facilitating osseointegration, and it is postulated that oxides with high dielectric constants inhibit the movement of cells to implant surfaces.

The Ti-6Al-4V alloy has a 60% greater strength than pure titanium, but it is more expensive. Both materials have complex, heterogeneous surface oxides. There may be differences in cell adhesion, and tissues may be in closer proximity to pure titanium surfaces than to alloy surfaces. However, there does not seem to be any difference in implant function, and there is no clear rationale for choosing pure titanium over titanium alloy.

The mechanical properties of titanium-based materials are well established. Microstructures with a small (<20 µm) α-grain size, a well-dispersed second (β)-phase, and a small α/β interface area, such as equiaxed microstructures, resist fatigue crack initiation best and have the best high-cycle fatigue strength (approximately 500 to 700 MPa). Lamellar microstructures, which have a greater α/β interface area and more oriented phase colonies, have lower fatigue strengths (approximately 300 to 500 MPa). Surface roughening, whether through screw threading or deposition of coatings, results in a reduced strength compared to smooth-surfaced implants.

Ceramics

The initial rationale for using ceramics in dentistry was based upon the relative biological inertness of ceramics compared to that of metals. Ceramics are fully oxidized materials and therefore chemically stable. Thus, ceramics are less likely to elicit an adverse biological response than metals, which only oxidize at their surface. Two types of "inert" ceramics of interest are carbon and alumina (Al_2O_3). Recently, a greater emphasis has been placed on bioactive and bioresorbable ceramics, materials that not only elicit normal tissue formation, but may also form an intimate bond with bone tissue and even be replaced by tissue over time. While inert ceramics elicit a minimal tissue response, bioactive ceramics are partially soluble, enabling ion transfer and the formation of a direct bond between implant and bone. Bioresorbable or biodegradable ceramics have a higher degree of solubility than bioactive ceramics, gradually resorb and integrate into the surrounding tissue, and are used as bone augmentation materials. Bioactive ceramics are primarily used as scaffold materials or as coatings on more structurally sound metal substrates.

The concept of bioactivity was originally introduced with respect to bioactive glasses via the following hypothesis: The biocompatibility of an implant material is optimal if the material elicits the formation of normal tissues at its surface, and, in addition, if it establishes a contiguous interface capable of supporting the loads that normally occur at the site of implantation. Important examples of these materials are bioactive glasses, glass ceramics, and calcium-phosphate ceramics. Bioactive glasses and glass ceramics include Bioglass, which is a synthesis of several glasses containing mixtures of silica, phosphate, calcia, and soda; Ceravital, which has a different alkali oxide concentration from that of Bioglass; and glass ceramic A-W, a glass ceramic containing crystalline oxyapatite and fluorapatite [$Ca_{10}(PO_4)_6(O,F_2)$] and β-wollastonite (SiO_2-CaO) in a MgO-CaO-SiO_2 glassy matrix. The calcium-phosphate ceramics are ceramic materials with varying calcium-to-phosphate ratios, depending on processing-induced physical and chemical changes. Among them, the apatite ceramics, one of which is hydroxyapatite, have been studied most and are the focus of this section.

The impetus for using synthetic hydroxyapatite as a biomaterial stems from the perceived advantage of using a material similar to the mineral phase in bone and teeth for replacing these materials. As such, better tissue bonding is expected. Additional perceived advantages of bioactive ceramics include low thermal and electrical conductivity, elastic properties similar to those of bone, control of in vivo degradation rates through control of material properties, and the possibility of the ceramic functioning as a barrier to metallic corrosion products when it is coated onto a metal substrate.

However, processing-induced phase transformations provoke a change in in vitro dissolution behavior, and the different structures and compositions alter the biological response. Given the range of chemical compositions available in bioactive ceramics and the fact that pure hydroxyapatite is rarely used, the broader term *calcium-phosphate ceramics* (CPC) should be used in lieu of the more specific *hydroxyapatite*. Each individual CPC is defined by its own unique set of chemical and physical properties.

Mixtures of hydroxyapatite, tricalcium phosphate, and tetracalcium phosphate may evolve as a result of plasma-spraying deposition processes onto metals. Physical properties of importance to the functioning of calcium phosphate ceramics include:

1. Powder particle size and shape
2. Pore size, shape, and distribution
3. Specific surface area
4. Phases present
5. Crystal structure and size
6. Grain size
7. Density
8. Coating thickness, hardness, and surface roughness

There are variable and conflicting data with respect to implant/tissue bond strength, solubility, and overall in vivo function. In addition, long-term stabilization and fixation strength do not depend on the ceramic coating. The ceramic/metal bond fails before the ceramic/tissue bond and is the "weak link" in the system. Thus, there is reason for concern about the weak ceramic/metal bond and integrity of that interface over a lengthy service life of functional loading.

Problems/future directions

Although there is no consensus regarding methods of evaluating dental implants and what parameters are most important, clinical evaluations have generally shown that dental implants are successful in about 75% of cases 5 years postimplantation. Despite advances in materials synthesis and processing, surgical technique, and clinical protocols, clinical failures do occur, at rates of approximately 2% to 5% per year. Causes of failure and current problems with dental implants include:

1. Early loosening, stemming from a lack of initial osseointegration
2. Late loosening, or loss of osseointegration
3. Bone resorption
4. Infection
5. Fracture of the implant and/or abutment
6. Delamination of the coating from the bulk implant

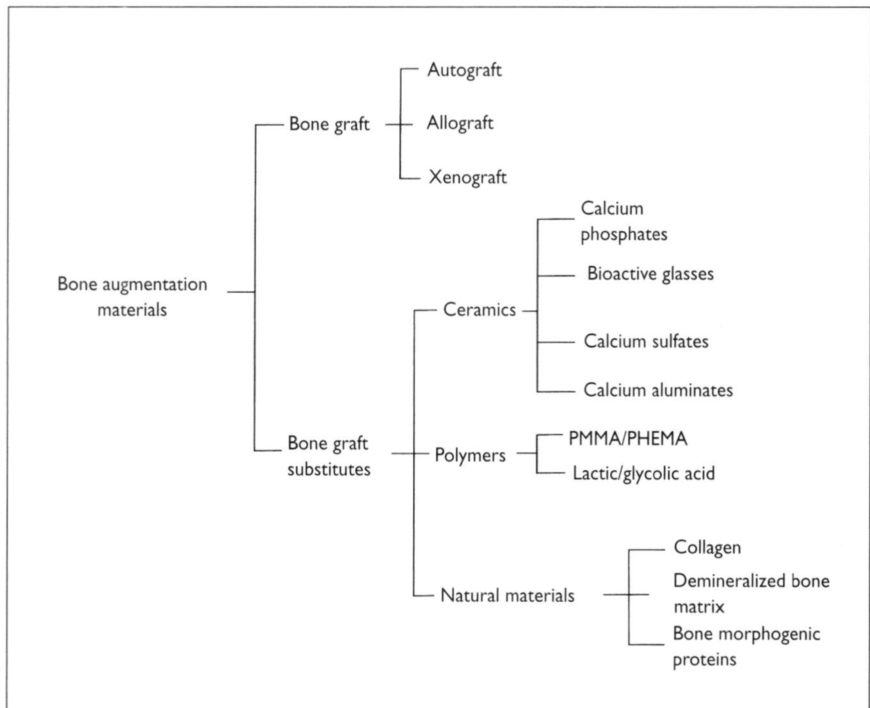

Fig 23-9 Classification of bone augmentation materials.

The most common failure mechanism with endosseous implants is alveolar crest resorption, leading to progressive periodontal lesions, decreased areas of supporting tissues, and ultimately implant loosening. Aseptic failures are most often the cumulative result of more than one of the above-mentioned factors.

As a result of these clinical problems, basic and clinical research should focus on the complete characterization of materials, including bulk and surface properties, development of new materials, more engineering-based designs for both existing and new materials, fundamental aspects and quantification of stresses and stress transfer between implant and tissue, mechanical and biological responses of tissues, and host response to these foreign materials.

Future materials

Although titanium and, to a lesser extent, ceramic and ceramic-coated implants have an excellent clinical record in implant dentistry, these materials are not necessarily end-stage materials. Continuing developments in the materials and biomedical fields can be expected in the next decade. Because one of the long-term problems with dental implants is stress shielding, or mechanically mediated bone resorption, which is due in part to the elastic mismatch between metal and bone, polymer and composite implants that offer reduced moduli are being considered. The motivation for using composite materials for implants is based on several concepts. Composite materials can be very strong, because materials in fiber form exhibit strengths near the theoretical values. As a result, advanced composites can be as strong as metals and, in some cases, more flexible. The properties of composites can be more easily tailored than those of metals. A specific example is that of the modulus of composites, which can be tailored to some extent to be near that of bone. The rationale for designing "isoelastic" implants, or implants with the same modulus as bone, is based on observations of bone resorption in the presence of stiff metal implants. This rationale is based on the hypothesis that an implant that matches the elastic properties of the mandible will result in a more physiological stress distribution than can be attained with higher modulus metallic implants.

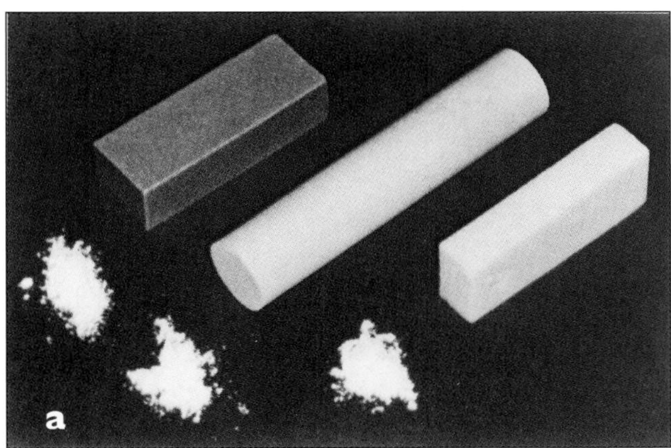

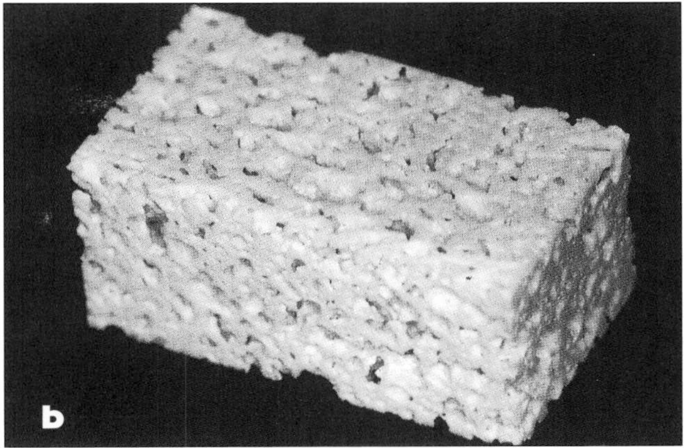

Fig 23-10 (a) Dense hydroxyapatite ceramic augmentation material with starting powders. (From Denissen et al, 1985, with permission.) (b) Porous hydroxyapatite augmentation material, 44 mm x 18 mm x 16 mm; porosity = 45%. (From Osborn, 1985.)

Augmentation materials

One of the oldest biomaterials problems has been the search for materials that can repair or replace bone defects. The standard materials, historically, have been bone grafts. However, given the morbidity associated with autogenous grafts and recent concern about transmission of live viruses with allogenic grafts, increased research into alternative substitute materials, such as ceramics, polymers, composites, bone derivatives, and natural materials, is underway (Fig 23-9). Examples of dense and porous calcium-phosphate ceramics are shown in Figs 23-10 and 23-11.

The three primary application areas for augmentation materials in dentistry are intramucosal, endodontic, and bone-substitute materials. An ideal bone substitute material should be biocompatible; easy to fabricate, sterilize, and shape intraoperatively; inexpensive; osteoinductive (ie, cause the conversion of mesenchymal cells preferentially to bone progenitor cells); and osteoconductive (ie, act as a scaffold for new bone formation). It should also offer mechanical integrity over a lengthy service life.

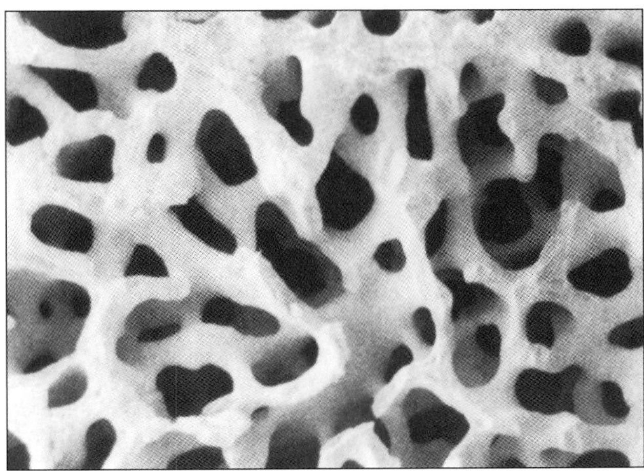

Fig 23-11 Porous coralline hydroxyapatite ceramic augmentation material: Pro Osteon Implant 500, Interpore Orthopaedics, Inc., West Caldwell, NJ (with permission).

Glossary

calcium phosphate ceramics A class of ceramics with varying calcium-to-phosphate ratios, which can form a direct bond with bone.

interfacial zone The thin zone at the surface of an implant, which includes the surface oxides, protein layers, and connective tissue.

osseointegration A direct structural and functional connection between ordered, living bone and the surface of a load-carrying implant.

osteoconductive material A material that acts as a scaffold for new bone formation.

osteoinductive material A material that causes the conversion of mesenchymal cells preferentially to bone progenitor cells.

titanium The "material of choice" in dentistry, primarily because of its excellent biocompatibility (as a result of its stable oxide layer), mechanical properties, and, in implantology, its proven ability to achieve osseointegration.

Discussion questions

1. What are the properties (bulk and surface) of titanium that make this material attractive for use as a dental implant?
2. What is/are the rationale(s) for using bioactive ceramics (eg, hydroxyapatite) as coatings on dental implants?
3. What is the importance of implant/tissue interfacial stability, and what are current methods of accelerating osseointegration such that the time between first and second stage implant surgery may be reduced?
4. What are the physical, mechanical, and biological parameters affecting the clinical success of dental implants?

Questions and answers

1. **What is osseointegration?** A working definition of osseointegration is a direct structural and functional connection between ordered, living bone and the surface of a load-carrying implant.
2. **What materials are used for osseointegrated implants?** Commercially pure titanium, titanium alloy (Ti-6Al-4V), bioactive glasses and glass ceramics, and calcium-phosphate ceramics.
3. **What factors dictate the effectiveness of osseointegration?** Surgical technique, bone quality, minimization of interfacial motion, surface chemistry, among other factors.
4. **What parameters influence implant success?** Materials and material processing; mechanisms of implant/tissue attachment; mechanical properties; implant design; loading type; tissue properties; stress analysis; initial stability and mechanisms of enhancing osseointegration; biocompatibility of the implant materials; surface chemistry, mechanics, and bone-bonding ability of the implant.

Recommended reading

Adell R, Lekholm U, Rockler B, Brånemark PI. A 15-year study of osseointegrated implants in the treatment of the edentulous jaw. Int J Oral Surg 10:387–416, 1981.

Albrektsson T, Brånemark PI, Hansson HA, Kasemo B, Larsson K, Lundstrom I, et al. The interface zone of inorganic implants in vivo: titanium implants in bone. Ann Biomed Eng 11:1–27, 1983.

Brånemark PI, Hansson BO, Adell R, Breine U, Lindstrom J, Hallen O, et al. Osseointegrated implants in the treatment of the edentulous jaw. Experience from a 10-year period. Stockman: Alnquist and Wiksell International, 1977.

Brånemark PI, Zarb GA, Albrektsson T. Tissue-Integrated Protheses—Osseointegration in Clinical Dentistry. Chicago: Quintessence, 1987.

Brunski JB, Hipp JA. In vivo forces on endosteal implants: a measurement system and biomechanical considerations. J Prosthet Dent 51:82–90, 1984.

Brunski JB, Moccia AF, Pollack SR, Korostoff E, Trachtenberg DI. The influence of functional use of endosseous dental implants on the tissue-implant interface. I. histological aspects. J Dent Res 58(10):1953–1969, 1979.

Chehroudi B, Gould TRL, Brunette DM. Effects of a grooved titanium-coated implant surface on epithelial cell behaviour in vitro and in vivo. J Biomed Mater Res 23:1067–1085, 1989.

Damien CJ, Parsons JR. Bone graft and bone graft substitutes: a review of current technology and applications. J Appl Biomat 2:187–208, 1991.

Daniels AU, Chang MKO, Andriano KP, Heller J. Mechanical properties of biodegradable polymers and composites proposed for internal fixation of bone. J Appl Biomat 1:57–78, 1990.

Denissen H, Mangano C, Venini G. Hydroxylapatite Implants. Padua, Italy: Piccin, 1985.

Ducheyne P. Bioceramics: material characteristics versus in vivo behavior. J Biomed Mater Res: Appl Biomat 21(A2):219–236, 1987.

Ducheyne P, Healy KE. Surface spectroscopy of calcium phosphate ceramic and titanium implant materials. In Ratner B (ed). Surface Characterization of Biomaterials. Amsterdam: Elsevier, 175–192, 1988.

Hale TM, Boretsky BB, Scheidt MJ, McQuade MJ, Strong SL, Van Dyke TE. Evaluation of titanium dental implant osseointegration in posterior edentulous areas of microswine. J Oral Implantol 17:118–124, 1991.

Healy KE, Ducheyne P. The mechanisms of passive dissolution of titanium in a model physiological environment. J Biomed Mater Res 26:319–338, 1992.

Hench LL, Splinter RJ, Allen WC, Greenlee TK Jr. Bonding mechanisms at the interface of ceramic prosthetic materials J Biomed Mater Res Symp 2:117–141, 1972.

Kasemo B. Biocompatibility of titanium implants: surface science aspects. J Prosthet Dent 49:832–837, 1983.

Koeneman J, Lemons J, Ducheyne P, Lacefield W, Magee F, Calahan T, Kay J et al. Workshop on characterization of calcium phosphate materials J Appl Biomat 1:79–90, 1990.

Kohn DH. Overview of factors important in implant design. J Oral Implantol 18:204–219, 1992.

Kohn DH, Ducheyne P. Materials for bone, joint and cartilage replacement. In DF Williams (ed). Medical and Dental Materials. Vol 14. In RW Cahn, P Haasen, EJ Kramer (eds). Materials Science and Technology—A Comprehensive Treatment. Germany: VCH Verlagsgesellschaft, 1992;29–109.

Kohn DH. Structure-property relations of biomaterials for hard tissue replacement. In DL Wise (ed). Handbook of Biomaterials and Applications. Matawan, NJ: Marcel Dekker, 1995; 83–122.

Kohn DH, Ko CC, Hollister SJ. Localized mechanics of dental implants. In NA Langrana, MH Friedman, ES Grood (eds). Bioengineering Conference, BED-Vol. 24. American Society of Mechanical Engineers, New York: 1993; 331–334.

Lacombe P. Corrosion and oxidation of Ti and Ti alloys. In JC Williams, AF Belov (eds). Titanium and titanium alloys. New York: Plenum Press, 1982; 847–880.

Lemons JE. Dental implant retrieval analyses. J Dent Ed 52:748–756, 1988.

Listgarten MA, Lang NP, Schroeder HE, Schroeder A. Periodontal tissues and their counterparts around endosseous implants. Clin Oral Impl Res 2:1–19, 1991.

Maniatopoulos C, Pilliar RM, Smith DC. Threaded versus porous-surfaced designs for implant stabilization in bone-endodontic implant model. J Biomed Mater Res 20:1309–1333, 1986.

Nakamura T, Yamamuro T, Higashi S, Kokubo T, Ito S. A new glass-ceramic for bone replacement: evaluation of its bonding to bone tissue. J Biomed Mater Res 19:685–698, 1985.

National Institutes of Health Consensus Development Conference statement on dental implants June 13–15, 1988 J Dent Ed 52:824–827, 1988.

Osborn JF. Implantatwerkstoff Hydroxylapatitkeramik. Berlin: Quintessence, 1985.

Ratner B, Johnston AB, Lenk TJ. Biomaterial surfaces. J Biomed Mater Res: Appl Biomat 21(A1):59–90, 1987.

Schnitman PA, Schulman LB. Dental implants: benefit and risk. In US Dept HHS, Pub. # 81-1531. Washington DC: US Government Printing Office, 1980.

Taylor TD. Dental Implants: are they for me? Chicago: Quintessence, 1990.

Williams DF, (ed). Biocompatibility of Clinical Implant Materials. Vol I. Boca Raton, FL: CRC Press, 9–44, 1981.

Worthington P, Bolender CL, Taylor TD. The Swedish system of osseointegrated implants: problems and complications encountered during a 4-year trial period. Int J Oral Maxillofac Imp 2:77–84, 1987.

Appendix

A

Tabulated Values of Physical and Mechanical Properties

Bond strengths between restorative materials and tooth structures . . . 332
Brinell hardness number . . . 333
Coefficient of friction, μ . . . 334
Coefficient of thermal expansion (linear), α . . . 335
Colors of dental shade guides . . . 337
Contact angle, θ (liquid phase) . . . 339
Contact angle, θ (solid surface) . . . 341
Creep of amalgam . . . 342
Critical surface tension, γ_c . . . 343
Density, ρ . . . 344
Dynamic modulus . . . 346
Elastic modulus, *E* . . . 347
Flow . . . 352
Heat of fusion . . . 354
Heat of reaction, ΔH . . . 354
Impact strength, *IZOD* . . . 355
Index of refraction, χ . . . 355
Knoop hardness number, *KHN* . . . 356
Melting temperatures and ranges . . . 359
Mohs hardness . . . 360
Penetration coefficient, *PC* . . . 360
Percent elongation (Ductility), *n* . . . 361
Permanent deformation . . . 363
Poisson's ratio, υ . . . 365
Proportional limit, *PL* . . . 366
Shear strength, *S* . . . 367
Shore A hardness . . . 368
Solubility and disintegration in water . . . 369
Specific heat, C_p . . . 370
Strain in compression . . . 371
Surface free energy, γ_s . . . 373
Surface tension, γ . . . 373
Tear energy . . . 374
Tear strength . . . 375
Thermal conductivity, *K* . . . 377
Thermal diffusivity, Δ . . . 379
Transverse strength, *T* . . . 381
Ultimate compressive strength, *C* . . . 383
Ultimate tensile strength, *UTS* . . . 387
Vapor pressure, *P* . . . 392
Vickers hardness, *VHN* . . . 393
Viscosity, η . . . 395
Water sorption . . . 396
Yield strength, *YS* . . . 397
Zeta potential, ζ . . . 399
References . . . 400

Bond strengths between restorative materials and tooth structures

Adhesion of restorative materials to tooth structures has been studied since 1955. The bond strength is the load required to fracture the bond divided by the cross-sectional area of the bond. Bond strengths are measured either in shear or tension. Many factors, including the dentin substrate, the storage conditions, and the test method, affect the bond strength values.

			Shear bond strength		
Substrate	Adhesive	Adherend	psi x 10^3	MPa	Reference
Dentin	Dentin bonding system	Composite	3.2–5.1	22–35	238
Dentin	No smear layer	Light-cured hybrid			238
		glass-ionomer	1.5–1.7	10–12	238
Enamel	Enamel bonding system	Composite	2.6–3.2	18–22	238
Enamel	Amalgam bonding system	Composite	1.5–1.7	10–12	238
Enamel	Amalgam bonding system	Amalgam	0.3–0.9	2–6	238
Enamel	No smear layer	Traditional glass-ionomer	1.2–1.7	8–12	238
Enamel	Enamel bonding system	Orthodontic bracket	2.6–2.9	18–20	238

			Tensile bond strength		
Substrate	Adhesive	Adherend	psi x 10^3	MPa	Reference
Dentin	Polyurethane	Composite	0.1–0.9	1–6	147
Dentin	Polyacrylic acid	Composite	0.3–0.6	2–4	147
Dentin	Organic phosphonates	Composite	0.4–1.4	3–10	147
Dentin	4-META*	Composite	0.4–1.0	3–7	147
Dentin	HEMA + GA†	Composite	1.6–2.4	11–17	147
Dentin	NPG-GMA/PMDM‡	Composite	0.6–1.8	4–12	147
Dentin		Glass-ionomer	0.6	4	147
Dentin		Zinc polycarboxylate	0.4–0.6	3–4	147
Dentin		Adhesive resin cement	0.6	4.1	147
Dentin		Conventional resin cement	0.0	0.0	147
Etched enamel		Fine composite	2.4–2.8	17–20	147
Etched enamel		Microfine composite	1.4	10	147
Enamel		Glass-ionomer	0.7	5	147
Etched enamel		Adhesive resin cement	2.2	15	147
Etched enamel		Conventional resin cement	1.5	10	147

* 4-META-4-methyloxyethyl-trimellitic anhydride.
† HEMA - hydroxyethyl methacrylate.
GA - glutaraldehyde.
‡ NPG-GMA - N-phenyl glycine - glycidyl methacrylate.
PMDM - pyromellitic acid diethylmethacrylate.

Brinell hardness number, *BHN*

The Brinell hardness test depends upon the resistance offered to the penetration of a steel ball (1.6-mm diameter) when subjected to a weight of 12.6 kg. The resulting hardness value is computed as the ratio of the applied load to the area of the indentation produced.

Material	Product	BHN (kg/mm²)	Reference
Cobalt-chromium alloy	Genesis II	265	9
Gold (condensed)			
Foil		69	33
Mat		40	33
Powdered	Goldent	46	33
Gold alloys			
Type I	Ney-Oro A	45	7
Type II	Ney-Oro A-1	95	7
Type III, soft	Ney-Oro B-2	110	7
Type III, hard	Ney-Oro B-2	120	7
Type IV, soft	Ney-Oro G-3	140	7
Type IV, hard	Ney-Oro G-3	220	7
40% Au-Ag-Cu, soft	Forticast	175	9
40% Au-Ag-Cu, hard	Forticast	265	9
10-15% Au-Ag-Pd, soft	Paliney No. 4	150	7
10-15% Au-Ag-Pd, hard	Paliney No. 4	205	7
Au-Pd	Olympia	200	9
Porcelain-fused-to-metal	Jelenko O	165	9
Palladium-based dental alloy	Microstar	240	9
Silver-palladium alloys			
Crown-and-bridge, soft	Albacast	130	9
Crown-and-bridge, hard	Albacast	140	9
Porcelain-fused-to-metal	Jel-5	170	9

Coefficient of friction, μ

The coefficient of friction is defined as the ratio of tangential force to normal load during a sliding process.

Material couples	μ Dry	μ Wet	Reference
Amalgam on:			
Amalgam	0.19–0.35		95
Bovine enamel		0.12–0.28	95
Composite resin		0.10–0.18	95
Gold alloy		0.10–0.35	95
Porcelain	0.06–0.12	0.07–0.15	95
Bone on:			
Metal (bead-coated)	0.50		203
Metal (fiber mesh-coated)	0.60		203
Metal (smooth)	0.42		203
Bovine enamel on:			
Acrylic resin	0.19–0.65		95
Amalgam	0.18–0.22		95
Bovine dentin	0.35–0.40	0.45–0.55	95
Bovine enamel	0.22–0.60	0.50–0.60	95
Chromium-nickel alloy	0.10–0.12		95
Gold	0.12–0.20		95
Porcelain	0.10–0.12	0.50–0.90	95
Composite resin on:			
Amalgam	0.13–0.25	0.22–0.34	95
Bovine enamel		0.30–0.75	95
Gold alloy on:			
Acrylic	0.6–0.8		95
Amalgam	0.15–0.25		95
Gold alloy	0.2–0.6		95
Porcelain	0.22–0.25	0.16–0.17	95
Hydrogel-coated latex on:			
Hydrogel		0.054	204
Latex on:			
Glass		0.470	204
Hydrogel		0.095	204
Metal (bead-coated) on:			
Bone	0.54		203
Metal (fiber mesh-coated) on:			
Bone	0.58		203
Metal (smooth) on:			
Bone	0.43		203
Prosthetic tooth materials:			
Acrylic on acrylic	0.21	0.37	94
Acrylic on porcelain	0.23	0.30	94
Porcelain on acrylic	0.34	0.32	94
Porcelain on porcelain	0.14	0.51	94

Coefficient of thermal expansion (linear), α

The coefficient of thermal expansion (linear) is the change in length per unit length of material for a 1°C change in temperature.

Material	Product	α [(°C^{-1}) x 10^6]	Temperature range (°C)	Reference
Alumina (recrystallized)		6.2	0–200	20
Amalgam		22.1–28.0	20–50	147
Cement				
Unmodified ZOE		35	25–60	91
Cobalt-chromium alloys	Master Tec	14.7	25–500	222
	Novarex	14.1	25–500	223
Denture resins				
Acrylic		76	5–37	59
Polystyrene	Jectron	67.3	20–37	46
Polyvinylacrylic	Luxene 44	69.2	20–37	46
Gold Alloys				
Au-Pd	Olympia	14.1	25–500	9
Au-Pt-Pd	TPW	15.48	200–700	196
Porcelain-fused-to-metal	Jelenko O	14.71	40–500	134
	SMG-2	15.73	40–500	134
	Williams-Y	14.83	40–500	134
Gutta percha		54.9	23–38	114
Impression materials				
Silicone, addition	Exaflex			
	light	142	22–40	225
	medium	128	22–40	225
	Permagum			
	light	184	22–40	225
	medium	158	22–40	225
	heavy	147	22–40	225
	putty	132	22–40	225
	President			
	light	156	22–40	225
	medium	144	22–40	225
	heavy	120	22–40	225
	putty	109	22–40	225
	Reflect	152	22–40	225
	Reprosil			
	light	154	22–40	225
	medium	152	22–40	225
	heavy	136	22–40	225
	putty	109	22–40	225
	Xantogum	160	22–40	225
Mercury		60.6	20–50	147
Nickel-chromium alloys	Biobond C & B	14.27	40–500	134
	Ceramalloy II	14.63	40–500	134
	NP-2	15.28	40–500	134
	Pentillium	14.14	40–500	134

* Range is for 1–7 firing cycles. Values of the coefficients are not necessarily related to the specific firing cycle.

Coefficient of thermal expansion (linear), α (continued)

Material	Product	α [(°C^{-1}) x 10^6]	Temperature range (°C)	Reference
Nickel-chromium alloys (continued)	Unimetal	15.68	200–700	196
Palladium-based dental alloys	Microstar	14.3	25–500	9
	Spartan	14.2	25–500	222
	W-1	15.2	25–500	222
Pit and fissure sealants				
Self-cured	Delton	90.3–97.1	0–60	148
	Kerr	70.9–78.2	0–60	148
	White	93.7–99.1	0–60	148
Light-cured	Nuva Seal	78–80	0–60	148
Porcelains				
Feldspathic		6.4–7.8	0–200	20
Body	Biobond	13.59–14.82*	40–500	134
	Ceramco	12.93–13.07*	40–500	134
	Microbond	14.59–15.28*	40–500	134
	Neydium	14.04–15.93*	40–500	134
	Vita (VMK-68)	12.73–14.45*	40–500	134
	Will-Ceram	15.94–16.23*	40–500	134
Opaque	Biobond	13.10–14.35*	40–500	134
	Ceramco	12.70–14.23*	40–500	134
	Microbond	12.38–14.80*	40–500	134
	Neydium	13.25–14.23*	40–500	134
	Vita (VMK-68)	14.29–16.03*	40–500	134
	Will-Ceram	14.68–15.45*	40–500	134
Pure metals				
Gold		14.4	20–50	147
Platinum		8.9	Near 20	130
Silver		19.2	20–50	147
Titanium		11.9	23	126
Restorative materials				
Acrylic	Sevriton	92.0	24–88	42
Composite resin	Adaptic	39.4	24–88	42
		35.8–40.1	0–60	148
	Adaptic (radiopaque)	32.2–39.0	0–60	148
	Concise	39.6–43.4	0–60	148
	Nuva Fil	28.3–30.2	0–60	148
	Simulate	28.2–31.6	0–60	148
	Vytol	26.5–27.8	0–60	148
Ti-6Al-4V alloy		12.43	200–700	196
Tooth structures				
Crown		11.4	20–50	147
Root		8.3	20–50	66
Vitreous carbon		2.2	0–100	117
Waxes				
Inlay casting, hard	Kerr blue hard	320	22–37	29
Inlay casting, soft	Kerr blue regular	260	22–37	29

Colors of dental shade guides

The colors of shade guide teeth were determined using a methodology developed for a reflectance spectrophotometer.[149] The spectral reflectance of each shade tab was measured using a dual-beam spectrophotometer equipped with an integrating sphere and a beam-reducing accessory. Relative reflectance measurements were converted to absolute reflectance. Tristimulus coordinates were determined for each sample by use of the CIE standard observer function and standard illuminant source C. The tristimulus coordinates were then converted to the CIE L*a*b* and Munsell Color Systems.

Bioform shade-guide colors[149]

	Munsell notation		Chromaticity coordinates			CIE L* a* b*		
Shade	H	V C	Y	x	y	L*	a*	b*
B-59	3.5Y	7.80/2.0	55.72	0.3407	0.3502	79.49	–1.10	15.26
B-51	3.2Y	7.80/2.2	55.24	0.3432	0.3525	79.21	–0.99	16.31
B-91	2.4Y	7.45/1.9	49.57	0.3406	0.3484	75.84	–0.42	14.14
B-62	3.1Y	7.45/2.3	49.92	0.3454	0.3539	76.05	–0.64	16.53
B-66	2.8Y	7.55/2.8	51.21	0.3534	0.3615	76.84	–0.42	20.18
B-52	3.6Y	7.50/2.1	50.42	0.3451	0.3553	76.36	–1.28	16.94
B-53	2.1Y	7.40/2.5	49.39	0.3499	0.3559	75.72	0.33	17.76
B-92	3.0Y	7.35/2.0	48.67	0.3429	0.3514	75.28	–0.66	15.27
B-63	1.7Y	7.45/2.8	50.00	0.3548	0.3594	76.10	0.87	19.64
B-54	2.0Y	7.40/2.7	49.15	0.3532	0.3589	75.58	0.46	19.13
B-65	1.1Y	7.30/3.1	49.14	0.3606	0.3629	75.57	1.73	21.48
B-93	2.2Y	7.15/2.6	45.01	0.3526	0.3584	72.93	0.40	18.34
B-55	2.9Y	7.30/2.9	47.10	0.3558	0.3639	74.28	–0.39	20.69
B-69	2.6Y	6.95/2.6	42.49	0.3545	0.3614	71.24	0.03	19.11
B-94	3.0Y	6.95/2.7	42.30	0.3548	0.3627	71.11	–0.32	19.48
B-95	2.6Y	6.85/2.4	41.22	0.3502	0.3570	70.36	0.03	17.07
B-67	2.5Y	7.20/3.2	46.26	0.3614	0.3681	73.74	0.14	22.66
B-56	2.0Y	7.30/2.9	47.80	0.3581	0.3633	74.73	0.66	21.00
B-77	2.3Y	7.05/2.8	44.09	0.3572	0.3628	72.32	0.50	20.16
B-81	1.5Y	6.60/2.8	38.82	0.3588	0.3616	68.65	1.43	19.24
B-96	1.9Y	6.55/2.9	37.05	0.3610	0.3641	67.34	1.31	19.93
B-83	1.3Y	7.00/3.6	43.25	0.3693	0.3701	71.52	2.25	23.94
B-84	0.9Y	6.65/3.2	37.98	0.3663	0.3653	68.01	2.74	21.21
B-85	1.8Y	6.65/4.1	38.24	0.3811	0.3794	68.23	2.91	27.38

H hue.
V value.
C chroma.
Y lightness.
x and y hue and chroma.
L* lightness.
a* hue and chroma on a red/green scale.
b* hue and chroma on a yellow/blue scale.

Vita shade-guide colors

Shade	Munsell notation[151]		Chromaticity coordinates[152]			CIE L*a*b*[151]		
	H	V C	Y	x	y	L*	a*	b*
A1	4.5Y	7.80/1.7	55.92	0.3352	0.3459	79.57	–1.61	13.05
A2	2.4Y	7.45/2.3	49.95	0.3468	0.3539	76.04	–0.08	16.73
A3	1.3Y	7.40/2.9	48.85	0.3559	0.3593	75.36	1.36	19.61
A3.5	1.6Y	7.05/3.2	44.12	0.3627	0.3657	72.31	1.48	21.81
A4	1.6Y	6.70/3.1	38.74	0.3633	0.3658	68.56	1.58	21.00
B1	5.1Y	7.75/1.6	54.76	0.3336	0.3447	78.90	–1.76	12.33
B2	4.3Y	7.50/2.2	50.97	0.3437	0.3549	76.66	–1.62	16.62
B3	2.3Y	7.25/3.2	46.91	0.3611	0.3669	74.13	0.47	22.34
B4	2.4Y	7.00/3.2	43.38	0.3620	0.3678	71.81	0.50	22.15
C1	4.3Y	7.30/1.6	47.16	0.3361	0.3462	74.29	–1.26	12.56
C2	2.8Y	6.95/2.3	42.12	0.3487	0.3563	70.95	–0.22	16.72
C3	2.6Y	6.70/2.3	39.11	0.3499	0.3569	68.83	–0.01	16.68
C4	1.6Y	6.30/2.7	33.77	0.3600	0.3622	64.78	1.59	18.66
D2	3.0Y	7.35/1.8	48.71	0.3391	0.3473	75.27	–0.54	13.47
D3	1.8Y	7.10/2.3	44.48	0.3482	0.3534	72.55	0.62	16.14
D4	3.7Y	7.05/2.4	43.45	0.3492	0.3591	71.86	–1.03	17.77

H hue.
V value.
C chroma.
Y lightness.
x and y hue and chroma.
L* lightness.
a* hue and chroma on a red/green scale.
b* hue and chroma on a yellow/blue scale.

Contact angle, θ (liquid phase)

The angle of contact between a liquid and a solid is a measure of the tendency for the liquid to spread over or wet the solid surface. The lower the contact angle, the greater the tendency for the liquid to wet the solid, until complete wetting occurs at an angle of zero degrees.

Material	Product	Liquid phase	θ (degrees)	Reference
Amalgam	New True Dentalloy	Water	77	58
Bacteria				
A. odontolyticus A7-1		Water	41	200
A. viscosus C7-4		Water	35	200
S. mutans C7-3		Water	12	200
S. salivarius B3-4		Water	24	200
S. sanguis C7-2		Water	48	200
Cement				
Orthodontic	Concise	Water	30	215
Denture resins				
Acrylic		Alcohol	0	57
		Saliva	73	57
		Water	75	57
Acrylic (modified)	Hydrocryl	Water	78	112
Polystyrene		Saliva	79	50
		Water	86	50
Glass		Water	14	58
Gold alloy				
Porcelain-fused-to-metal	Ceramco No. 1	Porcelain	40*	56
Impression materials				
Polyether	Impregum			
	Untreated	Dental stone mix	55–58	236
			40.4	237
	30 min. in Clorox	Dental stone mix	59–60	236
	30 min. in Sporicidin	Dental stone mix	81–93	236
	Impregum F	Water	42.6	216
	Permadyne			
	light	Water	43.1	216
	heavy	Water	43.9	216
Polysulfide	Permlastic			
	Untreated	Water	42.1	216
		Dental stone mix	76–82	236
	30 min in Clorox	Dental stone mix	78–82	236
	30 min in Sporicidin	Dental stone mix	43–47†	236
Silicone, addition	Examix			
	Untreated	Dental stone mix	71–74	236
	30 min in Clorox	Dental stone mix	90–92	236
	30 min in Sporicidin	Dental stone mix	94–95	236
	Express			
	light	Water	104.9	216
	putty	Water	101.7	216

* Measured at 1038° C.

† "The polysulfide appeared to have reacted with the 0.5% sodium hypochlorite."[236]

Contact angle, θ (liquid phase) (continued)

Material	Product	Liquid phase	θ (degrees)	Reference
Impression materials				
Silicone, addition (continued)	Express Hydrophilic			
	light	Water	19.7	216
	medium	Water	78.3	216
		Dental stone mix	64.4	237
	putty	Water	63.8	216
	Imprint Hydrophilic			
	medium	Water	46.3	216
	Mirror 3 Extrude			
	light	Water	33.9	216
	medium	Water	57.7	216
	putty	Water	98.4	216
	President			
	Untreated	Dental stone mix	92–96	236
	30 min in Clorox	Dental stone mix	98–99	236
	30 min in Sporicidin	Dental stone mix	94–98	236
	Unosil	Dental stone mix	75.0	237
Silicone, condensation	Citricon			
	light	Water	81.7	216
	putty	Water	90.7	216
	Rapid			
	light	Water	95.2	216
	putty	Water	102.6	216
	Xantopren	Dental stone mix	89.1	237
Polymers				
Poly (butyl cyanoacrylate)		Water	69	217
Poly (ether urethane)		Water	80	202
Poly (ethyl cyanoacrylate)		Water	65	217
Poly (2-hydroxyethyl methacrylate)				
Atactic		Water	17	217
Isotactic		Water	13	217
Poly (2-hydroxyethyl methacrylate-methoxyethyl methacrylate) (1:1)		Water	22	217
Poly (methoxyethyl methacrylate)		Water	46	217
Poly (methyl cyanoacrylate)		Water	57	217
Poly (methyl methacrylate)		Water	62–73	217
Polystyrene		Water	66	217
Poly (tetrafluoroethylene)	Teflon	Water	110	58
Poly (vinyl chloride)		Water	69	202
Silicone		Water	110	202
Restorative materials				
Acrylic	Bonfil	Water	38	58
Composite resin	Addent	Water	51	58
Silicate	Improved Filling Porcelain	Water	12	58
Wax, paraffin		Water	109	50

Contact angle, θ (solid surface)

Material	Product	Solid surface	θ (degrees)	Reference
Bonding agents	Adaptic Bonding Agent	Enamel	0	133
	Concise Enamel Bond	Enamel	0	133
Fluoride gels	Flura-Gel	Enamel	30	132
	Luride	Enamel	31	132
	Predent	Enamel	36	132
	Rafluor	Enamel	38	132
Fluoride solutions	Rafluor	Enamel	0	132
	NaF Rinse	Enamel	0	132
Glaze	Adaptic Glaze	Enamel	0	133
Pit and fissure sealants				
Light-cured	Nuva-Seal	Enamel	28	133
Self-cured	Delton	Enamel	0	133

Creep of amalgam

Creep is a measure of the viscoelastic properties of a material. In the dynamic creep method, a compressive load is applied to a specimen to produce a fluctuating stress which is cycled from 500 to 10,000 psi (3.45 to 69.0 MPa) at a rate of 1800 times/minute. In the static creep method, a constant compressive stress of 5250 psi (36.2 MPa) is applied to the specimen. In the American National Standards Institute/American Dental Association's flow method,[73] the specimen is subjected to a compressive stress of 1450 psi (10.0 MPa). In each method the change in length of the specimen is measured and divided by the original length.

		Method			
Material	Product	Dynamic creep (%)	Static creep (%)	ADA flow (%)	Reference
Amalgams					
Admixed	Dispersalloy	0.86	0.76	0.50	53
			0.67		214
			0.3		143
	Dispersalloy				
	fast set		0.41*		142
			0.32†		142
	regular set		0.46*		142
			0.37†		142
	non zinc		1.01		214
	Optaloy II		1.77		214
			1.47*		142
			1.08†		142
	Valiant PhD		0.21		171
Lathe-cut	ANA 68 Dental Alloy		2.1		143
	ANA 2000 Nongamma 2		0.15		143
	Aristoloy		3.77		214
	Caulk Fine Cut		1.56*		142
			1.57†		142
	New True Dentalloy	1.85	2.36	0.65	53
			1.53		214
	Revalloy		1.2		143
	20th Century Micro	8.76	8.37	3.91	53
Spherical	Cupralloy Esp		0.37*		142
			0.25†		142
	Indiloy		0.34*		142
			0.15†		142
	Sybraloy		0.10		214
			0.10*		142
			0.05†		142
	Tytin		0.20		171
			0.08		214
	Valiant		0.06		171

* Hand triturated.
† Mechanically triturated.

Critical surface tension, γ_c

The critical surface tension is the surface tension of a liquid that would completely wet the solid of interest.

Material	Product	γ_c (dynes/cm)	Reference
Amalgam	Argos Alloy	48.1	52
Co-Cr-Mo, as polished	Vitallium*	22.3	137
Co-Cr-Mo, plasma cleaned	Vitallium*	>72	137
Glass	Pyrex	170	71
Gold	AB Adelmetall	57.4	52
Impression materials			
Polyether	Impregum	27.9	169
Silicone, addition	Express Hydrophilic	53.8	169
	Imprint Hydrophilic	52.4	169
	President	21.2	169
	Provil	20.2	169
Silicone, condensation	Xantopren	14.4	169
Paraffin		22–26	71
Polymers			
Polyetherurethane	Pellethane 80A	19.3	170
	Pellethane 55D	22.1	170
	Pellethane 75D	35.7	170
Polyetherurethane urea	Biomer	23.0	170
Polyethylene		31–33	71
Poly(methyl methacrylate)		39.0	71
Polystyrene		33–43	71
Poly(tetrafluoroethylene)	Teflon	18	71
Tooth structure, enamel		38.5–40†	51
		31.5‡	51

* Surgical.
† 23°C, 50% relative humidity.
‡ 37°C, 100% relative humidity.

Density, ρ

Density is the concentration of matter as measured by the mass per unit volume. The specific gravity of a substance is the ratio of the density of the substance to that of water

Material	Product	ρ (g/cm³)	Reference
Amalgam		11.6	220
Bonding agent	Silux Enamel Bond	1.20	221
Bones			
Cancellous		1.3	192
Cortical		1.3	192
Cements			
Calcium hydroxide	Dycal	1.91	206
	Life	1.88	206
Glass-ionomer	Base cement	2.13§	205
	Dentin cement	2.02§	205
	Ketac-cem	2.16§	205
Polymer-modified ZOE	IRM	2.29*	24
Resin	CBA 9080	2.02	109
Unmodified ZOE	Cavitec	2.05	206
Zinc phosphate	Tenacin	2.59‡	24
Zinc polycarboxylate		2.19	124
Cobalt-chromium alloys	Genesis II	8.8	9
	Master Tec	8.1	222
	Novarex	8.75¶	223
	Vitallium	8.5	220
Denture resin, acrylic		1.19	59
Fluorapatite, mineral	Durango, Mexico	3.215	40
Gold (condensed)			
Foil		17.22	33
Mat		16.44	33
Powdered	Goldent	17.36	33
Gold alloys			
Type II		16.4	97
Type III		15.5	220
40% Au-Ag-Cu	Forticast	12.5	9
10%-15% Au-Ag-Pd	Paliney No. 4	12.3	7
Au-Pd	Olympia	13.7	9
Porcelain-fused-to-metal	Jelenko O	18.2	9
Gypsum	Moldablaster	1.9–2.0	224
Hydroxyapatite		3.1	192
Impression materials (polymerized)			
Polyether	Impregum	1.06	207
Silicone, addition	Baysilex	1.37	207
	Provil		
	medium	1.40	207
	high	1.43	207

* Powder/liquid ratio, 5.0 g/mL
† Powder/liquid ratio, 3.0 g/mL
‡ Powder/liquid ratio, 2.5 g/mL
§ Powder/liquid ratio 1.0.
¶ Specific gravity.

Density, ρ (continued)

Material	Product	ρ (g/cm³)	Reference
Mercury		13.55	130
Monomers (crown and bridge resins)			
Methyl methacrylate		0.9374	128
Ethylene glycol dimethacrylate		1.055	129
1,3-butylene glycol dimethacrylate		1.02	129
Triethylene glycol dimethacrylate		1.072	129
Nickel-chromium alloys			
Crown-and-bridge	Howmedica III	7.9	10
Porcelain-fused-to-metal	Ultratek	8.0	6
Palladium-based dental alloys	Microstar	10.8	9
	Spartan	10.6	222
	W-1	11.1	222
Pit and fissure sealant	Delton	1.23	127
Porcelain, feldspathic		2.4	20
Pure metals			
Chromium		7.19	130
Copper		8.96	130
Gold		19.3	130
Nickel		8.9	130
Palladium		12.02	130
Platinum		21.45	130
Silver		10.49	130
Titanium		4.51	130
Zinc		7.13	130
Restorative materials			
Composite resin			
All-purpose	Heliomolar Radiopaque	1.84	221
	Herculite XR	2.09	221
Anterior	Silux Plus	1.61	221
Posterior	Ful Fil	2.14	221
	Visiomolar	2.38	221
Silicate	Improved Filling Porcelain†	2.01†	24
Silver-palladium alloys			
Crown-and-bridge	Albacast	10.6	9
Porcelain-fused-to-metal	Jel-5	10.9	9
Ti-6 Al-4V alloy		4.5	220
Tooth structures			
Cementum		2.03	44
Dentin (deciduous)		2.18	43
Dentin (permanent)		2.14	44
Enamel (deciduous)		2.95	43
Enamel (permanent)		2.97	44
Vitreous carbon		1.47	117
Water (4°C)		1.00	1

Dynamic modulus

The dynamic modulus is defined as the ratio of stress to strain for small cyclic deformations at a given frequency and at a particular point on the stress-strain curve.

Material	Product	Dynamic modulus		Reference
		psi x 10^3	MPa	
Maxillofacial materials				
Polyurethane	Dermathane 100	0.444*	3.06*	38
Polyvinyl chloride	Sartomer Resins	0.364*	2.51*	38
Silicone rubber	Silastic 382	0.435*	3.00*	38
	Silastic 399	0.554*	3.82*	38
Mouth protector material				
Polyvinyl acetate-polyethylene	Proform	3.07*	21.2*	37
	Sta-Guard	1.36*	9.39*	37
Restorative materials				
Composite resin				
Anterior	Silar	372.6†	2569†	219
	Silux	374.5†	2582†	219
Posterior	P10	1218†	8396†	219
	P50	1399†	9645†	219
	Profile	1147†	7911†	219
	Profile TLC	1274†	8786†	219

* Measured at 37°C.
† Dynamic sheer modulus, measured wet at 40°C.

Elastic modulus, *E*

The elastic modulus of a material represents the relative stiffness of the material within the elastic range and can be determined from a stress-strain curve by calculating the ratio of stress to strain. Unless indicated otherwise, values were determined in tension.

Material	Product	E		Reference
		psi x 10^6	GPa	
Alumina	De Trey	60.6*	418*	21
Amalgams (7d)				
Admixed	Dispersalloy	7.60*	52.4*	186
	Valiant PhD	8.05*	55.5*	186
Spherical	Indiloy	7.56*	52.1*	186
	Logic	7.82*	53.9*	186
	Sybraloy	8.72*	60.1*	186
	Tytin	7.64*	52.7*	186
	Valiant	8.54*	58.9*	186
Bones				
Cancellous		0.071	0.49	192
Cortical		2.1	14.7	192
Long bones				
Femur		2.49	17.2	172
Humerus		2.49	17.2	172
Radius		2.70	18.6	172
Tibia		2.63	18.1	172
Vertebrae				
Cervical		0.033	0.23	172
Lumbar		0.023	0.16	172
Cements (base consistency, 24 h)				
Polymer-modified ZOE	B & T	0.310†	2.14†	2
Zinc phosphate	Zinc Cement Improved	3.25†	22.4†	2
Zinc polycarboxylate	Durelon	0.718†	4.95†	2
Cements (luting consistency, 24 h)				
EBA-alumina ZOE	Opotow	0.787†	5.43†	2
		0.45‡	3.1‡	145
Glass-ionomer	ASPA	1.4‡	9.8‡	145
	Fuji	0.58‡	4.0‡	145
	Ketac-cem	0.91*	6.3*	178
Noneugenol zinc oxide	Nogenol	0.0257†	0.177†	2
Polymer-modified ZOE	Fynal	0.441†	3.04†	2
		0.17‡	1.2‡	145
Zinc phosphate	Zinc Cement Improved	1.99†	13.7†	2

* Measured in bending.
† Measured in compression with optical strain gauge.
‡ Measured in compression.
§ As cast.
¶ Heat treated.
# Cord modulus in tension at 5% strain.
** Measured with Shearheometer at setting time.

Elastic modulus, *E* (continued)

Material	Product	E psi x 10^6	E GPa	Reference
Cements				
(luting consistency, 24 h) (continued)				
Zinc polycarboxylate	Carboxylon	0.35‡	2.4‡	145
	Durelon	0.638†	4.40†	2
		0.46‡	3.2‡	145
	Durelon (thin liquid)	0.44‡	3.0‡	145
Cements (liners, 24 h)				
Calcium hydroxide				
Light-cured	VLC Dycal	0.087*	0.6*	178
Self-cured	Dycal	0.32*	2.2*	178
	Life	0.29*	2.0*	178
Glass-ionomer				
Light-cured	Vitrabond	0.16*	1.1*	179
	XR Ionomer	0.35*	2.4*	179
Self-cured	GC Lining Cement	0.42*	2.9*	178
	Ketac Bond	0.68*	4.7*	178
Resin	Cavalite	0.38*	2.6*	179
	Timeline	0.25*	1.7*	179
Unmodified ZOE	Cavitec	0.0406†	0.280†	2
Cobalt-chromium alloys	Advantage§	18.2	125	198
	Advantage¶	21.6	149	198
	Cobond§	21.8	150	198
	Cobond¶	23.0	159	198
	Genesis II§	30.6	211	198
	Genesis II¶	22.8	157	198
	Master Tec§	21.2	146	198
	Master Tec¶	22.8	157	198
	Novarex§	22.4	154	198
	Novarex¶	26.3	181	198
	Novarex II§	23.8	164	198
	Novarex II¶	21.8	150	198
	Vi-Comp§	21.6	149	198
	Vi-Comp¶	22.8	157	198
	Vitallium	31.6	218	61
Crown-and-bridge resins				
Acrylic	Biotone	0.327†	2.26†	23
Polyester	Mer-Don 7	0.267†	1.84†	23
Polyvinyl acrylic	Luxene	0.410†	2.83†	23
Denture resins				
Cold-cured	PERform	0.236	1.63	218
Heat-cured	Lucitone 199	0.154	1.06	218
	Paragon	0.426	2.94	209
	Perma-cryl 20	0.193	1.33	218
Light-cured	Triad	0.306	2.11	218

Elastic modulus, *E* (continued)

Material	Product	E psi x 10^6	E GPa	Reference
Duplicating material				
Agar	Nobiloid	70×10^{-6}	0.48×10^{-3}	60
Fluorapatite, mineral	Durango, Mexico	21.4	148	40
Gold alloys				
Type I	Special Inlay	11.2†	77.2†	4
Type III	Sjoding C-3	14.5	100	144
Type IV	Ney-Oro G-3	14.4†	99.3†	4
	Sjoding D	13.8	95	144
64% Au-Ag-Cu	Begolloyd	11.5	79	144
48% Au-Ag-Cu	Midigold	14.5	100	144
Au-Ag-Pd		11.4	78	192
Au-Pd	Olympia§	14.9	103	199
	Olympia¶	15.7	108	199
Porcelain-fused-to-metal	Ceramco O	12.5	86.2	6
Gutta-percha	Indian Head	0.027	0.186	28
	Mynol	0.022	0.152	28
Gypsum				
Improved stone	Velmix	2.1*	14.5*	83
Hydroxyapatite		5.0	34	192
Impression materials				
Agar	Surgident	200×10^{-6}†	1.38×10^{-3}†	60
Alginate, 6 min	Jeltrate	38×10^{-6}#	0.26×10^{-3}#	27
Polyether	Impregum F	51×10^{-6}**	0.35×10^{-3}**	187
	Permadyne	59×10^{-6}**	0.41×10^{-3}**	187
Polysulfide	Permlastic			
	light	2×10^{-6}**	0.013×10^{-3}**	187
	heavy	17×10^{-6}**	0.12×10^{-3}**	187
Silicone, addition	Provil			
	light	45×10^{-6}**	0.31×10^{-3}**	187
	putty	51×10^{-6}**	0.35×10^{-3}**	187
Silicone, condensation	Rapid			
	light	13×10^{-6}**	0.088×10^{-3}**	187
	putty	38×10^{-6}**	0.26×10^{-3}**	187
Iron-chromium alloys				
Crown-and-bridge	Dentillium C-B	25.7	177	61
Partial denture	Dentillium P-D	29.3	202	61
Maxillofacial material				
Silicone rubber	Silastic 382	297×10^{-6}	2.05×10^{-3}	39
Nickel-chromium alloys	Ceramalloy II §	27.2	188	199
	Ceramalloy II ¶	23.1	159	199
	Micro-Bond N-P2§	21.1	145	199
	Micro-Bond N-P2¶	21.1	145	199
	Pentillium	24.9	172	136
	Ticon §	25.6	177	199
	Ticon ¶	24.8	171	199

Elastic modulus, E (continued)

Material	Product	E psi x 10^6	E GPa	Reference
Nickel-chromium alloys (continued)				
Porcelain-fused-to-metal	Ultratek	29.4	203	6
Crown-and-bridge	Howmedica III	26.0	179	110
Palladium-based dental alloys	Microstar §	19.5	134	199
	Microstar ¶	17.9	123	199
	Spartan §	15.8	109	199
	Spartan¶	15.0	103	199
	W-1§	16.9	117	199
	W-1¶	16.8	116	199
Polymers				
Polyetherurethane	Pellethane2363-80A	0.0023	0.016	182
Polyetherurethane urea	Biomer	0.0016	0.011	182
Poly (methyl methacrylate)		0.345	2.38	183
Porcelains				
Alumina-reinforced	Vitadur-N(Core)	15.5	107	231
Castable ceramic	Dicor	10.7	74	231
Ceramic-whisker-reinforced	Mirage II	10.0	69	231
Feldspathic	Excelco	8.7	60	231
	Vita VMK 68	10.2	70	231
	Vita VMK 68-N	10.0	69	231
	Will-Ceram	9.1	63	231
Leucite-reinforced	Optec HSP	9.1	63	231
Restorative materials				
Composite resin				
All-purpose	Brilliant	2.41	16.6	158
	Charisma	2.04	14.1	158
	Conquest DFC	2.54	17.5	158
	Heliomolar Radiopaque	1.41	9.8	158
	Herculite XR	2.33	16.0	158
	Herculite XRV	1.38	9.5	211
	Marathon	2.95	20.3	158
	P-50 APC	3.63	25.0	158
	Pertac Hybrid	2.18	15.1	158
	Prisma APH	1.98	13.6	158
	True Vitality	0.78	5.4	211
	Z-100	3.05	21.0	158
Anterior	Durafill	0.88	6.1	158
	Helio Progress	1.32	9.1	158
	Multifil VS	1.14	7.8	158
	Prisma Fil	2.07	14.3	158
	Prisma Microfine	0.83	5.7	158
	Silar	1.32	9.1	158
	Silux	1.36	9.4	158
	Silux Plus	1.37	9.5	158
	Valux	2.86	19.7	158

Elastic modulus, *E* (continued)

Material	Product	E psi x 10^6	E GPa	Reference
Restorative materials				
Composite resin				
Anterior (continued)	Visio Dispers	1.56	10.8	158
	Visio Fil	3.15	21.7	158
Posterior	Clearfil Photo Posterior	3.68	25.3	158
	Ful Fil	2.10	14.5	158
	Heliomolar	1.54	10.6	158
	Occlusin	3.45	23.8	158
	P-10	3.64	25.1	158
	Post Comp II LC	2.33	16.1	158
Glass-ionomer	Ketac-fil	1.57	10.8	188
Metal-reinforced glass-ionomer	Ketac-Silver	0.62*	4.3*	178
Silicate	Improved Filling Porcelain	3.25†	22.4†	4
Silver-palladium alloys	Alborium	14.4	99	144
	Hvitstøp	15.2	105	144
	Palliag H	15.8	109	144
Titanium		17.0	117	126
Tooth structures				
Dentin (bovine)				
Demineralized		0.036	0.25	185
Mineralized		1.99	13.7	185
Dentin (human)				
Demineralized		0.038	0.26	185
Mineralized		2.13	14.7	185
Enamel		12.2†	84.1†	4
		18.9	130	192
Peridontal membrane (young calf)		172×10^{-6}	1.18×10^{-3}	65
Vitreous carbon		3.5	24.1	117
Waxes				
Inlay casting, hard	Kerr blue hard	0.092†	0.634†	30
Inlay casting, soft	Kerr blue regular	0.101†	0.696†	30

Flow

Flow is defined as the permanent strain of an elastic impression material when it is loaded in compression at a fixed stress (100 g on 12.7 x 19 mm cylinder) for 15 minutes at 1 hour after mixing. The method of testing is described in American National Standards Institute/American Dental Association Specification No. 19.[73]

Material	Product	Flow (%)	Reference
Bite registration material	Correct-Bite	0.00	155
Impression materials			
Alginate			
normal consistency	Jeltrate	3.6*	27
thin consistency	Jeltrate	6.3*	27
thick consistency	Jeltrate	2.7*	27
Polyether	Impregum F	0.02	156
	Permadyne		
	light	0.03	156
	heavy	0.02	156
	Polyjel NF	0.02	156
Polysulfide	Coeflex		
	light	0.45	156
	medium	0.45	156
	heavy	0.42	156
Silicone, addition	Absolute		
	light	0.03	156
	medium	0.02	156
	heavy	0.02	156
	putty	0.03	156
	Baysilex	0.04	156
	Exaflex Hydrophilic		
	light	0.05	156
	medium	0.03	156
	Examix Hydrophilic		
	light	0.03	156
	medium	0.01	156
	monophase	0.00	155
	Express Hydrophilic		
	light	0.03	156
	medium	0.02	156
	putty	0.09	156
	Hydrosil	0.02	156
	Imprint	0.03	156
	Mirror 3 Extrude		
	light	0.03	156
	medium	0.02	156
	putty	0.03	156

* Measured at 6 min.

Flow (continued)

Material	Product	Flow (%)	Reference
Impression materials			
Silicone, addition (continued)	Omnisil		
	light	0.02	156
	medium	0.02	156
	putty	0.07	156
	Permagum		
	light	0.00	155
	medium	0.00	155
	heavy	0.02	155
	President		
	light	0.01	156
	heavy	0.01	156
	putty	0.01	156
	Reprosil Hydrophilic		
	light	0.02	156
	medium	0.02	156
	heavy	0.02	156
	putty	0.02	156
Silicone, condensation	Coltex		
	light	0.11	156
	medium	0.15	156
	Coltoflax	0.08	156
	Cuttersil		
	light	0.02	155
	medium	0.04	155
	Elasticon		
	light	0.03	155
	heavy	0.00	155
	Rapid		
	light	0.01	155
	putty	0.01	155

Heat of fusion

The heat of fusion is the heat in calories required to convert 1 g of a material from the solid to the liquid state at the melting temperature. The equation for the calculation of heat of fusion is $L = Q/m$, where Q is the total heat absorbed and m is the mass of the substance.

Material	Product	L (cal/g)	Temperature (°C)	Reference
Gutta-percha (pure)		45.2	74	111
Ice		79.7	0	1
Mercury		2.8	–38	130
Pure metals				
Chromium		96	1875	130
Copper		50.6	1083	130
Gold		16.1	1063	130
Nickel		73.8	1453	130
Palladium		34.2	1552	130
Platinum		26.9	1769	130
Silver		25	961	130
Zinc		24.09	420	130
Waxes				
Beeswax	Ross Co.	42.8	62.8	67
Carnauba	Ross Co.	45.5	82.8	67
Inlay casting	Kerr blue hard	45.9	60.0	67
Paraffin	Ross Co.	42.4	52.0	67

Heat of reaction, ΔH

The heat of reaction represents the difference in the enthalpies of the reaction products and reactants at constant pressure and at a definite temperature, with every substance in a definite physical state. If heat is liberated in the reaction, the process is said to be exothermic and ΔH is a negative number. If heat is absorbed, the process is endothermic and ΔH is a positive number.

Material	Reaction	ΔH (kcal/g-mol)	Reference
Denture resin, acrylic	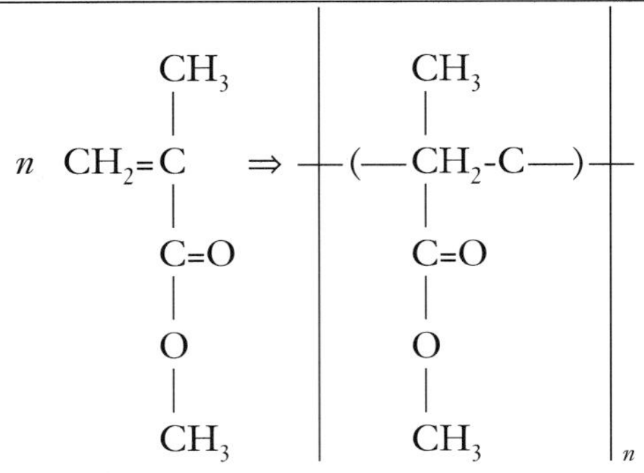 $n\ CH_2{=}C(CH_3)(C{=}O{-}O{-}CH_3) \Rightarrow \left[{-}(CH_2{-}C(CH_3)(C{=}O{-}O{-}CH_3)){-}\right]_n$	–13.9	88
Gypsum	$CaSO_4{\cdot}\frac{1}{2}\ H_2O + 1\frac{1}{2}\ H_2O \Rightarrow CaSO_4{\cdot}2H_2O$	–3.9	87

Impact strength, *IZOD*

Impact strength is a measure of the energy required to cause a material to fracture when struck by a sudden blow (high rate of deformation).

Material	Product	IZOD (J/m)	Reference
Denture resins			
Cold-cured	PERform	15	218
Heat-cured	Lucitone 199	27–31	218
	Perma-cryl 20	14	218
Light-cured	Triad	13	218

Index of refraction, χ

The index of refraction for any substance is the ratio of the velocity of light in a vacuum to its velocity in the substance. The extraordinary and ordinary indices of refraction are denoted as χ_e and χ_o, respectively.

Material	χ_e	χ_o	Reference
Filler particles for dental composites			
Barium borosilicate		1.554	158
Quartz		1.540	158
Strontium glass		1.550	158
Ytterbium trifluoride		1.530	158
Zirconium glass		1.520	158
Fluorapatite, synthetic	1.630	1.633	103
Hydroxyapatite, synthetic	1.643	1.649	104
Monomers			
Bisphenol-A-glycidyl dimethacrylate		1.545	168
2-Hydroxyethyl methacrylate		1.448	168
Triethyleneglycol dimethacrylate		1.457	168
Urethane dimethacrylate		1.481	168
Porcelain, feldspathic		1.504	147
Quartz		1.544	147
Tooth structure, enamel		1.655	105
Water		1.333	1

Knoop hardness number, *KHN*

The Knoop hardness test is a micro-indentation method. A load is applied to a diamond indenting tool and the dimensions of the resulting indentation are measured. The Knoop hardness number is the ratio of the applied load to the area of the indentation.

Material	Product	KHN (kg/mm²)	Reference
Abrasives			
Aluminum oxide	E.C. Moore Co.	2100	70
Flint (quartz)	E.C. Moore Co.	820	70
Garnet	E.C. Moore Co.	1360	70
Silicon carbide	E.C. Moore Co.	2480	70
Cements (luting consistency)			
Resin	C&B Metabond	12	160
	Panavia EX	53	160
Cements (liners)			
Calcium hydroxide			
Light-cured	VLC Dycal	2.4	161
Glass-ionomer			
Light-cured	Vitrabond	1.7	161
	XR Ionomer	0.1	161
	Zionomer	14–16	161
Self-cured	GC Lining Cement	2.8	161
Resin	Cavalite	15	161
	TimeLine	7.3	161
Cobalt-chromium alloys	Advantage*	356	198
	Advantage†	360	198
	Cobond*	406	198
	Cobond†	424	198
	Genesis II*	329	198
	Genesis II†	345	198
	Master Tec*	345	198
	Master Tec†	363	198
	Niranium N/N	391	61
	Novarex*	349	198
	Novarex†	375	198
	Novarex II*	352	198
	Novarex II†	368	198
	Vi-Comp*	386	198
	Vi-Comp†	399	198
	Vitallium	415	61
Denture resins			
Cold-cured	PERform	16.2	218
Heat-cured	Lucitone 199	14.0	218
	Perma-cryl 20	16.5	218
Light-cured	Triad	17.6	218

* As cast.
† Heat treated.

Knoop hardness number, *KHN* (continued)

Material	Product	KHN (kg/mm²)	Reference
Denture teeth			
Acrylic	Dura-Blend	19.9	36
Gold (condensed)			
Foil	Morgan, Hastings & Co.	69	32
Mat	Williams	52	32
Powdered	Goldent	55	32
Gold-alloy			
Au-Pd alloy	Olympia*	206	199
	Olympia†	226	199
Iron-chromium alloys			
Crown-and-bridge	Dentillium C-B	331	61
Partial denture	Dentillium P-D	335	61
Nickel-chromium alloys	Ceramalloy II*	314	199
	Ceramalloy II†	270	199
	Micro-Bond N-P2*	207	199
	Micro-Bond N-P2†	153	199
	Ticon*	328	199
	Ticon†	256	199
Palladium-based dental alloys	Microstar*	259	199
	Microstar†	247	199
	Spartan*	371	199
	Spartan†	362	199
	W-1*	232	199
	W-1†	228	199
Pit and fissure sealants (24 h)			
Light-cured	Delton LC	18	176
	Helioseal	21	176
	Pentra-Seal	19	176
	Visioseal	16	176
Self-cured	Delton	14	176
Porcelain			
Feldspathic	B.F. Vacuum	591	100
Restorative materials			
Composite resin			
All-purpose	Brilliant	57	211
	Charisma	43	211
	Conquest DFC	63	211
	Herculite XRV	69–71	162
	Pertac Hybrid	60	211
	Prisma APH	26	164
	True Vitality	28	211

Knoop hardness number, *KHN* (continued)

Material	Product	KHN (kg/mm^2)	Reference
Restorative materials			
Composite resin (continued)			
Anterior	Helio Progress	46–48	162
	Prisma Microfine	25	164
	Silux Plus	28	163
	Valux	46	163
	Visio Dispers	27	163
	Visio Fil	45	163
Posterior	Clearfil Photo Posterior	45	211
	P 50	60	163
	Visio Molar	64	163
Glass-ionomer	Chelon-Fil	31	165
	Chemfil II	18	165
	Fuji Ionomer II	18	165
Metal-reinforced glass-ionomer	Chelon Silver	24	166
	Miracle Mix	14	166
Tooth structures			
Calculus (on teeth)		86	12
Cementum		40	12
Dentin		68	11
Enamel (bovine)			
Etched		60–161	167
Softened		79–145	167
Sound		339–418	167
Enamel (human)			
Etched		88–171	167
Softened		149–179	167
Sound		355–431	167
Vitreous carbon		820	117

Melting temperatures and ranges

The temperature at which a single element or compound transforms from a solid to a liquid is the melting temperature. Materials that are mixtures or alloys generally do not melt at a single temperature but possess a melting range. The lower temperature of the range is the solidus temperature, below which the material is solid. The higher temperature is the liquidus, above which the material is liquid. Within the melting range, both solid and liquid are present.

Material	Product	°F	°C	Reference
Cobalt-chromium alloys	Genesis II	2415–2550	1325–1400	9
	Master Tec	2215–2380	1215–1300	222
	Novarex	2425–2475	1330–1357	223
Gold alloys				
Type I	Ney-Oro A	1825–1900	996–1038	7
Type II	Ney-Oro A-1	1650–1775	899–968	7
Type III	Ney-Oro B-2	1650–1775	899–968	7
Type IV	Ney-Oro G-3	1630–1740	888–949	7
40% Au-Ag-Cu	Forticast	1555–1665	846–907	9
10-15% Au-Ag-Pd	Paliney No. 4	1670–1810	910–988	7
Au-Pd	Olympia	2213–2380	1210–1304	9
Au-Pt-Pd	TPW	2012–2282	1100–1250	196
Porcelain-fused-to-metal	Jelenko O	2034–2206	1112–1208	9
Mercury		–37	–38	130
Nickel-chromium alloy	Unimetal	2098–2282	1148–1250	196
Palladium-based dental alloys	Athenium	2120–2330	1160–1277	197
	Legacy	2020–2360	1104–1293	197
	Liberty	2020–2280	1104–1249	197
	Microstar	2156–2336	1180–1280	9
	PTM-88	2120–2340	1160–1282	197
	Protocol	2320–2390	1271–1310	197
	Spartan	2040–2120	1116–1160	197
	W1	2165–2320	1185–1270	222
Pure metals				
Chromium		3407	1875	130
Copper		1981	1083	130
Gold		1945	1063	130
Nickel		2647	1453	130
Palladium		2826	1552	130
Platinum		3217	1769	130
Silver		1761	961	130
Titanium		3035	1668	130
Zinc		787	420	130
Silver-palladium alloys				
Crown-and-bridge	Albacast	1870–2010	1021–1099	9
Porcelain-fused-to-metal	Jel-5	2116–2341	1158–1283	9
Titanium-6Al-4V alloy		3002	1650	196
Waxes				
Beeswax	Ross Co.	93–158	34–70	68
Carnauba	Ross Co.	127–189	53–87	68
Inlay casting	Kerr blue hard	122–176	50–80	68
Paraffin	Ross Co.	111–140	44–60	68

Mohs hardness

A material's Mohs hardness value indicates the material's resistance to scratching. Diamond has a maximum Mohs hardness of 10.

Material	Mohs hardness	Reference
Abrasives		
Aluminum oxide	9	1
Boron carbide	9–10	1
Chalk ($CaCO_3$)	3	1
Cuttlebone	7	238
Diamond	10	1
Garnet	6.5–7	1
Gypsum	2	1
Pumice	6	1
Quartz	7	1
Silicon carbide	9–10	1
Talc	1	1
Tungsten carbide	9	1
Zirconium silicate	7.5	1
Amalgam	4–5	238
Gold	2.5–3	1
Porcelain, feldspathic	6–7	238
Restorative materials		
Composite resin	5–7	238
Tooth structures		
Dentin	3–4	238
Enamel	5	238

Penetration coefficient, *PC*

Definition: rate of penetration of a liquid into a capillary space. Units are cm/s.

$$PC = \frac{\gamma \cos \theta}{2\,\eta}$$

where γ is the surface tension of the liquid, η is the viscosity, and θ is the contact angle.

Material	Product	PC	Reference
Fluoride gels	Flura-Gel	0.0508	132
	Luride	0.217	132
	Predent	0.0870	132
	Rafluor	0.115	132
Fluoride solutions	NaF Rinse	2,350	132
Pit and fissure sealants			
Light-cured	Delton	5.18	176
	Helioseal	1.72	176
	Pentra-Seal	2.67	176
	Visioseal	2.21	176
Self-cured	Delton	4.90	176

Percent elongation (Ductility), *n*

Elongation is the deformation that results from the application of a tensile force and is calculated as the change in length divided by the original length. It is usually measured over a 5-cm gauge length.

Material	Product	*n* % in 5-cm gauge length	Reference
Cobalt-chromium alloys	Advantage*	3	198
	Advantage†	4	198
	Cobond*	4	198
	Cobond†	3	198
	Genesis II*	7	198
	Genesis II†	6	198
	Master Tec*	2	198
	Master Tec†	3	198
	Novarex*	2	198
	Novarex†	1	198
	Novarex II*	2	198
	Novarex II†	2	198
	Vi-Comp*	5	198
	Vi-Comp†	4	198
	Vitallium	1.5‡	61
Denture liners (resilient)			
Polyphosphazene fluoroelastomer	Novus	240	153
Silicone	Molloplast-B	325	153
Gold (999.9 fine)	Wilkinson Co.	60.1§	96
Gold alloys			
Type I	Ney-Oro A	29.5	7
Type II	Ney-Oro A-1	32	7
Type III, soft	Ney-Oro B-2	35	7
Type III, hard	Ney-Oro B-2	34	7
Type IV, soft	Ney-Oro G-3	24	7
Type IV, hard	Ney-Oro G-3	6.5	7
40% Au-Ag-Cu, soft	Forticast	18	9
40% Au-Ag-Cu, hard	Forticast	3	9
10%–15% Au-Ag-Pd, soft	Paliney No. 4	17	7
10%–15% Au-Ag-Pd, hard	Paliney No. 4	7	7
Au-Pd	Olympia*	8	199
	Olympia†	12	199
Au-Pt-Pd	TPW	9.2	196
Porcelain-fused-to-metal	Jelenko O	5	9
Impression material			
Alginate	Krompan	38¶	81

* As cast
† Heat treated.
‡ Measured on 2.5-cm gauge length.
§ Measured on 0.64-cm gauge length.
¶ Measured on 10-cm gauge length; head speed, 50 cm/min.
\# Measured on 1.5-cm gauge length.

Percent elongation (Ductility), *n* (continued)

Material	Product	*n* % in 5-cm gauge length	Reference
Iron-chromium alloys			
Crown-and-bridge	Dentillium C-B	8.5‡	61
Partial denture	Dentillium P-D	9.0‡	61
Maxillofacial materials			
Polyurethane	Epithane-3	224‡	210
Silicone rubber	A 102	130‡	210
	A-2186	480	154
	Cosmesil	588	154
	MDX 4-4210	438	154
	Medical Adhesive A	304‡	210
	Silastic 4-4515	476‡	210
Mouth protector materials			
Polyvinyl acetate-polyethylene	Proform	1000	125
	Sta-Guard	1150	125
Nickel-chromium alloys	Ceramalloy II*	6	199
	Ceramalloy II†	11	199
	Micro-Bond N-P2*	29	199
	Micro-Bond N-P2†	35	199
	Ticon*	4	199
	Ticon†	12	199
	Unimetal	12.2	196
Palladium-based dental alloys	Athenium	25#	197
	Liberty	20#	197
	Legacy	20#	197
	Microstar*	6	199
	Microstar†	18	199
	Protocol	34#	197
	PTM-88	25#	197
	Spartan*	2	199
	Spartan†	9	199
	W-1*	6	199
	W-1†	10	199
Silver-palladium alloys			
Crown-and-bridge, soft	Albacast	10	9
Crown-and-bridge, hard	Albacast	8	9
Porcelain-fused-to-metal	Jel-5	25	9
Titanium		13	131
Titanium-6 Al-4V alloy		5	131

Permanent deformation

Permanent deformation is the lack of recovery from deformation of an elastic impression or duplicating material compressed at a fixed strain, usually for 30 seconds. The method of testing is described in American National Standards Institute/American Dental Association Specification Nos. 11, 18, 19, and 20.[73] The trend is to report percent recovery rather than permanent deformation. Therefore a material with a permanent deformation of 1% has a 99% recovery.

Material	Product	Permanent deformation(%)*	Reference
Bite registration material	Correct-Bite	0.7	155
Duplicating material			
Agar	Nobiloid	2.4†	60
Impression materials			
Agar	Sugident	1.8†	60
Alginate, 6 min	Jeltrate	2.2	27
Polyether	Impregum F	1.10	156
	Permadyne		
	light	1.52	156
	heavy	1.70	156
	Polyjel NF	0.99	156
Polysulfide	Coeflex		
	light	4.13	156
	medium	4.39	156
	heavy	5.55	156
	Permlastic		
	light	2.90	157
	medium	2.28	157
	heavy	2.81	157
Silicone, addition	Absolute		
	light	0.26	156
	medium	0.22	156
	heavy	0.27	156
	putty	0.40	156
	Baysilex	0.17	156
	Exaflex Hydrophilic		
	light	0.29	156
	medium	0.43	156
	Examix Hydrophilic		
	light	1.23	156
	medium	0.63	156
	monophase	0.14	155
	Express Hydrophilic		
	light	0.42	156
	medium	0.25	156
	putty	0.51	156
	Hydrosil	0.50	156
	Imprint	0.41	156

* Fixed strain, 12%, for 30 s.
† Tested for 1 min.

Permanent deformation (continued)

Material	Product	Permanent deformation(%)*	Reference
Impression materials			
Silicone, addition (continued)	Mirror 3 Extrude		
	light	0.23	156
	medium	0.18	156
	putty	0.30	156
	Omnisil		
	light	0.17	156
	medium	0.26	156
	putty	0.35	156
	Permagum		
	light	0.13	155
	medium	0.11	155
	heavy	0.12	155
	President		
	light	0.05	156
	medium	0.04	156
	heavy	0.01	156
	putty	0.24	156
	Reprosil Hydrophilic		
	light	0.18	156
	medium	0.16	156
	heavy	0.15	156
	putty	0.15	156
Silicone, condensation	Coltex		
	light	1.18	156
	medium	1.50	156
	Coltoflax	1.41	156
	CutterSil		
	light	1.20	155
	medium	1.39	155
	Elasticon		
	light	0.84	155
	heavy	0.47	155
	Rapid		
	light	1.73	155
	putty	1.09	155

Poisson's ratio, υ

Poisson's ratio is a measure of the simultaneous change in elongation and in cross-sectional area within the elastic range during a tensile or compressive test. During a tensile test, the reduction in cross-sectional area is proportional to the increase in length in the elastic range by the dimensionless factor, υ.

Material	Product	υ	Reference
Amalgam		0.35*	63
		0.334*	113
Cements			
Zinc phosphate	Tenacin	0.35*	54
Zinc silicophosphate	Dorcate	0.30*	54
Fluorapatite (mineral)		0.28*	55
Gold alloys			
Au-Ag-Pd		0.33	192
Au-Pd		0.33	193
Hydroxyapatite (synthetic)		0.28*	55
Impression materials			
Polyether	Impregum	0.13‡	194
Silicones, addition	Baysilex Monophase	0.41‡	194
	Provil		
	medium	0.19‡	194
	heavy	0.44‡	194
Nickel-chromium alloys	Ceramalloy	0.27	136
	Micro-Bond N-P2	0.24	136
	Pentillium	0.32	136
Polymers			
Acrylic		0.37-0.45§	102
Polycarbonate		0.41-0.44§	102
Polyethylene		0.54-0.61§	102
Porcelain	Ceramco	0.19	135
	Vita	0.19	135
Restorative materials			
Acrylic	Sevriton	0.35*	116
Composite resins	Adaptic	0.24*	116
Silicate	Syntrex	0.30*	54
Titanium		0.33	192
Tooth and supporting structures			
Bone			
Cancellous		0.30	195
Cortical		0.30	195
Cementum		0.31	195
Dentin		0.31	195
Enamel		0.33	195
Periodontal ligament		0.45	195

* Measured by ultrasonic method.
§ Measured in tension with transverse strain gauge extensometers.
‡ Measured by dynamic method.

Proportional limit, *PL*

The proportional limit is defined as the greatest stress that a material will sustain without a deviation from the law of proportionality of stress to strain. Unless indicated otherwise, values are for tests in tension.

Material	Product	PL		Reference
		psi x 10^3	MPa	
Crown-and-bridge resins				
Acrylic	Biotone	6.9*	47.6*	23
Polyester	Mer-Don 7	4.95*	34.1*	23
Polyvinyl acrylic	Luxene	8.12*	56.0*	23
Duplicating material				
Agar	Nobiloid	0.051†	0.35†	60
Gold alloys				
Type I	Ney-Oro A	10	69	7
Type II	Ney-Oro A-1	27.5	190	7
Type III, soft	Ney-Oro B-2	32.0	221	7
Type III, hard	Ney-Oro B-2	38.0	262	7
Type IV, soft	Ney-Oro G-3	41.5	286	7
Type IV, hard	Ney-Oro G-3	83.0	572	7
10%–15% Au-Ag-Pd, soft	Paliney No. 4	63.5	438	7
10%–15% Au-Ag-Pd, hard	Paliney No. 4	84.5	583	7
Porcelain-fused-to-metal	Ceramco O	60.8	419	6
Impression materials				
Agar	Surgident	0.095†	0.66†	60
Nickel-chromium alloys				
Crown-and-bridge	Howmedica III	28.0	193	110
Porcelain-fused-to-metal	Ultratek	9.0#	545	6
Silicate	Improved Filling Porcelain	19.6‡	135‡	4
Tooth structures				
Dentin		24.2§	167§	4
Enamel (cusp)		51.2§	353§	4
Waxes				
Inlay casting, hard	Kerr blue hard	0.501¶	3.46¶	30
Inlay casting, soft	Kerr blue regular	0.634¶	4.37¶	30

* Tested in compression, head speed 0.05 cm/min.
† Tested in compression, head speed 25 cm/min.
‡ Tested in compression, head speed 0.04 cm/min.
§ Tested in compression.
¶ Tested in compression, head speed 0.50 cm/min.

Shear strength, *S*

The shear strength is defined as the maximum stress that a material can withstand before failure in shear. Calculation of shear strength depends upon the test method.

Material	Product	S* psi x 10^3	S* MPa	Reference
Amalgam	New True Dentalloy	27.3	188	93
Cement (base consistency)				
Polymer-modified ZOE	B & T	1.85	12.7	76
Cements (luting consistency)				
Polymer-modified ZOE	Fynal	1.85	12.7	76
Unmodified ZOE		0.60	4.1	91
Zinc phosphate		1.90	13.1	91
		9.17	63.4	139
Zinc polycarboxylate	Durelon	3.96	27.4	139
	Poly F	4.44	30.7	139
Denture resins				
Acrylic	Kallodent	17.8	122	93
Porcelains				
Feldspathic	Ceramco Opaque	18	128	120
Aluminous	Vita Aluminous	24	165	120
Tooth structures				
Dentin		20.0	138	93
Vital		17.1	118	138
Vital, constrained		19.4	134	138
Non-vital (endodontically treated)		14.8	102	138
Enamel		13.1	90.2	93

* Tested by punch method.

Shore A hardness

The relative hardness of elastic materials, such as rubber or soft plastics, can be determined with an instrument called a Shore A durometer. If the indenter completely penetrates the sample, a reading of 0 is obtained, and if no penetration occurs, a reading of 100 results. The reading is dimensionless.

Material	Product	Shore A hardness	Reference
Denture liners (resilient)			
Polyphosphazene fluoroelastomer	Novus	50	153
Silicone	Molloplast-B	43	153
Impression materials			
Polyether	Impregum	58.0*	150
Polysulfide	Permlastic		
	light	13.0*	150
	medium	24.2*	150
	heavy	34.2*	150
Silicone, addition	President		
	medium	62.5*	150
	putty	77.4*	150
	Provil		
	light	43.7*	150
	heavy	59.3*	150
Silicone, condensation	Optosil Plus	66.0*	150
	Xantopren blue	43.9*	150
Maxillofacial materials			
Polyurethane	Epithane-3	46.6*	210
Silicone rubber	A-102	38.3*	210
	A-2186	24.6*	154
	Cosmesil	30.4*	154
	MDX 4-4210	24.0*	154
	Medical Adhesive A	29.4*	210
	Silastic 4-4515	50.2*	210
Mouth protector materials			
Polyvinyl acetate-polyethylene	Proform	82	37
	Sta-Guard	67	37

* Measured at 24 h.

Solubility and disintegration in water

Solubility and disintegration are measured by suspending two disks 20 mm in diameter, representing approximately 1260 mm^2 of exposed surface, in distilled water at 37°C.

Material	Product	Mass loss (%)	Solubility (mg/cm^2)	Reference
Denture liners (resilient)				
Polyphosphazene fluoroelastomer	Novus		0.03‡	226
Silicone	Molloplast-B		0.13‡	226
Cement (base consistency)				
Polymer-modified ZOE	B & T	0.06*		76
Cements (luting consistency)				
EBA-alumina ZOE		0.05*		79
Glass-ionomer	Fuji I	0.08*		228
	Ketac-Cem	0.40*		228
Polymer-modified ZOE	Fynal	0.08*		76
Resin	Comspan	0.017*		233
Unmodified ZOE	Temporary Cement	0.10*		79
	Temporary Cement		0.39*	74
Zinc hydrophosphate	New Calmix	0.4*		75
Zinc phosphate	Flecks Cement	0.025*		233
	Flecks Cement		0.82†	77
Zinc polycarboxylate	Durelon	<0.04*		78
	Durelon		0.81†	77
Zinc silicophosphate	Kryptex Improved	1.0‡		62
Cements (liners)				
Glass-ionomer				
Light-cured	Vitrebond	3.6*		229
	XR Ionomer	1.5*		229
Self-cured	GC Lining Cement		0.50*	228
	Ketac-cem	0.023*		223
Periodontal dressings	Barricaid	0.54		232
	COEpak	1.5		232
	PerioCare	2.7		232
Pit and fissure sealants				
Light-cured	Nuva-Seal		0.5‡	115
Self-cured	9075		0.2‡	115
Restorative materials				
Glass-ionomer	Fuji II		0.07*	228
	Ketac-Fil		0.10*	228
Metal-reinforced glass-ionomer	Ketac-Silver		0.12*	228
Silicate	New Improved Filling Porcelain		2.09*	74

* Stored for 1 day.
† Stored for 5 days.
‡ Stored for 7 days.

Specific heat, C_p

The specific heat of a substance is the quantity of heat needed to raise the temperature of a unit mass of the substance 1°C. Water usually is chosen as a standard substance and 1 g as a standard mass.

Material	Product	C_p [cal/(g°C)]	Reference
Bones			
Cancellous		0.44	192
Cortical		0.44	192
Cements			
Calcium hydroxide	Dycal	0.429	206
	Life	0.346	206
Glass-ionomer	Base cement	0.273*	205
	Dentin cement	0.275*	205
	Ketac-Cem	0.293*	205
Polymer-modified ZOE	IRM	0.178†	24
Unmodified ZOE		0.138‡	24
	Cavitec	0.421	206
Zinc phosphate	Tenacin	0.122§	24
Gold alloy			
Au-Ag-Pd alloy		0.03	192
Hydroxyapatite		0.21	192
Impression materials (polymerized)			
Polyether	Impregum	0.502	207
Silicone, addition	Baysilex	0.229	207
	Provil		
	medium	0.256	207
	high	0.227	207
Mercury		0.033	130
Pure metals			
Chromium		0.11¶	130
Copper		0.092¶	130
Gold		0.0312#	130
Nickel		0.105¶	130
Palladium		0.0584**	130
Platinum		0.0314**	130
Silver		0.0559**	130
Titanium		0.124¶	130
Zinc		0.0915¶	130
Restorative materials			
Acrylic	Bonfil	0.280	24
Composite resin	Adaptic	0.197	24
Silicate	Improved Filling Porcelain	0.167‡	24
Tooth structures			
Dentin		0.28	14
		0.31	206
		0.38	41
Enamel		0.18	14
Vitreous carbon		0.30	117
Water		1.00	1
Zinc oxide	USP grade	0.095	24

* Powder/liquid ratio, 1.0 g/mL.
† Powder/liquid ratio, 5.0 g/mL.
‡ Powder/liquid ratio, 3.0 g/mL.
§ Powder/liquid ratio, 2.5 g/mL.
¶ At 20°C.
\# At 18°C.
** At 0°C.

Strain in compression

Strain in compression or flexibility of an elastomeric impression or duplicating material is measured between stresses of 100 and 1000 g/cm^2 (ca. 0.01 and 0.1 MPa). The method of testing is described in American National Standards Institute/American Dental Association Specification Nos. 11, 18, 19, and 20.[73]

Material	Product	Strain in compression (%)	Reference
Bite registration material	Correct-Bite	0.9–1.3	155
Duplicating materials			
Agar	Multi-Gel	14.5	80
Impression materials			
Alginate			
normal consistency	Jeltrate	13.4	27
thin consistency	Jeltrate	18.5	27
thick consistency	Jeltrate	10.1	27
Polyether	Impregum F	1.93	156
	Permadyne		
	light	3.31	156
	heavy	2.91	156
	Polyjel NF	2.65	156
Polysulfide	Coeflex		
	light	13.5	156
	medium	13.9	156
	heavy	11.1	156
	Permlastic		
	light	11.8	157
	medium	10.2	157
	heavy	6.2	157
Silicone, addition	Absolute		
	light	3.59	156
	medium	2.42	156
	heavy	2.64	156
	putty	1.55	156
	Baysilex	4.60	156
	Exaflex Hydrophilic		
	light	5.17	156
	medium	4.65	156
	Examix Hydrophilic		
	light	5.77	156
	medium	5.25	156
	monophase	2.81	155
	Express Hydrophilic		
	light	5.32	156
	medium	4.64	156
	putty	5.90	156
	Hydrosil	1.88	156
	Imprint	2.71	156

Strain in compression (continued)

Material	Product	Strain in compression (%)	Reference
Impression materials			
Silicone, addition (continued)	Mirror 3 Extrude		
	light	5.76	156
	medium	4.0	156
	putty	2.53	156
	Omnisil		
	light	4.95	156
	medium	4.72	156
	putty	1.62	156
	Permagum		
	light	2.94	155
	medium	2.06	155
	heavy	2.44	155
	President		
	light	3.5	156
	medium	2.6	156
	heavy	2.2	156
	putty	1.7	156
	Reprosil Hydrophilic		
	light	4.1	156
	medium	3.6	156
	heavy	2.6	156
	putty	1.7	156
Silicone, condensation	Coltex		
	light	11.1	156
	medium	5.66	156
	Coltoflax	2.13	156
	CutterSil		
	light	3.66	155
	medium	6.29	155
	Elasticon		
	light	6.37	155
	heavy	7.77	155
	Rapid		
	light	4.98	155
	putty	1.66	155

Surface free energy, γ_s

The surface free energy is defined as the work required to increase the area of a substance by 1 cm^2.

Material	Product	γ_s (ergs/cm^2)	Reference
Bacteria			
A. odontolyticus A7-1		106	200
A. viscosus C7-4		111	200
S. mutans C7-3		128	200
S. salivarius B3-4		113	200
S. sanguis C7-2		99	200
Polymers			
Polyethylene		33.5	71
Poly(methyl methacrylate)		36.5	71
Polystyrene		38.0	71
Poly(tetrafluoroethylene)	Teflon	24.0	71
Tooth structures			
Dentin		92	200
Enamel		87	200
Wax			
Paraffin		25.0	71

Surface tension, γ

Surface tension is a measure of the surface free energy of a liquid and is defined as the force acting along the surface of a liquid at right angles to any line 1 cm in length.

Material	Product	γ (dynes/cm)	Temperature (°C)	Reference
Blood		55.5–61.2		85
Mercury		483.5	25	49
Polymers				
Polyetherurethane	Pellethane 80A	24.0		170
	Pellethane 55D	24.8		170
	Pellethane 75D	32.3		170
Polyetherurethane urea	Biomer	33.9		170
Porcelain	Ceramco Undercoat A	366	1038	47
Saliva		53	37	48
Water		72.3	25	50

Tear energy

The tear energy is a measure of the energy per unit area of newly torn surface and is calculated from the load required to propagate a tear in a trouser-shaped specimen.

Material	Product	Tear energy (M ergs/cm^2)	Reference
Denture liners (resilient)			
Polyphosphazene fluoroelastomer	Novus	23*	153
Silicone	Molloplast - B	1.4*	153
Impression materials			
Alginate	Tissutex	0.4	98
		0.066	18
Polyether	Impregum F‡	0.81*	213
	Permadyne§	0.45*	213
	Polyjel NF ‡	0.85*	213
Polysulfide	Coe-flex	1.89*	213
	Permlastic§	0.71*	213
Silicone, addition	Absolute§	0.52*	213
	Baysilex¶	1.50*	213
	Express§	0.65*	213
	Extrude§	0.78*	213
	Hydrosil‡	0.63*	213
	Panapren‡	0.81*	213
	Permagum§	0.64*	213
	Reprosil§	0.60*	213
	Unosil‡	0.47*	213
Maxillofacial materials			
Polyurethane	Dermathane 100	1.8†	16
Polyvinyl chloride	Sartomer Resins	11†	16
Silicone rubber	Silastic 382	0.66†	16
	Silastic 399	0.61†	16

* Head speed, 5 cm/min.
† Head speed, 2 cm/min.
‡ Medium viscosity, monophase.
§ Low viscosity.
¶ High viscosity, monophase.

Tear strength

The tear strength is a measure of the resistance of a material to tear forces. The tear strength of a notched specimen is calculated by dividing the maximum load by the thickness of the specimen. A specimen suitable for measuring tear strength is described in American National Standards Institute/American Dental Association Specification No. 20.[73]

Material	Product	Tear strength		Reference
		lb/in	kg/cm	
Denture liners (resilient)				
Polyphosphazene fluoroelastomer	Novus	54*	9.7*	153
Silicone	Molloplast-B	33*	5.9*	153
Duplicating material				
Agar	Nobiloid	1.3†	0.232†	60
Impression materials				
Agar, tray	Surgident	5.68†	1.01†	27
Alginate	Jeltrate	3.0†	0.536†	27
Polyether	Impregum F	26.8‡	4.80‡	156
	Permadyne			
	light	10.1‡	1.80‡	156
	heavy	16.8‡	3.00‡	156
	Polyjel NF	19.6‡	3.50‡	156
Polysulfide	Coeflex			
	light	18.4‡	3.29‡	156
	medium	19.9‡	3.56‡	156
Silicone, addition	Absolute			
	light	15.7‡	2.80‡	156
	medium	19.6‡	3.50‡	156
	Baysilex	21.6‡	3.86‡	156
	Exaflex Hydrophilic			
	light	15.9‡	2.84‡	156
	medium	16.2‡	2.90‡	156
	Examix Hydrophilic			
	light	15.7‡	2.80‡	156
	medium	16.2‡	2.90‡	156
	monophase	18.8‡	3.36‡	155
	Express Hydrophilic			
	light	18.5‡	3.30‡	156
	medium	18.5‡	3.30‡	156
	Hydrosil	13.4‡	2.40‡	156
	Imprint	21.8‡	3.90‡	156
	Mirror 3 Extrude			
	light	12.3‡	2.20‡	156
	medium	26.3‡	4.70‡	156

* Head speed, 50 cm/min.
† Head speed, 25 cm/min.
‡ Head speed, 30 cm/min.

Tear strength (continued)

Material	Product	Tear strength		Reference
		lb/in	kg/cm	
Impression materials				
Silicone, addition (continued)	Omnisil			
	light	14.6[‡]	2.60[‡]	156
	medium	10.4[‡]	1.85[‡]	156
	Permagum			
	light	10.4[‡]	1.85[‡]	155
	medium	28.4[‡]	5.07[‡]	155
	heavy	29.5[‡]	5.26[‡]	155
	President			
	light	15.1[‡]	2.70[‡]	156
	medium	30.8[‡]	5.50[‡]	156
	Reprosil Hydrophilic			
	light	14.3[‡]	2.56[‡]	156
	medium	17.4[‡]	3.10[‡]	156
Silicone, condensation	Coltex			
	light	8.96[‡]	1.60[‡]	156
	medium	14.6[‡]	2.61[‡]	156
	Cuttersil			
	light	15.1[‡]	2.70[‡]	155
	medium	13.0[‡]	2.33[‡]	155
	Elasticon			
	light	15.5[‡]	2.76[‡]	155
	heavy	24.5[‡]	4.37[‡]	155
	Rapid			
	light	18.3[‡]	3.26[‡]	155
Maxillofacial materials				
Polyurethane	Epithane-3	45[*]	8.1[*]	210
Silicone rubber	A-102	23[*]	4.1[*]	210
	A-2186	203[*]	36.2[*]	210
		40[*]	7.1[*]	154
	Cosmesil	44[*]	7.8[*]	154
	MDX 4-4210	23[*]	4.1[*]	154
	Medical Adhesive A	70[*]	12.4[*]	210
	Silastic 4-4515	104[*]	18.6[*]	210
Mouth protector materials				
Polyvinyl acetate-polyethylene	Proform	160[†]	28.6[†]	125
	Sta-Guard	120[†]	21.4[†]	125

Thermal conductivity, *K*

The thermal conductivity of a substance is the quantity of heat in cal/s passing through a body 1 cm thick with a cross section of 1 cm² when the temperature difference between the hot and cold sides of the body is 1°C.

Material	Product	K mcal/s(cm²)(°C/cm)	Reference
Amalgam		54.0	13
Alumina (recrystallized)		38.7	20
Bones			
Cancellous		1.4	192
Cortical		1.4	192
Cement (base consistency)			
Zinc phosphate	Tenacin	3.1	13
Cements (luting consistency)			
Glass-ionomer	Ketac-cem	1.5*	205
Zinc phosphate	Tenacin	2.5	13
Cements (liners)			
Calcium hydroxide	Dycal	1.5	206
	Life	1.2	206
Glass-ionomer	Base cement	1.6*	205
	Dentin cement	1.3*	205
Unmodified ZOE		1.4†	24
	Cavitec	0.7	206
Denture resins			
Acrylic		0.37	82
Polystyrene		0.22	82
Gold alloy			
Au-Ag-Pd alloy		300	192
Gypsum		3.1	147
Hydroxyapatite		3.0	192
Impression materials (polymerized)			
Polyether	Impregum	2.3	207
Silicone, addition	Baysilex	1.0	207
	Provil		
	medium	1.4	207
	high	0.72	207
Mercury		19.6‡	130
Porcelain (feldspathic)		2.39	20
Pure metals			
Chromium		160§	130
Copper		941§	130
Gold		710§	130
Nickel		220¶	130

* Powder/liquid ratio, 1.0 g/mL.
† Powder/liquid ratio, 3.0 g/mL.
‡ At 0°C.
§ Near 20°C.
¶ At 25°C.
# At 18°C.
** At 17°C.

Thermal conductivity, *K* (continued)

Material	Product	K mcal/s/cm²/(°C/cm)	Reference
Pure metals (continued)			
Palladium		1680#	130
Platinum		165**	130
Silver		1000‡	130
Titanium		10.0	192
Zinc		270¶	130
Restorative materials			
Acrylic	Bonfil	0.38	24
Composite resin	Adaptic	2.61	24
		3.27	109
Silicate	Improved Filling Porcelain	1.78–1.86	13
		0.82†	24
Tooth structures			
Dentin		1.36	41
Enamel		2.23	41
Vitreous carbon		15	117
Water		1.42**	1

Thermal diffusivity, Δ

The thermal diffusivity is a measure of transient heat flow and is defined as the thermal conductivity divided by the product of specific heat times density.

Material	Product	Δ (mm^2/s)	Reference
Amalgam	Caulk Fine Cut	9.6	141
Cements			
Calcium hydroxide	Dycal	0.187	206
		0.240	140
	Life	0.186	206
Glass-ionomer			
Light-cured	Vitrabond	0.184	208
	XR Ionomer	0.194	208
	Zionomer	0.290	208
Self-cured	Base cement	0.266*	205
	Dentin cement	0.232*	205
	Fuji	0.262	139
	Ketac-Bond	0.205	208
	Ketac-Cem	0.239*	205
Resin	Time Line	0.174	208
Unmodified ZOE		0.389†	24
		0.471‡	140
	Cavitec	0.086	206
Zinc phosphate	Tenacin	0.290‡	24
	Stratford Cookson	0.308§	140
Zinc polycarboxylate	Poly-C	0.332	140
Gold (pure)		118	141
Impression materials			
Dental compound	Kerr	0.226	34
Polyether	Impregum	0.43	207
Silicone, addition	Baysilex	0.32	207
	Provil		
	medium	0.38	207
	high	0.22	207
Poly(methyl methacrylate)	Lucite	0.124	140
Restorative materials			
Acrylic	Bonfil	0.123	24
	Sevriton	0.125	140
Composite resin	Adaptic	0.675	24
		0.655	140
	Adaptic¶	0.725	139
	Concise	0.338	139
	Cosmic	0.310	139
	Isopast	0.191	139
	Profile	0.283	139

* Powder/liquid ratio, 1.0 g/mL.
† Powder/liquid ratio, 3.0 g/mL.
‡ Powder/liquid ratio, 2.5 g/mL.
§ Powder/liquid ratio, 1.85 g/mL.
¶ Radiopaque.

Thermal diffusivity, Δ (continued)

Material	Product	Δ (mm^2/s)	Reference
Restorative materials (continued)			
Glass-ionomer	Fuji Type II	0.216	208
	Improved Fuji Type II	0.228	208
Metal-reinforced glass-ionomer	Ketac Silver	0.516	208
	Miracle Mix	0.407	208
Silicate	Improved Filling Porcelain	0.243†	24
	Silicap	0.275	140
Tooth structures			
Dentin		0.183	41
		0.258	206
Enamel		0.469	41

Transverse strength, *T*

The transverse strength, modulus of rupture, or flexure strength is obtained by supporting a bar or beam at each end, and loading it in the middle. This test is called a three pointing bending (3PB) test.

Material	Product	T psi x 10^3	T MPa	Reference
Alumina (recrystallized)		55.0	379	20
Amalgams (7 days)				
Admixed	Dispersalloy	17.7	122	186
	Valiant PhD	20.6	142	186
Spherical	Indiloy	19.5	134	186
	Lojic	17.2	118	186
	Sybraloy	17.3	119	186
	Tytin	21.4	148	186
	Valiant	21.1	146	186
Cements (luting consistency, 24 h)				
Glass-ionomer	Fuji I	0.39	2.7	173
	Ketac-cem Radiopaque	0.42	2.9	173
Cements (liners, 24 h)				
Calcium hydroxide	Dycal	0.61	4.2	178
	Life	0.38	2.6	178
Glass-ionomer				
Light-cured	Vitrabond	3.51	24.2	179
	XR Ionomer	2.55	17.6	179
Self-cured	Baseline	1.68	11.6	173
	Baseline in Caps	1.71	11.8	173
	GC lining cement	0.20	1.4	173
	Ketac-bond	0.45	3.1	173
	Ketac-bond Capsule	0.96	6.6	173
	3M Glass ionomer liner	0.45	3.1	173
Resin	Cavalite	8.41	58.0	179
	Timeline	9.27	63.9	179
Denture resins				
Cold-cured	PERform	12	84	218
Heat-cured	Lucitone 199	11	78	218
	Perma-cryl 20	12	86	218
Light-cured	Triad	12	80	218
Gold (condensed)				
Foil	Morgan, Hastings & Co.	42.3	292	32
Mat	Williams	23.0	159	32
Powdered	Goldent	23.6	163	32
Gypsum				
Improved stone	Velmix	2.40	16.6	83
Investment				
Ethyl silicate, 23-1000°C	Hartex	0.071	0.49	84
Gypsum-bonded, 23°C	Kerr Model	0.355	2.45	84
Gypsum-bonded, 600°C	Kerr Model	0.014	0.10	84

Transverse strength, T (continued)

Material	Product	T psi x 10^3	T MPa	Reference
Investment (continued)				
Phosphate bonded, 23°C		0.384	2.65	84
Phosphate bonded, 1000°C		1.10	7.64	84
Porcelains				
Alumina-reinforced	HiCeram (core)	20.2	139	146
	Vitadur-N (core)	17.9	123	146
Castable ceramic	Dicor	18.1	125	146
Ceramic-whisker-reinforced	Mirage	10	70	146
Feldspathic	Ceramco II	8.9	61	146
	Excelco	8.0	55	146
	Vitadur-N(dentin)	9.1	62	146
	Vita VMK 68	9.5	66	146
Leucited-reinforced	Optec HSP	15	104	146
Magnesia core				
Glazed		39	270	189
Untreated		19	130	189
Restorative materials				
Composite resin	Herculite XRV	14.5	99.8	190
	P-50	12.3	85.1	190
	Silux Plus	8.9	61.4	190
	Z-100	20.2	139.4	191
Glass-ionomer	Chelon-fil	1.09	7.5	173
	Chelon-silver	1.65	11.4	173
	Chemfil II	1.35	9.3	173
	Chemfil II in caps	3.63	25.0	173
	Fuji II	0.51	3.5	173
	Ketac-fil Capsule	1.49	10.3	173
	Ketac-silver Capsule	1.00	6.9	173
		4.76	31.8	191
Vitreous carbon		22	152	117

Ultimate compressive strength, *C*

The ultimate compressive strength is defined as the maximum stress that a material can withstand before failure in compression. It is determined by dividing the maximum load in compression by the original cross-sectional area of the test specimen.

Material	Product	C psi x 10^3	C MPa	Reference
Alumina (recrystallized)		316	2180	20
Amalgams (1h)				
Admixed	Valiant PhD	29.2	201	171
Spherical	Tytin	29.7	205	171
	Valiant	42.1	290	171
Amalgams (24 h)				
Admixed	Dispersalloy	61.3*	423*	3
	Dispersalloy, fast set	56.1†	387†	142
		64.5‡	445‡	142
	regular set	51.2†	353†	142
		62.8‡	433‡	142
	Optaloy II	46.8†	323†	142
		50.9‡	351‡	142
Lathe-cut	Caulk Fine Cut	45.0†	310†	142
		49.0‡	338‡	142
	New True Dentalloy	46.1*	318*	3
Spherical	Indiloy	59.0†	407†	142
		60.3‡	416‡	142
	Sybraloy	52.3†	361†	142
		57.4‡	396‡	142
Bones (human)				
Long bones				
Femur		24.2	167	172
Humerus		19.1	132	172
Radius		16.5	114	172
Tibia		23.1	159	172
Vertebrae				
Cervical		1.5	10	172
Lumbar		0.73	5	172
Cements (base consistency, 24 h)				
Polymer-modified ZOE	B & T	5.52*	38.1*	2
Zinc phosphate	Zinc Cement Improved	23.3*	161*	2
Zinc polycarboxylate	Durelon	11.5*	79.6*	2
	PCA	9.93§	68.5§	124
Cements (luting consistency, 24 h)				
EBA-alumina ZOE	Opotow	9.32*	64.3*	2
		9.53	65.7	79

* Head speed 0.02 cm/min.
† Head speed 0.025 cm/min hand triturated.
‡ Head speed 0.025 cm/min mechanically triturated.
§ Head speed 0.5 cm/min.
¶ Head speed 0.05 cm/min.
\# Head speed 0.01 cm/min.
** Head speed 0.1 cm/min.
†† Head speed 25 cm/min.
‡‡ Head speed 0.15 cm/min.
§§ Head speed 0.12 cm/min.

Ultimate compressive strength, *C* (continued)

Material	Product	C		Reference
		psi x 10^3	MPa	
Cements (luting consistency, 24 h)				
EBA-alumina ZOE (continued)				
		6.5[#]	45[#]	145
Glass-ionomer	Fuji I	17.4[¶]	120[¶]	173
	Ketac-cem Radiopaque	17.7[¶]	122[¶]	173
Non-eugenol zinc oxide	Nogenol	0.587[*]	4.05[*]	2
Polymer-modified ZOE	Fynal	7.31[*]	50.4[*]	2
		5.1[#]	35[#]	145
Resin	Panavia EX	25.9[¶]	178[¶]	174
Unmodified ZOE	Temporary Cement	1.20[*]	8.28[*]	74
Zinc hydrophosphate	New Calmix	9.56[¶]	66.0[¶]	75
Zinc phosphate	Flecks	9.01[¶]	62.1[¶]	174
	Modern Tenacin	11.2[¶]	77.5[¶]	174
Zinc polycarboxylate	Durelon	9.78[¶]	67.4[¶]	174
	Shofu	7.98[¶]	55.0[¶]	174
Zinc silicophosphate	Kryptex Improved	24.8	171	62
Cements (liners, 24 h)				
Calcium hydroxide				
Light-cured	VLC Dycal	20.0[**]	138[**]	175
Self-cured	Dycal	2.10[**]	14.5[**]	175
	Life	5.50	37.9	178
Glass-ionomer				
Light-cured	Fuji lining	24.7[**]	170.3[**]	235
	Vitrabond	19.0[**]	130.9[**]	235
		8.24[**]	56.8[**]	175
	XR Ionomer	9.28[**]	64.0[**]	175
		2.9[**]	20.0[**]	235
	Zionomer	6.67	46.0	178
Self-cured	Baseline	9.64[¶]	66.5[¶]	173
	Baseline in caps	20.0[¶]	138[¶]	173
	GC lining cement	8.44[¶]	58.2[¶]	173
	Ketac-bond	17.0[¶]	117[¶]	173
	Ketac-bond Capsule	20.6[¶]	142[¶]	173
	3M Glass ionomer liner	9.51[¶]	65.6[¶]	173
Resin	Timeline	22.2[**]	153[**]	175
Unmodified ZOE	Cavitec	0.798[*]	5.50[*]	2
Crown-and-bridge resins				
Acrylic	Biotone	11.8[¶]	81.4[¶]	23

Ultimate compressive strength, *C* (continued)

Material	Product	C psi x 10^3	C MPa	Reference
Crown and bridge resins (continued)				
Polyester	Mer-Don 7	8.65¶	59.6¶	23
Polyvinyl acrylic	Luxene	12.0¶	82.8¶	23
Duplicating material				
Agar	Nobiloid	0.052††	0.36††	60
Gypsum (dried)				
Improved stone	Velmix	11.7‡‡	80.7‡‡	31
Plaster	Calspar	3.40‡‡	23.4‡‡	31
Stone	Calestone	8.70‡‡	60.0‡‡	31
Impression materials				
Agar	Surgident	0.11††	0.76††	60
Alginate (6 min)	Jeltrate	0.12††	0.82††	27
Polysulfide (8 min)	Rubberjel	0.28††	1.93††	27
Porcelains				
Feldspathic	Trubyte Bioform 2100	21.6§§	149§§	22
Fused to metal	Ceramco Opaque	21.7§§	150§§	22
Restorative materials				
Composite resin				
All-purpose	Brilliant	40.6¶	280¶	211
	Charisma	42.5¶	293¶	211
	Conquest DFC	42.9¶	296¶	211
	Heliomolar Radiopaque	49.3	340	158
	Herculite XR	57.6	397	158
	Herculite XRV	35.7¶	246¶	211
	Marathon	43.4	299	158
	P-50 APC	57.3	395	158
	Pertac Hybrid	47.9¶	330¶	211
	Prisma APH	55.5	383	158
	True Vitality	27.4¶	189¶	211
	Z-100	65.0	448	158
Anterior	Durafill	67.2	463	158
	Helio Progress	47.9	330	158
	Prisma Microfine	38.0	262	158
	Silar	41.0	283	158
	Silux	49.9	344	158
	Valux	62.4	430	158
	Visio Dispers	66.0	455	158
	Visio Fil	50.8	350	158

Ultimate compressive strength, C (continued)

Material	Product	C psi x 10^3	C MPa	Reference
Restorative materials (continued)				
Composite resin				
Posterior	Clearfil Photoposterior	42.6¶	294¶	211
	Heliomolar	47.1	325	158
	Occlusin	50.5	348	158
	P10	56.6	390	158
	Post Comp II LC	50.0	345	158
Glass-ionomer	Chelon-fil	22.4¶	155¶	173
	Chemfil II	28.6¶	198¶	173
	Chemfil II in caps	19.7¶	136¶	173
	Fuji II	23.0¶	159¶	173
	Ketac-fil Capsule	22.1¶	152¶	173
Metal-reinforced glass-ionomer	Chelon-silver	18.1¶	125¶	173
	Ketac-silver Capsule	16.3¶	113¶	173
	Miracle mix	18.7¶	129¶	234
Tooth structures				
Dentin		43.1	297	5
Enamel (cusp)		55.7	384	4
Vitreous carbon		100	690	117
Waxes				
Inlay casting, hard	Kerr blue hard	0.94¶	6.48¶	30
Inlay casting, soft	Kerr blue regular	1.13¶	7.79¶	30

Ultimate tensile strength, *UTS*

The ultimate tensile strength is defined as the maximum stress that a material can withstand before failure in tension. Unless indicated otherwise, values were determined by an extension test.

Material	Product	UTS psi x 10^3	UTS MPa	Reference
Alumina (recrystallized)		17.2*	119*	20
Amalgams (7d)				
Admixed	Dispersalloy	6.94*	47.9*	53
	Phasealloy	3.96*	27.3*	177
	Valiant PhD	4.68*	32.2*	177
Lathe-cut	New True Dentalloy	7.93*	54.7*	53
Bones (human)				
Long bones				
Femur		17.5	121	172
Humerus		18.9	130	172
Radius		21.6	149	172
Tibia		20.3	140	172
Vertebrae				
Cervical		0.45	3.1	172
Lumbar		0.54	3.7	172
Cements (base consistency, 24 h)				
Polymer-modified ZOE	B & T	0.500*	3.45*	2
Zinc phosphate	Zinc Cement Improved	1.20*	8.3*	2
Zinc polyacrylate	Durelon	2.25*	15.5*	2
	PCA	1.00*	6.92*	124
Cements (luting consistency, 24 h)				
EBA-alumina ZOE	Opotow	1.03*	7.12*	2
Glass-ionomer	Fuji I	0.80*	5.5*	173
	Ketac-cem Radiopaque	0.65*	4.5*	173
Non-eugenol zinc oxide	Nogenol	0.157*	1.08*	2
Polymer-modified ZOE	Fynal	0.603*	4.16*	2
Resin	Panavia EX	6.54*	45.1*	174
Zinc phosphate	Flecks	1.35*	9.3*	174
	Modern Tenacin	1.38*	9.5*	174
Zinc polycarboxylate	Durelon	2.19*	15.1*	174
	Shofu	1.57*	10.8*	174
Cements (liners, 24 h)				
Calcium hydroxide	Dycal	0.33*	2.3*	178

* Values determined from diametral compression test.
† Head speed, 5 cm/min.
‡ Head speed, 50 cm/min.
§ Head speed, 1.27 cm/min.
¶ Head speed, 25 cm/min.
\# Head speed, 0.005 cm/min.
** Head speed, 0.1 cm/min.
†† As cast
‡‡ Heat treated.
§§ Head speed, 0.05 cm/min.
¶¶ Head speed, 0.85 cm/min.

Ultimate tensile strength, *UTS* (continued)

Material	Product	UTS psi x 10^3	UTS MPa	Reference
Cements (liners, 24h)				
Calcium hydroxide (continued)	Life	0.35*	2.4*	178
Glass-ionomer				
Light-cured	Fuji Lining LC	2.06*	14.2*	235
	Vitrabond	1.83*	12.6*	179
	XR Ionomer	1.07*	7.4*	179
		0.32*	2.2*	235
	Zionomer	0.55*	3.8*	178
Self-cured	Baseline	0.90*	6.2*	173
	Baseline in caps	1.52*	10.5*	173
	GC lining cement	0.57*	3.9*	173
	Ketac-Bond	0.84*	5.8*	173
	Ketac-Bond Capsule	1.60*	11.0*	173
	3M Glass ionomer liner	0.33*	2.3*	173
Resin	Cavalite	3.33*	23.0*	179
	Timeline	2.04*	14.1*	179
Unmodified ZOE	Cavitec	0.062*	0.43*	2
Cobalt-chromium alloys	Advantage††	99.4§§	685§§	198
	Advantage‡‡	95.7§§	660§§	198
	Cobond††	111.9§§	772§§	198
	Cobond‡‡	113.9§§	785§§	198
	Genesis II††	93.9§§	647§§	198
	Genesis II‡‡	86.9§§	599§§	198
	Master Tec††	103.0§§	710§§	198
	Master Tec‡‡	108.9§§	751§§	198
	Novarex††	97.7§§	674§§	198
	Novarex‡‡	101.8§§	702§§	198
	Novarex II††	93.4§§	644§§	198
	Novarex II‡‡	95.4§§	658§§	198
	ViComp††	98.8§§	681§§	198
	ViComp‡‡	104.2§§	718§§	198
	Vitallium	126	869	61
Denture liners (resilient)				
Polyphosphazene fluoroelastomer	Novus	0.534‡	3.68‡	153
Silicone	Molloplast-B	0.634‡	4.37‡	153
Denture resins				
Acrylic	Kallodent 333	11.6†	80.4†	90
Polyvinylacrylic	Luxene T75	12.2†	84.3†	90
Gold (999.9 fine)	Wilkinson Co.	15.6	108	96
Gold (condensed)				
Foil		7.35	50.7	33
Mat		3.60	24.8	33
Powdered	Goldent	6.76	46.6	33
Gold alloys				
Type I	Ney-Oro A	32.0	221	7

Ultimate tensile strength, *UTS* (continued)

Material	Product	UTS psi x 10^3	UTS MPa	Reference
Gold alloys (continued)				
Type II	Ney-Oro A-1	55.0	379	7
Type III, soft	Ney-Oro B-2	61.0	421	7
Type III, hard	Ney-Oro B-2	65.0	448	7
	Sjoding C-3	66.3	457	144
Type IV, soft	Ney-Oro G-3	68.0	469	7
Type IV, hard	Ney-Oro G-3	110	759	7
	Sjoding D	101	699	144
64% Au-Ag-Cu, hard	Begolloyd G	80.5	555	144
48% Au-Ag-Cu, hard	Midigold	90.8	626	144
40% Au-Ag-Cu, soft	Forticast	85	586	9
40% Au-Ag-Cu, hard	Forticast	129	890	9
10-15% Au-Ag-Pd, soft	Paliney No. 4	81.0	559	7
10-15% Au-Ag-Pd, hard	Paliney No. 4	106	731	7
Au-Pd	Olympia[††]	88.6[§§]	611[§§]	199
	Olympia[‡‡]	97.5[§§]	672[§§]	199
Au-Pt-Pd	TPW	38.1	263	196
Porcelain-fused-to-metal	Jelenko O	73	503	9
Gutta-percha	Indian Head	2.80	19.3	28
	Mynol	2.40	16.6	28
Gypsum (dried)				
Improved stone	Velmix	1.11[*]	7.66[*]	31
Plaster	Calspar	0.600[*]	4.14[*]	31
Stone	Calestone	0.820[*]	5.66[*]	31
Impression materials				
Alginate	Krompan	0.034[‡]	0.24[‡]	81
Polyether	Impregum	0.300[‡]	2.07[‡]	180
	Reprosil			
	medium	0.287[‡]	1.98[‡]	180
	Permadyne			
	light	0.122[¶]	0.841[¶]	181
	heavy	0.180[¶]	1.24[¶]	181
Polysulfide				
Copper hydroxide cured	Omniflex	0.135[‡]	0.929[‡]	180
Lead dioxide cured	Coeflex	0.165[‡]	1.14[‡]	180
Silicone, addition	Express			
	light	0.174[¶]	1.20[¶]	181
	medium	0.269[¶]	1.85[¶]	181
	putty	0.092[¶]	0.634[¶]	181
	Mirror 3 Extrude			
	light	0.193[¶]	1.33[¶]	181
	medium	0.232[¶]	1.60[¶]	181
	putty	0.330[¶]	2.28[¶]	181
Silicone, condensation	Citricon			
	light	0.142[¶]	0.979[¶]	181

Ultimate tensile strength, *UTS* (continued)

Material	Product	UTS		Reference
		psi x 10^3	MPa	
Impression materials				
Silicone, condensation (continued)	putty	0.348[¶]	2.40[¶]	181
	Rapid			
	light	0.222[¶]	1.53[¶]	181
	putty	0.191[¶]	1.32[¶]	181
Iron-chromium alloys				
Crown-and-bridge	Dentillium C-B	134	924	61
Partial denture	Dentillium P-D	122	841	61
Maxillofacial materials				
Polyurethane	Epithane-3	0.12[¶¶]	0.83[¶¶]	210
Silicone rubber	A-102	0.28[¶¶]	1.9[¶¶]	210
	A-2186	0.73[‡]	5.0[‡]	154
	Cosmesil	0.73[‡]	5.0[‡]	154
	MDX 4-4210	0.57[‡]	4.0[‡]	154
	Medical Adhesive A	0.16[¶¶]	1.1[¶¶]	210
	Silastic 4-4515	1.38[¶¶]	9.5[¶¶]	210
Mouth protector materials				
Polyvinyl acetate-polyethylene	Proform	1.06[¶]	7.31[¶]	125
	Sta-guard	0.46[¶]	3.17[¶]	125
Nickel-chromium alloys	Ceramalloy II[††]	114.6[§§]	790[§§]	199
	Ceramalloy II[‡‡]	103.0[§§]	710[§§]	199
	Micro-Bond N-P2[††]	73.3[§§]	505[§§]	199
	Micro-Bond N-P2[‡‡]	71.5[§§]	493[§§]	199
	Ticon[††]	116.4[§§]	803[§§]	199
	Ticon[‡‡]	96.7[§§]	667[§§]	199
	Unimetal	119.9	827	196
Crown-and-bridge	Howmedica III	61.0	421	110
Partial denture	Ticonium 100	117	807	8
Porcelain-fused-to-metal	Ultratek	133	917	6
Palladium-based dental alloys	Microstar[††]	100.8[§§]	695[§§]	199
	Microstar[‡‡]	106.7[§§]	736[§§]	199
	Spartan[††]	165.5[§§]	1141[§§]	199
	Spartan[‡‡]	163.2[§§]	1125[§§]	199
	W-1[††]	103.6[§§]	714[§§]	199
	W-1[‡‡]	105.0[§§]	724[§§]	199
Polymers				
Polyetherurethane	Pellethane 2363-80A	7.21[§]	49.7[§]	182
Polyetherurethane urea	Biomer	7.28[§]	50.2[§]	182
Poly (methyl methacrylate)		8.48[**]	58.5[**]	183
Porcelains				
Feldspathic	Trubyte Bioform 2100	3.60	24.8	22
Fused to metal	Ceramco Opaque	5.40	37.2	22
Restorative materials				
Composite resin				
All-purpose	Brilliant	5.80[*]	40[*]	211
	Charisma	5.95[*]	41[*]	211

Ultimate tensile strength, *UTS* (continued)

Material	Product	UTS psi x 10^3	UTS MPa	Reference
Restorative materials				
Composite resin				
All-purpose (continued)	Conquest DFC	7.54*	52*	211
	Herculite XRV	5.66*	39.0*	184
	Pertac Hybrid	6.24*	43*	211
	True Vitality	4.64*	32*	211
	Z100	7.89*	54.4*	184
Anterior	Multifil VS	6.16*	42.5*	212
	Prisma Fil	8.47*	58.4*	212
	Silux Plus	5.86*	40.4*	212
Posterior	Clearfil Photo Posterior	6.53*	45*	211
	Coltene D1	6.54*	45.1*	212
	Ful Fil	8.67*	59.8*	212
	Heliomolar	5.99*	41.3*	212
	Marathon One	5.41*	37.3*	184
	P10	9.25*	63.8*	212
Glass-ionomer	Chelon-fil	1.46*	10.1*	173
	Chemfil II	1.80*	12.2*	173
	Chemfil II in caps	1.87*	12.9*	173
	Fuji II	1.26*	8.7*	173
	Ketac-fil Capsule	2.03*	14.0*	173
Metal-reinforced glass-ionomer	Chelon-silver	1.60*	11.0*	173
	Ketac-silver Capsule	1.87*	12.9*	173
	Miracle Mix	1.33*	9.2*	234
Silicate		0.630	4.34	92
Silver-palladium alloys				
	Alborium	88.6	611	144
	Hvitstøp	76.3	526	144
	Palliag M	59.6	411	144
Crown-and-bridge, soft	Albacast	63.0	434	9
Crown-and-bridge, hard	Albacast	68.0	469	9
Porcelain-fused-to-metal	Jel-5	105.0	724	9
Titanium		79.8	550	131
Titanium-6 Al-4 V alloy		134.9	930	131
Tooth structures				
Dentin (bovine)				
Demineralized		3.77**	26.0**	185
Mineralized		13.1**	90.6**	185
Dentin (human)				
Demineralized		4.29**	29.6**	185
Mineralized		15.3**	105.5**	185
Enamel (bovine)		3.00#	20.7#	92
Enamel (human)		1.50#	10.3#	92

Vapor pressure, *P*

Vapor pressure is the pressure exerted when a solid or liquid is in equilibrium with its own vapor.

Material	P (mm Hg)	Temperature (°C)	Reference
Mercury	0.0014	22	69
	0.0050	38	69
	0.26	100	69
Mercury (in dental amalgam)	10^{-8}	37	108
Monomers (crown-and-bridge resins)			
Methyl methacrylate	125	50	72
	760	100	72
Ethylene glycol dimethacrylate	8	100	72
1,3-butylene glycol dimethacrylate	1	100	72
Triethylene glycol dimethacrylate	0.01	100	72
Water	19.8	22	1
	47.1	37	1

Vickers hardness, *VHN*

The Vickers hardness test or the 136° diamond pyramid hardness test is a micro-indentation method. The indenter produces a square indentation, the diagonals of which are measured. The diamond pyramid hardness is calculated by dividing the applied load by the surface area of the indentation.

Material	Product	VHN (kg/mm^2)	Reference
Alumina (recrystallized)		1200	20
Amalgam			
Ag-Hg phase		120	86
Sn-Hg phase		15	86
Cements (liners)			
Glass-ionomer			
Light-cured	Fuji Lining LC	57	235
	Vitrabond	62	235
	XR Ionomer	38	235
Cobalt-chromium alloys	Genesis II	350	9
	Master Tec	390	222
	Novarex	350	223
Gold alloys			
Type I	Ney-Oro A	55	7
Type II	Ney-Oro A-1	105	7
Type III, soft	Ney-Oro B-2	125	7
Type III, hard	Ney-Oro B-2	135	7
Type IV, soft	Ney-Oro G-3	160	7
Type IV, hard	Ney-Oro G-3	250	7
40% Au-Ag-Cu, soft	Forticast	193	9
40% Au-Ag-Cu, hard	Forticast	292	9
10%–15% Au-Ag-Pd, soft	Paliney No. 4	170	7
10%–15% Au-Ag-Pd, hard	Paliney No. 4	230	7
Au-Pd	Olympia	220	9
Au-Pt-Pd alloy	TPW	104	196
Porcelain-fused-to-metal	Jelenko O	182	9
Gypsum	Moldablaster	12	224
Nickel-chromium alloys	Unimetal	395	196
Crown-and-bridge	Howmedica III	330	110
Porcelain-fused-to-metal	Ultratek	270	6
Palladium-based dental alloys	Athenium*	270	197
	Legacy*	270	197
	Liberty*	340	197
	Microstar	265	9
	Protocol*	235	197
	PTM-88*	235	197
	Spartan*	360	197
	W1*240	222	
	W1†285	222	
Porcelains			
Alumina-reinforced	Vitadur-N (core)	775	231
Castable ceramic	Dicor	449	231
Ceramic-whisker-reinforced	Mirage II	663	231
Feldspathic	Excelco	663	231
	Vita VMK 68	703	231

* Specimens subjected to the porcelain firing cycles.
† Oven hardened.

Vickers hardness, *VHN* (continued)

Material	Product	VHN (kg/mm^2)	Reference
Porcelains			
Feldspathic (continued)	Vita VMK 68-N	703	231
	Will-Ceram	611	231
Leucite-reinforced	Optec HSP	703	231
Restorative materials			
Composite resins			
All purpose	Charisma	81	158
	Conquest DFC	95	158
	Heliomolar Radiopaque	56	158
	Herculite XR	74	158
	Marathon	100	158
	P-50 APC	159	158
	Pertac Hybrid	126	158
	Prisma APH	77	158
	Z-100	120	158
Anterior	Durafill	48	158
	Helio Progress	50	158
	Multifil VS	55	158
	Prisma Fil	83	158
	Prisma Microfine	39	158
	Silux Plus	59	158
		41	159
	Valux	107	158
	Visio Dispers	63	158
	Visio Fil	160	158
Posterior	Clearfil Photo Posterior	159	158
	Ful Fil	97	158
	Heliomolar	61	158
	P-10	174	158
	Post Comp II LC	97	158
Glass-ionomer	Chemfil II	51	159
	Fujicap II	74	159
	Ketac-Fil	90	159
Metal-reinforced-glass-ionomer	Ketac-Silver	40	159
Silver-palladium alloys			
Crown-and-bridge, soft	Albacast	143	9
Crown-and-bridge, hard	Albacast	154	9
Porcelain-fused-to-metal	Jel-5	187	9
Titanium		210	131
Titanium-6 Al-4 V alloy		320	131
Tooth structures			
Dentin		60	158
		57	159
Enamel		408	158
		294	159

Viscosity, η

Viscosity is defined as the resistance of a substance to flow under stress. Units are g/(cm s) or poise. Centipoise (cp) is 10^{-2} poise.

Material	Product	η (cp)	Temperature(°C)	Reference
Cements				
Zinc phosphate	Modern Tenacin	43,200*	18	119
		94,700*	25	119
Zinc polycarboxylate	Durelon	101,000*	18	119
		109,800*	25	119
Impression materials				
Agar		281,000	45	99
Alginate	Jeltrate	252,000†	37	118
Impression plaster	Plastogum	23,800†	37	118
Polysulfide, light		109,000‡	36	99
	Permlastic	57,200†	37	118
Polysulfide, heavy		1,360,000‡	36	99
Silicone, addition				
medium	Hydrosil	1,294,000§	37	230
	Imprint	797,000§	37	230
	Omnisil	1,025,000§	37	230
heavy	Baysilex	689,000§	37	230
Silicone, condensation				
light		63,400‡	36	99
	Elasticon	95,000†	37	118
medium		420,000‡	36	99
Zinc oxide-eugenol	Luralite	99,600†	37	118
Mercury		1.554	20	101
Monomers (crown-and-bridge resins)				
Methyl methacrylate		0.52	25	128
Ethylene glycol dimethacrylate		3.40	25	129
1,3-butylene glycol dimethacrylate		3.5	25	129
Triethylene glycol dimethacrylate		7.5	25	129
Water		1.000	20	1

* Measured at 45 s after completion of mix and 5 rpm.
† Measured at 1.5 min from start of mix and 5 rpm.
‡ Measured at 2 min from start of mix.
§ Measured at 1 min from start of mix and 2.5 rpm.

Water sorption

Water sorption of a material represents the amount of water adsorbed on the surface and absorbed into the body of the material. The method of testing is described in American National Standards Institute/American Dental Association Specification Nos. 12 and 27.[73]

Material	Product	Water sorption (mg/cm2)	Reference
Denture liners (resilient)			
Polyphosphazene fluoroelastomer	Novus	4.01‡	226
Silicone	Molloplast-B	0.23‡	226
Denture resins			
Acrylic	Hy-Pro Lucitone	0.69*	45
Polystyrene	Jectron	0.36*	45
Polyvinylacrylic	Luxene 44	0.26*	45
Pit and fissure sealants			
Light-cured	Nuva-Seal	0.9‡	115
Self-cured	Delton	1.29†	127
	9075	1.8‡	115
Restorative materials			
Composite resin			
Posterior	Occlusin	0.71‡	227
	P-50	0.52‡	227

* Stored for 1 day.
† Stored for 30 days.
‡ Stored for 7 days.

Yield strength, *YS*

The yield strength is defined as the stress at which a material exhibits a specified limiting deviation from proportionality of stress to strain. The amount of permanent strain arbitrarily selected is referred to as the percent offset and is commonly 0.1%.

Material	Product	YS psi x 10^3	YS MPa	Reference
Cements (liners)				
Glass-ionomer				
Light-cured	Vitrabond	1.60	11.0	179
	XR Ionomer	3.15	21.7	179
Resin	Cavalite	8.99	62.0	179
	Timeline	4.31	29.7	179
Cobalt-chromium alloys	Advantage*	69.8†	481†	198
	Advantage‡	67.7†	467†	198
	Cobond*	71.8†	495†	198
	Cobond‡	66.0†	455†	198
	Genesis II*	68.4†	472†	198
	Genesis II‡	71.9†	496†	198
	Master Tec*	70.1†	483†	198
	Master Tec‡	73.8†	509†	198
	Novarex*	68.9†	475†	198
	Novarex‡	81.4†	561†	198
	Novarex II*	70.9†	489†	198
	Novarex II‡	75.5†	521†	198
	Vi-Comp*	77.3†	533†	198
	Vi-Comp‡	73.8†	509†	198
	Vitallium	93.4	644	61
Gold alloys				
40% Au-Ag-Cu, soft	Forticast	68†	469†	9
40% Au-Ag-Cu, hard	Forticast	125†	862†	9
Au-Pd	Olympia*	63.3†	436†	199
	Olympia‡	77.9†	537†	199
Porcelain-fused-to-metal	Jelenko O	72.5†	500†	9
Gutta-percha	Indian Head	1.70	11.7	28
	Mynol	1.20	8.28	28
Iron-chromium alloy				
Partial denture	Dentillium P-D	94.4	651	61
Nickel-chromium alloys	Ceramalloy II*	71.3†	492†	199
	Ceramalloy II‡	49.6†	342†	199
	Micro-Bond N-P2*	44.6†	308†	199
	Micro-Bond N-P2‡	34.0†	234†	199
	Ticon*	103.0†	710†	199
	Ticon‡	71.9†	496†	199
Palladium-based dental alloys	Athenium	76.1	525	197
	Legacy	95.5	658	197
	Liberty	115.5	796	197

* As cast.
† Percent offset of 0.2%.
‡ Heat treated.

Yield strength, *YS* (continued)

Material	Product	YS		Reference
		psi x 10^3	MPa	
Palladium-based dental alloys				
(continued)	Microstar*	76.8†	530†	199
	Microstar‡	70.7†	487†	199
	Protocol	68.7	474	197
	PTM-88	83.0	572	197
	Spartan*	153.7†	1060†	199
	Spartan‡	138.6†	956†	199
	W-1 *	76.1†	525†	199
	W-1 ‡	80.5†	555†	199
Restorative materials				
Acrylic	Sevriton	7.50	51.7	42
Composite resin	Adaptic	23.4	161	42
Silver-palladium alloys				
Crown-and-bridge	Albacast	42†	290†	9
Porcelain-fused-to-metal	Jel-5	70†	483†	9

Zeta potential, ζ

A charged particle suspended in an electrolytic solution attracts ions of opposite charge to those at its surface, where they form the Stern layer. To maintain the electrical balance of the suspending fluid, ions of opposite charge are attracted to the Stern layer. The potential at the surface of that part of this diffuse double layer of ions that can move with the particle when subjected to a voltage gradient is the zeta potential. This potential measured is very dependent upon the ionic concentration, pH, viscosity, and dielectric constant of the solution being analyzed.

Material	ζ, mV	Reference
Bacteria		
A. odontolyticus A7-1	–16.0*	200
A. viscosus C7-4	–11.1*	200
S. mutans		
C7-3	–7.1*	200
M4S	–13.7†	123
S. salivarius B3-4	–4.8*	200
S. sanguis C7-2	–12.4*	200
Bone	–7.01‡	201
Hydroxyapatite, synthetic	–10.9§	107
	–9.0†	123
Polymers		
Poly(ether urethane)	–17.3	202
Silicone	–98.5	202
Tooth structures		
Calculus	–15.3¶	106
Cementum, exposed	–6.96¶	106
Cementum, unexposed	–9.34¶	106
Dentin	–6.23¶	106
	+0.4*	200
Enamel	–10.3¶	106
	+0.9*	200

* Measured at 25°C in a physiological ionic strength ($\mu = 0.057$) medium, pH 7.0.
† Measured in distilled water.
‡ Measured in 0.145 M NaCl solution, pH 7.3.
§ Measured at 25°C at a solid/solution ratio of 0.1.
¶ Measured at 30°C in Hanks' balanced salt solution.

References

1. Lide DR, ed. CRC Handbook of Chemistry and Physics. 73rd ed. Boca Raton, Fla: The Chemical Rubber Co, 1992–1993.
2. Powers JM, Farah JW, Craig RG. Modulus of elasticity and strength properties of dental cements. J Am Dent Assoc 92(3):588–591, 1976.
3. Powers JM, Farah JW. Apparent modulus of elasticity of dental amalgams. J Dent Res 54(4):902, 1975.
4. Craig RG, Peyton FA, Johnson DW. Compressive properties of enamel, dental cements, and gold. J Dent Res 40(5):936–945, 1961.
5. Craig RG, Peyton FA. Elastic and mechanical properties of human dentin. J Dent Res 37(4):710–718, 1958.
6. Moffa JP, Lugassy AA, Guckes AD, Gettleman L. An evaluation of nonprecious alloys for use with porcelain veneers. Part I. Physical properties. J Prosthet Dent 30(4):424–431, 1973.
7. JM Ney Co, Bloomfield, Conn: 06002.
8. Asgar K, Allan FC. Microstructure and physical properties of alloys for partial denture castings. J Dent Res 47(2):189–197, 1968.
9. JF Jelenko & Co, Armonk, NY: 10504.
10. Austenal Dental, Inc, Chicago, Ill: 60632.
11. Craig RG, Peyton FA. The microhardness of enamel and dentin. J Dent Res 37(4):661–668, 1958.
12. Rautiola CA, Craig RG. The microhardness of cementum and underlying dentin of normal teeth and teeth exposed to periodontal disease. J Periodontol 32(2):113–123, 1961.
13. Craig RG, Peyton FA. Thermal conductivity of tooth structure, dental cements, and amalgam. J Dent Res 40(3):411–418, 1961.
14. Peyton FA, Simeral WG. The specific heat of tooth structure. University of Michigan School of Dentistry, Alumni Bull. p.33, 1954.
15. Craig RG, Gibbons P. Properties of resilient denture liners. J Am Dent Assoc 63(3):382–390, 1961.
16. Powers JM, Koran A. Unpublished data. Ann Arbor: University of Michigan School of Dentistry.
17. Lee H, Swartz ML. Evaluation of a composite resin crown and bridge luting agent. J Dent Res 51(3):756–766, 1972.
18. Webber RL, Ryge G. The determination of tear energy of extensible materials of dental interest. J Biomed Mater Res 2(3):281–296, 1968.
19. Sherrill CA, O'Brien WJ. Transverse strength of aluminous and feldspathic porcelain. J Dent Res 53(3):683–690, 1974.
20. McLean JW, Hughes TH. The reinforcement of dental porcelain with the ceramic oxides. Br Dent J 119(6):251–267, 1965.
21. Jones DW, Jones PA, Wilson HJ. The modulus of elasticity of dental ceramics. Dent Pract Dent Rec 22(5):170–173, 1972.
22. Leone EF, Fairhurst CW. Bond strength and mechanical properties of dental porcelain enamels. J Prosthet Dent 18(2):155–159, 1967.
23. Peyton FA, Craig RG. Current evaluation of plastics in crown and bridge prosthesis. J Prosthet Dent 13(4):743–753, 1963.
24. Civjan S, Barone JJ, Reinke PE, Selting WJ. Thermal properties of nonmetallic restorative materials. J Dent Res 51(4):1030–1037, 1972.
25. Mahler DB, Van Eysden J. Dynamic creep of dental amalgam. J Dent Res 48(4):501–508, 1969.
26. McLean JW. Physical properties influencing the accuracy of silicone and thiokol impression materials. Br Dent J 110(3):85–91, 1961.
27. MacPherson GW, Craig RG, Peyton FA. Mechanical properties of hydrocolloid and rubber impression materials. J Dent Res 46(4):714–721, 1967.
28. Friedman CE. The chemical composition and mechanical properties of gutta-percha endodontic filling materials. Master's Thesis. Chicago: Loyola University Medical Center, 1972.
29. Craig RG, Eick JD, Peyton FA. Properties of natural waxes used in dentistry. J Dent Res 44(6):1308–1316, 1965.
30. Craig RG, Eick JD, Peyton FA. Strength properties of waxes at various temperatures and their practical application. J Dent Res 46(1):300–305, 1967.
31. Earnshaw R, Smith DC. The tensile and compressive strength of plaster and stone. Aust Dent J 11(6):415–422, 1966.
32. Richter WA, Mahler DB. Physical properties vs clinical performance of pure gold restorations. J Prosthet Dent 29(4):434–438, 1973.
33. Mahan J, Charbeneau GT. A study of certain mechanical properties and the density of condensed specimens made from various forms of pure gold. Am Acad Gold Foil Operators J 8(1):6–12, 1965.
34. Braden M. Thermal properties of dental composition. J Dent Res 45(5):1453–1457, 1966.
35. Reisbick MH, Brodsky JF. Strength parameters of composite resins. J Prosthet Dent 26(2):178–185, 1971.
36. Martins EA, Peyton FA, Kingery RH. Properties of custom-made plastic teeth formed by different techniques. J Prosthet Dent 12(6):1059–1065, 1962.
37. Godwin WC, Koran A, Craig RG. Evaluation of the dynamic and static physical properties of mouth protectors. Microfilmed Paper no. 52. (Delivered at) the annual meeting of the International Association for Dental Research, Dental Materials Group, Atlanta, Ga, March 21–24, 1974.
38. Koran A, Craig RG. Dynamic mechanical properties of maxillofacial materials. J Dent Res 54(6):1216–1221, 1975.
39. Lontz JF, Schweiger JW, Burger AW. Modifying stress-strain profiles of polysiloxane elastomers for improved maxillofacial conformity. Microfilmed Paper no. 890. (Delivered at) the annual meeting of the International Association for Dental Research, Dental Materials Group, Atlanta, Ga., March 21–24, 1974.
40. Yoon HS, Newnham RE. Elastic properties of fluorapatite. Am Mineralogist 54:1193–1197, 1969.
41. Brown WS, Dewey WA, Jacobs HR. Thermal properties of teeth. J Dent Res 49(4):752–755, 1970.
42. Dennison JB, Craig RG. Physical properties and finished surface texture of composite restorative resins. J Am Dent Assoc 85(1):101–108, 1972.
43. Berghash SR, Hodge HC. Density and refractive index studies of dental hard tissues. III. Density distribution of deciduous enamel and dentin. J Dent Res 19(5):487–495, 1940.
44. Manly RS, Hodge HC, Ange LE. Density and refractive index studies of dental hard tissues. II. Density distribution curves. J Dent Res 18(3):203–211, 1939.
45. Chevitarese O, Craig RG, Peyton FA. Properties of various types of denture-base plastics. J Prosthet Dent 12(4):711–719, 1962.
46. Woelfel JB, Paffenbarger GC, Sweeney WT. Some physical properties of organic denture-base materials. J Am Dent Assoc 67(4):489–504, 1963.
47. O'Brien WJ, Ryge G. Relation between molecular force calculations and observed strengths of enamel-metal interfaces. J Am Ceram Soc 47(1):5–8, 1964.
48. Glantz P-O. The surface tension of saliva. Odontol Revy 21(2):119–127, 1970.
49. Nicholas ME, Joyner PA, Tessem BM, Olson MD. The effect of various gases and vapors on the surface tension of mercury. J Phys Chem 65(8):1373–1375, 1961.
50. Craig RG, Berry GC, Peyton FA. Wetting of poly(methyl methacrylate) and polystyrene by water and saliva. J Phys Chem 64:541–543, 1960.
51. Uy KC, Chang R. An approach to the study of the mechanism of adhesion to teeth. pp. 103–131 In Austin RH, Wilsdorf HGF, Phillips RW (eds). Adhesive Restorative Dental Materials. II. Proc. 2nd Workshop, Bio-Materials Research Advisory Committee, Public Health Service Publ. no. 1494, Washington, DC: US Government Printing Office, 1966.
52. Glantz P-O. On wettability and adhesiveness. A study of enamel, dentin, some restorative materials, and dental plaque. Odontol Revy 20(Suppl 17):1–132, 1969.

53. Mahler DB, Terkla LG, Van Eysden J, Reisbick MH. Marginal fracture vs mechanical properties of amalgam. J Dent Res 49(6):1452–1457, 1970.
54. Hall DR, Nakayama WT, Grenoble DE, Katz JL. Elastic constants of three representative dental cements. J Dent Res 52(2):390, 1973.
55. Grenoble DE, Katz JL, Dunn KL, Gilmore RS, Murty KL. The elastic properties of hard tissues and apatites. J Biomed Mater Res 6(3):221–223, 1972.
56. O'Brien WJ, Ryge G. Contact angles of drops of enamels on metals. J Prosthet Dent 15(6):1094–1100, 1965.
57. O'Brien WJ, Ryge G. Wettability of poly(methyl methacrylate) treated with silicon tetrachloride. J Prosthet Dent 15(2):304–308, 1965.
58. O'Brien WJ. Capillary penetration of liquids between dissimilar solids. Doctoral Dissertation. Ann Arbor: University of Michigan, 1967. Univ. Microfilm no. 6715666.
59. Chandler HH, Bowen RL, Paffenbarger GC. Physical properties of a radiopaque denture base material. J Biomed Mater Res 5(4):335–357, 1971.
60. Craig RG, Peyton FA. Physical properties of elastic duplicating materials. J Dent Res 39(2):391–404, 1960.
61. Morris HF, Asgar K. Physical properties and microstructure of four new commercial partial denture alloys. J Prosthet Dent 33(1):36–46, 1975.
62. Anderson JN, Paffenbarger GC. Properties of silico-phosphate cements. Dent Progress 2(2):72–75, 1962.
63. Grenoble DE, Katz JL. The pressure dependence of the elastic constants of dental amalgam. J Biomed Mater Res 5(5):489–502, 1971.
64. Lehman ML. Tensile strength of human dentin. J Dent Res 46(1):197–201, 1967.
65. Dyment MI, Synge JL. The elasticity of the periodontal membrane. Oral Health 25(3):105–109, 1935.
66. Souder WH, Paffenbarger GC. Physical properties of dental materials, Nat. Bur. Standards Circular no. C433, Washington, DC: US Government Printing Office, 1942.
67. Powers JM, Craig RG, Peyton FA. Calorimetric analysis of commercial and dental waxes. J Dent Res 48(6):1165–1170, 1969.
68. Craig RG, Powers JM, Peyton FA. Differential thermal analysis of commercial and dental waxes. J Dent Res 46(5):1090–1097, 1967.
69. Drake HJ. Mercury. pp. 143–156 In Grayson M (ed). Kirk-Othmer Encyclopedia of Chemical Technology. Vol 15. 3rd ed. New York: John Wiley & Sons, 1981.
70. Craig RG, O'Brien WJ, Powers JM. Dental Materials-Properties and Manipulation. St Louis: CV Mosby, 1992.
71. Lyman DJ, Muir WM, Lee IJ. The effect of chemical structure and surface properties of polymers on the coagulation of blood. I. Surface free energy effects. Trans Am Soc Artif Int Organs 11:301–306, 1965.
72. Cornell JA. Composite tooth and veneer gel composite formed of non-volatile dimethacrylate as the sole polymerizable constituent. US Patent 3,265,202 HD Justi Co, Div. Williams Gold-Refining Co, 1966.
73. Council on Dental Materials, Instruments, and Equipment. Certification programs of the Council on Dental Materials, Instruments and Equipment: ANSI/ADA specifications. Chicago: The Council on Dental Materials, Instruments and Equipment, 1990.
74. Norman RD, Swartz ML, Phillips RW, Virmini R. A comparison of the intraoral disintegration of three dental cements. J Am Dent Assoc 78(4):777–782, 1969.
75. Simmons FF, D'Anton EW, Hudson DC. Property studies of a hydrophosphate cement. J Am Dent Assoc 76(2):337–339, 1968.
76. Civjan S, Huget EF, Wolfhard G, Waddell LS. Characterization of zinc oxide-eugenol cements reinforced with acrylic resin. J Dent Res 51(1):107–114, 1972.
77. Phillips RW, Swartz ML, Rhodes B. An evaluation of a carboxylate adhesive cement. J Am Dent Assoc 81(12):1353–1359, 1970.
78. Smith DC. A review of the zinc polycarboxylate cements. J Can Dent Assoc 37(1):22–29, 1971.
79. Brauer GM, McLaughlin R, Huget EF. Aluminum oxide as a reinforcing agent for zinc oxide-eugenol-o-ethoxybenzoic acid cements. J Dent Res 47(4):622–628, 1968.
80. Lyon FF, Anderson JN. Some agar duplicating materials-An evaluation of their properties. Br Dent J 132(1):15–19, 1972.
81. Wilson HJ. Some properties of alginate impression materials relevant to clinical practice. Br Dent J 121(10):463–467, 1966.
82. Chen RYS, Barker RE Jr. Effect of pressure on heat transport in polymers used in dentistry. J Biomed Mater Res 6(3):147–154, 1972.
83. Combe EC, Smith DC. Some properties of gypsum plasters. Br Dent J 117(6):237–245, 1964.
84. Jones DW. The high temperature strength and thermal expansion of investment mould refractories. pp. 343–381 In Proc. 11th Int. Ceramic Congress, Madrid, 1968.
85. Altman PL, Dittmer DS. Blood and Other Body Fluids. Washington, DC: Fed Am Soc Exp Biol 12, 1961.
86. Wing G. Phase identification in dental amalgam. Aust Dent J 11:105–113, 1966.
87. Neville HA. Adsorption and reaction. I. The setting of plaster of paris. J Phys Chem 30:1037–1042, 1926.
88. Ekegren S, Ohrn O, Granath D, Kinell P-O. Heat of polymerization of chloroprene. Acta Chem Scand 4:126–139, 1950.
89. Braden M, Stafford GD. Viscoelastic properties of some denture base materials. J Dent Res 47(4):519–523, 1968.
90. Stafford GD, Smith DC. Some studies of the properties of denture base polymers. Br Dent J 125(8):337–342, 1968.
91. Civjan S, Brauer GM. Physical properties of cements, based on zinc oxide, hydrogenated rosin, o-ethoxybenzoic acid, and eugenol. J Dent Res 43(2):281–299, 1964.
92. Bowen RL, Rodriquez MS. Tensile strength and modulus of elasticity of tooth structure and several restorative materials. J Am Dent Assoc 64(3):378–387, 1962.
93. Smith DC, Cooper WEG. The determination of shear strength-A method using a micro-punch apparatus. Br Dent J 130(8):333–337, 1971.
94. Koran A, Craig RG, Tillitson EW. Coefficient of friction of prosthetic tooth materials. J Prosthet Dent 27(3):269–274, 1972.
95. Tillitson EW, Craig RG, Peyton FA. Friction and wear of restorative dental materials. J Dent Res 50(1):149–154, 1971.
96. Shell JS, Hollenback GM. Tensile strength and elongation of pure gold. J South Calif State Dent Assoc 34:219–221, 1966.
97. Shell JS. Some factors influencing specific gravity determinations on gold cast alloys. J Dent Res 45(2):337–342, 1966.
98. Braden M. Characterization of the rupture properties of impression materials. Dent Pract Dent Rec 14(2):67–71, 1963.
99. Reisbick MH. Effect of viscosity on the accuracy and stability of elastic impression materials. J Dent Res 52(3):407–417, 1973.
100. Miller GR, Powers JM, Ludema KC. Frictional behavior and surface failure of dental feldspathic porcelain. Wear 31(2):307–316, 1975.
101. Aylett BJ. Group IIB. pp. 187–328 In Trotman-Dickenson AF (ed). Comprehensive Inorganic Chemistry. Vol 3, Oxford:Pergamon Press, 1973.
102. Powers JM, Caddell RM. The macroscopic volume changes of selected polymers subjected to uniform tensile deformation. Polym Eng Sci 12(6):432–436, 1972.
103. Carlstrom D. Polarization microscopy of dental enamel with reference to incipient carious lesions. p. 277 In Staple PH (ed). Advances in Oral Biology. London: Academic Press, 1964.
104. Perloff A, Posner AS. Preparation of pure hydroxyapatite crystals. Science 124(3222):583–584, 1956.
105. Houwink B. The index of refraction of dental enamel apatite. Br Dent J 137(12):472–475, 1974.
106. Neiders ME, Weiss L, Cudney TL. An electrokinetic characterization of human tooth surfaces. Arch Oral Biol 15(2):135–151, 1970.

107. Leach SA. Electrophoresis of synthetic hydroxyapatite. Arch Oral Biol 3(1):48–56, 1960.
108. Reynolds CL Jr. Determination of mercury vapor pressure over amalgams from weight loss data. J Biomed Mater Res 8(6):369–373, 1974.
109. Brady AP, Lee H, Orlowski JA. Thermal conductivity studies of composite dental restorative materials. J Biomed Mater Res 8(6):471–485, 1974.
110. Caputo AA, Reisbick MH. Mechanical properties of a non-precious type III alloy. J Dent Res 54(2):428, 1975.
111. Mandelkern L, Quinn FA Jr, Roberts DE. Thermodynamics of crystallization in high polymers: Gutta percha. Am Chem Soc J 78:926–932, 1956.
112. Winkler S, Ortman HR, Ryczek MT. Improving the retention of complete dentures. J Prosthet Dent 34(1):11–15, 1975.
113. Dickson G, Oglesby PL. Elastic constants of dental amalgam. J Dent Res 46(6):1475, 1967.
114. Price WA. Report of laboratory investigations on the physical properties of root filling materials and the efficiency of root fillings for blocking infection from sterile tooth structures. Natl Dent Assoc J 5(12):1260–1280, 1918.
115. Dennison JB, Thompson WH. Unpublished data. Ann Arbor: University of Michigan School of Dentistry.
116. Nakayama WT, Hall DR, Grenoble DE, Katz JL. Elastic properties of dental resin restorative materials. J Dent Res 53(5):1121–1126, 1974.
117. Benson J. Elemental carbon as a biomaterial. J Biomed Mater Res 5(6):41–47, 1971.
118. Koran A, Powers JM, Craig RG. Apparent viscosity of materials used for making edentulous impressions. J Am Dent Assoc 95(1):75–79, 1977.
119. Vermilyea SG, Powers JM, Craig RG. Rotational viscometry of a zinc phosphate and a zinc polyacrylate cement. J Dent Res 56(7):762–767, 1977.
120. Johnston WM, O'Brien WJ. Shear strength of dental porcelain. J Dent Res 59(8):1409–1411, 1980.
121. O'Brien WJ, Fan PL, Apostolides A. Penetrativity of sealants and glazes. Oper Dent 3:51–56, 1978.
122. Faust JB, Grego GN, Fan PL, Powers JM. Penetration coefficient, tensile strength and bond strength of thirteen direct bonding orthodontic cements. Am J Orthod 73(5):512–525, 1978.
123. O'Brien WJ, Fan PL, Loesche WJ, Walker MC, Apostolides A. Adsorption of *Streptococcus mutans* on chemically treated hydroxyapatite. J Dent Res 57(9–10):910–914, 1978.
124. Barton JA Jr, Brauer GM, Antonucci JM, Raney MJ. Reinforced polycarboxylate cements. J Dent Res 54(2):310–323, 1975.
125. Going RE, Loehman RE, Chan MS. Mouthguard materials: their physical and mechanical properties. J Am Dent Assoc 89(1):132–138, 1974.
126. Bever MB (ed). Encyclopedia of Materials Science and Engineering. New York: Pergamon Press, 1059, 1986.
127. Fan PL, Edahl A, Leung RL, Stanford JW. Alternative interpretations of water sorption values of composite resins. J Dent Res 64(1):78–80, 1985.
128. Riddle EH. Monomeric Acrylic Esters. New York: Van Nostrand Reinhold Co, 13, 1954.
129. Sartomer Company. Sartomer Monomer Product Information Chart, West Chester, PA: 19380
130. Boyer HE, Gall TL (eds). Metals Handbook Desk Edition. Metals Park, Ohio: American Society for Metals, 1985.
131. Ida K, Togaya T, Tsutsumi S, Takeuchi M. Effect of magnesia investments in the dental casting of pure titanium or titanium alloys. Dent Mater J 1(1):8–22, 1982.
132. Strach EP, Fan PL, O'Brien WJ. Penetrativity and wetting of topical fluoride preparations: an in vitro study. J Clin Prev Dent 1(6):11–13, 1979.
133. Fan, PL, O'Brien WJ, Craig RG. Wetting properties of sealants and glazes. Oper Dent 4(3):100–103, 1979.
134. Whitlock RP, Tesk JA, Widera GEO, Holmes A, Parry EE. Consideration of some factors influencing compatibility of dental porcelains and alloys. Part I. Thermo-physical properties. pp. 273–282 In Proc. 4th Int. Precious Metals Conference, Toronto, June 1980. Willowdale, Ontario: Pergamon Press Canada, 1981.
135. Kase HR, Tesk JA, Case ED. Elastic constants of two dental porcelains. J Mater Sci 20:524–531, 1985.
136. Kase HR, Tesk JA. Elastic constants of nonprecious alloys at room and elevated temperatures. Microfilmed Paper no. 791. (Delivered at) the annual meeting of the International Association for Dental Research, Dental Materials Group, Dallas, Texas, March 15–18, 1984.
137. Carter JM, Flynn HE, Meenaghan MA, Natiella JR, Akers CK, Baier RE. Organic surface film contamination of Vitallium implants. J Biomed Mater Res 15(6):843–851, 1981.
138. Carter JM, Sorensen SE, Johnson RR, Teitelbaum RL, Levine MS. Punch shear testing of extracted vital and endodontically treated teeth. J Biomech 16(10):841–848, 1983.
139. Carter JM. Unpublished data. State University of New York at Buffalo, School of Dental Medicine.
140. Doctors M, Carter JM. Thermal properties of non-metallic dental restoratives. Microfilmed Paper no. 163. (Delivered at) the annual meeting of the International Association for Dental Research, Dental Materials Group, Chicago, March 18–21, 1971.
141. Carter JM. Thermal properties of dental restoratives. Microfilmed Paper no. 564. (Delivered at) the annual meeting of the International Association for Dental Research, Dental Materials Group, Las Vegas, March 23–26, 1972.
142. Iglesias AM, Sorensen SE, Carter JM, Wilko RA. Some properties of high-copper amalgam alloys comparing hand and mechanical trituration. J Prosthet Dent 52(2):194–198, 1984.
143. Holland RI, Jørgensen RB, Ekstrand J. Strength and creep of dental amalgam: The effects of deviation from recommended procedure. J Prosthet Dent 54(2):189–194, 1985.
144. Øilo G, Gjerdet NR. Dental casting alloys with a low content of noble metals: Physical properties. Acta Odontol Scand. 41(2):111–116, 1983.
145. Øilo G, Espevik S. Kompresjonsstyrke og deformering hos dentale sementer. Nor Tannlaegeforen Tid 88(11):500–503, 1978.
146. Seghi RR, Daher T, Caputo A. Relative flexural strength of dental restorative ceramics. Dent Mater 6:181–184, 1990.
147. Craig RG (ed). Restorative Dental Materials. 9th ed, St. Louis: Mosby-Year Book, 1993.
148. Powers JM, Hostetler RW, Dennison JB. Thermal expansion of composite resins and sealants. J Dent Res 58(2):584–587, 1979.
149. O'Brien WJ, Groh CL, Boenke KM. A one-dimensional color order system for dental shade guides. Dent Mater 5:371–374, 1989.
150. Finger W, Komatsu M. Elastic and plastic properties of elastic dental impression materials. Dent Mater 1:129–134, 1985.
151. O'Brien WJ, Groh CL, Boenke KM. A new, small-color-difference equation for dental shades. J Dent Res 69:1762–1764, 1990.
152. O'Brien WJ, Groh CL, Boenke KM. Unpublished data. Ann Arbor: University of Michigan School of Dentistry.
153. Dootz ER, Koran A, Craig RG. Comparison of the physical properties of 11 soft denture liners. J Prosthet Dent 67:707–712, 1992.
154. Dootz ER, Koran A, Craig RG. Physical properties of three maxillofacial materials as a function of accelerated aging. J Prosthet Dent 71:379–383, 1994.
155. Craig RG, Sun Z. Trends in elastomeric impression materials. Oper Dent 19:138–145, 1994.
156. Craig RG, Urquiola NJ, Liu CC. Comparison of commercial elastomeric impression materials. Oper Dent 15:94–104, 1990.

157. Rueggeberg FA, Paschal S. Proportioning effect on physical and chemical properties of polysulfide impression material. J Prosthet Dent 72:406–413, 1994.
158. Willems G, Lambrechts P, Braem M, Celis JP, Vanherle G. A classification of dental composites according to their morphological and mechanical characteristics. Dent Mater 8:310–319, 1992.
159. Forss H, Seppä L, Lappalainen R. In vitro abrasion resistance and hardness of glass-ionomer cements. Dent Mater 7:36–39, 1991.
160. White SN, Yu Z. Physical properties of fixed prosthodontic, resin composite luting agents. Int J Prosthodont 6:384–389, 1993.
161. Murchison DF, Moore BK. Influence of curing time and distance on microhardness of eight light-cured liners. Oper Dent 17:135–141, 1992.
162. Natho SA, Chmielewski MB, Kirkup RE. Effects of Colgate Platinum Professional Toothwhitening System™ on microhardness of enamel, dentin, and composite resins. Compend Contin Educ Dent 15(suppl 17):S627–S630, 1994.
163. Pilo R, Cardash HS. Post-irradiation polymerization of different anterior and posterior visible light-activated resin composites. Dent Mater 8:299–304, 1992.
164. Pagniano RP, Johnston WM. The effect of unfilled resin dilution on composite resin hardness and abrasion resistance. J Prosthet Dent 70:214–218, 1993.
165. Hotta M, Hirukawa H. Abrasion resistance of restorative glass-ionomer cements with a light-cured surface coating. Oper Dent 19:42–46, 1994.
166. Miyawaki H, Taira M, Toyooka H, Wakasa K, Yamaki M. Hardness and fracture toughness of commercial core composite resins. Dent Mater J. 12:62–68, 1993.
167. Collys K, Slop D, Cleymaet R, Coomans D, Michotte Y. Load dependency and reliability of microhardness measurements on acid-etched enamel surfaces. Dent Mater 8:332–335, 1992.
168. Asmussen E, Uno S. Solubility parameters, fractional polarities, and bond strengths of some intermediary resins used in dentin bonding. J Dent Res 72:558–565, 1993.
169. Vassilakos N, Fernandes CP. Effect of salivary films on the surface properties of elastomeric impression materials. Eur J Prosthodont Rest Dent 2(1):29–33, 1993.
170. Bordenave L, Baquey Ch, Bareille R, et al. Endothelial cell compatibility testing of three different Pellethanes. J Biomed Mater Res 27:1367–1381, 1993.
171. Chung K. Effects of palladium addition on properties of dental amalgams. Dent Mater 8:190–192, 1992.
172. Boeree NR, Dove J, Cooper JJ, Knowles J, Hastings GW. Development of a degradable composite for orthopaedic use: mechanical evaluation of an hydroxyapatite-polyhydroxybutyrate composite material. Biomaterials 14:793–796, 1993.
173. Cattani-Lorente, M-A, Godin C, Meyer JM. Early strength of glass ionomer cements. Dent Mater 9:57–62, 1993.
174. White SN, Yu Z. Compressive and diametral tensile strengths of current adhesive luting agents. J Prosthet Dent 69:568–572, 1993.
175. Lewis BA, Burgess JO, Gray SE. Mechanical properties of dental base materials. Am J Dent 5:69–72, 1992.
176. Lekka MP, Papagiannoulis L, Eliades GC, Caputo AA. A comparative in vitro study of visible light-cured sealants. J Oral Rehabil 16:287–299, 1989.
177. Bapna MS, Mueller HJ. Fracture toughness, diametrical strength, and fractography of amalgam and of amalgam to amalgam bonds. Dent Mater 9:51–56, 1993.
178. Tam LE, Pulver E, McComb D, Smith DC. Physical properties of calcium hydroxide and glass-ionomer base and lining materials. Dent Mater 5:145–149, 1989.
179. Tam LE, McComb D, Pulver F. Physical properties of proprietary light-cured lining materials. Oper Dent 16:210–217, 1991.
180. Klooster J, Logan GI, Tjan AHL. Effects of strain rate on the behavior of elastomeric impression. J Prosthet Dent 66:292–298, 1991.
181. Cullen DR, Sandrik JL. Tensile strength of elastomeric impression materials, adhesive and cohesive bonding. J Prosthet Dent 62:142–145, 1989.
182. Hergenrother RW, Wabers HD, Cooper SL. Effect of hard segment chemistry and strain on the stability of polyurethanes: in vivo biostability. Biomaterials 14:449–458, 1993.
183. Caycik S, Jagger RG. The effect of cross-linking chain length on mechanical properties of a dough-molded poly(methylmethacrylate) resin. Dent Mater 8:153–157, 1992.
184. Lee SY, Greener EH. Effect of excitation energy on dentine bond strength and composite properties. J Dent 22:175–181, 1994.
185. Sano H, Ciucchi B, Matthews WG, Pashley DH. Tensile properties of mineralized and demineralized human and bovine dentin. J Dent Res 73:1205–1211, 1994.
186. Bryant RW, Mahler DB. Modulus of elasticity in bending of composites and amalgams. J Prosthet Dent 56:243–248, 1986.
187. Jamani KD, Harrington E, Wilson HJ. Rigidity of elastomeric impression materials. J Oral Rehabil. 16:241–248, 1989.
188. Beatty MW, Pidaparti RMV. Elastic and fracture properties of dental direct filling materials. Biomaterials 14:999–1002, 1993.
189. O'Brien WJ. Magnesia ceramic jacket crowns. Dent Clin North Am 29:719–723, 1985.
190. Swift EJ Jr, LeValley BD, Boyer DB. Evaluation of new methods for composite repair. Dent Mater 8:362–365, 1992.
191. Dhummarungrong S, Moore BK, Avery DR. Properties related to strength and resistance to abrasion of VariGlass VLC, Fuji II L.C., Ketac-Silver, and Z-100 composite resin. ASDC J Dent Child 61:17–20, 1994.
192. Moroi HH, Okimoto K, Moroi R, Terada Y. Numeric approach to the biomechanical analysis of thermal effects in coated implants. Int J Prosthodont 6:564–572, 1993.
193. Anusavice KJ, Hojjatie B, Dehoff PH. Influence of metal thickness on stress distribution in metal-ceramic crowns. J Dent Res 65:1173–1178, 1986.
194. Pamenius M, Ohlson NG. The determination of elastic constants by dynamic experiments. Dent Mater 2:246–250, 1986.
195. Farah JW, Craig RG, Meroueh KA. Finite element analysis of three- and four-unit bridges. J Oral Rehabil 16:603–611, 1989.
196. Akagi K, Okamoto Y, Matsuura T, Horibe T. Properties of test metal ceramic titanium alloys. J Prosthet Dent 68:462–467, 1992.
197. Carr AB, Brantley WA. New high-palladium casting alloys: Part 1. Overview and initial studies. Int J Prosthodont 4:265–275, 1991.
198. Morris HF. Properties of cobalt-chromium metal ceramic alloys after heat treatment. J Prosthet Dent 62:426–433, 1989.
199. Morris HF. Veterans Administration Cooperative Studies Project No. 147/242. Part VII: The mechanical properties of metal ceramic alloys as cast and after simulated porcelain firing. J Prosthet Dent 61:160–169, 1989.
200. Weerkamp AH, Uyen HM, Busscher HJ. Effect of zeta potential and surface energy on bacterial adhesion to uncoated and saliva-coated human enamel and dentin. J Dent Res 67:1483–1487, 1988.
201. Walsh WR, Guzelsu N. Ion concentration effects on bone streaming potentials and zeta potentials. Biomaterials 14:331–336, 1993.
202. Fujimoto K, Minato M, Tadokoro H, Ikada Y. Platelet deposition onto polymeric surfaces during shunting. J Biomed Mater Res 27:335–343, 1993.
203. Shirazi-Adl A, Dammak M, Paiement G. Experimental determination of friction characteristics at the trabecular bone/porous-coated metal interface in cementless implants. J Biomed Mater Res 27:167–175, 1993.

204. Graiver D, Durall RL, Okada T. Surface morphology and friction coefficient of various types of Foley catheter. Biomaterials 14:465–469, 1993.
205. Inoue T, Saitoh M, Nishiyama M. Thermal properties of glass ionomer cement. J Nihon Univ Sch Dent. 35:252–257, 1993.
206. Fukase Y, Saitoh M, Kaketani M, Ohashi M, Nishiyama M. Thermal coefficients of paste-paste type pulp capping cements. Dent Mater J. 11:189–196, 1992.
207. Pamenius M, Ohlson NG. Determination of thermal properties of impression materials. Dent Mater 8:140–144, 1992.
208. Brantley WA, Kerby RE. Thermal diffusivity of glass ionomer cement systems. J Oral Rehabil 20:61–68, 1993.
209. Scherrer SS, de Rijk WG. The fracture resistance of all-ceramic crowns on supporting structures with different elastic moduli. Int J Prosthodont 6:462–467, 1993.
210. Haug SP, Andres CJ, Munoz CA, Okamura M. Effects of environmental factors on maxillofacial elastomers: Part III - Physical properties. J Prosthet Dent 68:644–651, 1992.
211. Eldiwany M, Powers JM, George LA. Mechanical properties of direct and post-cured composites. Am J Dent 6:222–224, 1993.
212. Covey DA, Tahaney SR, Davenport JM. Mechanical properties of heat-treated composite resin restorative materials. J Prosthet Dent 68:458–461, 1992.
213. Tam LE, Brown JW. The tear resistance of various impression materials with and without modifiers. J Prosthet Dent 63:282–285, 1990.
214. Mahler DB, Adey JD. Factors influencing the creep of dental amalgam. J Dent Res 70:1394–1400, 1991.
215. O'Kane C, Oliver RG, Blunden RE. Surface roughness and droplet contact angle measurement of various orthodontic bonding cements. Br J Orthod 20:297–305, 1993.
216. Cullen DR, Mikesell JW, Sandrik JL. Stability of elastomeric impression materials and voids in gypsum casts. J Prosthet Dent 66:261–265, 1991.
217. Arshady R. Microspheres for biomedical applications: preparation of reactive and labelled microspheres. Biomaterials 14:5–15, 1993.
218. Smith LT, Powers JM, Ladd D. Mechanical properties of new denture resins polymerized by visible light, heat, and microwave energy. Int J Prosthodont 5:315–320, 1992.
219. Papadogiannis Y, Lakes RS, Petrou-Americanos A, Theothoridou-Pahini S. Temperature dependence of the dynamic viscoelastic behavior of chemical-and light-cured composites. Dent Mater 9:118–122, 1993.
220. Lautenschlager EP, Monaghan P. Titanium and titanium alloys as dental materials. Int Dent J 43:245–253, 1993.
221. de Gee AJ, Feilzer AJ, Davidson CL. True linear polymerization shrinkage of unfilled resins and composites determined with a linometer. Dent Mater 9:11–14, 1993.
222. Ivoclar Williams, Amherst, NY: 14228.
223. Jeneric/Pentron Inc, Wallingford, Conn: 06492.
224. Li J, Alatli-Kut I, Hermansson L. High-strength dental gypsum prepared by cold isostatic pressing. Biomaterials 14:1186–1187, 1993.
225. Jørgensen KD. Thermal expansion of addition polymerization (Type II) silicone impression materials. Aust Dent J 27:377–381, 1982.
226. Kawano F, Dootz ER, Koran A, Craig RG. Sorption and solubility of 12 soft denture liners. J Prosthet Dent 72:393–398, 1994.
227. Tietge JD, Dixon DL, Breeding LC, Leary JM, Aquilino SA. In vitro investigation of the wear of resin composite materials and cast direct retainers during removable partial denture placement and removal. Int J Prosthodont 5:145–153, 1992.
228. Onose H. Properties and characteristics. Section 1: Physical and mechanical properties. In Katsuyama S, Ishikawa T, Fujii B (eds). Glass Ionomer Dental Cement - The Materials and Their Clinical Use. St. Louis: I Shiyaku EuroAmerica, 1993.
229. Nicholson JW, Anstice HM, McLean JW. A preliminary report on the effect of storage in water on the properties of commercial light-cured glass-ionomer cements. Br Dent J 173:98–101, 1992.
230. Kim KN, Craig RG, Koran A. Viscosity of monophase addition silicones as a function of shear rate. J Prosthet Dent 67:794–798, 1992.
231. Seghi RR, Denry I, Brajevic F. Effects of ion exchange on hardness and fracture toughness of dental ceramics. Int J Prosthodont 5:309–314, 1992.
232. von Fraunhofer JA, Argyropoulos DC. Properties of periodontal dressings. Dent Mater 6:51–55, 1990.
233. Gorodovsky S, Zidan O. Retentive strength, disintegration, and marginal quality of luting cements. J Prosthet Dent 68:269–274, 1992.
234. Roeder LB, Fulton RS, Powers JM. Bond strength of repaired glass ionomer core materials. Am J Dent 24:15–18, 1991.
235. Eliades G, Palaghias G. In vitro characterization of visible light-cured glass ionomer liners. Dent Mater 9:198–203, 1993.
236. DeWald JP, Nakajima H, Schneiderman E, Okabe T. Wettability of impression materials treated with disinfectants. Am J Dent 5:103–108, 1992.
237. Chong YH, Soh G, Setchell DJ, Wickens JL. The relationship between contact angles of die stone on elastomeric impression materials and voids in stone casts. Dent Mater 6:162–166, 1990.
238. Sturdevant CM, Roberson TM, Heyman HO, Sturdevant JR (eds). The Art and Science of Operative Dentistry. St. Louis: Mosby, 1995.

Appendix

B

Periodic Chart of the Elements

GROUP	I	II	3	4	5	6	7	8			1	2	III	IV	V	VI	VII	0
VALENCES / PERIOD	+1	+2	VARIABLE										+3	−4+4	−3+5	−2+6	−1+7	0
1	1 **H** 1.00797 ±0.00001																	2 **He** 4.0026 ±0.00005
2	3 **Li** 6.941 ±0.0005	4 **Be** 9.0122 ±0.00005											5 **B** 10.811 ±0.003	6 **C** 12.01115 ±0.00005	7 **N** 14.0067 ±0.00005	8 **O** 15.9994 ±0.0001	9 **F** 18.9984 ±0.00005	10 **Ne** 20.183 ±0.0005
3	11 **Na** 22.9898 ±0.00005	12 **Mg** 24.312 ±0.0005											13 **Al** 26.9815 ±0.00005	14 **Si** 28.086 ±0.001	15 **P** 30.9738 ±0.00005	16 **S** 32.064 ±0.003	17 **Cl** 35.453 ±0.001	18 **Ar** 39.948 ±0.0005
4	19 **K** 39.102 ±0.0005	20 **Ca** 40.08 ±0.005	21 **Sc** 44.956 ±0.0005	22 **Ti** 47.90 ±0.005	23 **V** 50.942 ±0.0005	24 **Cr** 51.996 ±0.001	25 **Mn** 54.9380 ±0.00005	26 **Fe** 55.847 ±0.003	27 **Co** 58.9332 ±0.00005	28 **Ni** 58.71 ±0.005	29 **Cu** 63.54 ±0.005	30 **Zn** 65.37 ±0.005	31 **Ga** 69.72 ±0.005	32 **Ge** 72.59 ±0.005	33 **As** 74.9216 ±0.00005	34 **Se** 78.96 ±0.005	35 **Br** 79.909 ±0.002	36 **Kr** 83.80 ±0.005
5	37 **Rb** 85.47 ±0.005	38 **Sr** 87.62 ±0.005	39 **Y** 88.905 ±0.0005	40 **Zr** 91.22 ±0.005	41 **Nb** 92.906 ±0.0005	42 **Mo** 95.94 ±0.005	43 **Tc** (99)	44 **Ru** 101.07 ±0.005	45 **Rh** 102.905 ±0.0005	46 **Pd** 106.4 ±0.05	47 **Ag** 107.870 ±0.003	48 **Cd** 112.40 ±0.005	49 **In** 114.82 ±0.005	50 **Sn** 118.69 ±0.005	51 **Sb** 121.75 ±0.005	52 **Te** 127.60 ±0.005	53 **I** 126.9044 ±0.00005	54 **Xe** 131.30 ±0.005
6	55 **Cs** 132.905 ±0.0005	56 **Ba** 137.34 ±0.005	57 *__La__ 138.91 ±0.005	72 **Hf** 178.49 ±0.005	73 **Ta** 180.948 ±0.0005	74 **W** 183.85 ±0.005	75 **Re** 186.2 ±0.05	76 **Os** 190.2 ±0.05	77 **Ir** 192.2 ±0.05	78 **Pt** 195.09 ±0.005	79 **Au** 196.967 ±0.0005	80 **Hg** 200.59 ±0.005	81 **Tl** 204.37 ±0.005	82 **Pb** 207.19 ±0.005	83 **Bi** 208.980 ±0.0005	84 **Po** (210)	85 **At** (210)	86 **Rn** (222)
7	87 **Fr** (223)	88 **Ra** (226)	89 †**Ac** (227)	104 (257)														

*Lanthanum Series

58	59	60	61	62	63	64	65	66	67	68	69	70	71
Ce	**Pr**	**Nd**	**Pm**	**Sm**	**Eu**	**Gd**	**Tb**	**Dy**	**Ho**	**Er**	**Tm**	**Yb**	**Lu**
140.12 ±0.005	140.907 ±0.0005	144.24 ±0.005	(147)	150.35 ±0.005	151.96 ±0.005	157.25 ±0.005	158.924 ±0.0005	162.50 ±0.005	164.930 ±0.0005	167.26 ±0.005	168.934 ±0.0005	173.04 ±0.005	174.97 ±0.005

†Actinium Series

90	91	92	93	94	95	96	97	98	99	100	101	102	103
Th	**Pa**	**U**	**Np**	**Pu**	**Am**	**Cm**	**Bk**	**Cf**	**Es**	**Fm**	**Md**	**No**	**Lw**
232.038 ±0.0005	(231)	238.03 ±0.005	(237)	(244)	(243)	(245)	(247)	(249)	(254)	(255)	(256)	(253)	(257)

Appendix C

Units and conversion factors

Unit	SI equivalent
Angstrom (Å)	1×10^{-10} meter (m)
Angstrom (Å)	1×10^{-1} nanometer (nm)
nanometer (nm)	1×10^{-9} meter (m)
micrometer (μm)	1×10^{-6} meter (m)
inch (in)	0.0254 meter (m)
inch (in)	2.54 centimeter (cm)
pound (lb)	0.4536 kilogram (kg)
dyne	1×10^{-5} newton (N)
pound force (lbf)	4.4482 newton (N)
erg	1×10^{-7} joule (J)
Calorie (Cal)	4.1868 joule (J)
Btu	1055.06 joule (J)
dyne/cm^2	1×10^{-1} newton/meter^2 (N/m^2)
atmosphere	1.013×10^5 N/m^2 (Pascal, Pa)
pound per square inch (psi)	6.895×10^3 N/m^2 (Pascal, Pa)
pound per square inch (psi)	6.895×10^{-3} MN/m^2 (MPa)
kg/cm^2	9.804×10^4 MN/m^2 (Pa)

1 pennyweight (dwt) (Troy) = 1.555 g
20 dwt = 1 ounce (Troy) = 1.097 ounce (Avoirdupois)

Photomicrograph distance: $\mu m/cm = \dfrac{10{,}000}{\text{magnification}}$

Temperature: $(°C \times 1.8) + 32 = °F$

$$\frac{(°F - 32)}{1.8} = °C$$

Prefixes for SI units

Multiply by this factor	Symbol	Prefix
10^{12}	T	tera
10^{9}	G	giga
10^{6}	M	mega
10^{3}	k	kilo
10^{2}	h	hecto
10	da	deca
10^{-1}	d	deci
10^{-2}	c	centi
10^{-3}	m	milli
10^{-6}	μ	micro
10^{-9}	n	nano
10^{-12}	p	pico
10^{-15}	f	femto
10^{-18}	a	atto

Appendix D

Longevity of Restorations Commonly Used in Dentistry

Gordon J. Christensen, DDS, MSD, PhD

Material / Estimated longevity	Indications	Contraindications	Strengths	Weaknesses
Aluminous porcelain crowns / 15 y	Restoration of teeth requiring good appearance and moderate strength	Heavy occlusal stress or other situations requiring maximum strength	Esthetics; moderate strength; lower cost than porcelain-fused-to-metal	Have only moderate strength; difficult to use for fixed prosthesis
Amalgam, silver / 14 y	Incipient, moderate-sized, and some large lesions in adolescents and adults	Large intracoronal restorations (cusp replacement); endodontically treated teeth	Good marginal seal; strength; longevity; manipulability; cariostatic activity	Tarnish; stains tooth; marginal breakdown
Cast gold (inlays, onlays, and crowns) / 20 y	Large lesions; teeth requiring additional strength; teeth used in rebuilding or changing occlusion	Adolescents; high caries activity; persons who object to gold display	Reproduces anatomy well; onlays and crowns may increase strength of tooth; longevity; wears occlusally similar to enamel	Cement margin; time required for placement; high fee; poor esthetics; thermal sensitivity
Compacted golds (gold foil, powdered gold, mat gold) / 24 y	Initial Class III and V lesions for patients of all ages	Periodontally unstable teeth; high caries activity; persons who object to gold display	Margin integrity; longevity	Time-consuming; high fee; poor esthetics
Composite resin (Class I, II) / 8 y	Class I and II areas of high esthetic need; patients sensitive to metal	Bruxers and clenchers; no enamel occlusal stops present	Esthetics; may strengthen tooth with acid-etch concept	Wear of restoration during service; no cariostatic activity; may create sensitive tooth
Composite resin (Class III, IV, V) / 10 y	Incipient to large Class III, IV, and V lesions	Teeth where coronal portion is nearly gone	Esthetics; ease of use; strength	Pulp irritant; margin breakdown over time
Glass-ionomer / 8 y	High caries activity; Class III, IV, and repairs	Areas of high esthetic need or areas of difficult moisture control	Cariostatic activity	Only fair esthetics; time-consuming to place
Porcelain-fused-to-metal crowns / 20 y	Teeth requiring full coverage and subject to heavy occlusal forces	Adolescents (because great amount of tooth reduction is necessary); potentially damaging to pulp	Strength; good marginal seal; esthetics	Appearance not as good as some others; wear of opposing teeth
Porcelain inlays and onlays (acid etched) / 10y	Class II and V locations where high esthetics is desired	Teeth that are grossly broken down requiring crowns	Esthetic potential extremely high; properly etched tooth and restoration increase strength of tooth	May create tooth sensitivity; may fracture during service
Porcelain jacket crowns / 13y	Anterior teeth requiring extensive coverage	Teeth subject to heavy occlusal forces	Esthetics	Lack of strength; poor marginal adaption

Index

Page numbers followed by "f" indicate figures; page numbers followed by "t" indicate tables.

A

Abrasion
  definition of, 115
  factors affecting rate of, 115–116, 116f, 116t
  handpiece instruments for, 118
Abrasive(s)
  dentifrices, 117
  denture cleaners, 117–118
  hardness of, 116t
  prophylaxis pastes, 117
Accelerators
  effect on setting, 56
  in gypsum-bonded investments, 61
Acid-etching, of enamel, 44, 45f, 106
Acids, for dentin conditioning, 45, 47f
Acrylic base(s)
  heat-cured
    advantages and disadvantages of, 84t, 86, 88
    composition and manufacture of, 83–85, 85f
    physical and mechanical properties of, 87–88
    spherical bead polymer in, 83
  high-impact
    heat-cure and phase inversion in manufacture of, 86
    rubber reinforced, 85–86, 86f
      advantages and disadvantages of, 84t
  polishing technique for, 119
Acrylic resin
  cements, 165
    modified, 165–166
  history of, 97
  soft liners
    advantages and disadvantages of, 90t
    plasticized, 91
  veneers
    polishing technique for, 119
Addition (vinyl) silicone impression materials. *See also* Condensation silicone rubber impression materials
  advantages and disadvantages of, 136
  composition of, 135
  vs condensation silicones, 135
  definition of, 143
  disinfection of, 136
  manipulation of, 129t, 136
    automatic mixers for, 136f
  mechanical properties of, 127t, 135–136
  troubleshooting of, 136
  use of, 135
Adhesion
  bonding mechanisms in, 43, 43f
  to dentin, 45, 46f, 47f
  to enamel, 44, 45f
  factors affecting bond strength in, 44
  of porcelain to metal, 290
    failure of, 291, 292f, 293
    promotion of, 291, 291f
  shrinkage and, 44, 44f
  tensile bond strengths between restoration materials and tooth substance, 48t
Adsorption, 41
Adventitious bursa
  definition of, 268
  from permanent implants, 266
Agar (reversible) hydrocolloid impression material
  advantages and disadvantages of, 129
  composition of
  disinfection of, 129
  handling properties of, 129t
  manipulation sequence for, 128
  mechanical properties of, 127, 127t
  specifications for, 124t
  storage of
    dimensional changes with, 128t
  troubleshooting of, 129
  uses for, 127
Alginate (irreversible) hydrocolloid impression materials
  advantages and disadvantages of, 131
  composition of, 130
  disinfection of, 132
  manipulation of, 129t, 130–131
  mechanical properties of, 130, 127t
  specifications for, 124t
  troubleshooting of, 131–132
  use of, 130
Alloy(s). *See also* Base metal alloy(s)
  base metal, 259–267
  castability of
    determination of, 242–243
  for crown-and-bridge restoration, 262t, 262–264, 263f
  gallium, 191, 191f
  hardening of
    heat treatment in, 181–182
  high-copper, 193
  high-gold
    American National Standards Institute/American Dental Association specifications and, 215
    composition ranges for, 217t, 218, 228–229

currently available, 215, 217t
disadvantages of, 229
heat treatment of, 219
in porcelain-fused-to-metal restorations, 228–229, 229t
properties of, 215, 217t, 218, 229t
role of alloying elements in, 215, 216t
homogenization of, 182
low-gold, 217t, 218
metals in
noble, 225–226
precious, 226
semiprecious, 226
for orthodontic wires, 275–279
palladium-silver, 218, 219f, 229–230
for porcelain-fused-to-metal restorations, 217t, 218–219
base metal, 231–232
biocompatibility, 228–229
classification of, 225, 225f
commercial, 226t
compatibility of porcelain-metal in, 228
composition of, 227t
gold-palladium, 230
gold-palladium-silver, 229
high-gold, 228–229, 229f
metal classification in, 225–226
palladium-cobalt, 231
palladium-copper, 230–231
palladium-silver, 229–230
physical and chemical properties of, 227–228, 229t
selection of, 225
criteria for, 232–234
thermal properties of, 228
titanium, 232
precious metal
cast microstructure of, 220, 221f
crystal structure of, 220, 220f
heat treatment of, 219
temperatures for, 175
titanium, 232, 267–268
for implants, 324
Alloy systems
equilibrium phase in, 180
phase diagrams of, 179f, 180f
solid solution phase of, 179
Amalgamators, 195
Amalgam(s)
biocompatibility of, 198–199
classification of, 187f, 187t
clinical performance of, 194–196
composition of, 187–188
correlations between laboratory properties and clinical data
for corrosion, 196–197, 197f
for creep, 196, 196f
corrosion of, 193t, 193–194
creep of, 192–193, 196, 196f, 199, 342
definition of, 199
gallium, 190, 199
clinical behavior of, 195
corrosion of, 194
structure of, 191, 191f
high-copper systems
biocompatibility of, 198
blended, 188–189, 189f
corrosion of, 193
definition of, 199
marginal fracture of, 194–195
palladium in, 193
setting reactions of, 190–191, 191f
single-composition, 189
history of, 187
investigational, 189
marginal breakdown of, 194, 194f
prevention of, 195
physical properties of, 192t, 192–193
polishing technique for, 118
traditional
lathe-cut, 188, 188f
setting reactions of, 190, 190f
spherical, 188, 189f
Amalgam restorations
adhesives vs cavity varnish under, 170
base under
glass ionomers vs zinc phosphate, 169
liner under
zinc oxide–eugenol vs calcium hydroxide, 169–170
American Dental Association (ADA)
specifications of
for dental impression materials, 123, 124t
for high-gold alloy, 215
American National Standards Institute (ANSI)
specifications of
for dental impression materials, 123–124, 124t
for high-gold alloy, 215
Annealing, 182, 183
Autopolymerizing denture base, 84t, 86

B

Base metal alloy(s)
chromium-containing
currently available commercial, 260t
mechanical properties of, 260–261
classification of, 259
cobalt-chromium, 259–260, 263–265
cobalt-chromium-nickel, 260
commercially pure titanium, 266–267
for crown-and-bridge, 262t 262–265
nickel-chromium, 260–262, 263
for partial dentures, 259–262
chemical properties of, 261
disadvantages of, 261–262
physical properties of, 260
for permanent implants, 265–266
for porcelain-fused-to-metal restorations, 231–232
titanium, 267–268
Basic materials
classification of, 1f
properties of, 1–2, 2t
selection of, 1–2
strengths of, 2–3
Benzoyl peroxide, in heat-cured acrylic manufacture, 83
Binders, in gypsum-bonded investments, 61, 61f, 62
Bioactivity, of bioactive glasses, 325
Biocompatibility
of amalgams, 198–199
of chromium-type alloys, 264
of composite systems, 106
of titanium, 268
Bleaching
dental office systems, 121
home systems, 120
side effects of, 121
Bonding agent, dentin, 106
Bonds, metallic, 6, 7f, 8f
Bond strengths
in porcelain-fused-to-metal restorations, 228
between restoration materials and tooth structure, 332
Bone
augmentation materials for, 326f, 327, 327f
applications of, 327
calcium-phosphate materials for, 327, 327f
classification of, 326f

Bridges, metal-ceramic, soldering of, 306–307
Brinell hardness number (BHN), 18, 333
Brittle fracture, 8, 8f

C

Calcination
- definition of, 71
- dry, 53, 55
- wet, 53, 53f, 54, 55

Calcium hydroxide chelate cements
- advantages and disadvantages of,161
- applications of, 160
- biologic effects of, 161
- composition and setting of, 160–161
- properties of, 161
- as pulp-capping material, 160, 160f

Calcium sulfate dihydrate, in gypsum products, 51
Capillary penetration
- capillary rise and, 42f, 42–43, 43f
- effect on
  - of contact angle, 42f
  - of gap distance, 42f
- penetration coefficient and, 43, 360

Cast gypsum
- facture surface of, 57f
- water/powder ratio effect on, 56–57, 57f

Casting
- accuracy of
  - for gold restorations, 244
  - with gypsum-bonded investments, 68–70
- for cobalt alloys, 244
- expansion requirements for, 238t
- gold
  - troubleshooting, 244–245
- lost wax process, 237, 237f
  - direct and indirect, 237
- machines for
  - with centrifugal force, 242–243
  - with pneumatic force, 242
- melting in, 241
  - electrical, 242
  - methods of, 241t
  - torch, 241f, 241–242
- shrinkage in
  - gold alloy, 238
  - wax, 238
- thermal expansion of investments in
  - high-heat technique and, 238, 238f, 239t
  - phosphate-bonded investment, 239
  - water-immersion (hygroscopic) technique, 238–239, 239t
- wax pattern in
  - spruing of, 237, 237f, 239–241, 240f

Casting-ring liner
- dry ceramic, 70, 70f
- wet
  - effect on thermal expansion, 67, 69, 69f

Castings
- cleaning of, 243
- polishing of, 243–244

Cavity varnish, effect on composite resins, 106
Cement(s)
- acrylic resins, 165
  - modified, 165–166
- applications of, 151
- for bases under amalgam restorations
  - glass ionomers vs zinc phosphate, 169
- calcium hydroxide chelate, 160f, 160–161
- classification of, 152, 152f, 152t
- clinical decision scenarios for, 167–171
- for crowns
  - glass ionomers vs zinc phosphate, 168
  - zinc phosphate vs resin, 168
- current brands of
  - composite restorative, 154t
  - permanent luting, 153t
  - temporary, 154t
- EBA and chelate, 159–160
- glass-ionomer, 151
- history of, 151–152
- for liners under amalgam
  - zinc oxide–eugenol vs calcium hydroxide, 169–170
- luting
  - current brands of, 153t
  - properties of, 154t
- phenolate-based, 157–161
- phosphate-based, 154–157
- polycarboxylate (carboxylate)-based, 151, 161–165
  - classification of, 152t
  - history of, 161
- polymer-based, 165–166
  - classification of, 152t
  - properties of, 154t
- poly(methyl methacrylate), 152
- selection and use of, 153t, 167
- selection of, 153
- two-paste systems, 151
- zinc oxide–eugenol, 157–158
- zinc oxide–eugenol
  - reinforced, 158–159

Ceramic, definition of, 11
Ceramic restorations
- milled
  - computer-assisted design and computer-assisted manufacture of, chairside, 297–298, 298f
  - copy milling, Celay system, 298f, 298 299f

Ceramics. *See also* Basic materials
- classification of, 1, 1f
- clinical applications of, 5
- fractures in, 4f, 5
- for implants
  - calcium-phosphate, 325
  - inert vs bioactive, bioresorbable, 324–325
- properties of, 2, 2t
- stress concentration effect on, 3, 4f, 5

Chromium-containing alloy(s). *See also named, eg, Cobalt-chromium alloy*
- advantages and disadvantages of, 281t, 282
- cobalt-chromium, 259–261, 263–266
- cobalt-chromium-nickel, 260–262, 276–278
- nickel-chromium, 231–232, 265–266

Cobalt alloys
- casting for, 244
- phosphate-bonded investment for, 244

Cobalt-chromium alloy
- casting for, 244
- ethyl silicate–bonded investments for, 261
- for partial dentures, 259–260, 260t
  - manipulation of, 261
- phosphate-bonded investments for, 249–250, 261
- surgical and for permanent implants
  - manipulation of, 265–266
  - mechanical properties of, 265, 265t

Cobalt-chromium-nickel alloy
- advantages and disadvantages of, 281t, 282
- mechanical properties of, 276t
- for orthodontic wire, 276t, 277–278
- for partial dentures, 260
- tempers of, 277–278

Cold working (work hardening), 181, 183

Colloids
  association, 42
  classification of, 41, 41t
  large molecules, 41–42
  lyophobic, 41, 41t
Color
  alloy composition and, 227
  of an object, 27–28
  detection by observer, 28, 28f
  illuminant and, 25–27
  matching of
    metamerism and, 30–31, 31f
  measurements of, 30–31
  observer and, 28
  reflected
    mixing of, 28
  shade guides for, 32, 337–338
  systems for
    Commission Internationale de l'Eclairage, 29f, 29–30
    Munsell, 28–29, 29f
Color fatigue, 28
Colorimeter(s)
  chromascan, 30f
  in color measurement, 30
  IDL Color-Eye, 30f
  Minolta Chroma-Meter, 30f
Color systems, clinical color-matching tolerances and, 29t, 29–30
Commission Internationale de l'Eclairage (CIE) color system, 29f, 29–30
Composite materials, microstructure of, 98f
Composite resin(s)
  vs amalgams
    for cores, 111
  for anterior restorations, 108
    light-cured vs chemically cured, 110
  clinical decision scenarios for, 110–111
  composition and reaction in, 98–100
  for cores
    composite vs amalgam, 111
  coupling agents in, 99, 111
  definition of, 97, 111
  filler composition in, 98–99
  fine-particle, 97, 108t, 111
  history of, 97
  hybrids, 98, 98f, 108t, 111
  inhibitors and stabilizers in, 100
  initiators and accelerators in, 99–100
  macrofills, 98, 99f, 108t, 112
  microfine, 97–98, 98f, 108t, 112
  organic matrix in, 99
  pigments in, 100
  polishing technique for, 110–120, 119f, 120f
  for posterior restorations, 107–108
  for restorations
    dentin adhesives vs glass ionomer liners under, 171
  selection of, 107–108, 108t
Composite system(s)
  biocompatibility of, 106
  color stability of, 103
  cure depth of, 105
  curing lights for, 101f
  finishing of, 107
  mechanical properties of, 103, 103t
  placement of, 106–107
  polymerization shrinkage in, 100-101
    correction of, 102, 102f
  properties of, 100–106
    comparison of average, 101t
  radiopacity of, 103
  sealing procedure for placement of, 106
  setting time for, 100
  single-paste, 100
    manipulation of, 107
  solubility of, 102
  thermal properties of, 102
  two-paste, 100
    manipulation of, 106
  water sorption of, 102, 396
  wear of, 103–104
    factors in, 104f, 104–105, 105f
Compressive strength
  of ethyl silicate–bonded investments, 252t
  of phosphate-bonded investments, 250t
Computer-assisted design and computer-assisted manufacture (CAD/CAM)
    inlay vs Empress inlays, 300–301
Computer-assisted design and computer-assisted manufacturer (CAD/CAM, Cerec) chairside system, 298f
  advantages and disadvantages of, 297–298
  utilization sequence with, 297
Condensation, of direct gold filling materials, 209, 210f
Condensation silicone rubber impression materials. *See also* Addition (vinyl) silicone impression materials
  advantages and disadvantages of, 134
  composition of, 134
  definition of, 143
  disinfection of, 135
  manipulation of, 129t, 143
  mechanical properties of, 127t, 134
  troubleshooting of, 134–135
  use of, 134
Conductivity, thermal, 19, 22
Contact angle
  capillary penetration effect on, 42f
  degree of wetting and, 40f, 40t, 40–41, 41f
  liquid phase, 339–340
  solid phase, 340
Contamination, in casting, 241
Core(s)
  composite vs amalgam, 111
  glass ionomer vs amalgam, 171
  spinel injection-molded, 294–296
Coring, 182
Corrosion
  eta prime phase reaction in, 193
  of gallium amalgams, 194
  galvanic
    clinical effects of, 196f, 196–197, 197f
  gamma 2 phase reaction in, 193
  of high-copper amalgams, 193
  marginal in traditional amalgam, 193, 193t
  mercury release during, 193–194
  surgical alloy resistance to, 265
Coupling agents
  in composite materials, 99
  wear and, 105
Crack propagation, 3, 4
  porcelain bonded to metal, 290, 290f
Creep
  of amalgams, 192–193, 199
    static and dynamic method of, 342
  correlation with marginal fracture for amalgam restorations, 196, 196f
Cristobalite
  in gypsum-bonded investments, 62, 63f
  in gypsum investment powder
    effect on thermal behavior, 63f
  thermal expansion of, 67, 67f, 238, 239f
Cross-linking agents, in heat-cured acrylic manufacture, 85
Crown-and-bridge alloy(s). *See also* Partial dentures
  biologic effects of
    with beryllium-containing, 264–265
    with chromium-type, 264
    with nickel-type, 264

casting shrinkage of, 264
chromium-type, 262t, 262–263
manipulation of, 264
properties of, 263–264
cobalt-chromium, 262
nickel- and chromium-based
advantages and disadvantages of, 265
nickel-chromium, 263, 263f
Crown(s)
all-ceramic, 293–294
castable porcelain, 295, 295f
cements for, 168
glass ionomers vs zinc phosphate for, 168
zinc phosphate vs resin cement for, 168
platinum-bonded alumina
electroformed die for, 310
porcelain-fused-to-metal
alloy selection for, 233
Crystal lattices
unit cells of, 175–176, 177f, 183
definition of, 175, 183
Crystallites, formation of, 176–177, 178f
Cure
depth of
in chemically activated systems, 105
in light-activated systems, 105

D

Dentifrices
composition of, 117
selection of, 117
Dentin
bonding agents for, 47f
bonding to, 45, 46f, 47f
composition of, 45
conditioners for, 45, 47f
conditioning and resin-impregnation for bonding, 45, 46f
Denture base polymer(s)
acrylic, 86
classification of, 83f
comparison of materials, 84t
composition and manufacture of, 83–86
autopolymerizing, 86
heat-cured acrylic, 83, 85, 85f
high-impact acrylic, 85–86, 86f
injection-molded plastic, 84t, 86
fabrication of
effect on physical and mechanical properties, 87–89
fiber-reinforcement of, 89–90
history of, 82–83
light-activated materials, 87
nylon, 87
physical and mechanical properties
light-activated fabrication and, 89
polycarbonate, 87
radiopacity of, 89
Dentures
bases for
future improvements in, 89–90
cleaners for
brushing with, 118
composition of, 117
investments for
strength of, 68
teeth in
acrylic, 287
porcelain, 287
Detail
loss of
in addition silicone cast, 136
in alginate hydrocolloid cast, 131
in condensation silicone rubber cast, 135
in polyether rubber cast, 138
in polysulfide rubber cast, 133
in zinc oxide–eugenol cast, 127
Dies
electroformed
construction procedures for, 309–310
for gold copings, 310
for platinum-bonded alumina crown, 310
vs stone dies, 310
stone, 51f, 52
Diffusion, in heat treatment, 182
Diffusivity, thermal, 19–20, 20f, 22
Dimensional change
in agar hydrocolloid impression material, 128t
in alginate hydrocolloid cast, 132
Dimethacrylate cements
advantages and disadvantages of, 167
applications of, 166
biologic effects of, 167
classification of, 152t
composition and setting of, 166
manipulation of, 166
properties of, 154t, 166–167
Direct gold filling (DGF) material(s)
advantages and disadvantages of, 204
alloyed, 208, 208f
classification of, 203, 204f
clinical advantages of, 203
clinical decision scenarios for, 211–212
clinical processing of, 208–209
alcohol flame method, 209, 209f
desorbing (annealing) in, 208
desorbing in, 208, 213
hot plate method, 208, 209
powdered gold method, 209
condensation of, 211
controlling factors in, 209
manual, 209, 210f
mechanical, 209, 210f
electrolytic precipitate (mat gold), 206–207
finishing of, 211
gold foil, 203, 205–206
vs composite restoration in anterior tooth, 212
platinized, 206
indications for, 204
manipulation of, 211
mat foil, 207
powdered gold, 207f, 207–208, 211
properties of, 205t
Disinfection
of addition (vinyl) silicone impressions, 136
of agar (reversible) hydrocolloid impressions, 129f
of alginate (irreversible) hydrocolloid impressions, 132
of condensation silicone rubber impressions, 135
of dental impression compound, 125
of gypsum casts, 60
of polyether rubber impressions, 138
of polysulfide rubber impressions, 133
of zinc oxide–eugenol impressions, 127
Disks, for polishing and finishing, 118, 121
Dislocation
in ceramic materials, 6, 7f
definition of, 11
ductility of metals and, 6
in intermetallic compounds, 7f, 8
in plastic deformation, 180–181, 181f
Distortion
of addition silicone cast, 136
of alginate hydrocolloid cast, 131
of condensation silicone rubber cast, 135
of impression compound cast, 125
of polyether rubber cast, 138
of polysulfide rubber cast, 133

troubleshooting
in gold casting, 244
of zinc oxide–eugenol cast, 127
Dough technique, in acrylic manufacture, 82–83
Ductility. *See also* Elongation
of metals
clinical applications of, 8, 8f
effect on stress concentration, 4f, 5
mechanism of, 5–6, 6f, 7f
Duplicating materials, 138
classification of, 138f

E

EBA. *See* Ethoxybenzoic acid (EBA) cement
Edentulous patient, problem of, 315
Elastic limit (proportional limit), 16, 16f, 366
Elastic modulus, 15f, 15–16
in polymers, 9, 9f
of various materials, 347–351
Elastic strain, 180
Electrical and electrochemical property(ies)
electrical resistivity, 22, 22t
electrode potentials, 20–21, 21t
Electrode potentials, 20–21, 21t
Electrolytic precipitate (mat gold)
advantages and disadvantages of, 208
condensation of, 211
finishing of, 211
manipulation of, 211
manufacture of, 206f, 206–207
properties of, 205t, 208
Electroplating
commercial products for, 310
of dies, 309. *See* Dies, electroformed
galvanic corrosion relationship with, 309
throwing power of solutions in, 309
Elements, metallic, 175t
Elgiloy (soft temper, chromium-cobalt-nickel alloy), 276t, 277
Elongation. *See also* Ductility
clinical importance of
in porcelain-fused-to-metal restorations, 227
definition of, 17, 22
percent of, 361–362
Empress inlays, computer-assisted design and computer-assisted manufacture (CAD/CAM) vs, 300–301
Enamel
acid-etching of, 44, 45f, 106
composition of, 44
Esthetic appearance
color and, 25–31
double layer effects on, 32, 33f
factors in, 25
fluorescence, 32, 35
gloss and, 31–32, 32f
interaction of illumination, object, observer in, 25f, 25–28
translucency and, 31
Ethoxybenzoic acid (EBA) cement, 159–160
Ethyl silicate–bonded investments
advantages of, 252–253
applications of, 251
composition of, 251–252
properties of, 252, 252t
disadvantages of, 253
Eugenol, effect on composite resins, 106
Excavating burs, for polishing and finishing, 118
Expansion
of gypsum-bonded investments
control of, 67–68, 68f
setting, 65–66, 66f
thermal, 66–67, 67f

F

Fatigue, curves for glass-filled composite resin, 17, 17f
Filler
in composites, 98–99, 99f
in gypsum-bonded investments, 60, 61–62, 64–65
wear and, 104, 104f, 105f
Finishing
of composites, 107
methods of
wear and, 105
Fluids, types and behavior of, 17
Fluorescence, 31, 35
Fluoride cements, 156
Fluxes and antifluxes, for soldering, 304, 310
Fracture
of amalgam restorations
prevention of marginal, 195
brittle, 8, 8f
of ceramics, 4f, 5
of high-copper alloys, 194–195
of metals, 179

G

Gallium alloys, 191, 191f
Gelation, of agar hydrocolloid impression material, 127, 128
Glass-ionomer cements
advantages and disadvantages of, 165
applications of, 163, 163f
biologic effects of, 165
classification of, 164
composition and setting of, 163–164
development of, 163
manipulation of, 164
properties of, 154t, 164–165
vs zinc phosphate for crown cementation, 168
Glass-ionomer vs amalgam, for cores, 171
Glass-transition temperature, of polymers, 82, 93
Gloss, 31–32, 32f
Gold alloy(s), 208, 208f
condensation of, 211
Electraloy RV, 208, 208f
finishing of, 211
manipulation of, 211
mat foil–calcium, 208
polishing technique for, 118–119
Gold coping, for porcelain-fused-to-metal restorations, 310
Gold foil
advantages and disadvantages of, 206
cohesive and noncohesive, 203
vs composite restoration in maxillary anterior tooth, 212
condensation of, 211
finishing of, 211
manipulation of, 211
manufacture of, 205, 205f
plastinized, 206, 211
properties of, 205, 205t
Gold-palladium alloys
advantages and disadvantages of, 230
for porcelain-fused-to-metal restorations
selection of, 233
silver content of, 230
Gold-palladium-silver alloys, 229
disadvantages of, 229
for porcelain-fused-to-metal restorations
selection of, 233
properties of, 229t
Gold solder
composition of, 304t
mechanical properties of, 306, 306t

melting ranges of, 304t
for postceramic soldering, 307
Grinding, definition of, 115, 115f
Gypsum-bonded investments
casting accuracy and, 68–70
shrinkage and, 68–70, 69t
classification of, 60, 61f
components of
binder, 61, 61f
effect on setting and thermal behavior, 61–64
modifiers, 61, 64
refractory, 60
expansion techniques in
hygroscopic, 65, 66f
thermal, 65, 67, 67f
properties of, 64–68
expansion, 65–68
particle size of powder, 64–65
setting rate, 65
setting expansion in, 65–66, 66f
setting rate for, 65
thermal expansion in
hygroscopic technique, 66, 66f
thermal expansion technique, 67, 67f
typical materials in, 61t
Gypsum casts
disinfection of, 60
facture surface of, 57f
water/powder ratio effect on, 56–57, 57f
Gypsum product(s). *See also* Cast gypsum; Gypsum-bonded investments
apparent density of, 54
casts
disinfection of, 60
chemistry of, 52
classification of, 51f, 51–52
control of, 58, 59f
definition of, 51
gypsum-bonded investments, 60–70
manufacture of, 51, 53–54
dry calcination in, 53
high-strength plasters, 54, 54f
wet calcination in, 53, 53f, 54
medium-strength plasters, 54
microstructure of cast gypsum, 56–57
plaster, 51f, 52, 52t
plaster of Paris, 53, 53f
setting expansion for, 58, 58t, 59f
immersion effect on, 58
setting process for, 54–56
additive effect on, 56
rate of setting reaction in, 55–56
setting reaction in, 54–55
stages in, 55
volume changes during, 55
water requirement for, 55
setting rate for
control of, 58
manipulation and setting times in, 57
solubility of, 60
stone, 51f, 52, 52t
storage of, 70–71
strength of, 59t, 59–60
typical, 52t

H

Halide salts, effect on thermal expansion, of gypsum-bonded investments, 64
Handpiece instruments, for polishing and finishing, 118
Hardening
of precious metal alloys, 219, 221
processes for
cold working, 181, 183
heat treatment, 181–182
precipitation, 181
Hardness
abrasion rate and, 115, 116t
clinical importance of
in porcelain-fused-to-metal restorations, 227
definition of, 18
scales of, 18–19
Brinell, 333
Knoop, 356–358
Mohs, 360
Rockwell, 268
Vickers, 393–394
Heat treatment(s), 181–182
annealing, 182
residual stress, 182
Homogenizing heat treatment, 219, 221
Hydrocolloid, definition of, 143
Hygroscopic expansion techniques
in setting expansion, 65, 66f
in thermal expansion, 66, 66f
of mold, 238–239, 239t
Hysteresis, of agar hydrocolloid impression material, 127, 143

I

Illuminant. *See also* Object
color content of, 25, 26f
color-rendering index of, 27, 27t
dispersion of, 25, 26f
effect on color and appearance, 25–27
intensity distributions of, 25, 26f
interaction with object, 27–30
representative spectral distributions of, 26, 26f
in shade matching, 33
Imbibition, 128, 143
Implants. *See also* Osseointegration
base metal, 265–266
commercially pure titanium, 324
contraindications to, 315
criteria for successful
biomaterial and biomechanical factors in, 320, 320f
implant design, 322–323
mechanical properties, 321–322
surface chemistry and biological response, 321
surgical parameters for, 320–321
edentulous patient problem and, 315
failure of, 325–326
feedback mechanisms in loosening, 322, 322f
interfacial zone in, 322–323
material in, 322
future materials for, 326
indications for, 315–316, 316t
materials for
ceramics, 324–325
classification of, 323f, 324
metals, 324
osseointegration of, 316–320, 318f
Impression compound
advantages and disadvantages of, 125
composition of, 124
disinfection of, 125
mechanical properties of, 124, 125f
specification for, 124t
thermal properties of, 124
troubleshooting, 125
types and applications of, 124
Impression material(s)
classification of, 123, 123f
clinical decision scenarios for, 138–143
elastic
agar (reversible) hydrocolloid, 127–129
alginate (irreversible) hydrocolloid, 130–132

condensation silicone rubber, 134–135
flow in, 352–353
polyether rubber, 136–138, 143
polysulfide rubber (mercaptan), 132–133, 143
specifications for, 127t
nonelastic
dental impression compound Types I and II, 124–125, 125f
impression plaster, 124
zinc oxide–eugenol, 125–127
plaster, 123
polysulfides vs addition silicones
in busy practice, 140
for full-arch impression, 142–143
in dental school clinic, 139
for triple tray, 141
specifications for
American National Standards Institute/American Dental Association, 124t
waxes, 148
Impression plaster (plaster of Paris), 123
Impression waxes, 148, 148f
Infrared light
for soldering, 307
Injection molding
of core for all-ceramic crown, 294–296
of dental base polymers, 84t, 86
of dental bases
effect on physical and mechanical properties of, 88–89
of high-leucite, 296, 297f
Intermetallic compound, definition of, 11
Interpenetrating polymer network (IPN), 87–88, 92
Investment(s)
ethyl silicate–bonded, 251–253
green strength of, 252, 255
gypsum-bonded, 60–70. *See also* Gypsum-bonded investments
high-temperature, 249–255
for titanium casting, 253, 253t
uses of, 249
phosphate-bonded, 239, 239t, 249–251
strength of, 68
IPS Empress inlay vs Vita InCeram, 300–301

K

Knoop hardness number (KHN), 19, 19f, 356–358

L

Laser welding, 308, 309
Liner(s). *See also* Denture based polymer(s)
with amalgam restorations, 198
dentin adhesives vs glass ionomer under composite restorations, 171
soft
acrylic, 91
comparison of, 90t
polymer, 83t
silicone, 91–92
temporary, 90t, 92
zinc oxide–eugenol vs calcium hydroxide
under amalgam restorations, 169–170
Liquidus temperature, 175
of chromium-type surgical alloys, 265
Lubricants, abrasion rate and, 116
Luster, 31, 32f

M

Magnesia
in high-expansion porcelain core material
spinel injection-molded, 295, 296f
in phosphate-bonded investments, 253t, 254
Mandible
mechanical properties of, 323
microstructure of, 323
Margins, troubleshooting in gold casting, 245
Mat gold. *See* Electrolytic precipitate (mat gold)
Mechanical property(ies). *See also* Physical property(ies)
of cements, 154t
of chromium-containing alloys, 260–261, 263–264
definition of, 22
elasticity, 15f, 15–16
fatigue, 17, 17f
hardness, 18, 19f
scales of, 18–19
plasticity, 16f, 16–17
of porcelain, 289–290, 290f
of porcelain-fused-to-metal restorations, 229t
of precious metal alloys, 217t
strain, 15, 22, 371–372
stress, 14–15, 22
of titanium, 267–268
viscoelastic behavior, 18, 18f
viscous flow, 17
Mercaptan. *See* Polysulfide rubber (mercaptan) impression materials
Mercury
blood levels in dental practitioners, 198–199
corrosion release of, 193–194
handling and disposal of, 199
uptake from amalgam restorations, 198, 198t
Metal(s), 175t. *See also* Basic materials
vs ceramics and intermetallic compounds, 6, 7f, 8
classification of, 1, 1f
clinical applications of, 8, 8f
correlations between laboratory properties and clinical data
sensitivity and amalgam bonding, 197–198
crystal lattices of, 175–176
definition of, 11
deformation of, 180–181
dislocation motion in, 180–181,
elastic strain in, 180
plastic, 180
diffusion in, 182
dissimilar in occlusion
galvanic effects of, 196–197
ductility of, 8, 8f
effect on stress concentration, 4f, 5
mechanism of, 5–6, 6f, 7f
fracture of, 179
grain size and properties of, 178–179
hardening of, 181–182, 183
noble, 225–225
nonprecious, 226
nucleation and polycrystalline grain structure of, 176–179
nucleation of, 177
polycrystalline grain structure of, 176–177, 178f
precious, 226
properties of, 1–2, 2t
semiprecious, 226
yield stress of, 178
Metamerism, 30–31, 31f
Microporosity
of cast gypsum, 56–57
Mohs hardness, 360
Munsell color system
chroma in, 29
coordinates in, 29f
hue in, 28
value in, 28

N

Nickel alloys
- carcinogenicity of, 264
- casting of, 244

Nickel-chromium alloys
- advantages and disadvantages of, 231, 232
- allergenicity and carcinogenicity of, 232
- biologic hazards with, 232
- for partial dentures
  - commercially available, 260t
  - composition of, 260
- phosphate-bonded investments for, 249–250
- in porcelain-fused-to-metal restorations, 231
- properties of, 229t

Nickel-chromium-beryllium alloy, properties of, 229t

Nickel-chromium-cobalt alloys
- surgical and for permanent implants
  - manipulation of, 265–266
  - mechanical properties of, 265t

Nickel-titanium (nitinol) alloy
- advantages and disadvantages of, 281t, 282
- bending properties of, 279, 280f
- comparison of
  - with Chinese NiTi, 279
  - with Japanese Sentalloy, 279
- composition of, 276t, 278
- important features of, 278–279
- mechanical properties of, 277t, 278–279
- for orthodontic wire, 278–280
- shape-memory characteristics of, 279, 283

Nitinol. *See* Nickel-titanium (nitinol) alloy

Nucleation
- heterogeneous, 177
- homogeneous, 177, 178f

Nucleation center
- definition of, 71

Nylon
- in dental bases, 87
- glass-fiber reinforced, 87

O

Object
- interactions with illuminant
  - absorption, 27–28
  - reflection, 27f, 27–28
  - transmission, 28

Organic matrix, in composite materials, 99

Orthodontic materials, commercial welders for, 309

Orthodontic wires
- alloys for, 276t
  - beta-titanium, 277
  - classification of, 273f, 274
  - cobalt-chromium-nickel, 277–278
  - nickel-titanium, 278–290
  - stainless steel, 275–277, 276t, 276–277, 277t
  - superelastic NiTi wire vs stainless steel wires, 283
- bending tests of
  - cantilever, 274
  - Olsen stiffness tester in, 274
- flexural yield strength of, 274
- manufacture of, 273–275
- mechanical properties of, 273–274, 276t, 277t
- nonmetallic
  - for arch, 282
- resistance modulus of, 275
- round, 273
- selection of
  - considerations in, 274, 280–282, 281t
- soldering of
  - free-hand, 305
- springback of, 275
- square, 273
- stiffness of, 274
  - factors in, 275
- working range of, 275

Osseointegration
- bioceramics and tissue attachment in, 319
- with commercially pure titanium, 318
- definitions of, 316–317
- ideal situation, 318–319
- implant surfaces and, 319–320
- mechanisms for achieving and enhancing, 317–320
- vs natural tooth, 318f
- requirements for, 317–318
- titanium-based, 324
- types of, 316, 316t, 317f
- in well-functioning vs failed, 317, 318f

P

Palladium-cobalt alloys, 231

Palladium-copper alloys
- composition of, 230–231
- for high-copper amalgams, 193
- for porcelain-fused-to-metal restorations
  - selection of, 233
- properties of, 229t

Palladium-silver alloys
- for cast restorations, 218, 219f
- color problem with, 230
- disadvantage of, 230
- for porcelain-fused-to-metal restorations
  - selection of, 233
- properties of, 229, 229t

Partial dentures. *See also* Crown-and-bridge alloy(s)
- alloys for
  - cobalt-chromium, 259–261
  - cobalt-chromium-nickel, 260
  - commercially available, 260t
  - nickel-chromium, 260
- fixed crown-and-bridge
  - porcelain-fused-to-metal in
    - alloy selection for, 233
- investment soldering of, 305

Particle shape
- abrasion rate and, 115–116, 116f

Particle size
- abrasion rate and, 115, 116f

Pattern waxes
- composition of, 148
- types of, 147–148

Penetration coefficient, 43, 43t, 360

Phosphate-bonded investments
- advantages and disadvantages of, 251
- for alloys in porcelain-fused-to-metal restorations, 249
- applications of, 249–250
- for casting, 239, 244
- for casting chromium-type crown-and-bridge alloys, 264
- composition of, 250
- magnesia in
  - for titanium and titanium alloy casting, 253t, 254
- properties of, 250t, 250–251
- for refractory die stones, 250, 250t

Physical property(ies). *See also named, eg, Mechanical property(ies)*
- classification of, 13, 13f
- electrical and electrochemical, 20–22
- mechanical, 13–19
- thermal, 19–20

Pickling solution, 243

Pigments
- in composites, 100

Pits
troubleshooting
in gold casting, 245
Plasticity, 16f, 16–17
Plasticizer
definition of, 93
in heat-cured acrylic manufacture, 83
Platinum-bonded alumina crown, electroformed die for, 310
Polishing
appearance and feel of polished surface, 117
of castings, 243–244
definition of, 115, 115f
preparation for, 117
techniques in, 118–120
Polyamides. *See* Nylon
Polycarbonate, in dental bases, 87
Polycarboxylate (carboxylate)-based cement(s), 151, 161–165
glass-ionomer, 163–165
zinc polycarboxylate, 161–163
Polyether rubber impression materials
advantages and disadvantages of, 137
composition of, 136–137
disinfection of, 138
manipulation of, 129t, 137
mechanical properties of, 127, 127t
troubleshooting of, 138
use of, 136–137
Polymer-based cement(s), 152t, 154t
acrylic resin, 165
modified, 165–166
dimethacrylate, 166–167
Polymerization
addition process in
definition of, 80, 92
stages of, 80, 81f
condensation process in, 80, 92
definition of, 79, 93
degree of, 79
and wear, 105
initiation of
in light-activated systems, 99–100
Polymer(s). *See also* Basic materials
addition silicone, 143
amorphous, 82
vs ceramics and metals, 8–10
chains in, 79, 80f
classification of, 1, 1f
clinical applications of, 10, 10f
composition of, 79
condensation silicone, 143
cross-linking of, 10
definition of, 11
denture base, 82–90. *See also* Denture base polymer(s)
fabrication effect on physical and mechanical properties, 87–89
flexibility of, 82
modulus of elasticity in, 9, 9f
molecular weight of, 79
polyether, 143
polymerization and, 80
polysulfide, 143
properties of, 2, 2t
silicone rubber, 143
spatial structure of, 79–80, 80f
strength of, 9, 10f
relation to molecular weight, 81, 81f
temperature and, 82, 82f
thermal expansion of, 9, 10f
thermoplastic, 80, 93
thermoset, 80, 93
warpage of, 82
water absorption by, 10
Poly(methyl methacrylate) (PMMA)
in heat-cured acrylic manufacture, 83, 85, 85f
in high-impact acrylic manufacture, 86
Poly(methyl methacrylate) (PMMA) cement, 152
Polysulfide rubber (mercaptan)
advantages and disadvantages of, 133
composition of, 132
disinfection of, 133
manipulation of, 129t, 133
mechanical properties of, 127t, 133
troubleshooting, 133
as two-paste system, 132, 132f
use of, 132
Porcelain. *See also* Ceramic restorations, milled
advantages of, 287
for all-ceramic crowns, 293–294
alumina-reinforced vs feldspathic, 294
classification according to composition, 293, 293f
failures of, 293
alumina core material
slip casting of, 296–297, 297f
bonded to metal
adhesion in, 290–293
advantages and disadvantages of, 293
composition of, 288, 288f, 288t
condensation and sintering of, 288–289, 289f
crack propagation in, 290, 290f
properties of, 289–290, 290f
strength of, 290, 290f, 301
vitreous structure of, 289–290, 290f
in castable ceramic crowns
calcium-phosphate glass-based, 295
centrifugal casting machine for, 295, 295f
fluorine mica silicate in, 295
manufacture of, 295
chemical analysis of, 288t
classification of, 287
clinical scenario for manufacture, 299–301
core material, spinel injection-molded
advantages and disadvantages of, 294–295
for all-ceramic crown, 294–296
alumina magnesia spinel ceramic in, 294
magnesia high-expansion, 295, 296f
manufacture of, 294
tooth preparation for, 294
for denture teeth
advantages and disadvantages of, 287
high-leucite
injection-molded, 296, 297f
magnesia-core crown
advantages and disadvantages of, 296
design of, 296f
mechanical properties of, 295
microstructure of, 296f
polishing technique for, 120
Porcelain-fused-to-metal (PFM) restoration
alloys used for, 217t, 218
double layer effects and, 32, 32f
properties of, 219
Porosity
in alginate hydrocolloid cast, 132
internal and external
of gold casting, 245
wear and, 105
Precipitation hardening, 181
Pressure, abrasion rate and, 116f, 116
Pressure welding
of gold, 308, 309
procedure in, 308
Processing waxes, types and applications of, 148
Prophylaxis pastes
in common use, 117
selection of, 117

Proportional limit. *See* Elastic limit (proportional limit)
Pulp, calcium hydroxide chelate cement capping for, 160
Pyramid hardness number (DHN). *See* Vickers hardness number (VHN)

Q

Quartz
in gypsum-bonded investments, 62, 63f
thermal expansion of, 67, 67f, 238, 239f

R

Radiopacity
in polymeric denture bases, 89
Refractory filler
in gypsum-bonded investments, 60
effect on setting and thermal behavior, 61–62
particle size of, 64–65
Resilience, definition of, 17
Restoration materials, history of, 97
Retarders
effect on setting, 56
in gypsum-bonded investments, 61
Rockwell hardness, 19
Rockwell superficial hardness scale (R-30N), definition of, 268
Roughness, troubleshooting in gold casting, 245
Rubber wheels, for polishing and finishing, 118, 121

S

Sealants
fluoride-containing, 109f
penetration of, 109f
pit and fissure, 109
Sensitivity, with high-copper spherical amalgams, 197–198
Setting expansion
definition of, 255
of ethyl silicate-bonded investments, 252t
of phosphate-bonded investments, 250
Setting time, definition of, 172
Shade
communication to laboratory, 34, 34f, 337–338
dental guides for, 32, 337–338
matching in office, 33
recommendations for, 33
Shear stress, dislocation from, 6, 7f
Shore A durometer, 19
Shore A hardness, 19, 368
Shrinkage
casting accuracy and
of gypsum-bonded investments, 68–70, 69t
of composites, 100–101
correction of, 102, 102f
of gold casting, 69, 69f, 69t
Silica
in gypsum-bonded investments, 61, 62
in gypsum investment powder
effect on setting and thermal behavior, 62, 63f, 64
Silicate cement, 97
Silicone(s)
addition. *See* Addition (vinyl) silicones
condensation. *See* Condensation silicone rubber
Silicone soft liners
advantages and disadvantages of, 90t
heat-cured, 91
room-temperature vulcanized, 91
Silicophosphate cements
advantages and disadvantages of, 157
applications of, 156
biologic effects of, 157
classification of, 152t
composition and setting of, 156–157
properties of, 154t, 157
Silver solder, use of, 304
Sintering
definition of, 40, 48, 207, 213
of gold, 207
of porcelain-fused-to-metal, 289, 289f
Solder
gold, 304t, 306t, 306–307
properties of, 306
selection of, 304
tensile properties of gold, 306t
Soldering
antifluxes for, 304, 310
cleaning for, 304–305
commercial materials for, 307
composition of alloys for, 303–304, 304t
defective
causes of, 305–306
fluxes for, 304
free-hand, 305
infrared, 307
investment soldering procedure in, 305
melting ranges for, 304t
of metal ceramic bridges, 306–307
of orthodontic wires, 305
of partial dentures, 305
postceramic, 307
preceramic, 303, 306
technique in, 303
uses of, 303
Soldering fixtures, phosphate-bonded investments for, 250, 251
Solidus temperature, 175
Space lattice, 176, 177f, 183
Spectrophotometers, in color measurement, 30
Speed, abrasion rate and, 116
Spot welding
diagram of welder for, 308f
manipulation in, 309
procedure in, 307–308
Spruing
orientation of pattern in mold, 237f, 240
point of attachment in, 240
purpose of, 239
ring liner in, 240–241
sprue selection in, 240
sprue size and design in, 240, 240f
Stainless steel wire alloy
advantages and disadvantages of, 281t, 282
composition of, 276t, 275–276
mechanical properties of, 276t, 276–277, 277t
Stones, for polishing and finishing, 118, 121
Strain, 15, 22
in compression, 371–372
Strength
of amalgams, 192, 192f
of polymers, 9, 9f
Stress
tensile, 14f
types of, 14
Stress concentration
ductility effect on, 4f, 5
effect on ceramics, 3, 4f, 5
Stress raiser, 3, 4f, 5, 11
Substrates, hardness of abrasives and, 116t
Surface chemistry and structure, in implant osseointegration, 321
Surface energy
definition of, 39, 48
sintering and, 40
vacancies and attraction in, 39, 39f, 40f
of various substances, 39, 40t

Surface free energy, 373
Surface phenomena. *See also named, eg, Adhesion*
adhesion, 43–48
adsorption, 41
capillary penetration, 42–43
colloids, 41t, 41–42
surface energy, 39–40
wetting, 40–41
Surgical alloy(s)
advantages and disadvantages of, 266
adventitious bursa formation from, 266
biologic effects of, 266
chemical responses to, 266
cobalt-chromium, 265t, 265–266
manipulation of, 265–266
mechanical properties of, 265, 265t
nickel-chromium-cobalt, 265t, 265–266

T

Tear energy, of various materials, 374
Tearing
of alginate hydrocolloid cast, 131
in polyether rubber cast, 138
Tear strength, of various materials, 375–376
Temper, of cobalt-chromium-nickel wire, 277–278, 283
Thermal expansion, 20, 20f
definition of, 255
of ethyl silicate-bonded investments, 252t
of gypsum-bonded investments
hygroscopic technique, 66, 66f
thermal expansion technique, 67, 67f
of phosphate-bonded investments, 250
of polymers, 9, 10f
in porcelain-fused-to-metal restorations, 228, 290, 291f
techniques of, 67, 67f
high-heat, 238, 238f 239t
hygroscopic, 238–239, 239t
Thermal property(ies)
conductivity, 19, 22, 377
diffusivity, 19–20, 20f, 22, 379–380
heat flow through material, 19–20
thermal expansion, 20, 20f
Thermoplasticity, of dental impression compound, 80
Thermoplastic polymer, 80, 93
Thermoset polymer, 80, 93
Tissue conditioners. *See* Denture based polymers
advantages and disadvantages of, 90t
composition and manufacture of, 92
Titanium
alloys
benefits of, 267
for dental prostheses, 267
for implants, 324
for orthodontic wire
advantages and disadvantages of, 281t, 282
composition of, 276t, 278
mechanical properties of, 277t, 278
for porcelain-fused-to-metal restorations
selection of, 232
properties of, 267–268, 324
biologic effects of, 268
commercially pure
vs chromium-type alloys, 266
elastic modulus of, 267
for implants, 318, 324
problems with, 266–267
properties of, 267
corrosion resistance of, 268
in dentistry, 327
interactions with atmospheric gases, 267
investments for
ethyl silicate-bonded vs phosphate-bonded, 253t, 254
high-temperature, 253t, 253–254, 254t
phosphate-bonded, magnesia-modified, 253t, 254
Torch melting
air/acetylene, 241, 242
oxygen/acetylene, 241, 242
zones of flame in, 241f
Toughness, definition of, 17
Translucency
definition of, 31
measurements of, 31
Trituration, 190, 199
mechanical, 195

V

Vickers hardness number (VHN), 18, 393–394
Viscoelastic behavior, 18, 18f
Viscous flow, 17
Vita InCeram inlay, IPS Empress vs, 300–301
Voids, in polysulfide rubber cast, 133

W

Water/powder (W/P) ratio
definition of, 71
in setting
in expansion control, 58, 59f
rate of, 57
Wax(es)
classification of, 147–148, 148f
commercial materials, 149
composition of, 147
definition of, 147
distortion of, 149, 149f
impression, 148
natural, 147
pattern, 147–148
processing, 148
properties of, 149
synthetic, 147
Welding
commercial orthodontic welders, 309
laser, 308, 309
pressure, 308, 309
properties of welds, 309
spot, 307–308, 308f, 309
Wetting
contact angle in, 40, 40f, 40t, 48
definition of, 40
hydrophobic substances and, 41, 41f
Work hardening. *See* Cold working (work hardening)
definition of, 16
Working time, definition of, 172

Y

Yield strength, 16, 22
of alloys and cements, 397–398
clinical importance of
in porcelain-fused-to-metal restorations, 227–228

Z

Zinc oxide–eugenol cement(s)
advantages and disadvantages of, 158
classification of, 152t
ethoxybenzoic acid–containing
advantages and disadvantages of, 160
applications of, 159
biologic effects of, 160
composition and setting of, 159
manipulation of, 159
properties of, 160
properties of, 154t

reinforced
advantages and disadvantages of, 159
applications of, 158–150
biologic effects of, 159
composition and setting of, 158
manipulation of, 158–159
properties of, 159
simple
applications of, 157
biologic effects of, 158
composition and setting of, 157–158
manipulation of, 158
properties of, 158
Zinc oxide–eugenol impression materials
advantages and disadvantages of, 126
composition of, 126
disinfection of, 127
manipulation of, 126
mechanical properties of, 126
specification for, 124t
troubleshooting, 127
use of, 125–126
Zinc phosphate cements, 153t
advantages and disadvantages of, 156
applications of, 154
biologic effects of, 156
classification of, 152t
composition and setting of, 154–155, 155f
manipulation of, 155
modified, 156
properties of, 154t, 155–156
vs resin cement
for crown cementation, 168
Zinc polycarboxylate cement
advantages and disadvantages of, 163
applications of, 161
biologic effects of, 162–163
composition and setting of, 161–162
manipulation of, 162, 162f
properties of, 154t, 162